Role Development for
Doctoral Advanced
Nursing Practice

H. Michael Dreher, PhD, RN, FAAN, is Associate Professor with Tenure and Chair, Doctoral Nursing Department, Drexel University, Philadelphia (appointed 2004). His PhD is in Nursing Science from Widener University (2000) and AS (1984), BSN (1988), and MN (1991) from the University of South Carolina, Columbia. His dissertation was *The Effect of Caffeine Reduction on Sleep and Well-being in Persons with HIV* (published in the *Journal of Psychosomatic Research* 2003) under the supervision of the late Dr. Susan Kun Leddy, author of six editions of *Leddy and Pepper's Conceptual Bases of Professional Nursing* (LWW/2009). Dreher is a dynamic leader, innovator, and educator. He has led Drexel to the forefront of doctoral nursing education and spearheaded the Drexel DNP Conferences on DNP Education in Annapolis in 2007 and in Hilton Head Island, SC in 2009 (the 3rd conference is scheduled for Fall 2011). In 2007 he established the first mandatory doctoral study abroad program in nursing (London/Dublin). His clinical nursing experience (1984–2000) has focused primarily on Adult Health/Coronary Care/Home Care of Cardiac Patients and he completed his postdoctoral research in sleep and respiratory neurobiology at the University of Pennsylvania (2001–2003). He has participated in the Harvard Macy Institute Program for Leading Innovation in Healthcare & Education (Harvard Business School/Medical School—2007) and established the first MSN in Innovation (2007). Dr. Dreher has published over 70 journal articles and has been PI or Co-PI on more than 20 funded projects. His current scholarship has focused on innovation, "boomer health," professional/practice doctorate issues and in expanding his Model of Practice Knowledge Development. He recently presented two papers at the first International Conference on Professional Doctorates in London (11/2009) and was the invited endnote speaker at the Southern Universities Alliance for Doctoral Education's Professional Doctorate Conference at the University of Brighton, UK (4/2009). Dr. Dreher conceived and has taught NURS 716: *The Structure of Scientific Knowledge in Nursing* to Drexel DrNP students for several years and is coauthor of a recent text from Springer on *Philosophy of Science for Nursing Practice: Concepts and Application* with Michael D. Dahnke, PhD.

Mary Ellen Smith Glasgow, PhD, RN, ACNS-BC, is Dean and Professor at Duquesne University School of Nursing. Dr. Glasgow received her BSN from Gwynedd-Mercy College, MSN from Villanova University, and PhD from Duquesne University, School of Nursing, and obtained additional graduate course work at The Catholic University of America. She developed the BSN Co-op Program, BSN Accelerated Career Entry Program, RN-BSN Online Program, Pathway to Health Professions Program, and other forward-thinking educational programs in her former position at Drexel University. As an early driver and adopter of innovation, Dr. Glasgow incorporated the cooperative education model, envisioned and implemented the use of online courses, standardized patients and simulation in the nursing and undergraduate health professions curricula, e-books, as well as implemented the use of handheld technology. Additionally, she had overall responsibility for the Division of Continuing Nursing Education (CNE). She completed a fellowship at Bryn Mawr College and HERS, Mid-America Summer Institute for Women in Higher Education Administration. In 2010, she was honored with the Villanova University College of Nursing Alumni Medallion for Distinguished Contribution to Nursing Education. She served as the Associate Editor for *Oncology Nursing Forum* and was responsible for the Leadership and Professional Development Feature from 2008–2012. Dr. Glasgow was a Trustee of Princeton HealthCare System and was selected as a 2009 Robert Wood Johnson Foundation Executive Nurse Fellow. She has over 70 publications, 120 national and international presentations, and recently coauthored two books, *Role Development for Doctoral Advanced Nursing Practice* (2011), the recipient of the 2012 AJN Book of the Year Award, and *Legal Issues Confronting Today's Nursing Faculty: A Case Study Approach* (2012). She has secured over 2 million dollars in funding. Her research interests include safety and interprofessional simulation, and leadership development in nursing.

Role Development for
Doctoral Advanced
Nursing Practice

H. Michael Dreher, PhD, RN, FAAN

Mary Ellen Smith Glasgow, PhD, RN, ACNS-BC

Foreword
by
Bernadette Mazurek Melnyk, PhD, RN, CPNP/PMHNP, FNAP, FAAN

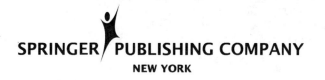

SPRINGER PUBLISHING COMPANY
NEW YORK

Contents

Contributors

Susan Baseman, DrNP, APRN, NEA-BC, Vice-President of Patient Quality and Disease Management, Cooper University Hospital, Camden, NJ

Sandra Bellini, DNP, NNP-BC, APRN, Assistant Clinical Professor, Coordinator, DNP Program, School of Nursing, University of Connecticut, Storrs, CT and Neonatal Nurse Practitioner, Connecticut Children's Medical Center, Hartford, CT

Joan Rosen Bloch, PhD, CRNP, Assistant Professor, Doctoral Nursing Department, College of Nursing and Health Professions and Joint Appointment, Department of Epidemiology and Biostatistics, School of Public Health, Drexel University, Philadelphia, PA

Victoria M. Bradley, DNP, RN, CPHIMS, FHIMSS, Assistant Professor, Adjunct Faculty, College of Nursing, University of Kentucky, Lexington, KY and President, American Nursing Informatics Association—ANIA-CARING™

Marie Annette Brown, PhD, ARNP, FNP-C, FAAN, Professor and Group Health Endowed Term Professorship in Chronic Illness Care, School of Nursing, University of Washington, Seattle, WA and Primary Care Nurse Practitioner, University of Washington Medical Center Women's Health Care Clinic, Seattle, WA

Geraldine M. Budd, PhD, CRNP, FNP-BC, FAANP, Associate Professor and Assistant Dean—Harrisburg Campus, Widener University School of Nursing, Chester, PA

Sharon Byrne, DrNP, CRNP, NP-C, AOCNP, Assistant Clinical Professor and FNP MSN Track Coordinator, Department of Nurse Practitioner Programs, College of Nursing and Health Professions, Drexel University and Advanced Practice Nurse, Cancer Screening Project, Cancer Institute of New Jersey at Cooper University Hospital, Camden, NJ

Grant Charles, PhD, Associate Principal (Research) of the College of Health Disciplines and Associate Professor, School of Social Work, University of British Columbia, Vancouver, BC, Canada

Gary M. Childs, MS, Education/Reference Librarian, Drexel University Libraries, Philadelphia, PA

Michael E. Conti, Assistant Clinical Professor, Department of Nurse Anesthesia, College of Nursing and Health Professions, Drexel University, Philadelphia, PA and PhD student, Villanova University, Villanova, PA

Frances H. Cornelius, PhD, MSN, RN, CNE, RN-BC (Informatics), Associate Clinical Professor, Chair, MSN Advanced Role Department, College of Nursing and Health Professions, Drexel University, Philadelphia, PA

Regina M. Cusson, PhD, NNP-BC, APRN, FAAN, Professor and Associate Dean Academic Affairs and Advanced Practice, School of Nursing, University of Connecticut, Storrs, CT

Sheila M. Davis, DNP, RN, ANP-BC, FAAN, Clinical Assistant Professor, School of Nursing, MGH Institute of Health Professions, Boston, MA

Sheila P. Davis, PhD, RN, FAAN, Professor of Nursing, University of Southern Mississippi School of Nursing, Hattiesburg, MS *Editor-Online Journal of Health Ethics*

Robin Donohoe Dennison, DNP, RN, CCNS, Associate Professor of Clinical Nursing, University of Cincinnati College of Nursing, Cincinnati, OH

Sister Rosemary Donley, PhD, APRN-BC, FAAN, Donley Professor, Jacques Laval Endowed Chair for Justice for Vulnerable Populations, Duquesne University School of Nursing, Pittsburgh, PA

Gloria F. Donnelly, PhD, RN, FAAN, Professor and Dean, College of Nursing and Health Professions, Drexel University, Philadelphia, PA

Lynne M. Dunphy, PhD, FNP-BC, Routhier Chair of Practice and Professor of Nursing, College of Nursing, University of Rhode Island, Kingston, RI, Center Director, Rhode Island Center for Nursing Excellence (RICNE) and Robert Wood Johnson Executive Nurse Fellow

M. Christina R. Esperat, PhD, RN, FAAN, Associate Dean for Research and Clinical Services and CH Foundation Regents Professor in Rural Health Disparities, Texas Tech Health Science Center, School of Nursing, Lubbock, TX

Rosario P. Estrada, DNP, RN, BC, CPN, Assistant Professor/Track Coordinator, Nursing Informatics MSN Program, University of Medicine and Dentistry of New Jersey, School of Nursing, Newark, NJ

Joyce J. Fitzpatrick, PhD, MBA, RN, FAAN, Elizabeth Brooks Ford Professor of Nursing at the Frances Payne Bolton School of Nursing, Case Western Reserve University, Cleveland, OH

Marcia R. Gardner, PhD, RN, CPNP, CPN, Assistant Professor, Department of Nursing, Camden College of Arts and Sciences, Rutgers University-Camden, NJ

Cynthia Gifford-Hollingsworth, DrNP (c), MSN, CRNP, CPNP, Surgical Research Nurse Supervisor, Department of Surgery, College of Medicine, Drexel University, Philadelphia, PA

Elizabeth W. Gonzalez, PhD, APRN-BC, Associate Professor, Doctoral Nursing Department, College of Nursing and Health Professions, Drexel University, Philadelphia, PA

Cheryl Holly, EdD, RN, Associate Professor, Chair, Department of Capacity Building Systems and Director, Doctor of Nursing Practice Program and Co-Director of the New Jersey Center for Evidence-Based Practice, University of Medicine and Dentistry of New Jersey, School of Nursing, Newark, NJ

Sandra N. Jones, DrNP (c), PMHCNS-BC, Director, A Systems Approach and Licensed Independent Nurse Psychotherapist, Pikesville, MD

Margo A. Karsten, PhD, MSN, RN, Assistant Professor, Loretto Heights School of Nursing, Regis University, Denver, CO and former VP and COO, Exempla Saint Joseph Hospital, Denver, CO

Karen Kaufman, MS, President and Co-Founding Principal, The Kaufman Partnership, Ltd, Philadelphia, PA

Vicki D. Lachman, PhD, MBE, APRN, Associate Clinical Professor and Track Coordinator, MSN in Innovation & Intra/Entrepreneurship in Advanced Practice Nursing, Department of MSN Advanced Roles, College of Nursing and Health Professions, Drexel University, Philadelphia, PA

Rosalie O. Mainous, PhD, ARNP, NNP-BC, Associate Dean for Graduate Programs & Research, School of Nursing, Associate Faculty, Birth Defects Center, School of Dentistry, University of Louisville, Louisville, KY and Robert Wood Johnson Nurse Executive Fellow

Lucy N. Marion, PhD, RN, FAAN, Professor and Dean, School of Nursing, Medical College of Georgia, Augusta, GA

Diane J. Mick, PhD, RN, CNS, GNP, FNAP, Associate Professor, Wegmans School of Nursing, St. John Fisher College, Rochester, NY

Jason E. Miller, Esq., JD, PAHM, Provider Contracts Team Lead, Highmark Inc., Pittsburgh, PA

Kym A. Montgomery, DrNP, WHNP-BC, Assistant Clinical Professor and WHNP MSN Program Track Coordinator, Department of Nurse Practitioner Programs, College of Nursing and Health Professions, Drexel University and WHNP Dept. OB/GYN, College of Medicine, Drexel University, Philadelphia, PA

Owen C. Montgomery, MD, Chair of Department of Obstetrics and Gynecology, Drexel University College of Medicine, Philadelphia, PA

Deena Nardi, PhD, PMHCNS-BC, FAAN, Professor and Director, Doctor of Nursing Practice Program, University of St. Francis College of Nursing, Joliet, IL

Julie Cowan Novak, DNSc, RN, CPNP, FAANP, Associate Dean for Practice and Crow Endowed Professor, University of Texas Health Science Center San Antonio School of Nursing, San Antonio, TX

David G. O'Dell, DNP, FNP-BC, Associate Professor, College of Nursing, South University, Royal Palm Beach, FL and Founding Member of Doctors of Nursing Practice, LLC, Jupiter, FL

Ann L. O'Sullivan, PhD, FAAN, CRNP, Dr. Hildegarde Reynolds Endowed Term Professor of Primary Care Nursing, University of Pennsylvania School of Nursing, Philadelphia, PA

Scott Oldfield, DrNP(c), MSN, CRNP, Instructor, Department of Nursing, Bloomsburg University, Bloomsburg, PA and FNP, Geisinger Medical Center, Vascular Surgery Clinic, Danville, PA

Bobbie Posmontier, PhD, CNM, CNS, Assistant Professor, Doctoral Nursing Department, College of Nursing and Health Professions, Drexel University, Philadelphia, PA

Suzanne S. Prevost, RN, PhD, COI, Professor and Associate Dean for Practice and Community Engagement, College of Nursing, University of Kentucky, Lexington, KY, President-Elect, Sigma Theta Tau International and Robert Wood Johnson Nurse Executive Fellow

Courtney Reinisch, DNP, APN-BC, DCC, Assistant Professor of Clinical Nursing, School of Nursing, Columbia University, New York, NY

Marlene Rosenkoetter, RN, PhD, FAAN, Professor, School of Nursing, Medical College of Georgia, Augusta, GA

Albert Rundio, PhD, DNP, RN, APRN, NEA-BC, DPNAP, Associate Clinical Professor, Department of MSN Advanced Roles, College of Nursing and Health Professions, Drexel University, Philadelphia, PA

Carol Savrin, DNP, CPNP, FNP, BC, FAANP, Associate Professor and Director of MSN Programs, Frances Payne Bolton School of Nursing, Case Western Reserve University, Cleveland, OH

Linda D. Scott, PhD, RN, NEA-BC, FAAN, Professor and Associate Dean for Graduate Programs, Kirkhof School of Nursing, Grand Valley State University, Grand Rapids, MI

Janice Smolowitz, DNP, EdD, DCC, ANP-BC, Professor of Clinical Nursing, Senior Associate Dean, Columbia University School of Nursing, New York, NY

Graham Stew, DPhil, MA, Cert Ed, DipN, RGN, RMN, RNT, FHEA, Principal Lecturer, Professional Doctorate in Health and Social Care, University of Brighton, Brighton, UK

Tukea L. Talbert, RN, DNP, Chief Nursing Officer, Clark Regional Medical Center, Winchester, KY

Jeannine Uribe, PhD, RN, Assistant Clinical Professor, Department of Baccalaureate Nursing, College of Nursing and Health Professions, Drexel University, Philadelphia, PA

Cheryl M. Vermey, EdD, RN, CPCC, ACC, President and CEO EnVision Coaching, Inc., West Chester, PA, and Member, Global Board of Directors, International Coach Federation

Roberta Waite, EdD, RN, APRN, CNS-BC, Associate Professor, Doctoral Nursing Department, College of Nursing and Health Professions, Drexel University, Philadelphia, PA

Louise S. Ward, CRNP, PhD, Assistant Clinical Professor, Department of MSN Advanced Roles, College of Nursing and Health Professions, Drexel University, Philadelphia, PA

Beth Weinstock, PhD, Independent Consultant, Philadelphia, PA

Ann Bartley Williams, EdD, RNC, FAAN, Professor of Nursing, UCLA School of Nursing, Los Angeles, CA and Guest Professor, Faculty of Nursing Xiangya School of Medicine, Central South University Changsha, PRC

Linda Wilson, RN, PhD, CPAN, CAPA, BC, CNE, Assistant Clinical Professor and Assistant Dean for Special Projects, Simulation, and CNE Accreditation, Drexel University, Philadelphia, PA

Ruth Wittmann-Price, PhD, RN, CNS, CNE, Professor and Chair, Department of Nursing, Frances Marion University, Florence, SC

Debra L. Woda, DNP, APRN, CNM, Clinical Associate Professor, College of Nursing, University of South Carolina, Columbia, SC

Patricia S. Yoder-Wise, RN, EdD, NEA-BC, ANEF, FAAN, Professor, Anna Thigpen Perry School of Nursing, Texas Tech University Health Sciences Center, Lubbock, TX and Texas Woman's University, Houston, TX

Connie L. Zak, DNP, MBA, FNP-BC, Clinical Assistant Professor and Director of the Doctor of Nursing Practice Program, College of Nursing, University of Illinois-Chicago, Chicago, IL

Rick Zoucha, PhD, PMHCNS-BC, CTN, Associate Professor and Coordinator, MSN Psychiatric/ Mental Health CNS Program and Transcultural/International Nursing Post-Masters Certificate, School of Nursing, Duquesne University, Pittsburgh, PA

Eileen H. Zungolo, RN, EdD, CNE, FAAN, ANEF, Professor and Dean, School of Nursing, Duquesne University, Pittsburgh, PA

Patti Rager Zuzelo, EdD, RN, ACNS-BC, ANP-BC, CRNP, Professor of Nursing, DNP Program Director and CNS Track Coordinator La Salle University School of Nursing and Health Sciences, Philadelphia, PA and President, National Association of Clinical Nurse Specialists

Foreword

"Nothing happens unless first a dream!" This particular quote by Carl Sandburg could not be truer, especially when it comes to doctoral preparation of nurses and the recent evolution of the Doctor of Nursing Practice (DNP) degree. A key element that is often missed in the transformation of any profession or system is how critical the vision or dream is to the accomplishment of any endeavor. The dream of elevating advanced nursing practice to the doctoral degree was bold and met with controversy throughout the nursing and medical communities when it was first proposed. However, with risk-taking and persistence through many "character-builders" by nurse leaders across the nation, the dream is now realized as hundreds of academic institutions throughout the United States have implemented, or are planning to implement, the DNP degree. There is no doubt that even more institutions will follow this trend with the recent recommendation by the Institute of Medicine Report that at least 10% of baccalaureate program graduates enter master's or doctoral degree programs within five years of graduation.

As with all new degrees, there is often a period of uncertainty regarding the curriculum, competencies, and role of the graduates as they enter the workforce with new knowledge and skills. Although competencies exist for the DNP degree, there is still much variation in preparation of the DNP graduate by academic programs across the nation. Unlike the PhD graduate who has been prepared to generate external evidence through rigorous research, the DNP graduate should be an expert in translating the best evidence from rigorous research into clinical practice for the ultimate purpose of improving the quality and cost of health care as well as patient outcomes. In addition, the DNP graduate should be an expert at generating internal evidence through quality improvement, outcomes management, and evidence-based practice projects in order to develop new knowledge and interventions for clinical practice within their own practice settings. However, there is still uncertainty about the curriculum in DNP programs throughout the United States as many institutions have taken courses from traditional PhD programs and infused them into the curriculum for the DNP, which will likely lead to role confusion for the graduates as well as for employers who hire DNP graduates.

Findings from a body of research have indicated that implementation of evidence-based practice (EBP) throughout our health system results in higher-quality care, reduced costs, and improved patient outcomes. However, it is currently well recognized that the majority of health care decisions are not evidence based and that it often takes well over a decade to translate findings from research into clinical practice to improve health-care quality. It is truly unfortunate that many interventions that have been supported as efficacious through rigorous research are never used in clinical practice to enhance patient outcomes. In order to stimulate a higher and more consistent level of EBP, insurers and third-party payers have begun to incentivize health care providers and institutions to deliver evidence-based care. From their academic preparation, DNP graduates should be well equipped with the knowledge and skills needed to be the "transformers" of health care quality, safety, and patient outcomes through their expertise as evidence-based practitioners, EBP mentors, and professionals who are capable of influencing health and health care organizational policies as well as positively leading change in health care systems based on sound evidence. Although DNP-prepared nurses can certainly contribute to generating external evidence through rigorous research as part of teams, they should be the nursing professionals who are experts at generating internal evidence and practice knowledge for use within their own clinical settings for the ultimate purpose of improving quality of care and enhancing their patients' outcomes.

As the role of the doctoral advanced practice nurse continues to evolve, it will be critical to conduct research that documents the impact that the role of the doctoral advanced practice nurse is making on health care delivery and patient outcomes. Failure to document outcomes for the clinical nurse specialist years ago resulted in many of these health professionals losing their positions in health care institutions throughout the country. We must not let this happen to the role of the DNP. Data-driven or evidence-based decisions must be the paradigm from which we consistently operate now and into the future.

Individuals with DNPs who enter academia to teach, mentor students, and generate clinical scholarship need to be recognized for their expertise and integrated into transdisciplinary teams to improve the quality of advanced practice education, health care services, and health policy. DNPs who choose to remain in clinical practice must be provided with opportunities to spearhead initiatives that will improve the health of populations and systems of health care. Finally, DNPs who are executives in healthcare systems must model evidence-based leadership and innovation as well as provide the necessary resources and culture for clinicians to professionally flourish and deliver the highest quality of evidence-based care.

This outstanding and thought-provoking book by Drs. H. Michael Dreher and Mary Ellen Smith Glasgow not only provides the knowledge to understand the issues and role-related challenges of doctoral advanced nursing practice, but also the inspiration to embrace the role and become a transformer of health care. Dr. Dreher and Dr. Glasgow's expertise in leading transformational change through the DNP has resulted in a unique book that presents the issues in a relatable and thought-provoking manner. The content in this book covers all salient points for the doctoral advanced practice role with informative chapters on how doctoral-level advanced practice roles differ from master's-level advanced practice nursing roles, as well as content on the roles of the clinical executive, clinical scholar, and clinical educator. In addition, the use of reflective responses throughout the chapters by national DNP scholars, practitioners, and experts is a gift to the field. The chapters that focus on using technology and developing negotiation and mentorship skills are especially exciting and necessary for advanced nursing practice at the doctoral level. I have no doubt that readers of this book will be challenged to evolve their roles to a higher level in order to transform health care, health systems, and academic curriculums.

Peter F. Drucker said that "the best way to predict the future is to create it." Let us continue to create an exciting future for doctoral advanced practice nurses with demonstrated outcomes that indicate they truly are transformers of health care and leaders of systems reengineering that result in high-quality, safe and low-cost care for all Americans.

Bernadette Mazurek Melnyk, PhD, RN, CPNP/PMHNP, FNAP, FAAN
Dean and Distinguished Foundation Professor
Arizona State University College of Nursing and Health Innovation,
Phoenix, AZ
Member, United States Preventive Services Task Force
Associate Editor, *Worldviews on Evidence-based Nursing*

Preface

Functioning as both a graduate textbook and a professional resource, *Role Development for Doctoral Advanced Nursing Practice* explores the historical and evolving role of the new Doctoral Advanced Practice Registered Nurse, termed "DAPRN," to describe DNP-educated nurse practitioners, nurse midwives, nurse anesthetists, and clinical nurse specialists. Similarly, this text addresses roles for nurses engaged in Doctoral Advanced Nursing Practice, termed "DAPNs," to describe the role of the clinical executive, educator, and the other diverse roles that the DNP graduate may assume. There is a growing literature on the domain of *practice* "beyond the MSN" and this text specifically focuses on this emerging discussion. Because the role of the DNP graduate is evolving, the primary authors and contributing authors of this text present positions and reflective responses that represent a wide range of current views on the DNP role and the diverse "ideals" of what the role of the DAPRN and DAPN should be. This is also the first text that exclusively examines the evolving and expanding *role functions* of the DNP graduate.

Too often, nursing texts offer the sole view of the author. This text uniquely offers the views of many diverse faculty, executives, practitioners, and scholars. The distinctive feature of this text is the two-part chapter organization that presents the chapter content followed by one or more *Reflective Responses*, which provide commentaries that may counter or support the opinions of each chapter author or authors. Each Reflective Response is written by well-known DNP leaders representing the diverse roles and experience of academics, administrators, and practitioners, including graduates from different doctor of nursing practice programs. This innovative chapter presentation is bound to enhance classroom discussion. The work in its entirety is hopefully stimulating and provocative, and a well-rounded presentation of issues germane to DNP education, core competencies, and unfolding role development. We believe this is a "must have" text in DNP role development courses and courses covering contemporary DNP degree issues.

Each of the textbook's sections thoroughly covers important aspects of *role development*:

- Section I provides background information on the evolution of the DNP degree, essential content on role theory, what nursing "roles" are and how they evolved, and a discussion of how master's versus doctoral-level advanced nursing practices differ.
- Section II focuses on the four basic roles of the DNP graduate which currently predominate: practitioner, clinical executive, educator, and clinical scientist who is engaged mostly in the clinical trials industry; as well as the role of the clinical scholar, something each graduate is expected to embrace as stewards of the discipline.
- Section III covers the diverse skills that comprise the doctoral APRN and doctoral APN role; including leadership content, negotiation skills, and leveraging technology to support doctoral advanced level practice; debate over the DNP Exam; discussion of DNP graduates using the title "Dr."; inclusion of doctoral global health competencies

with mandatory study abroad; and how the DAPRN/DAPN can use their new competencies to function at a higher level.

There has always been debate in nursing about the direction of the profession. We have witnessed the evolution of our practice-focused disciplinary trajectory from first our earliest nursing curricula in the 19th century, to the predominance of the diploma-educated nurse, and now to current forces attempting to supplant the MSN in favor of the DNP for entry-level advanced practice. This text aims to honor our history of diverse discourse and add to the growing literature about the evolution of nursing "practice" now emerging at the doctoral level.

H. Michael Dreher
Mary Ellen Smith Glasgow

Acknowledgments

We want to acknowledge some of the individuals who really made this book happen. The editing of Drs. Barbara Granger and Michael Dahnke, a social work and philosophy scholar both very familiar with our nursing world, was a godsend. We will take a structural editing over simple copy editing any day. We have borrowed some excellent figures from Dr. Dahnke and Dr. Dreher's recently published book *Philosophy of Science for Nursing Practice*, and the Drexel undergraduate graphic design student Joseph Dunphy, who designed them, professionally took tons of emails that read "No, fix this. Enlarge that. No, more bold, less that... etc." Jasmine Tun, my Drexel co-op research assistant and pre-physical therapy health sciences major, literally did anything I requested with grace and precision. Last, we want to particularly thank the chapter contributors and reflective response contributors who took our endless emails and heard our tired, but hopefully pleasant, pleas about publisher deadlines. Without the practitioners, scholars, and deeply concerned individuals who made this book happen, the doctor of nursing practice degree, at this time, could not have undergone such diverse discourse as it moves into its first decade.

H. Michael Dreher
Mary Ellen Smith Glasgow

List of Reviewers

Katherine Kaby Anselmi, JD, PhD, FNP-BC, WHNP-BC, Assistant Clinical Professor & Assistant Dean for MSN, On Line, and RN/BSN Programs College of Nursing and Health Professions, Drexel University, Philadelphia, PA

Dorit G. Breiter, DNP, ARNP, PMHNP-BC, Assistant Clinical Professor, Psychiatric Nurse Practitioner MSN Program Track Coordinator, Department of Nurse Practitioner Programs, Drexel University College of Nursing and Health Professions, Philadelphia, PA

Sharon K. Byrne, DrNP, CRNP, NP-C, AOCNP, Assistant Clinical Professor and FNP MSN Track Coordinator, Department of Nurse Practitioner Programs, College of Nursing and Health Professions, Drexel University, Philadelphia, PA and Advanced Practice Nurse, Cancer Screening Project, Cancer Institute of New Jersey at Cooper University Hospital, Camden, NJ

Joan E. Dacher, PhD, RN, GNP, Associate Professor, Director Doctor of Nursing Science Program, The Sage Colleges, Troy, NY

Ellen Daroszewski, PhD, APRN, DNP Program Director, College of Graduate Nursing, Western University of Health Sciences, Pomona, CA

Joan Engebretson, DrPH, AHN-BC, RN, Professor, School of Nursing, Department of Integrated Nursing Care, University of Texas Health Science Center-Houston, Houston, TX

Karyn Holt, PhD, CNM, Assistant Clinical Professor, Department of MSN Advanced Roles, College of Nursing and Health Professions, Drexel University, Philadelphia, PA

Alicia Huckstadt, PhD, ARNP, FNP-BC, GNP-BC, Professor and Graduate Programs Director, School of Nursing, Wichita State University, Wichita KA

Rose Marie E. Kunaszuk, DrNP, CNM, Nurse Midwife, Neighborhood Health Services, Plainfield NJ, Adjunct Nursing Faculty, Immaculata University, Immaculata, PA

Jean S. MacFadyen, PhD, MSEd, BA, BSN, Assistant Clinical Professor, Department of MSN Advanced Roles, College of Nursing and Health Professions, Drexel University, Philadelphia, PA

Anne C. Mohan, RN, DrNP(c), NEA-BC, Director, Professional Practice and Ambulatory Nursing Patient Safety Officer, Nursing Department, Children's Hospital of Philadelphia, Philadelphia, PA

Judith Reishtein, PhD, RN, Assistant Professor, Doctoral Nursing Department, Drexel University College of Nursing and Health Professions, Philadelphia, PA

Ruth Wittmann-Price, PhD, RN, CNS, CNE, Professor and Chair, Department of Nursing, Frances Marion University, Florence, SC

I. Historical and Theoretical Foundations for Role Delineation in Doctoral Advanced Nursing Practice

INTRODUCTION

H. Michael Dreher and Mary Ellen Smith Glasgow

Although the doctor of nursing practice (DNP) degree was introduced by one pioneering program in 2001, the degree first came into prominence in 2005 when a group of schools implemented several diverse models of doctor of nursing practice degree curricula (AACN, 2010; Fulton & Lyon, 2005). Today, there are 121 DNP programs and 1 DrNP program (as of September 2010). Led primarily by the American Association of Colleges of Nursing (AACN) and the National Organization of Nurse Practitioner Faculties (NONPF), the momentum toward the DNP degree model has been swift. However, in this early wave of momentum, the other primary nursing specialty organizations (representing nurse anesthetists, nurse midwives, and clinical nurse specialists) were on the periphery of the substantive discussion. Over time, there has been considerable outreach to the specialty organizations regarding the 2015 goal of endorsing the DNP degree as the entry-level degree for advanced practice nursing. In 2010, we see extensive dialogue and enormous progress with the doctor of nursing practice degree movement. Indeed, the DNP degree is projected to surpass the PhD in Nursing/Nursing Science in total number of programs in 2010 (Smith Glasgow, Dreher, Cornelius, & Bhattacharya, 2009). However, none of the leading advanced practice nursing organizations have endorsed the DNP degree for entry level into advanced practice nursing by 2015 as the AACN had envisioned in 2004.

In early 2010, the American Nurses Association (ANA) published a draft of their position statement on the Doctor of Nursing Practice degree. The organization is now in a period of public comment and we await their stand. Despite the reluctance to formalize doctoral entry into advanced practice nursing and begin the slow process of modifying 50 State Nurse Practice Acts, changing regulatory requirements on the federal, state, accrediting organizational and specialty practice level, there is enormous enthusiasm for this degree among nurse educators and DNP graduates who have graduated from the earliest founded programs. The primary authors of this text nevertheless believe that the ultimate success of this degree will be largely affected by the marketplace as well as the data-driven outcomes of these graduates. Therefore, it is critical, especially in a time of health-care upheaval and an economy with limited resources still recovering from the Great Recession, that DNP degree outcome research be conducted and data disseminated (Krugman, 2009).

This text explores the intricately complex historical trajectory of the discipline toward the nursing "practice doctorate" with an emphasis on the evolution of doctoral nursing practice roles. This new quest to prepare nurse clinicians (the four traditional APRN roles) and the nurse executive at the doctoral level is progressive, to some exhilarating, and still to others, regressive and unwelcome. Mainly, the real opposition to the DNP degree has waned, and the discussion is now, "what is the future of the doctor of nursing practice degree?" and "how does the degree need to be refined?" These authors hope that a more meaningful discussion about knowledge development occurs as the doctor of nursing practice degree evolves, especially because many senior nurse scientists are retiring and PhD enrolments are remaining flat. If the profession does not formally embrace DNP-generated "practice knowledge development," we are left to worry about the scientific basis of our discipline, which clinicians will need to practice safely and expertly. For a degree in its seminal stages of development, the doctoral nursing community needs to continue to debate and discuss the vision and essential competencies of this degree.

The first doctoral degree in nursing was an EdD in Nursing Education at Teacher's College, Columbia University in 1933 (Roy, 2007). Remarkably, despite its innovation, this degree model was never again replicated in the profession. The first PhD in Nursing was founded at New York University in 1934, and yet it was 20 years before the next PhD at the University of Pittsburgh was founded in 1954 (AACN, 2009). This text actually may be the first to declare that the first doctorate in nursing, the EdD, was actually *a practice doctorate*. Since the EdD degree is classified globally as a professional doctorate (Maxwell, 2003; Townsend, 2002) and the term "professional doctorate" has become mostly synonymous with "practice doctorate"[1] (the influential *Carnegie Project on the Education Doctorate* [n. d.] calls the EdD a "professional practice doctorate"), the DNP may simply be a doctoral degree that returns us to the practice roots of our profession and discipline. Thus, some may even consider the DNP degree "an awakening" and a welcome departure from our recent emphasis on the science of nursing at the expense of its art of practice. Alas, even the often used term *the practice of medicine* is still defined and described as both "art" and "science" (Tucker, 1999). The DNP degree will certainly undergo further metamorphosis and we have no idea what it will ultimately look like in 20 years. The anticipated transformation of the DNP degree is actually what makes graduate and doctoral nursing education so fascinating today.

We embrace debate, discourse, and difference in this text. The concept "difference" in many ways is naturally associated with "innovation" and indeed the statement made by Collinge, Burfitt, and MacNeill (2006) that "'Innovation' is the process of bringing 'novelty' into being, but to analyse this a little further it is useful to recognise that novelty is a kind of 'difference'" (p. 4). For this reason, as this degree moves into its first real decade, differences in doctor of nursing practice programs ought not to be the focus. Premature conformity in any industry (including education) can stamp out innovation and that is why "disruptive innovators" generally burst onto the scene with success (Christenson, 1997). What may be the better focus is to examine (1) of what is there much consensus? and (2) of what is there less? This might allow the discipline to spend less time on issues with the practice doctorate such as "whether we should have this degree" or whether "doctoral nursing practice is better than masters practice" (we contend it is more advanced, but the literature does not yet support it is better) and focus more on "what is the role of the DNP graduate with regard to knowledge development" and "how will DNP graduates be socialized to be more engaged stewards of the discipline than masters graduates"? We aver that DNP graduates *must* advance the discipline, even if some traditional PhD-degree focused faculty remain skeptical. After all, Lee S. Shulman (2010), President Emeritus of the Carnegie Foundation for the Advancement of Teaching and Professor of Education Emeritus at Stanford University, recently stated "Doctoral education shouldn't be a marathon" (p. 1).

The great advances of this degree for the profession include: (1) giving nurses a doctoral degree option other than the PhD; (2) more degree parity for highly educated nurse clinicians, nurse executives, and others; (3) enhanced credibility and prestige of DNP graduates in the corridors of the health practice environment and at the tables of health policy; and (4) more refined skills in knowledge management and in the translating and dissemination of evidence for healthcare utilization. However, unresolved issues remain: (1) how much research belongs in the practice doctorate?; (2) should DNP graduates become leaders in practice knowledge development derived by generating practice-based evidence (versus evidence-base practice)?; (3) is 1,000 total clinical hours for the DNP degree reasonable and sound?; (4) should there be any crossover coursework between DNP and PhD students?; and (5) should the PhD and DNP degrees ultimately be the only nursing doctorates offered? and (6) whether the EdD, DNS, and DrNP degree models, which only a few schools offer, be valid alternatives. As these issues are debated and hopefully resolved, it is still likely that the DNP degree may ultimately look different at research-intensive universities than at colleges where teaching is more of an emphasis. We, and the multiple contributors to this text, write with great optimism, but also with circumspect and critical analyses about the doctor of nursing practice degree. We view this approach to this text as a strength.

This text is divided into three sections. The first section is titled "Historical and Theoretical Foundations for Role Delineation in Doctoral Advanced Nursing Practice." In this section, the historical and political evolution of the doctor of nursing practice degree is traced and an analytical view of the "state of the degree" is presented. This section continues with a historical orientation of professional roles in nursing as the discipline slowly emerged from simply "work" to a "field" and then ultimately to a "discipline." Role theory and a perspective on the meaning of nursing roles, from professional to advanced, to doctoral advanced practice, are offered. The concluding chapters in this section trace the historical evolution of advanced practice nursing roles (including nurse practitioner, nurse midwife, nurse anesthetist, and clinical nurse specialist), and ends with an opening discussion by two doctor of nursing practice graduates, who discuss how their doctoral advanced practice roles differ from their previous master's roles.

The second section is titled "Primary and Secondary Contemporary Roles for Doctoral Advanced Nursing Practice." Here the contributing authors first discuss the two primary roles of the DNP degree that the American Association of Colleges of Nursing has endorsed—practitioner and clinical executive. It would, however, be neglectful not to address roles that other DNP or DrNP graduates are working in, and so the secondary roles of the educator and the clinical scientist chiefly working in the clinical trials/ pharmaceutical industry are also explored. This section concludes with an important discussion on the roles of both DAPRNs and DAPNs as clinical scholars. One of the assumptions of this text is that there is a domain of practice beyond the MSN degree (or why else obtain a practice doctorate?) and that with the doctoral credential the graduate is empowered and obliged to be a greater steward to the discipline. Part of this enhanced stewardship is a commitment to both the conduct and dissemination of clinical scholarship in its multiple forms.

The final section is titled "Operationalizing Role Functions of Doctoral Advanced Nursing Practice." This critical section of the text addresses the multifaceted aspects of the role of DAPRNs and DAPNs as they claim their new roles and enact them in the workplace. Smith Glasgow and Zoucha begin this section with a study of the roles of new doctor of nursing practice graduates. It is this kind of empirical data that the discipline will need in increasing volume in order to best understand the competencies and outcomes of this new critical mass of nurses who possess a practice doctorate. Career development is particularly important for DNPs, and since there are few role models, the first graduate cohorts will eventually become the mentors of the future. Chapters 11 and 16 both discuss this important topic. DNP graduates are educated to assume higher levels of leadership with enhanced skills, and therefore with doctoral preparation much more is expected from them. Chapter 12 specifically addresses leadership preparation for the DNP-educated clinical executive and Chapters 13 and 15 outline the benefits of coaching for DNP students and the art of negotiation, two important aspects of any diverse DNP role. DNP student and graduate skills at knowledge management are critical and discussed in Chapter 14. While there has been great emphasis recently on BSN and MSN student technology competencies, there needs to be equivalent (and perhaps more) emphasis on how the DNP graduate can leverage technology to enhance their doctoral practice role.

Chapter 17 examines the necessity for more interprofessional collaboration between DAPRNs/DAPNs and their peer health professions colleagues. Having a critical mass of new nurse clinicians with doctoral preparation will likewise be very new for other disciplines who will be working with and alongside these new graduates. Chapter 18 calls attention to what is expected of this new graduate—a higher level of expert advocacy. One of the positive aspects of this new role is that its graduates are expected to exert greater influence on health practice and health policy. Chapters 19 and 22 address two very controversial issues with the nursing practice doctorate—the use of the title "Dr" by new DNP/DrNP graduates, and the very controversial DNP exam. Because these two issues are so volatile, this text has reflective responses both supporting and opposing the chapter authors' arguments.

Among the concluding chapters in this text is Chapter 20, which proposes that the DAPRN must engage in more reflective practice in order to enhance the doctoral practitioner role. And finally, Chapter 21 outlines why DNP/DrNP clinical scholars ought to have more real educational experiences in global health, and why a mandatory study abroad program is one way to achieve this. The final two chapters are designed to leave the doctor of nursing practice student with thought of the present and future. Bloch, with her some 30 years as a veteran nurse practitioner, has wise counsel and advice, particularly for MSN-prepared NPs who are heading back to graduate school and perhaps wondering how their doctoral degree might really improve their already fine-tuned practice. The text concludes with some futuristic thoughts about the doctor of nursing practice degree by the text's two primary authors. We provide a summary of the text's discussion of the practitioner, clinical executive, educator, and clinical scientist role; we also present projections of how we see these roles evolving in the future.

After each of these chapters, reflective responses are provided by leading academics, administrators, and practitioners, including graduates from different doctor of nursing practice programs. These contributions by leading nursing scholars are one great innovation of this text. Sometimes these additional viewpoints complement, sometimes contradict, but mostly add additional insight and perspective. The concluding reflective response is by Dr. Suzanne Prevost, President Elect of Sigma Theta Tau International. In the end, we are certain these reflective responses will markedly enhance the discussion that will likely take place in the classroom or online as these multiple positions are evaluated. Each chapter also has 10 critical thinking questions which we highly recommend as discussion points, paper topics, debates, or even as weekly written assignments. We mostly hope they will be fodder for "tussling in the doctoral classroom," which is what the late Dr. Susan K. Leddy (Dr. Dreher's dissertation chair and former Dean at Widener University) said should occur in doctoral study. She had little affinity for polite or convenient agreement. Having completed a postdoctoral research fellowship late in her career, Dr. Leddy told us she did not feel that conformist thinking advanced science much. She embraced vigorous debate, but she always required doctoral nursing students to provide principled rationales for their arguments.

We are both indebted to the many contributors to this text who are all paving the way for an improved doctor of nursing practice degree that will ultimately gain its proper place and foothold in the discipline. In many ways, this text *could not* have been written earlier. Only now, after five years, have the substantive issues with the degree begun to surface in a constructive and perhaps less political way. This degree is alive and thriving and it is up to you, your faculty, and all other stakeholders (and there are many) to move forward, advance the nursing discipline, and improve the health of this nation and the globe.

NOTE

1. Many revisionists considered the ND degree the first "practice nursing doctorate," when in reality, the title "practice doctorate" was not yet in the common vernacular nor a recognized term when the degree was first offered at Case Western Reserve University in 1979 (Schlotfeldt, 1978).

REFERENCES

American Association of Colleges of Nursing (AACN). (2004a). *AACN position statement on the practice doctorate in nursing October 2004.* Retrieved from http://www.aacn.nche.edu/DNP/pdf/DNP.pdf

American Association of Colleges of Nursing (AACN). (2006). *The essentials of doctoral education for advanced nursing practice.* Retrieved from http://www.aacn.nche.edu/DNP/pdf/Essentials.pdf

American Association of Colleges of Nursing (AACN). (2009). *Institutions offering doctoral programs in nursing and degrees conferred.* Retrieved from http://www.aacn.nche.edu/IDS/pdf/DOC.pdf

American Association of Colleges of Nursing (AACN). (2010). *Doctor of nursing practice (DNP) programs.* http://www.aacn.nche.edu/DNP/DNPProgramList.htm

Carnegie Project on the Practice Doctorate (n.d.). Resource Library. Retrieved from http://cpcdinitiative.org/resource-library

Christensen, C. (1997). *The innovator's dilemma: When new technologies cause great firms to fail.* Cambridge: Harvard Business Press.

Collinge, C., Burfitt, A., & MacNeill, S. (2006). The impossibility of innovation: Towards a knowledge-based approach to Eurodite. *Paper presented at the EURODITE, Regional Trajectories to the Knowledge Economy Meeting, DG Research, European Commission,* Brussels, Belgium, March 30–31.

Fulton, J., & Lyon, B. (2005). The need for some sense making: Doctor of nursing practice. *Journal of Issues in Nursing, 10*(3), Manuscript 3. Retrieved from www.nursingworld.org/MainMenu-Categories/ANAMarketplace/ANAPeriodicals/OJIN/TableofContents/Volume102005/No3Sept05/tpc28_316027.aspx

Krugman, P. (2009). The Great Recession versus the Great Depression. *New York Times.com* Retrieved from http://krugman.blogs.nytimes.com/2009/03/20/the-great-recession-versus-the-great-depression/

Maxwell, T. (2003). From first to second generation professional doctorate. *Studies in Higher Education, 28*(3), 279–291.

Roy, C. (2007). Advances in nursing knowledge and the challenge for transforming nursing practice. In C. Roy, & D. A. Jones (Eds.), *Nursing knowledge development and clinical practice* (pp. 3–38). New York, NY: Springer.

Schlotfeldt, R. M. (1978). The professional doctorate: Rationale and characteristics. *Nursing Outlook, 26,* 302–311.

Shulman, L. S. (2010). Doctoral education shouldn't be a marathon. *The Chronicle Review of Higher Education,* April 4, 2010 Retrieved from http://chronicle.com/article/Doctoral-Education-Isnt-a/64883/

Smith Glasgow, M. E., Dreher, H. M., Cornelius, F., & Bhattacharya, A. (2009). *A preliminary report on a national study of doctoral faculty (both PhD and DNP) and succession planning.* Paper presented at the Second National Conference on The Doctor of Nursing Practice: The Dialogue Continues. . ., Hilton Head Island, SC, March 24–27, 2009.

Townsend, B. K. (2002). *Rethinking the Ed.D., or what's in a name.* Paper presented at the Annual Meeting of the Association for the Study of Higher Education, Sacramento, CA, November 21–24, 2002.

Tucker, N. H., III. (1999). President's message—Medicine: Art versus Science. *Jacksonsville Medicine, 15*(12), December.

CHAPTER ONE

The Historical and Political Path of Doctoral Nursing Education to the Doctor of Nursing Practice Degree

H. Michael Dreher

INTRODUCTION

This opening chapter will examine the history of the Doctor of Nursing Practice degree in the United States. It is the historical and sociological evolution of the degree and its reception in our health system labor market that will ultimately shape the role of this new *doctoral advanced practice nurse* or the nurse who engages in *doctoral advanced nursing practice* (Dreher & Montgomery, 2009). The chapter will draw upon contexts, both historical and political, that illustrate the progress of the degree—from the earliest attempts, the failures and successes in our discipline—to first create a professional doctorate (EdD), then a research doctorate (PhD), a clinical doctorate (DNSc), another professional doctorate (ND), and finally a practice doctorate (DNP), including other various degree iterations splattered along the way—DSN, DNS, and DrNP.[1] Some of the important benefits and largely unresolved issues with this still relatively new DNP degree will also be summarized. Finally, this chapter will conclude with final points on how the American iteration of the DNP degree interfaces with the prevalent international professional doctorate degree model, highlighting how today's global health issues can impact anyone anywhere, and the need for the health professions', education that advances health best for all.

A new doctorate in any discipline is rarely created without some controversy. The doctor of nursing practice degree is no different. However, the largely subsided controversy today is more "Where do we go from here?" Some of the earliest programs are now about 5 years old, and curriculum evaluation and revision are underway in many of these institutions with some already having performed the perfunctory initial tweaks. Different from most historical analyses in nursing education, this chapter will attempt to provide an honest and objective (as much as possible) narrative critique of both the problems and progress of this new nursing doctorate as it has emerged over this last decade. This author was not at the table of the American Association of Colleges of Nursing (AACN) when members (restricted to College and Schools of Nursing Deans only) cast a very narrow vote in 2004 to require the DNP degree instead of the MSN degree for advanced practice registered nurses[2] (APRNs) by 2015. However, this author has nonetheless been a keen observer of the practice doctorate movement from the beginning and even prior to 2004 (AACN, 2004a; Dreher, 2005; Dreher, Donnelly, & Naremore, 2005; Smith Glasgow & Dreher, 2010).

My own university sponsored what was the very first national conference on the practice nursing doctorate in Annapolis, Maryland, in 2007 titled *The Practice Doctorate: Where Is It Headed? The First National Conference on the Doctor of Nursing Practice: Meanings and Models* and the third held in Hilton Head Island, South Carolina, in 2009 titled *The Doctor of Nursing Practice: The Dialogue Continues . . . .* The next Drexel DNP Conference is being planned for fall 2011. At each of these venues, many of the contemporary discussion points were highly visible in the podium papers, poster sessions, and in the conversations and networking that took place among faculty, some of the first graduates with the degree in the country, and current students. Actually, as the Conference Chair for each of those conferences, one of the primary objectives of the organizing committee was to attempt to provide a safe platform for nursing scholars with diverse points of view. We thought that the profession was in need of more critical discourse about the DNP degree, especially from a broader subset of doctoral nursing faculty who were not necessarily academic administrators or not tied more publically to the mission or position statements of various nursing organizations.

Internal debate, nonetheless, is nothing new to nursing. We only have to look at our profession's failure, now about 35 years and counting, to require the BSN degree for entry into professional nursing for example (Donley & Flaherty, 2008). Labor historian Barbara Melosh (1982), in her outstanding sociological analysis of nursing in *The Physician's Hand: Work, Culture and Conflict in American Nursing*, calls the history of nursing a battle between the "professionalizers" and the "traditionalists." The battle lines again appear to be drawn (although more meekly or perhaps less visibly these days) between those perceived to be the most in favor of requiring the practice doctorate for advanced practice by 2015—the professionalizers (nursing academics), and those against—the traditionalists (the masses of currently practicing advanced practice nurses). This divide exists since APRNs, despite being only master's prepared (and without a DNP degree), astutely know the literature which touts their outstanding outcomes is widely acknowledged (Horrocks, Anderson, & Salisbury, 2002; Mundinger et al., 2000). Of course, this description is partly an oversimplification, as these lines are not so black and white. There are indeed nursing faculty who oppose the DNP degree (increasingly fewer it seems) and APRNs who support it (increasingly more it seems). And of course, if you are a DNP student reading this book, you are likely matriculating in a DNP program of your own volition, and therefore absolutely not a traditionalist! Nonetheless, discourse, debate, and critique are very healthy for our discipline. Absolute division is not. Maybe with the surge of the DNP degree (and make no mistake, nursing education has *never* seen a degree captivating the profession so quickly), professionalizers and traditionalists can learn from each other. It would be helpful in the spirit of egalitarianism (not elitism) and continuous improvement, however, if the nursing profession's members could work more cohesively toward the broader benefit of increased access to health services and ultimately to the improvement of health in our nation.

Hopefully, as we reflect on from where we have come, we can emphasize graduate nursing education policy that is both evidence based and does not do what Melosh says happened in our earlier history when "Nurses on the job were sometimes threatened by the strategies leaders adopted, for the rising standards of professionalization often meant downgrading or even eliminating current practitioners" (1982, p. 5). Dracup and Bryan-Brown (2005) also express these concerns, stating "We also worry that the current advanced practice nurses who hold MS degrees will feel disenfranchised" (p. 280).

And in very frank language, Dracup and Bryan-Brown echo much of Melosh's early analysis:

> When nursing education moved from the hospital to the university or college setting, diploma nurses found themselves with an education that provided little or no college credit. We had an entire generation of embittered nurses who saw nursing academics as out of touch with clinical practice ... "
>
> — *2005, p. 280*

We implore the nursing profession not to forget its history and, this time, to learn from some of these very painful growing pains in our discipline, and respond differently in the future. As Dracup and Bryan-Brown beseech, we must avoid disenfranchising a large number of nurse practitioners, nurse midwives, nurse anesthetists, and clinical nurse specialists who believed they were properly prepared for their roles when they entered advanced practice with a master's degree.

BACKGROUND

This book may be the first to have ever declared that the first doctorate in nursing, the EdD in Nursing Education at Teacher's College, Columbia University in 1933, was actually a professional (or practice) doctorate.[3] Globally, the EdD degree is viewed as the professional doctorate in education, whereas the PhD in Education is viewed as the research degree (Maxwell, 2003; Townsend, 2002). Herein lies one of the issues that still plague the nursing academy with the DNP degree. The EdD graduate also completes a dissertation (like the PhD graduate), but the EdD dissertation is more practice oriented and work based. Some even view the EdD as a research degree, too, but it is worth noting that Harvard does not offer the PhD in Education; it offers only the EdD (Baez, 2002; Courtenay, 1988). And like Harvard's DBA degree (Doctor of Business Administration), both are viewed as professional doctorates but include practice-oriented, rigorous research (Fink, 2006). The DNP degree, however, is very similar to other professional doctorates that do not normally include an original research project—the Doctor of Medicine (MD), the Doctor of Pharmacy (PharmD), and the Doctor of Physical Therapy (DPT), for example. Nonetheless, in 2010, this question remains one of the most contentious discussion points among doctoral nursing educators (both DNP and PhD): What is the role of research in the DNP degree, and should DNP students and graduates generate *new nursing knowledge* or be restricted to expertly translating and disseminating what is currently known? We will revisit this issue later in this chapter as we discuss the central unresolved issues with the degree. Nevertheless, maybe what we are attempting now with the largely DNP degree, is simply a return to nursing's orientation as a practice discipline in the way the EdD was first created to advance nursing education practice. Some would applaud this return to our disciplinary roots, whereas others would see this as a diversion.

As there was very sluggish growth of doctoral programs in nursing after the Teacher's College experiment in 1933, it is noteworthy that three of the next four doctoral nursing programs were aimed at clinical specialization in the discipline rather than a doctorate awarded in the general discipline of nursing itself. The first PhD (Doctor of Philosophy) program in Nursing was started at New York University in 1934. There is not a lot written about this very early PhD and this author has wondered "Who taught in this program?" Further, because nursing was often not allowed to offer a PhD degree by many university faculties beginning in the 1960s and into the 21st century,[4] with other disciplines arguing "is nursing a *real* science?," it is remarkable that the New York University faculty was progressive enough to position itself at the literal forefront of nursing as a recognized academic discipline (Meleis & Dracup, 2005). It would take until the mid-1980s, at least 50 years, before nursing science would clearly evolve into a scientific discipline (Dreher, 2010a); and as stated in a recent issue of *The Academic Nurse* (2010), "In late 1985 . . . In nursing schools where faculty were active in moving the profession forward, research was now becoming a significant part of the academic role, while at the same time faculty clinical practice was falling out of favor" (p. 21). The third and fourth doctorates in nursing were developed with a clinical focus. The PhD in Nursing at the University of Pittsburgh was started in 1954 with a clinical nursing and clinical research emphasis and the DNSc (Doctor of Nursing Science) at Boston University in 1960 with a psychiatric-mental health focus (Grace, 1989; Nichols & Chitty, 2005). Two important distinctions should be made about these two programs, as they both created two distinctive pathways to nursing science knowledge development and shaped doctoral nursing education differently.

First, it is the historic inability of the profession to truly develop a widely viewed "clinical doctorate" for the profession as an alternative to the research-intensive PhD that has led to the surge of the DNP degree. Fitzpatrick (2003) made a very strong case for the clinical doctorate in nursing in 2003 (prior to the 2004 AACN vote), even advocating a clinical doctorate for teachers. Over the years, much has been written about the DNSc, DSN (Doctor of Science in Nursing), and DNS (Doctor of Nursing Science) degrees. While all three were initially designed to be clinically oriented doctorates, the profession has come to view them all as *de facto* PhD degrees (AACN, 2006; Carlson, 2003). To that measure, in 2010 almost all of them have now converted to a PhD mostly in the last decade (except for one DNSc degree at the University of Tennessee Health Sciences Center, which oddly converted to a DNP program perhaps because they already had a PhD degree). See Table 1.1 below; it lists most of the schools that attempted the Clinical Doctorate and also traces one school's history from its earliest nursing education, to the conversion of their clinical doctorate (DNS) to a PhD, and finally to approval of the DNP degree (Exhibit 1.1).

The unanswered question is why did the profession ultimately abandon the idea of a clinical doctorate? The discipline of psychology faced this very issue in the 1960s when many felt the PhD in Psychology had become too research oriented, too experimental,

TABLE 1.1
The First Quest for an Alternative Nursing Doctorate to the PhD

Iteration #1: The "Doctor of Nursing Science" degree: DNSc	First at Boston University 1960, later at UCSF, Penn, Columbia, Yale, Catholic, Rush, Widener, etc. . . . all phased out now
Iteration #2: The "Doctor of Science of Nursing" degree: DSN	First at the University of Alabama-Birmingham 1975, later at East Tennessee State, U Texas Health Sciences-Houston, West Virginia, etc. . . . all phased out now
Iteration #3: The "Doctor of Nursing Science" degree: DNS	First at Indiana University 1976, later at Arizona State, LSU Health Sciences Center (LSUHSC), University of Buffalo, etc . . . all of these are phased out except LSUHSC, The City University of New York (CUNY), Kennesaw State University, and the Sage Colleges

EXHIBIT 1.1   The Indiana University Nursing Story

University-based nursing education began in 1914

Sigma Theta Tau founded in 1922 by 6 educators from Indiana University Training School for Nurses

BSN curricula first established 1932

MS first offered 1945

MSN first offered 1966

DNS approved 1976

First DNS degree awarded 1981

Planning for PhD began 1990

DNS converts to PhD 1996

DNP degree approved 2009

and not client focused. As a result, the Doctor of Psychology degree (PsyD) was first started in 1968 as a clinical doctorate (Murray, 2000). The PsyD degree, however, did not eliminate the research enterprise in the new degree, only de-emphasized it, and its founders developed a clinical dissertation model in lieu of the traditional PhD dissertation, which is still integral to the degree (Sayette, Mayne, & Norcross, 2010). Peterson (1997), in referring to the PsyD degree versus the PhD, succinctly said that it is not that science and practice do not belong in the same program, but that it is a matter of emphasis. The AACN, however, is quite precise in stating that the DNP degree should not be described as a clinical doctorate but a "practice doctorate" stating: "The Task Force recommends that the terminology, practice doctorate be used instead of clinical doctorate" (2004a, p. 4). Is the reason for this distinction (i.e., calling the DNP a "practice" doctorate and not a "clinical" doctorate) the realization that our earlier clinical doctorate nursing models did include both a clinical and research emphasis (and the desire, at least by the AACN leadership at the time, was to move away from this type of degree model)? We will later revisit two universities that have tried to resurrect different models of the "clinical doctorate" in 2005, but their curricular innovations have not been adopted by others (Dreher et al., 2005; Mundinger, 2009).

Second, the arrival of the PhD at the University of Pittsburgh in 1954 was perhaps better timed than the PhD at NYU in 1934 for the slow maturation of the field of nursing to a discipline. The profession's first research journal, *Nursing Research*, was founded in 1952, and this author discusses at length the early struggles of the journal to attract enough high-level, true research-oriented submissions in chapter 15 in *Philosophy of Science for Nursing Practice* (Dreher, 2010a). The profession also benefited, especially the specialty of psychiatric-mental health nursing, with the publication and work of Dr. Hildegard Peplau's *Interpersonal Relations in Nursing* in 1952. Her work spurred interest in this specialty, and indeed the editor of *Nursing Research* at one early point emphasized (or complained about?) the overrepresentation of articles specific to psychiatric-mental health nursing (Bunge, 1962). Nevertheless, the momentum was slowly growing toward nursing as a scientific discipline. With the first federal research grants in nursing established in 1955 through a new research and fellowship branch within the federal Division of Nursing Resources (founded in 1948) and the first grants awarded that fall, and with the later implementation of the Nurse-Scientist Training Program in 1961, the growing need for nurses with a doctorate was emerging (Gortner, 1986,

TABLE 1.2
First Doctoral Nursing Programs in the United States

Rank	Institution	Degree	Year
1	Teacher's College, Columbia University	EdD	1933
2	New York University	PhD	1934
3	University of Pittsburgh	PhD	1954
4	Boston University	DNSc	1960
5	University of California San Francisco	DNSc	1964
6	Catholic University	DNSc	1967
7	Texas Woman's University	PhD	1971
8	Case Western Reserve University	PhD	1972
9	University of Pennsylvania	DNSc	1974
	University of Texas-Austin	PhD	1974
10	University of Alabama-Birmingham	DSN	1975
	University of Illinois-Chicago	PhD	1975
	University of Michigan	PhD	1975
	Wayne State University	PhD	1975
	University of Arizona	PhD	1975

2000). Interestingly, with so few doctoral programs in nursing in 1961 (there were only three), this innovative research training program prepared nurses for PhDs in *other fields besides nursing*. The idea was that hopefully these early nurse scientists from the fields of sociology, anthropology, and psychology, for example, would graduate and then pursue nursing scientific inquiry and establish new doctoral programs in nursing. Table 1.2 lists the first 10 doctoral programs in nursing, and the prevalence of the PhD degree or the clinical doctorate (the DNSc in particular) should be noted. What is perhaps fascinating is why the Teacher's College degree model EdD in Nursing Education was never again replicated. There have recently been new PhDs in Nursing Education (the University of Northern Colorado established in 2004), but they are rare.[5]

It is obvious, especially with the further establishment of the First Division of Nursing Field Research Center founded in San Francisco in 1962, that nursing was aiming toward a scientific orientation (Vreeland, 1964).[6] Whether that would evolve at the expense of the discipline's original practice orientation is another question. This author would add that it is the failure of the discipline to bridge its two disciplinary orientations, what Peplau aptly called the "art and science [*or art versus science*] of nursing" (1988, p. 8), that has led many practicing nurses (both professional and advanced) to view the "nursing ivory tower" as too removed from practice (and its realities) and, in some eyes, even irrelevant.

THE EVOLUTION OF THE NEED FOR THE NURSE WITH A DOCTORATE

With the first step in the movement of nursing into the university setting—which included various landmark events such as: (1) the first constituted nursing school in a university (albeit under Medicine) at the University of Minnesota in 1909; (2) the first individual (Professor Adelaide Nutting) appointed as a nursing professor at Teacher's College in 1910; and (3) the first independent nursing school at Yale University in 1924—nursing began its slow path to perceiving the need for the profession to produce nurses with doctorates (Donohue, 1996). If nurses were indeed going to be full members of the academy (a rather oblique term which includes the members of the formal academic community) with other disciplines, this would be essential. The Flexner Report on the state of medical education in 1910 also had implications for nursing education (Flexner, 1910). Although this report was in many ways very critical of institutionalized medicine,[7] medicine's dominance over nursing was under way (Hiatt, 1999). Further, and perhaps most importantly, the derision of medicine did not elevate nursing or the status of nurses. This widely publicized report on medicine also made it obvious to nursing leaders that they would likewise need to evaluate the state of nursing education even as the profession was in its early formative years. A subsequent 1912 report titled *The Educational Status of Nursing* (Nutting, 1912), which became the first comprehensive survey of schools of nursing, was likewise critical of the about 1,100 schools of nursing that responded. Of this report Melosh (1982) writes, "... 315 schools, or nearly 45 percent, reported that they did not have a single paid instructor, and 299 did not maintain a library. Instead the nursing 'curriculum' in many hospitals consisted of two or three years of ward work" (1982, p. 41).

THEN: THE DOCTORAL-PREPARED NURSE EMERGES FROM A MINISCULE POOL

The ultimate movement of nursing into the college and university from the hospital-based diploma settings has taken place ever so slowly in the past 100 years (diploma programs are still widespread in Pennsylvania and Ohio and sparingly elsewhere). And while the average nurse today is first educated in a college or university (more than 95% of all new nurse graduates), it is certain that the early nursing leaders who sought the increasing professionalism of nursing did not intend that nursing education should be from a community college rather than from a university or other 4-year degree granting institution (National League for Nursing [NLN], 2007). Among the 1.4 million nurses who entered the profession between 1970 and 1994 with either an Associate Degree (AD) or BSN, 59% entered with an AD and 41% a BSN (Aiken, Cheung, & Olds, 2009). More recently, NLN data from 2006 to 2007 indicate that 60% of new graduates are AD prepared and 31% BSN prepared (2007). Further, in California, our largest and sometimes called the most progressive state, about 70% of all RNs have an AD (Dreher, 2008a). Because only 6% of nurses who first get an AD go on to higher education and advanced practice (the master's degree), this trend toward a community college nursing education continues to have an enormous negative impact on the profession, as it continues to face a shortage of RNs (despite the Great Recession), a shortage of nursing faculty (with doctorates), and a shortage of nurse scientists with the projected retirements of so many senior faculty (Aiken, Cheung, & Olds). Further, the movement to end advanced practice at the master's degree, or at least the transition away from the MSN to the DNP, has caused some to warn that this move may cause a drop in the number of new nurse practitioners each year (Bloch, 2007; Dreher & Gardner, 2009; Ford, 2008). As the expense and time commitment to skip the MSN can be burdensome and can take longer than obtaining the MSN, the Great Recession that began in the Bush administration and continued into the Obama administration is already impacting the employer-based tuition reimbursement system that so many RNs who seek higher education have always relied on (Azam, 2010; Babcock, 2009; Krugman, 2009). Bloch warns that nurse practitioners, particularly those who work with vulnerable professions, may see declining numbers, and this would be tragic, especially now that about 30 million or more individuals will be transitioning into the health care system in the next 5 years and will need primary care (National Association of Community Health Centers, 2009). We mention this in particular because the 2004 AACN vote must be placed in this context—the vote occurred *before* this substantial economic downturn and this author wonders whether it would still pass today?

Likely, and partly due to economic factors that have impacted the United States since the 2004 AACN vote (2004a), we are seeing that while more schools are offering the post-master's DNP degree, they are increasingly reticent about closing their MSN advanced practice tracks out of fear of potential declining enrollments and loss of tuition revenue. We now hear of schools indicating that they plan to offer both options (MSN and DNP entry), and at the recent 2010 National Organization of Nurse Practitioner Faculties (NONPF) meeting, the sense was that both degrees would continue and be supported at least for the time being (*Academic Nurse*, 2010). Despite offering a post-master's DrNP degree (and a BSN-to-DrNP option that does not prepare APRNs), my own college has actually expanded its MSN nurse practitioner offerings recently. Further, there is no current plan to phase them out, but to perhaps add an option for doctoral entry. Further, the greater Philadelphia region is saturated with nursing schools, and yet only in fall 2010 will the first nursing school in this region offer a BSN-to-DNP program for nurse practitioners. In a 2009 article in *The American Nurse*, Dean and Professor Linda Cronenwett of the School of Nursing at the University of North Carolina Chapel Hill was quoted stating, "I support the DNP essentials outlined by AACN and the important emphasis on quality and safety competencies, but I think society would be better served by a post-master's DNP" (Trossman, 2009, p. 8).

So the question remains: Does the profession really need nurses with doctorates? The answer is unequivocally "yes." In our history, the burden of a burgeoning discipline has always necessitated that nurses posess doctorates to achieve parity with other faculty in other disciplines in colleges and universities (the academy). Superimposed on this need for nurses with doctorates with research skills was the realization that if the scientific basis of nursing was going to grow, the profession would need them in larger numbers, and thus we saw mostly new PhD and DNSc programs opening in the 1970s. Certainly, this supply would have to grow in order for more rigorous nursing science to be conducted and for our science to be perceived more as a "real science" by others. We should mention that as the science of nursing slowly evolved, there was initially a focus on nursing administration and nursing education research and an absence of focus on clinical research. Indeed, with the founding of the Association of Collegiate Schools of Nursing in 1935, with its mission to promote nursing education in the collegiate/university environment and away from the hospital-based programs, one of the aims of the new organization was "to promote study and experimentation in nursing service and nursing education" (Goodrich, 1936, p. 767). This may very well have been one of the earliest visible policy statements to encourage nursing research. And yet, over time, while nursing administration research has been aligned with health services research, the predominance of clinical research over all other types (with the devaluation of nursing education research), the debate has largely waned, and clinical research, favoring quantitative methods, now predominates as it has more and more extensive funding sources (Hutchinson, 2001; Werley & Westlake, 1985). Despite significant advances in nursing education, however, education-focused research in the discipline has unfortunately suffered, and this author believes that this did not need to happen. For example, nursing health systems research (oriented toward the administrative indirect care role in nursing) has grown in sophistication over the decades. One only has to look at the extensive work of Dr. Linda Aiken, Claire M. Fagin Leadership Professor in Nursing, Professor of Sociology, and Director of the Center for Health Outcomes and Policy Research at the University of Pennsylvania School of Nursing, to see the kind of high impact that nursing health system research can make. Nursing education research, however, has suffered from a lack of innovation and too many education-oriented dissertations that have focused on minor issues of importance inside and outside the profession. Maybe this will change as the NLN slowly ramps up its nursing education funding, and *if* DNP faculty scholars and graduates seriously conduct and publish outcome data.

Severely complicating this early drive to the doctorate were data in 1965 indicating that only approximately 22% of all nurses had been prepared in academic programs (this included AD graduates) (Nelson, 2002). As mentioned earlier, the American Nurses Association (ANA) in 1965 first tried to change this percentage by mandating that nursing education should take place in a college or university setting, and that the BSN be required for entry into professional nursing (Donley & Flaherty, 2008). Today, this percentage has grown to about 45%; hence, although the mandate was never realized, perhaps there has been some success at upgrading the overall preparation of registered nurses (Aiken et al., 2009). Next, the emergence of the nurse practitioner role at the University of Colorado, Denver, in 1965 and the rise of nurse practitioner programs offering MSN degrees in the 1970s increased the need for the doctoral credential for faculty nurse practitioners, as nurses without common university credentials (typically the PhD) were marginalized in academia (Dunphy, Smith, & Youngkin, 2009; Silver, Ford, & Day, 1968). What is not known, however, is how broadly current faculty nurse practitioners (or other advanced practice nursing faculty) are indeed prepared at the doctoral level. This author's cursory review of many nursing school websites across the country indicates that there are still a plethora of nurse practitioner track coordinators, particularly nurse anesthesia program coordinators, who do not possess the doctorate. Perhaps the DNP degree will help alleviate this.

NOW: THE DWINDLING SUPPLY OF NURSING FACULTY WITH THE PhD

More contemporary, in 2008, the AACN published a white paper *The Preferred Vision of the Professoriate in Baccalaureate and Graduate Nursing Programs* indicating that nurses who teach in university settings (not the community college) should have a doctorate degree at minimum (AACN, 2008). Unfortunately, in challenging economic times, the profession faces two issues on this front to accomplish this: (1) how to attract more nurses to doctoral study and to the educator role; and (2) how can we help the masses of MSN-prepared faculty across the country complete a doctorate? These two issues are critically important since it is the nursing faculty role that most drives the need for nurses with doctorates. For instance, DNP programs would not be offered, nor would you be sitting in your classroom (or behind your computer), if there were not a faculty member in front of you or online.[8] Similarly, it will likely take time for the consumer health care market to expect the nurse clinician (CRNP, CRNA, CNM, or CNS) to have a doctorate in the same way that it is expected in academia.

The complete answer to the first question above—how to attract more nurses to doctoral study and to the educator role—is beyond the scope of this chapter. There is, however, a protracted nursing faculty shortage that has now existed for over a decade and is predicted to persist (AACN, 1999, 2005a; Aiken et al., 2009). The reasons why the shortage is likely to continue include the following:

- A predicted surge in faculty retirements that will exceed predicted replacements (Smith Glasgow & Dreher, 2010);
- Lack of competitive salaries for nursing professors versus what they can earn in industry (Smith & Dreher, 2003);
- Lack of adequate role modeling in undergraduate nursing education to foster pursuing the doctorate and a teaching career (Potempa, Redman, & Anderson, 2008); and
- Perhaps even gender bias in the academy that disenfranchises nursing schools, largely composed of women, from their full exercise of power, influence, and benefit in many colleges and universities (Smith & Dreher, 2003).

One example of the above, with regard to gender bias,[9] is the low comparative research start-up packages reported for tenure-track nursing faculty versus start-up packages for business, law, medicine, and engineering faculty (Valian, 2005). While Rudy and Grady (2005) reported that among 31 biological nurse scientists engaged mostly in animal-model research (48% had formal postdoctoral training and all had received previous NINR funding), their mean research start-up package was for $50,000 (in the range from $2,000 to $105,000); this author has heard numerous doctoral faculty at the annual AACN Doctoral Nursing Education meeting complain about their comparative research start-up packages in their own universities.[10] Further, administrative stipends for nursing administrators pale in comparison to stipends for faculty administrators from the disciplines mentioned above and perhaps others (Kirkpatrick, 1994). While Kirkpatrick in 1994 reported stipends as low as $1,000 for the nursing department chair, this type of data admittedly is hard to substantiate, because the university power structure that favors one discipline (for whatever reason) over another has reason to keep these data hidden. Nevertheless, this author (and others) have had multiple confirmations of this practice, and there is no reason to believe that this inequity has been rectified in the last 15 years. This critique of the "status of the nurse in the academy" is not meant to discourage readers from the professoriate, but to identify some of the challenges that the current generation and next generation of nursing professors will face. A critical mass of DNP faculty educators in particular, whose own entrance into the academy is going to spark a multitude of additional issues, may be particularly vulnerable.

The second item, encouraging MSN-prepared faculty to pursue the doctorate, is equally problematic. I am reminded of Melosh's (1982) and Dracup and Bryan-Brown's (2005) critiques of the disenfranchisement of nurses in an earlier generation (and the risk to current MSN-prepared APRNs), and of the current lack of flexible transitioning to the next degree as the profession suddenly mandates a doctorate for all university nursing professors (AACN, 2008). On the surface, this is a realistic expectation—that nurses who teach in a university setting should possess a doctorate. But again, as a practice profession, is this realistic? Foremost, what is needed most in undergraduate and advanced practice nursing education is to have faculty who are current and competent. I recall very vividly in my own master's education in the late 1980s how a very talented pathophysiology instructor (with an MSN) was removed from the roster in favor of a faculty member with a doctorate who had very little background or currency in the topic. We literally taught ourselves each week with class presentations. Most current MSN-prepared nursing faculty have no aim to be nurse scientists, and thus the PhD option (which takes an average of 8.3 years to complete post a master's degree!) for many reasons is not attractive (Valiga, 2004). Further, many nursing schools prohibit nurses from matriculating in internal doctoral nursing programs (they must go to another university for the nursing doctorate or attend a non-nursing, internally offered doctorate). And even in those universities that do permit internal matriculation, "faculty-as-students" face conflicts of interest when nursing faculty attend classes taught (and graded) by their peers and colleagues (Anselmi, Dreher, Smith Glasgow, & Donnelly, 2010). If the PhD is not an option, then what other nursing degree can faculty attend?

The DNP degree is being increasingly suggested as a solution to the nursing faculty shortage, but strangely, the nursing educator role is not a role supported by the AACN within the confines of the normal DNP curriculum (AACN, 2006; Fitzpatrick, 2008). Authors in this text will argue for this to change, especially because Zungolo (2009) indicates that more than 30% of all DNP graduates *are going into academia.* This more than supports earlier data from Loomis, Willard, and Cohen (2006) indicating that 55% of a sample of current DNP students ($N = 69$) had intentions of pursuing a career in nursing education post graduation. The fear is that these graduates may be unprepared for the faculty role and may experience even more inequities in the academy. McKenna (2005) has similarly suggested that "However, a word of warning; without an adequate background in the knowledge and skills necessary for teaching and scholarship, these people [graduates from practice doctorate programs] may be set up for failure in the University setting" (p. 246). The AACN (2006) has suggested that DNP graduates may take *extra courses* to add the educator role to the DNP degree. Again, this seems reminiscent of Melosh's (1982) earlier critique of nursing leadership's professionalizers. The NLN (2007), however, has indicated some displeasure with the DNP degree being promoted as a solution to the nursing faculty shortage, especially as the NLN has a central mission to conduct nursing education research and most DNP graduates are not educated to do this. In their *Reflection and Dialogue* web series, they write:

> However, foundational essentials for DNP curriculum design do not include courses related to pedagogy, evaluation, academic role issues and elements, and educational theory, and the NLN fears that graduates of such programs will lack the complex and specialized knowledge intrinsic to the advanced practice role of nurse educator.
>
> —*NLN, 2007, p. 1*

More recently, the NLN (2010) has clearly pronounced that "Advanced practice nurses must have in-depth clinical knowledge of nursing practice; similarly, both part- and full-time faculty must have an in-depth knowledge of nursing education and nursing practice" (p. 1). This indicates that the proper preparation for the nursing faculty role is to have coursework and practica in the teaching role to ensure the effectiveness of the graduate. Our continued concern is whether the move to properly and expertly prepare the DNP graduate for the academic role will nonetheless result in the burden of extra coursework at an additional cost.

What, then, is the solution? Certainly, the answer is not to create easy doctorates that MSN-prepared nurse educators can complete. Nor can work experience be credited to the awarding of the doctorate. Anselmi and colleagues (2010) suggest nursing faculty exchange programs (e.g., "you take two of our MSN faculty for free and we will take two of yours for free") and mention that internal matriculation of nursing faculty in their own doctoral nursing program could be allowed reputably if the potential conflicts of interest can be minimized. This is where nursing innovation is needed and where accreditors too often become the barriers to innovation (Dreher, 2008a; Melnyk & Davidson, 2009; Neal, 2008; Stewart, 2009). Last, large numbers of MSN faculty are not going to return for the doctorate with the likelihood of only marginal increases in compensation. Both the AACN and NLN need to be more proactive (like the Association to Advance Collegiate Schools of Business) and include adequate compensation to their review criteria. And with any new white paper, suggesting or mandating a change in educational requirements should be accompanied by clear policy recommendations to ensure its equitable, realistic, and fair implementation.

THE SECOND PROFESSIONAL DOCTORATE IN NURSING: THE ND DEGREE

To be completely true to history, Case Western Reserve University's initiation of the extraordinarily innovative ND (Doctor of Nursing) degree in 1979 was never called nor classified as a "practice" doctorate. Indeed, it was called a "professional doctorate" (p. 308) by its founder, Dean Rozella Schlotfeldt of the Frances Payne Bolton School of Nursing at Case Western Reserve University (1978). Only now do revisionists call it the "first practice doctorate" (AACN, 2006; Hathaway, Jacob, Stegbauer, Thompson, & Graff, 2006; Lenz, 2005). Again, the 1970s was a time of rapid growth in nursing education. The DSN and DNS clinical doctorates were initiated, more PhD and DNSc programs were founded, MSN nurse practitioner programs began to flourish, and the ANA was still battling to require the BSN for professional nursing (Nelson, 2002). Then Schlotfeldt (1978), followed by Dean Luther Christman (1980) of the Rush University School of Nursing in Chicago, affirmed this vision that the doctorate should be the entry-level degree for nursing (Nelson, 2002). If there were ever a larger gap in the nursing profession between the professionalizers and the masses of practitioners or traditionalists, it was at this time. The ND degree at Case Western was designed after the MD (Doctor of Medicine) degree. Students entered the doctoral nursing program with any basic college degree (just like medicine) and then completed a 3-year full-time curriculum including the completion of a ND thesis (somewhat differentiated from the university's PhD dissertation). Without a doubt, this was a professional doctorate model, and graduates initially were not prepared for advanced practice roles. This changed in 1990 when alternate pathways to the ND were created, including a post-master's option for nurses with an MSN, and indeed graduates at this time were prepared for advanced practice roles (Dr. Joyce Fitzpatrick, personal communication, April 13, 2010). Technically, this degree modification *could* be termed "a practice doctorate" (entry level versus advanced practice), but again the term *practice doctorate* was not yet part of the nursing vernacular. In the end, the ND was a failure of innovation and only three other schools ever adopted the degree model (Rush University in 1987, the University of Colorado in 1990, and the University of South Carolina in 1999). All four of these programs subsequently closed and transitioned to Doctor of Nursing Practice programs in 2004 and 2005.

One day someone will write the history of the ND degree and why it failed. Was it the unrealistic initial concept that any nurse needed a doctorate for entry into practice? In hindsight, and with apologies to Christman, a true pioneer in nursing, retrospectively this idea seems absurd or, more kindly, extremely idealistic. For whatever reason, the first working group on the clinical doctorate established by the AACN in 2002 did not see much of a future for the degree. Were the initials "ND" perhaps too foreign? Was the degree confusing to some outside the discipline who thought it was a Doctor of

Naturopathy—also a ND degree as the AACN has noted (AACN, 2004a)? Certainly, the post-master's ND model was an alternative doctorate model to the PhD. But this author thinks it was more properly a "second generation clinical doctorate" (the DNSc, DSN, and DNS degrees were the first generation), in that its graduates did complete a ND thesis and were generating evidence for the discipline.[11] In other words, this post-master's model emphasized practice and practice-based research. And in the transition from the ND to the DNP it is perplexing why the practice mission of the degree was retained but the practice-evidence-generating mission eliminated.

THE CONTEMPORARY PRACTICE DOCTORATE MOVEMENT: DNP (MOSTLY) AND DrNP

The contemporary practice doctorate movement can be largely attributed to the innovators at Columbia University School of Nursing and its Dean, Mary Mundinger (who just retired in 2010). In the late 1990s, a team of investigators conducted a randomized clinical trial to determine whether, under comparable primary care protocols, MSN-prepared nurse practitioners and doctorally prepared physicians would have similar or different patient outcomes? In 2000, Mundinger and colleagues published their findings in the prestigious *Journal of the American Medical Association* (*JAMA*) and indeed reported that the outcomes were equivalent. This was certainly a landmark study for the nursing profession and caused quite a controversy in medicine. This author, if possible, would give a special courage award to the physician investigators and participants who even agreed to participate in the study (at seemingly some risk to the prestige of their discipline and the superiority of physician practice). The first outcome of this study set the stage for an innovative comprehensive care practice by Columbia University faculty nurse practitioners (Rubenstein, 2009). With this evidence, they gained admitting privileges (albeit with great passionate, political maneuvering by Dean Mundinger) to hospitals, and participated in the first model of comprehensive care where the nurse practitioner sees and follows patients throughout their hospital stays, and not just seen by the APRN in the confines of a primary care clinic (Mundinger, 2005).

The second outcome of this study was the initiation of the doctor of nursing practice (DrNP) degree model. While the inventors first described this as a "clinical doctorate" and a "Doctor of Nursing Practice in Primary Care," they later dropped the primary care emphasis, largely out of the realization that many of their APRNs were not practicing *just primary care* and they embraced their comprehensive care model more explicitly (Dreher et al., 2005; Mundinger, 2005). They have since retained the idea that their degree is a clinical doctorate, as the overwhelming emphasis in their curriculum is on direct clinical practice and focuses on Essential VII: Advanced Practice from the AACN's *Essentials of Doctoral Education for Advanced Practice* (2006) (Dr. Janice Smolowitz, personal communication, June 25, 2010). This author is in a quandary whether this iteration is really a clinical doctorate. It does not have the thesis or dissertation knowledge generation model that the earlier clinical doctorates all had. Instead, they have implemented a DNP Portfolio that is innovative, but does not have an emphasis on generating new practice knowledge; rather, it emphasizes translation of evidence to practice (which is technically more in line with the AACN conception of the DNP degree as a non-research degree) (Honig & Smolowitz, 2009). Nonetheless, there is no doctor of nursing practice program in the United States that has more emphasis on clinical practice, and it even includes a 1-year full-time practicum in the second year of study. For whatever reason, the Columbia DrNP degree model has never been replicated and indeed they changed their initials to "DNP" in 2009, probably in order to be accredited by the Commission on Collegiate Nursing Education (CCNE), which has elected to only accredit doctor of nursing practice programs that subscribe to the "DNP" initials (AACN, 2005b). Consequently, is this degree model a clinical doctorate as the profession has traditionally defined this term? As this author is aware that some Columbia graduates are actually assuming primary investigator roles and obviously going to be at the forefront of creating new evidence for the profession, the conclusion is yes, the Columbia DNP model with its intensive emphasis on clinical practice is a new type of third-generation clinical doctorate (despite the use of the DNP degree initials).

Historically, credit for the first DNP degree (Doctor of Nursing Practice) degree in 2001 belongs to the faculty of the University of Kentucky. However, this DNP focused on the Clinical/Executive Management role and *not advanced practice.* As Montgomery and Byrne detail in chapter 4, it is perplexing why the AACN membership chose to endorse the Kentucky DNP model that did not emphasize advanced clinical practice, instead of the Columbia DrNP degree model that did. It is also unfortunate that the inventors of the Kentucky DNP model did not publish the reasoning behind their new degree in the peer-reviewed literature. Thus, we are left only with the Dean's deliberations at the AACN membership to ascertain why the DNP degree model was preferred and why it was altered (from the Kentucky degree model) to include the *traditional advanced practice role* in the organization's first endorsement of the degree (AACN, 2004a). Interestingly, the addition of the clinical executive role[12] (termed Aggregate/Systems/Organizational Focus) was only done after minor language in the AACN draft document was changed from the January 2004 *AACN Draft Position Statement on the Practice Doctorate in Nursing* (AACN, 2004b). From the January 2004 draft, it states in Recommendation 8:

> The practice doctorate should eventually be identified as the preferred graduate degree for APN preparation in the four current roles: clinical nurse specialist, nurse anesthetist, nurse midwife, and nurse practitioner (p. 10).
>
> —*AACN, 2004b, p. 10*

Two months later, in the March 2004 *AACN Draft Position Statement on the Practice Doctorate in Nursing* in Recommendation 10 (originally Recommendation 8), the language changed to:

> The practice doctorate should eventually be identified as the preferred graduate degree for *advanced nursing practice preparation, but not limited to* [italics my emphasis] the four current roles: clinical nurse specialist, nurse anesthetist, nurse midwife, and nurse practitioner.
>
> —*AACN, 2004c, p. 12*

The change in language from *advanced practice nursing* (APN) to *advanced nursing practice* is important, because the administrative role could never technically be equated with the advanced practice roles of the four traditional APRN roles. But if it were under the umbrella of advanced nursing practice, it could. This inclusion of the clinical executive role, however, was not widely realized or perhaps promoted (again we reaffirm the clinical executive has been granted an advanced role by this definition, but not the advanced role of the educator). Even in the October 27, 2004 press release by the AACN titled *AACN Adopts a New Vision for the Future of Nursing Education and Practice,* the AACN states:

> In a historic move to help shape the future of nursing education and practice, the American Association of Colleges of Nursing (AACN) has adopted a new position which recognizes the

Doctor of Nursing Practice degree as the highest level of preparation for *clinical practice"* [italics my emphasis].

—AACN, 2004d, p. 1

Further in the press release, the AACN states:

> Currently, advanced practice nurses (APNs), including Nurse Practitioners, Clinical Nurse Specialists, Nurse Mid-wives, and Nurse Anesthetists, are prepared in master's degree programs that often carry a credit load equivalent to doctoral degrees in the other health professions. AACNs newly adopted Position Statement on the Practice Doctorate in Nursing calls for educating APNs and *other nurses seeking top clinical roles* [italics my emphasis] in Doctor of Nursing Practice (DNP programs).
>
> *—AACN, 2004d, p. 1*

Certainly, this is just a press release and not the official policy of the AACN, but the reader is left to believe that APRNs are the target and who are the "other nurses seeking top clinical roles"? That is indeed a very odd way to describe the job description of a Chief Nursing Officer or Vice President for Nursing. These are not clinical roles. All the indirect functions in nursing (e.g., administration, teaching, clinical trials management) are classified differently from direct care roles, and the point made here is that the nursing professor who oversees students in the clinical area is as close to *clinical* as the administrator in charge of clinical services. Ultimately, the clinical executive role was made explicit in the AACN's 2006 *Essential for Doctoral Education for Advanced Practice*.

A further examination of the final 2004 AACN Position Statement document does indicate that there was no consensus over endorsing only the DNP degree initials, but the argument that multiple degree initials would create confusion and perhaps lead to the DNSc, DNS, and DSN conundrum again apparently won (AACN, 2004a). It is largely unknown, however, how the practice of the nurse executive was deemed "advanced practice" by the AACN in 2006, but the practice of the nurse educator was excluded. The authors of chapter 7 and indeed the reflective response in chapter 12 by Dr. Joyce Fitzpatrick, former Dean at Case Western Reserve University, raise this issue This author has covered this unfolding history in detail, mostly because it is unrealistic to assume that increased PhD enrollment is going to alleviate the nursing faculty shortage. Throughout this book, and especially in the last chapter, the very erratic enrollments and graduations from PhD programs noted do not look promising. For instance, in 2008 there were only 3 net new PhD graduates in the United States with an overall increase of 0.1%, while there was an increase of 5.1% in 2009 with 201 net new graduates (AACN, 2009a; Fang, Tracy, & Bednash, 2010). Nevertheless, what is worrisome is whether even this 5.1% increase in 2009 will exceed actual retirements from the professoriate. Already, according to a 2010 press release from the Tri-Council of Nursing[13] (July 14, 2010):

> Even though 444,668 nurses received their license to practice from 2004 through 2008, the U.S. nursing workforce only grew by 153,806 RNs during this timeframe providing the first clear indication of the large scale retirements which the aging nursing profession has begun and will continue to experience. Given the demographics of the nursing workforce, this pattern is expected to continue over the next decade. (p. 3)

Because the DNP degree is the "sizzling hot nursing degree" (simply based on numbers and new programs), a re-engineered curriculum that allows at least some schools to embrace the educator role without penalizing students with extra coursework seems to be one realistic option.

THE AACN'S EARLY DEVELOPMENTAL WORK ON THE DNP DEGREE

While Columbia started down one track toward what they called a new clinical doctorate (DrNP), which would ultimately become a practice doctorate, and with Kentucky boldly introducing a practice doctorate (DNP) that did not actually emphasize clinical practice, we should trace the third track by the AACN that in the end had the most influence. In March of 2002, the AACN Board of Directors charged a Task Force to examine the current status of clinical or practice doctoral programs and other related charges (AACN, 2004b). What is interesting about this 2004 document is that the Task Force reported they had established a collaborative relationship with the National Organization of Nurse Practitioner Faculties (NONPF), and therefore there was a strong faculty-nurse practitioner connection in these early deliberations. Yet, there was also no liaison to the major practicing APRN organizations including the American College of Nurse Midwives (ACNM), the American Association of Nurse Anesthetists (AANA), the National Association of Clinical Nurse Specialists (NACNS), the American Academy of Nurse Practitioners (AANP), or the American College of Nurse Practitioners (ACNP). Further, none of the ten External Reaction Panel members invited by the AACN to comment on deliberations represented these organizations, and the formal exclusion of the ANA is noteworthy (AACN, 2004c). This lack of diversity of decision makers and formal consultants to the exclusion of organizations representing members (and future members) who would be the most impacted by any proposed change in educational requirements led to early criticism of the AACN for not fully vetting its proposal with audiences not inclined to agree with them. As Fulton and Lyon wrote back in 2005, "In proposing the practice doctorate AACN has engaged only a limited number of stakeholders in meaningful dialogue" (Fulton & Lyon, 2005, p. 3).

For this reason, as of July of 2010 none of the advanced practice organizations excluded above have endorsed the AACN's 2015 mandate for the entry-level DNP for advanced practice. The ACNM Accreditation Commission for Midwifery Education has gone on record of endorsing the DNP but not to the exclusion of its other educational entry-level degree options for nurse midwives (ACNM, 2009). Recently, they stated in response to the ANA's call for comment on the DNP that ". . . our overall position [is] that a graduate degree is required for entry to practice, however we do not support the practice doctorate as a requirement for entry to practice at this time" (ACNM, 2010). The AANA has endorsed doctoral-level entry for CRNAs starting from 2025, but new CRNAs can obtain *any doctorate*, not just the DNP degree (AANA, 2007). The NACNS has remained neutral on the DNP degree, neither endorsing it nor discouraging it for future Clinical Nurse Specialists (NACNS, 2009). Part of the NACNS argument was a study presented at the 2007 DNP Conference in Annapolis, Maryland; the study indicated significant duplication of curriculum outcomes between MSN and DNP degrees, and thus the need for another degree was questioned (Jacobson et al., 2007). Further, since many Clinical Nurse Specialist positions have a strong research role component (and many have a PhD), this author wonders whether a degree that de-emphasizes the conduct of research was seen as problematic (Fulton, 2010; McNett, 2006). Finally, many of the major nurse practitioner specialty organizations have endorsed the *NP DNP Education, Certification and Titling: A Unified Statement* (Nurse Practitioner Roundtable, 2008), which states:

> Current master's and higher degree nurse practitioner programs prepare fully accountable clinicians to provide care to well individuals, patients with undifferentiated symptoms, and those with acute, complex chronic and/or critical illnesses. The DNP degree more accurately reflects current clinical competencies and includes preparation for the changing health

care system. It is congruent with the intense rigorous education for nurse practitioners. This evolution is comparable to the clinical doctoral preparation for other health care professions.
—*Nurse Practitioner Roundtable, 2008, p. 1*

This unified statement is actually quite progressive. It does not appear to disenfranchise current MSN-prepared NPs (I note the emphasis on "current" however), while acknowledging that they endorse the evolution of clinical doctoral preparation for nurse practitioners.

After the constitution of the AACN Task Force on the Clinical Doctorate in 2002, NONPF and the AACN co-hosted the National Forum on the Practice Doctorate in December of 2003. What is interesting about the Executive Summary of this document is the following: (1) The constituent attendees identified that "practice" might encompass the clinical role, administrator, educator, or informaticist; (2) "Also clinically expert, doctorally prepared faculty will have to be recognized and have parity with other doctorally prepared faculty" (p. 3); and (3) "If the scope of practice remains unchanged, certification could accommodate an evolution from master's to doctoral preparation" (National Forum on the Practice Doctorate, p. 4). While this forum had much more representation than the AACN Task Force, it still had only 51 attendees plus the invited speakers, and it appears that concerns expressed about moving forward with an acute nursing shortage and aging population, as reported by Hawkins-Walsh (2004), went unheeded. Along with Hawkins-Walsh, this author and colleagues Donnelly and Naremore in 2005 also questioned why the AACN undertook a new doctorate for advanced practice and a new generalist master's degree role (i.e., Clinical Nurse Leader) when there were already two more critical nursing issues facing the nation: (1) a protracted nursing shortage; and (2) a nation that was woefully preparing for an aging population with a meager production of geriatricians and gerontological nurse practitioners (Dreher et al., 2005; Dreher, 2008b). Both physician and nursing leadership can be faulted for this poor health policy planning. What is also interesting about this meeting was that the seeds were already planted that this degree would not be for practitioners only. On the conference's second point, DNP faculty unfortunately will not receive parity with PhD faculty in academia as long as they are denied tenure-track positions in most universities. This is very likely to continue in research-intensive universities, but small liberal arts colleges may be more accommodating.

Finally, with regard to scope of practice, even the AACN in 2004a stated "Master's prepared advanced practice nurses identify additional knowledge that is needed for a higher level of advanced practice" (2004a, p. 7) and "A new and higher level of preparation for advanced practice nursing is justified if and only if it results in sufficient knowledge and skill above that already included at the master's level" (p. 12). Even NONPF (2008) states: "The practice doctorate for the nurse practitioner (NP) includes additional competencies that are to be combined with the existing Domains and Core Competencies of Nurse Practitioner Practice" (p. 1). It is for this reason that the term "doctoral advanced practice" is used to refer to practice by nurses with the DNP or DrNP to differentiate their practice from master's-prepared advanced practice nurses (Dreher & Montgomery, 2009). Extending this definition, we now suggest that the term "DAPRN" be used for "doctoral advanced practice registered nurse" instead of simply "APRN." For nonclinicians, the term suggested is "DANP" for "doctoral advanced nursing practice" instead of "ANP" (advanced nursing practice). *This issue of the doctoral advanced nursing practice role is actually the focus of this text.* Much has been written about master's-level advanced practice nursing, but with so few graduates and so few outcome data, these authors and contributors thought that it is time to focus on this new level of practice, with an emphasis on the role. Other books have begun to conflate DNP role development with DNP-related issues. We thought that a particular emphasis on *role* was essential, especially because the success of this degree will depend on how the role of the DNP graduate evolves and is embraced or rejected by other health professions and the health care market. Despite the degree's surge in popularity, there is no guarantee that the degree will enact all that it was intended to do. Only with conscientious attentiveness and concern by stakeholders for the degree, professional development of graduates in their new roles, and the elevated stewardship of its graduates to the discipline *beyond* what master's degree preparation has historically provided, will the degree's future success be ensured. If the degree becomes watered down and "quick to get," it is doomed. If the degree, however, helps improve the health care delivery system (and with opportunities for us to prove its worth with some 33 million additional individuals soon needing primary care) and simultaneously advance the profession, then the degree's creation will have been a triumph.

These two groups, the AACN and NONPF, therefore, became the drivers of the DNP degree. And as reported to this author by attendees at various subsequent AACN meetings (remember that only Deans could vote and only recently have nonvoting Associate Deans been invited to attend if the Dean were in attendance), it was evident that the PharmD and DPT degree models were being promoted over the research-oriented hybrid professional doctorates like the PsyD. This decision was likely made by conference conveners to perhaps better differentiate a new practice doctorate from the PhD. But in retrospect, the decision to exclude empirical research or some form of "dissertation" was for some nursing academics a reactionary overreach. This decision, left unchallenged, may ultimately harm nursing knowledge development unless this issue of the place of the conduct of research in the practice doctorate is revisited. Good nursing scholars, however, can disagree on this point. And while some feel the degree should be made more accommodating to practice scholars who have every right to conduct research, others feel just as strongly that this is precisely what the PhD is for. Thus, with the train headed toward a nonresearch DNP, the dialogue at open meetings leading up to the 2004 vote and the post vote "team building" nevertheless, for some, seemed unstoppable.

THE AACN'S 2015 POSITION AND THE RUSH BEGINS

As we reflect on the history that both Columbia University and the University of Kentucky have provided to the contemporary practice doctorate, it is also important to examine the first critical mass of schools that began doctor of nursing practice programs in 2005. At this time, despite the October 25, 2004, vote[14] by the AACN to require the Doctor of Nursing Practice degree for all advanced practice nurses—NPs, CRNAs, CNMs, and CNSs—by 2015, the landscape and the curricula of the doctor of nursing practice degree had not yet evolved. Table 1.3 lists the doctor of nursing practice programs (both DNP and DrNP) as of August 1, 2005.

Right after Columbia University introduced their DrNP model in early 2005, Drexel University developed its own DrNP degree model in March of 2005 and labeled it a "clinical research doctor of nursing practice degree." It combined both advanced practice and the conduct of practical clinical research, concluding with a clinical dissertation. The degree was modeled after the PsyD and DrPH degrees (both professional doctorates that include a research emphasis), and the authors detailed their new degree model in *The Journal of Online Issues in Nursing* in 2005 (Dreher et al., 2005). As the chair of the

TABLE 1.3
Inaugural Doctor of Nursing Practice Programs in the
United States (as of August 1, 2005)

University	Year Founded	Type of Program	Notes
Case Western Reserve University	2005	DNP	Founded as ND and converted to DNP
Columbia University	2005	DrNP	Founded as DrNP and converted to DNP in 2008. Founders still refer to degree as a "clinical doctorate"
Drexel University	2005	DrNP	A hybrid professional doctorate combining the practice doctorate and the academic research doctorate. Founders refer to degree as a "clinical research doctor of nursing practice degree"
Rush University	2005	DNP	Founded as ND and converted to DNP in Leadership and the Business of Health Care (only)
Tri-College University Nursing Consortium[a]	2005	DNP	NDSU left consortium in 2007; consortium disbanded in 2008
University of Colorado, Denver	2005	DNP	Founded as ND and converted to DNP
University of Kentucky	2001	DNP	First DNP—Clinical Leadership (only)
University of South Carolina	2005	DNP	Founded as ND and converted to DNP. First school to offer the BSN-to-DNP option to prepare entry level nurse practitioners
University of Tennessee, Memphis	2005	DNP	Founded as DNSc and converted to DNP

[a]Concordia College; Minnesota State University, Moorhead; North Dakota State University.

Note: Modified from *Philosophy of Science for Nursing Practice*, M. D. Dahnke & H. M. Dreher, 2010, New York, NY: Springer.

doctoral nursing program development committee, I can say that our faculty group began working on our degree model in 2000 in our own quest to find a practice-oriented degree as an alternative to the PhD. However, the Drexel nursing faculty felt very strongly that the research mission of the degree should only de-emphasize the PhD degree's focus on conducting research and creating new knowledge, not eliminate it. Certainly, since 2005 the Drexel program has been an outlier, but it has maintained its commitment to what we now call a "hybrid professional doctorate degree." All hybrid doctorates in the health professions complete a research project, usually in the form of a dissertation (Dreher, Fasolka, & Clark, 2008; Hawkins & Nezat, 2009; Smith Glasgow & Dreher, 2010). Figure 1.1 indicates that the DrNP degree is theoretically designed to fall in between the PhD and the DNP degree. Lastly, as our DrNP degree model includes four roles (practitioner, clinical executive, educator, and clinical scientist), it is interesting to note that 50% of the 16 current Drexel graduates who *entered the doctoral program in a role other than as an educator* (most were full-time practicing certified nurse practitioners) have gone into academia post graduation, and 56% of the graduates are in full-time

FIGURE 1.1

Practice/nonresearch, practice/research-oriented, and research-focused nursing doctorates

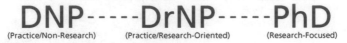

academic appointments.[15] We suggest that this degree model has a high rate of producing new full-time nursing faculty (three of which have even procured tenure-track positions) and the average time from matriculation to graduation is approximately 3.29 years.

The hybrid degree is particularly facile in academia, because all students complete a clinical dissertation and therefore have common research skills. And although their research skills are not typically as extensive as that of the PhD graduate, they are nonetheless comparable. Other health professions have also dealt with the realities of professional doctorates and the difficult transition of their graduates into academic roles, particularly when the degree emphasis was on practice, not scholarly productivity. For this reason, physical therapy and occupational therapy both developed a hybrid professional degree *after* their introduction of their DPT and OTD or DOT (Doctor of Physical Therapy and Occupational Therapy Doctorate or Doctor of Occupational Therapy) degrees respectively, with the DScPT and DSc degrees (Doctor of Science in Physical Therapy and Doctor of Science), and in occupational therapy, the DrOT degree (Doctor of Occupational Therapy). Table 1.4 identifies other health professions that have hybrid doctorates and indicates the differences between the research, hybrid professional, and professional doctorates.

TABLE 1.4

Types of Doctorates for Health Professions Disciplines in the United States

Academic Research Doctorate (*research-intensive emphasis*)	Hybrid Professional Doctorates (*practice/ research-oriented emphasis*)	Professional Doctorates (*practice/nonresearch emphasis*)
PhD—doctor of philosophy	DrPH—doctor of public health	MD/DO—doctor of medicine, doctor of osteopathy
ScD—doctor of science	DSc—doctor of science	DPT—doctor of physical therapy
DNS—doctor of nursing science	PsyD—doctor of psychology	PharmD—doctor of pharmacy
DSN—doctor of science in nursing	DSW—doctor of social work	DNP—doctor of nursing practice
DNSc—doctor of nursing science	DScPT—doctor of science in physical therapy	DDS/DMD—doctor of dental surgery, *Dentariae Medicinae Doctoris*
	DrNP—doctor of nursing practice	DVM/VMD—doctor of veterinary medicine, *Veterinariae Medicinae Doctoris*
	DCN—doctor of clinical nutrition	DOT—doctor of occupational therapy

Note: Modified from "The Future of Oncology Nursing Science: Who Will Generate the Knowledge?" by M. E. Smith Glasgow & H. M. Dreher, 2010, *Oncology Nursing Forum, 37*(4), 393–396.

What is interesting is that the National Institute of Health (NIH) has now opened up research funding (at least in the Parent K23 mechanism) to both graduates of "doctoral nursing research and nursing practice" programs (NIH, 2009a, Section 1.B) and a few schools are revisiting the role of research in the DNP; in one case, the University of Connecticut has added courses in research methods that they previously did not have and now require a clinical practice dissertation that was previously only a project (Dr. Regina Cusson, personal communication, June 25, 2010). In some ways, it seems un-egalitarian to say that one doctoral nursing graduate will create the evidence and the other will then translate and disseminate it. Good science, especially science grounded in practice, is not really conducted that way. That is part of the critique that Florczak (2010) has recently provided stating "just how and where one could arbitrarily uncouple the practice of nursing from nursing research" (p. 16).

With the University of Washington School of Nursing faculty's promotion of "practice inquiry" (adopted by some schools), which does not prohibit the conduct of nursing research but only frames it for a practice orientation[16] (Magyary, Whitney, & Brown, 2006), to a call to revisit the research mission of the DNP (Bellini & Cusson, in press; Reel, 2009; Smith Glasgow & Dreher, 2010; Webber, 2008) now that the degree is some 5 years old and the *Essentials* (AACN, 2006) are now 4 years old, what lies ahead is unknown. This author has studied DNP curricula intensely for years. Having chaired two national conferences on the practice doctorate and presented at the first *International Conference on Professional Doctorates* in London in 2009, this author has come to hypothesize that the DNP graduate may be best positioned to create "Practice Knowledge" for the profession (Dreher, 2010b). In my view, it is in the focus on creating practice-based evidence where DNP graduates may excel, even beyond the PhD graduate, who if trends continue with BSN-to-PhD programs will produce future graduates that are going to be less clinically competent and have less a frame of reference to know what questions should be asked.

In my own proposed *Model of Scientific Inquiry in Nursing* (see Figure 1.2), I suggest that it is Practice Knowledge or Mode 2 knowledge (represented by the right circle of the Venn diagram) that the DNP graduate is most prepared to conduct (Dreher, 2010b). This knowledge is created through practice-based research and inquiry that leads to

FIGURE 1.2
A model of scientific inquiry in nursing. From "*Philosophy of Science for Nursing Practice*," by M. D. Dahnke & H. M. Dreher, 2010, New York, NY: Springer. Figure may be copied/reprinted only with permission of author H. M. Dreher.

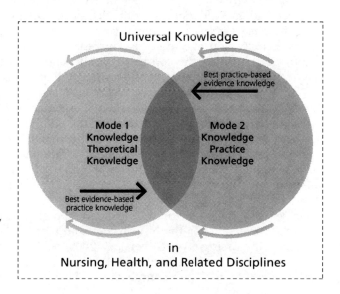

practice-based evidence (Barkham & Mellor-Clark, 2003; Hellerstein, 2008; San Francisco AIDS Foundation, 2008). The left circle represents Theoretical Knowledge or Mode 1 knowledge, and it is here where the PhD student is more prepared to conduct theoretical knowledge and generate evidence-based practice knowledge using larger data sets. The knowledge emanating from the best DNP programs, however, would be more practice oriented, closely connected to the work or clinical environment, and likely conducted in real time. Then, after rigorous but efficient analysis, the findings are translated into practice on a smaller scale until larger, more empirical work (evidence-based practice) can be conducted. Indeed, this drive for practice-based evidence should not be construed as a lesser research function. Some new or novel phenomena are just not ready for multi-site, clinical trial investigation, or even multivariate analysis. The practitioner or clinical executive scholar closest to practice is in the best position to identify new clinical problems that need clinical investigation. The intersection of the two circles in the Venn diagram represents research that is highly contextualized to both practice-based evidence and evidence-based practice domains. Here the final research project (whatever it is called), whether PhD or DNP, is simply indistinguishable. Here lies the rigor of the best DNP programs and the PhD programs where clinical practice problem solving is the overwhelming emphasis. We also believe that this is where the hybrid professional doctorate (DrNP) lies, as these graduates are working both with large and small data sets, with some clinical dissertations more focused on practice-based evidence and others on creating knowledge for evidence-based practice. A more complete description of this model (Figure 1.2) can be found in chapter 16, "Next Steps Toward Practice Knowledge Development: An Emerging Epistemology in Nursing," in Dahnke and Dreher's recently published (2010) *Philosophy of Science for Nursing Practice*.

WHERE WE STAND NOW: A NEW DEGREE, PROGRESS, AND UNRESOLVED ISSUES

Progress

This chapter will conclude with a short overview of some of the progress and central challenges or unresolved issues that the doctor of nursing practice degree now faces. Resolving these is essential as this relatively new degree tries to gain a foothold in academic nursing circles and into the consciousness of the health care market that includes peer health professionals, the consumer public, and individuals from all walks of life who have substantive policy input and authority that impacts nursing. Certainly, three Institute of Medicine (IOM) reports, *To Err is Human: Building a Safer Health System* (1999), *Crossing the Quality Chasm, A New Health System for the 21st Century* (2001), and *Health Professions Education: A Bridge to Quality* (2003), influenced the AACN leadership in their deliberations about moving forward with the DNP degree. Florczak (2010), however, writes creatively and extensively about the influence of the IOM reports and concludes "she remained somewhat confused about the link between the IOM reports and the push toward the DNP" (p. 15). Perhaps a more influential report was by the National Academy of Sciences (NAS) (2005), which called for nursing to consider developing a nonresearch clinical doctorate to prepare expert practitioners who could also serve as faculty. However, even the NAS recognized that "the concept of a nonresearch clinical doctorate in nursing is controversial" (2005, p. 7).

The first of the chief positive outcomes of the doctor of nursing practice degree is the realization that with the complexity of health care today, there is indeed curricular content and specialized knowledge *beyond the MSN* to give DNP graduates additional, enhanced skills. This has been detailed earlier both by the AACN (2004a) and NONPF (2008). There will continue to be resistance, however, to claiming that there is a domain of practice and a skill set above and beyond basic advanced practice. Whether the DNP degree ultimately changes the scope and practice of the advanced practice nurse is another question. While the AACN (2009b) says, "No, transitioning to the DNP will not alter the current scope of practice for APRNs" (p. 1), it is somewhat illogical to require additional skills and competencies for more advanced nursing practice and then assume that the scope of practice will not change. Maybe that is actually what the American Medical Association (AMA) fears the most: not nurses using the title "Dr." but real fears about the possibility that the scope and boundaries of their practice will expand (AMA, 2009). Nevertheless, if there was ever an argument against the DNP, it would be a situation in which MSN programs simply added a few credits and called the degree a "doctorate" without any forthright attention to educating a more highly prepared practitioner.

A second positive outcome is that there is now a widely established nursing doctorate that gives nurses an alternative to the PhD (Sperhac & Clinton, 2008). For decades, nurses only had a research-intensive degree, clinical doctorates that were *de facto* research-intensive degrees, and 1 lone EdD and 4 NDs—degree models that never gained a foothold within the profession. Whether it really is in the interest of nursing for there to be only one alternative to the PhD, the DNP, with the CCNE's refusal to recognize hybrid DrNP programs that generate knowledge for the discipline but in a different way than the PhD, is still debatable (AACN, 2005b). However, because of the power and influence of the AACN and CCNE, they are not likely to endorse a third doctorate at this time. The National League for Nursing Accrediting Commission (NLNAC) has indicated a more progressive stance on titling, however, stating in their *NLNAC Statement on Clinical Practice Doctorates* (2005):

> Other health care professionals such as dentists (DDS and DMD), psychologists (PhD and PsyD), and physicians (MD and DO) are able to define their roles, qualifications, and expertise to their patients and the public with more than one type of degree. We have confidence that doctorally prepared advanced practice nurses will be able to do so as well.
>
> —*NLNAC, 2005, p. 1*

Nevertheless, in graduate nursing education circles, the AACN and CCNE seem to be more influential in some ways. In the end, often the determining factor of influence is whether it is the CCNE or NLNAC that is accrediting the individual nursing school and sometimes it is both.

A third positive outcome of this doctoral option gives doctoral advanced practice nurses more parity with other health professionals (O'Sullivan, 2005). While this was one of the goals for the creation of this degree, it really should not be a leading reason for individuals to seek it. The incentive to be called "Dr." ought to be driven more by what the doctorate adds to the master's-prepared practitioner to warrant the higher degree. Further, the doctorate ought to be credible, have rigor, and, and must be seen by others as legitimate. This happens with every new doctorate: Public critical analyses by degree supporters, detractors, and skeptics, and not just toward the DNP. Further, with a new degree, some DAPRNs are going to experience some difficulty in the workplace while working alongside master's-prepared APRNs who may feel resentment or deny that there is any difference in practice. Doctoral-prepared physical therapists, working alongside master's-prepared physical therapists, have already experienced this, and it is likely to happen in nursing, too (Salzman, 2010). But parity is important. It allows us to sit at the table as an equal contributor. Suzanne Gordon (2005) has written about the "invisibility of nursing" (p. 184). Maybe the DNP degree can help increase our visibility and permit our practitioners and clinicians (and others) to be seen as full partners in both practice and policy.

A final positive outcome (and surely there are others) is that this degree was designed to emphasize the translation and dissemination of research findings (AACN, 2006). While this author and others believe that generating practice knowledge through practice inquiry (Dreher, 2010b; Magyary et al., 2006) should be incorporated into the degree, the opportunity this degree presents the profession is nonetheless unique. Magyary and colleagues write of the DNP student's role in practice inquiry:

> How to frame researchable questions generated from clinical observations and discourse is an essential practice inquiry competency. Clinical observations discrepant with habitual ways of knowing and doing may reveal new insights into clinical phenomena that have received limited or no empirical inquiry. These types of revelations may generate questions that beg to be answered through rigorous scientific investigation.
>
> —*Magyary et al., 2006, p. 144*

Further, if properly and rigorously educated, the DNP degree graduate should be a skilled professional who should be able to data-mine (even skillfully scour) the endless databases that warehouse the enormous amount of research conducted every year in nursing and the health sciences. These graduates should be experts in knowledge management, poised to extract information and apply it in a novel or utilitarian way, and then efficiently translate and disseminate this new conceptualization of the evidence (Dreher, 2009). However, this theoretical rubric for what this graduate can be trained and educated to do can only be accomplished *if* the DNP student is exposed to coursework that indeed enables the student to truly participate credibly in this kind of practice inquiry. Philosophy of Science courses are unusual in DNP programs, although this content is sometimes dispersed or integrated into other courses. But how else will these doctoral students understand the concepts of evidence, causation, empirical data, deduction, induction, probability, bias, scientific truth, and other important concepts all necessary to practice inquiry and the evaluation of evidence, if this content is absent in curricula? How can a student perform a meta-analysis or secondary analysis of existing data, conduct outcomes research, or engage in basic interpretive inquiry if the student does not have the advanced research methods courses (beyond the master's degree) to prepare one for this level of inquiry? The DNP student will likely be at the forefront of making the impractical practical and Fink (2006) suggests that the professional doctorate graduate should be well prepared for the knowledge economy simply based on the very practice orientation of the degree.

DNP graduates should also help broaden the definition of evidence through their work-based problem solving. Very traditional definitions of "what is evidence in the health professions" is now being challenged by Pearson, Wiechula, Court, and Lockwood (2007) at the Joanna Briggs Institute at the University of Adelaide in Adelaide, Australia, and American DNP (and PhD) nursing faculty would benefit from exploring this literature. Pearson and colleagues describe four different types of clinical evidence that are posited based on a clinical question: (1) evidence of feasibility; (2) evidence of appropriateness; (3) evidence of meaningfulness; and (4) evidence of effectiveness. Also, the generation of Mode 2 knowledge, which is work based, practice oriented, and often derived differently and disseminated differently than Mode 1 knowledge (which is mostly

FIGURE 1.3

Path of practice knowledge generation in an emerging nursing epistemology. Modified from *"Philosophy of Science for Nursing Practice,"* by M. D. Dahnke & H. M. Dreher, 2010, New York, NY: Springer. Figure may be copied/reprinted only with permission of author H. M. Dreher.

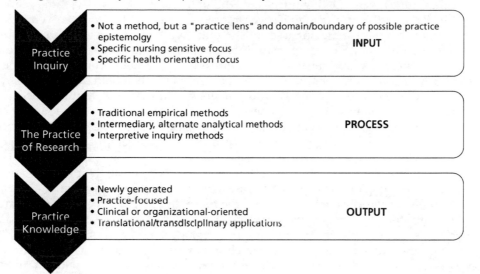

traditional, empirical, theoretical and disseminated very typically according to academy norms), is where the professional/practice doctorate graduate should excel (Gibbons et al., 1994; Nowotny, Scott, & Gibbons, 2001; Reed, 2006; Smith Glasgow & Dreher, 2010). This author has proposed that the DNP graduate generates practice knowledge (output) through the lens of practice inquiry (input) and by utilizing practice research methods (process) (Dreher, 2010b). This is illustrated in Figure 1.3.

Unresolved Issues

The chief unresolved issues surrounding the DNP degree can be summarized as follows:

1. Controversy over the mandate that the DNP degree does not require (or even permit?) an empirical research project or dissertation;
2. Disagreement over the required number of clinical hours necessary for the degree, particularly for post-master's students;
3. Controversy over the mandate that the DNP degree does not formally prepare educators; and
4. A burgeoning discussion over whether PhD and DNP students should share any common coursework.

Some of these issues, particularly the first and third, will be discussed at length in this text by various authors, and because this chapter has addressed these to some degree already, only a few summary points will be made here.

The issue over the role of research in the DNP degree is likely to continue. Our inclination is to predict that ultimately the doctor of nursing practice degree may look different at research-extensive and research-intensive universities where knowledge generation and scholarship is central to the mission. DNP programs that reside in colleges where the teaching mission and scholarship are emphasized, however, may be less inclined to design curricula that generate practice knowledge. However, these generalizations need not be used indiscriminately to prevent practice inquiry or even formal empirical inquiry by any DNP student anywhere. If we are honest, the same reality is present in PhD Nursing/Nursing Science programs all across the country. While some PhD programs emphasize the nurse scientist model (with a focus on generating nursing science), other PhD programs emphasize teaching and education research, and are less focused on generating graduates for research careers. The DNP degree should be no different. It will continue to evolve, and it will evolve best when both doctoral advanced nursing practitioners who simply want to practice and those who want to practice *and* generate practice knowledge (e.g., generate primary care, clinical, or organizational nursing knowledge) are both seated at the table and can respect the role each wants to play as stewards of the discipline. Medicine is actually no different as many practicing physicians are not involved in research or have no interest in it. They simply want to practice the art of medicine. Other physicians, however, see problems in their practice and are interested in initiating or participating in research related to these problems.

The other previously discussed issue—the role of the DNP degree in the preparation of nurse educator—will be discussed further by Wittman-Price, Waite, and Woda in chapter 7. As mentioned earlier, there are unfortunately no aggressive strategic plans by nursing's current leadership to adequately replenish the supply of retiring nursing professors and nurse scientists. This is most unfortunate, because without nursing faculty, we cannot admit more nursing students and help alleviate the long-term nursing shortage. It seems highly unlikely, however, that we can increase the number of PhD students and graduates in the critical mass that is needed. The only solution that seems plausible is to re-engineer the DNP graduate, especially those interested in teaching in MSN and DNP programs, for pathways that include a specific curriculum focus on teaching doctoral advanced practice. The creation of more hybrid degrees that seem to do this very effectively and are more welcomed in academia is another option, but one that the AACN or CCNE is unlikely to support in the near future. Maybe, as one of our faculty members said recently, we need to "wait until we have a critical mass of 100 DrNP graduates and the profession sees what they are contributing."

The last two unresolved issues (the 2nd and 4th listed above) are not discussed sufficiently in this text, so they will be addressed here. First, there continues to be debate over the required number of clinical hours necessary for the degree, particularly for post-master's students. However, it seems many programs have interpreted the statement from the AACN *Essentials* (2006) "In order to achieve the DNP competencies, programs should provide a minimum of 1,000 hours of practice post-baccalaureate as part of a supervised academic program" (p. 19) very, very liberally. Even the usually supportive NONPF has not fully endorsed the mandate that every post-master's clinical DNP student needs 400 more hours of actual practice (if the original MSN degree in pediatrics, for example, had 600 hours). According to NONPF (2006), "The evidence for the AACN recommendation for 1,000 clinical hours for all practice doctorate students has not been presented" (p. 1). This issue was debated at length at the 2007 DNP Conference in Annapolis, Maryland. For some it seemed unrealistic that part-time students (who work full-time) would need a total of 1,000 clinical hours (including whatever was earned for the master's degree), plus coursework (and still remain fully employed, particularly if they were receiving employer-based tuition benefits), to complete the degree. At Drexel, almost all of our students work full-time and attend doctoral study as part-time students, and they barely seem able to complete the rigorous intense curriculum that is structured year round (4 quarters) over 3 years (the third year is devotedly exclusively to the completion of the clinical dissertation). The Drexel program does not require 1,000 hours, but it focuses more on the quality of the two required doctoral practice practica and not the quantity of hours. Supposedly, students are not allowed to count work (paid hours) or portfolio assessment toward the minimum number of required hours. So this author is in a quandary to explain how so many DNP programs with an overwhelming majority of part-time students meet this CCNE requirement. Interestingly, the clinical hour requirement does not appear to be required of DNP students enrolled in Clinical Executive Tracks. Many of these students did not complete hundreds of hours during their MSN degrees in Nursing Administration, and therefore it would be exorbitant to require them to complete 1,000 total hours for the degree. This is not logical. One DNP track requires 1,000 hours and one does not? There is an inequity here. This absolute requirement needs revisiting given NONPF's lack of enthusiasm for this requirement, stating "The NONPF Board has significant concern in establishing a random standard" [of required number of clinical hours] (2006, p. 1).

The last issue—shared coursework between the two degree programs—was debated extensively by attendees in one session focusing on the future of the PhD at the January 2009 AACN Doctoral Nursing Education Conference in Coronado Island, California. From this author's point of view, there seem to be two camps of nursing faculty perspectives. One camp firmly believes that students from both degrees can learn from each other and therefore support some joint coursework between the two programs. The other camp is firmly against crossover between the two curricula fearing dilution of the PhD degree and the slow trajectory to one day "the DNP becoming the same as the PhD." Interestingly, I have not heard DNP faculty similarly state they do not want their DNP students taking courses with PhD students. It appears, however, that across the country there is some minimal coursework that students in the two degrees share. For administrators, it is also more cost effective to offer some courses to both groups, especially if the class size (usually the PhD class these days) is small. Our own newly approved PhD in Nursing Science curriculum does include DrNP and PhD students sharing two courses (Nurs 703: The Politics of Health: Implications for Nursing Practice; Nurs 819: Qualitative Methods for Clinical Nursing Inquiry),[17] but also sharing some common workshops during summer residencies and study abroad. If, however, admission standards vary considerably between the two programs, there may be a risk to DNP student performance in PhD coursework. However, absolute separatism also might foster elitism among PhD students and in PhD programs (or even among faculty), and indeed we fear this. Deans and Chairs need to actively promote collegiality among students (and faculty) in both cohorts, and if these students are going to be involved in PhD/DNP translational research teams, as some are now suggesting, then what better time to begin to work together than during doctoral study (Cacchione, 2007; Hastings, Mitchell, & Loud, 2010)?

One important point, however, needs to be emphasized. "Translation of research" and "translational research" are not the same thing. The NIH has very clear definitions of what constitutes translational research, indicating:

> Translational research includes two areas of translation. One is the process of applying discoveries generated during research in the laboratory, and in preclinical studies, to the development of trials and studies in humans. The second area of translation *concerns research* [italic mine] aimed at enhancing the adoption of best practices in the community. Cost-effectiveness of prevention and treatment strategies is also an important part of translational science.
>
> —*NIH, 2009b, Section 1.1*

The AACN *Essentials* (2006) document is clear that "translational research" is not what they are referring to when it states:

> ... the scholar applies knowledge to solve a problem via the scholarship of application (referred to as the scholarship of practice in nursing). This application involves the *translation of research* [italics mine] into practice and the dissemination and integration of new knowledge, which are key activities of DNP graduates.
>
> —*AACN Essentials, 2006, p. 11*

The nuance is nevertheless very clear. Translational research involves very formal traditional methods of scientific inquiry (Rubio et al., 2010). Supporting this in their description of practice inquiry, Magyary and colleagues (2006) at the University of Washington School of Nursing indicate, "Practice inquiry entails a wide spectrum of designs, methods and statistical approaches. Emerging conceptual and technological advances in clinical epidemiology and informatics provide APNs the instruments to identify and monitor clinical patterns over time" (p. 145). To this author at least, the skill set of the DNP graduate described here is different from the more narrow focus of the scholarship of application. Therefore, until there is more clarity about the direction of the scholarship focus of the DNP degree, we are likely to see individual DNP programs undertaking very different forms of scientific and practice inquiry.

INTERNATIONAL IMPLICATIONS FOR THE DOCTOR OF NURSING PRACTICE DEGREE

Finally, this chapter concludes with some thoughts about the DNP degree in the larger professional doctorate and larger universal doctoral nursing community.[18] With the exception of medicine, dentistry, and veterinary medicine, there are no doctoral programs outside of the United States that do not include the conduct of research. Indeed, the European Union (EU) in their Bologna Third Doctoral Cycle deliberations are trying to establish some uniformity among EU nations to better standardize both the PhD and the professional doctorate so that the transferability of scholars' credentials across borders is not an issue (Bologna Process, 2010; Davies, 2008). First, it may not be common knowledge, but professional nursing doctorates have existed globally, particularly in Australia, Northern Ireland and Great Britain, since the 1990s (Ellis & Lee, 2005; McKenna & Cutcliffe, 2001). What is common among them (and professional doctorates in all other disciplines aside from those disciplines identified above) is that the conduct of research is an integral part of their core competencies. Graham Stew, author of chapter 20, and his colleagues from the University of Brighton indicate the difference between the PhD and the professional doctorate is that the PhD prepares the "professional researcher" and the professional doctorate prepares the "researching professional" (2009). But does the DNP degree fit into this international professional nursing doctorate degree model? The answer is that some do, but that most do not. However, what the DNP and other U.S.-based professional doctorates do that the international professional doctorate largely do not[19] is to emphasize and actually require additional practice hours beyond the MSN or other health professions master's degree. Even as I attended the first *Professional and Practice-Focused Doctoral Research Special Interest Group* meeting in London in July of 2010 as the only U.S. attendee, I queried a fellow colleague who indicated that their professional doctorate graduates do gain advanced practice hours at their work site, although absolute hours are not required. I argued that it would be controversial (even open the university to liability, which I understand is less prevalent in the British legal system) to award credit in the United States for actual work the student completed as the agent of the employer (hospital) and not primarily as the agent of the university. Further, I am skeptical that one can prepare a more advanced practitioner just by gaining more clinical research skills that can be applied in the practice environment. Nevertheless, especially with the emerging codified language from the Bologna Third Cycle, it is very unlikely that a nursing doctorate without a research project would be accepted outside the United States. Therefore, any American DNP nurse who might seek a teaching position outside the United States should be aware of this expectation. On the other hand, the proximity of Canada to the United States has already got Canadian nursing scholars wondering how the DNP might impact the Canadian nursing educational system (Brar, Boschma, & McCuaig, 2010; Joachim, 2008). Further, this author was informed that a DNP program is indeed nearing the implementation stage at the University College Cork (UCC) in Ireland; however, it appears that UCC will be including the conduct of research in this degree based on the Case Western Reserve University DNP Thesis model or something similar (Dr. Joyce Fitzpatrick, personal communication, March 17, 2010). So I conclude by writing humorously that I did warn my mostly British colleagues in London recently that they should not ignore what is happening in the United States with the professional doctorate or with the DNP degree. Our ideas, both good and bad, can easily make a transatlantic voyage or flight.

SUMMARY

As the DNP degree continues to evolve, 10 years since the first DNP degree and some 5 years since the first large cohort of programs were first established, it is now time to take a deep breath and evaluate how far we have come and what direction this degree should now take. It is only recently, in the spring of 2010, that the ANA has undertaken its first analysis of the doctor of nursing practice degree and taken public comment. It will likely be a 2-year process before the ANA House of Delegates votes on this degree and either: (a) endorses it; (b) offers cautionary approval or suggests a slower period of transition (rather than 2015); or (c) possibly rejects the idea that all advanced practice nurses one day must have an entry-level doctorate. But more realistically, the ANA's ultimate position may not be determinative. This degree has arrived and graduates are going out into the professional work force and starting to make their mark. New DNPs, and yes a handful of DrNPs, are working in roles the health care system has never seen before. Some PhD nursing graduates have unfairly, but sometimes fairly, had their relevance to the clinical practice environment questioned (Wilkes & Mohan, 2008). The clinical practice environment, however, is fertile ground for the DNP graduate, and it is here where they are educated to excel.

This author has tried to provide an accurate analysis of the trajectory of this degree. Sometimes history is ugly, but mostly it is complex. In the end, the history of the DNP degree can be summarized as follows: Initially there was great opposition to the DNP degree, but the opposition was largely quelled quickly. Now what we have left is the fine tuning of the degree and a need to generate outcome data that will help enable our graduates to better define and "live" this new role so that nursing's mission to improve health and alleviate suffering can advance.

NOTES

1. To be completely historically accurate, we can add two nurse anesthesia-oriented doctorates developed recently: DNAP degree (Doctor of Nurse Anesthesia Practice) at Virginia Commonwealth University and the DMPNA degree (Doctor of Management Practice of Nurse Anesthesia) at Marshall University. Further, the since degree initials "DNP" and "DrNP" are both Doctor of Nursing Practice degrees, for simplification (and because the DNP degree model is far more prevalent), the initials "DNP" will be used in most cases in this chapter and text except when the difference between the two is noted.
2. Certified Registered Nurse Practitioners (CRNPs) Certified Nurse Midwives (CNMs), Certified Registered Nurse Anesthetists (CRNAs), and Clinical Nurse Specialists (CNSs).
3. Because "professional doctorate" and "practice doctorate" are nearly synonymous, for simplicity we will use the work "practice doctorate' to include both. Where the nuance between each is indeed important, we will use the terms separately and indicate why.
4. Why did some university faculties not allow the PhD in Nursing? Certainly, for many, the issue was prejudice against nursing as a discipline as Meleis and Dracup (2005) affirm. Senior faculty (who often predominate in conservative university faculty senates), were often the elected members who viewed nursing disparagingly as a scientific discipline. In other cases, like Widener University, the university charter did not permit the awarding of any PhD, and so an alternate doctorate (DNSc) was offered. Many of those charter restrictions have been modified over the years.
5. This author has always thought that PhD programs that emphasize the nurse scientist model should be titled PhD in Nursing Science, and other PhD programs that emphasize the teaching or other mission in nursing should be titled PhD in Nursing.
6. Two examples of the kinds of research projects that were funded by this new field research division was a study that examined pre–post knowledge of diabetic patients after teaching and another that looked at classifying patients and distributing nursing staff according to patients' nursing needs (American Journal of Nursing, 1965).
7. Examples of his critique of institutionalized medicine among the 155 graduate and 12 postgraduate medical schools in the United States and Canada he claimed to have visited included findings of equipment at one school "dirty and disorderly beyond description" (Flexner, 1910, p. 190) and another institution had "in place of laboratories, laboratory signs" (p. 165). Additionally, Flexner was actually criticized for being *too* critical and his methods of data collection came under heavy fire (Hiatt, 1999).
8. Moreover, scholarship such as this text needs to be better recognized by nursing Deans and traditional tenure and promotion committees because, again, if there are no nursing texts, then there is no nursing curricula period, and ultimately no tuition revenue.
9. Even a recent report found that female law partners at elite law firms made on average $66,000 less than their male counterparts, and this disparity was largely attributed to stereotyping, gender bias, and even bullying and intimidation (Williams & Richardson, 2010).
10. I cannot help but also mention that when these discussions of "research start-up packages" takes place, there are always gasps among other nursing faculty who received zero research support upon hire. What is more typical is nursing faculty have *no idea* how equitable their packages are respective to other faculty in other departments in their universities.
11. Similarly, with the EdD at Teacher's College a first generation professional doctorate, the initial ND degree at Case Western could also be termed a second-generation professional nursing doctorate.
12. The original Kentucky DNP degree model.
13. Tri-Council for Nursing represents leaders from the American Association of Colleges of Nursing, the National League for Nursing, the American Nurses Association, and the American Organization of Nurse Executives.
14. The actual vote was 162 yes, 101 no, 13 abstain, and no proxy or in absentia votes were permitted. Indeed, the power and influence of 162 individuals is substantial (Dreher et al., 2005).

15. The Drexel DrNP degree was fully approved by the Pennsylvania Department of Education (PDOE) on April 29, 2010. As it includes a clinical dissertation, it was classified as a research degree by the PDOE.

16. They, however, have not called it a practice dissertation, DNP thesis, or clinical practice dissertation, but a clinical investigative project, even though the faculty workload of supervising one of these projects can be near that of a dissertation (Dr. Marie-Annette Brown, personal communication, July 24, 2010). Will this become a trend in academia (especially at research universities) where faculty are assigned or expected to chair more DNP Final Projects because they are not "dissertations?"

17. Our rationale for having both students take the qualitative methods course is that in most doctoral nursing programs the first qualitative methods course is usually a survey course. They will not share quantitative methods courses.

18. This issue is discussed thoroughly in Dreher, H.M., & Smith Glasgow, M.E. (in press). Global perspectives on the professional doctorate. Int. J. Nurs. Stud. 2010. doi:10.1016/j.ijnurstu.2010.09.003.

19. The DCPsych degree is one exception. This professional doctorate in counseling psychology uniformly requires additional practicum hours to complete the degree. But this degree is an exception among professional doctorates globally outside the United States.

REFERENCES

Academic Nurse. (2010). Ten years of progress: The Council for the Advancement of Care. *The Academic Nurse: The Journal of Columbia University School of Nursing and Its Alumni*, Spring, 21–27.

Aiken, L. H., Cheung, R. B., & Olds, D. M. (2009). Education policy initiatives to address the nurse shortage in the United States. *Health Affairs, 28*(4), 646–656.

American Association of Colleges of Nursing. (1999). *Faculty shortages intensify nation's nursing deficit.* Retrieved from http://www.aacn.nche.edu/publications/issues/IB499WB.htm

American Association of Colleges of Nursing. (2004a). *AACN Position Statement on the Practice Doctorate in Nursing October 2004.* Retrieved from http://www.aacn.nche.edu/DNP/pdf/DNP.pdf

American Association of Colleges of Nursing. (2004b). *AACN Draft Position Statement on the Practice Doctorate in Nursing January 2004.* Washington, DC: Author.

American Association of Colleges of Nursing. (2004c). *AACN Position Statement on the Practice Doctorate in Nursing March 2004.* Washington, DC: Author.

American Association of Colleges of Nursing. (2004d). *AACN Adopts a New Vision for the Future of Nursing Education and Practice.* Retrieved from http://www.aacn.nche.edu/Media/NewsReleases/DNPRelease.htm

American Association of Colleges of Nursing. (2005a). *Faculty shortages in baccalaureate and graduate nursing programs: Scope of the problem and strategies for expanding the supply.* Retrieved from http://www.aacn.nche.edu/publications/pdf/05FacShortage.pdf

American Association of Colleges of Nursing. (2005b). *Commission on Collegiate Nursing Education moves to consider for accreditation only practice doctorates with the DNP degree title.* Retrieved from http://www.aacn.nche.edu/Media/NewsReleases/Archives/2005/CCNEDNP.htm

American Association of Colleges of Nursing. (2006). *The essentials of doctoral education for advanced nursing practice.* Retrieved from http://www.aacn.nche.edu/DNP/pdf/Essentials.pdf

American Association of Colleges of Nursing. (2008). *The preferred vision of the professoriate in baccalaureate and graduate nursing programs.* Retrieved from http://www.aacn.nche.edu/Publications/pdf/PreferredVision.pdf

American Association of Colleges of Nursing. (2009a). *2008–2009 Enrollment and graduations in baccalaureate and graduate programs in nursing.* Washington, DC: Author.

American Association of Colleges of Nursing. (2009b). *Frequently asked questions, position statement on the practice doctorate in nursing.* Retrieved from http://www.aacn.nche.edu/DNP/dnpfaq.htm

American Association of Nurse Anesthetists. (2007). *AANA position on doctoral preparation of nurse anesthetists June 2007.* American Association of Nurse Anesthetists, Park Ridge, IL: Author.

American College of Nurse Midwives. (2009). *ACNM Division of Accreditation (now the Accreditation Commission for Midwifery Education) Statement on Midwifery Education.* Retrieved from http://www.midwife.org/siteFiles/DNPstatementedited.doc

American College of Nurse Midwives. (2010). *ACNM response to ANA position statement on the DNP.* Retrieved from http://www.midwife.org/documents/ACNMonDNP.pdf

American Journal of Nursing. (1965). *The Division of Nursing USPHS, 65*(7), 82–85: Author.

American Medical Association. (2009). *AMA scope of practice data sets: Nurse practitioners.* Chicago, IL: Author.

Anselmi, K. K., Dreher, H. M., Smith Glasgow, M. E., & Donnelly, G. F. (2010). Faculty colleagues in your classroom as doctoral students: Does a conflict of interest exist? *Nurse Educator, 35*(5), 213–219.

Azam, M. S. (2010). Fewer employers paying for tuition, corporate training. *Orlando Business Journal.com* Retrieved from http://orlando.bizjournals.com/orlando/stories/2010/04/19/focus1.html

Babcock, P. (2009). Always more to learn. *Society for Human Resource Management.org* Retrieved from http://www.shrm.org/Publications/hrmagazine/EditorialContent/Pages/0909babcock.aspx://www.shrm.org/Publications/hrmagazine/EditorialContent/Pages/0909babcock.aspx

Baez, B. (2002). *Degree of distinction: The Ed.D. or the Ph.D. in education.* Paper presented at the Annual Meeting of the Association for the Study of Higher Education, Sacramento, California, November 21–24, 2002.

Barkham, M., & Mellor-Clark, J. (2003). Bridging evidence-based practice and practice-based evidence: Developing a rigorous and relevant knowledge for the psychological therapies. *Clinical Psychology and Psychotherapy, 10*(6), 319–327.

Bellini, S., & Cusson, R. (in press). The role of the practitioner. In H. M. Dreher & M. E. Smith Glasgow, *Role development for doctoral advanced nursing practice.* New York, NY: Springer.

Bloch, J. R. (2007). *The DNP/DrNP degree as entry into NP practice: Is this nursing's answer to eliminate disparities in health care access for vulnerable populations?* Paper presented at the First National Conference on The Doctor of Nursing Practice: Meanings and Models, Annapolis, Maryland, March 28–30, 2007.

Bologna Process. (2010). *Third cycle: Doctoral education.* Retrieved from http://www.ond.vlaanderen.be/hogeronderwijs/bologna/actionlines/third_cycle.htm

Brar, K., Boschma, G., & McCuaig, F. (2010). The development of nurse practitioner preparation beyond the master's level: What is the debate about? *International Journal of Nursing Education Scholarship, 7*(1), Article 9, 1–15.

Bunge, H. (1962). The first decade of 'Nursing Research.' *Nursing Research, 11*(3), 132–138.

Cacchione, P. Z. (2007). What is clinical nursing research? *Clinical Nursing Research, 16*(3), 167–169.

Carlson, L. H. (2003). The clinical doctorate—Asset or albatross? *Journal of Pediatric Health Care, 17*(4), 216–218.

Christman, L. (1980). Leadership in practice. *Image: Journal of Nursing Scholarship, 12,* 31–33.

Courtenay, B. C. (1988). Eliminating the confusion over the EdD and PhD in colleges and schools of education. *Innovative Higher Education, 13*(1), 11–20.

Dahnke, M. D., & Dreher, H. M. (2010). *Philosophy of science for nursing practice: Concepts and applications.* New York, NY: Springer.

Davies, R. (2008). The Bologna process: The quiet revolution in nursing higher education. *Nurse Education Today, 28,* 935–942.

Donley, R., & Flaherty, M. J. (2008). Revisiting the American Nurses Association's first position on education for nurses: A comparative analysis of the first and second position statements on the education of nurses. *The Online Journal of Issues in Nursing, 13*(2). Retrieved from http://www.nursingworld.org/MainMenuCategories/ANAMarketplace/ANAPeriodicals/OJIN/TableofContents/vol132008/No2May08/ArticlePreviousTopic/EntryIntoPracticeUpdate.aspx

Donohue, P. (1996). *Nursing the finest art: An illustrated history* (2nd ed.). St. Louis, MO: Mosby.

Dracup, K., & Bryan-Brown, C. (2005). Doctor of nursing practice—MRI or total body scan? *American Journal of Critical Care, 14*(4), 278–281.

Dreher, H. M. (2005). The doctor of nursing practice: Has this train left the station? If so, just where is it going? *The Pennsylvania Nurse, 60*, 17–19.

Dreher, H. M. (2008a). Innovation in nursing education: Preparing for the future of nursing practice. *Holistic Nursing Practice, 22*(2), 77–80.

Dreher, H. M. (2008b). A dearth of geriatric specialists: Will invention and gerotechnology save us? *Holistic Nursing Practice, 22*(5), 255–260.

Dreher, H. M. (2009). How do RNs today best stay informed? Do we need "knowledge management?" *Holistic Nursing Practice, 23*(5), 263–266.

Dreher, H. M. (2010a). The path to nursing science today, 1910–2010. In M. D. Dahnke, & H. M. Dreher, *Philosophy of science for nursing practice: Concepts and applications*. New York, NY: Springer.

Dreher, H. M. (2010b). Next steps toward practice knowledge development: An emerging epistemology in nursing. In M. D. Dahnke, & H. M. Dreher, *Philosophy of science for nursing practice*. New York, NY: Springer.

Dreher, H. M., & Gardner, M. (2009). *With the rise of the DNP, who will conduct primary care research?* Paper presented at the Second National Conference on the Doctor of Nursing Practice: The Dialogue Continues..., Hilton Head Island, South Carolina, March 24–27, 2009.

Dreher, H. M., & Montgomery, K. E. (2009). Let's call it "doctoral" advanced practice nursing. *The Journal of Continuing Nursing Education, 40*(12), 530–531.

Dreher, H. M., Donnelly, G., & Naremore, R. (2005). Reflections on the DNP and an alternate practice doctorate model: The Drexel DrNP. *Online Journal of Issues in Nursing, 11*(1), Retrieved from www.nursingworld.org/ojin/topic28/tpc28_7.htm

Dreher, H. M., Fasolka, B., & Clark, M. (2008). Navigating the decision to pursue an advanced degree. *Journal of Men in Nursing, 3*(1), 51–55.

Dunphy, L. M., Smith, N. K., & Youngkin, E. Q. (2009). Advanced practice nursing: Doing what has to be done—Radicals, renegades, and rebels. In L. Joel, *Advanced practice nursing: Essentials for role development* (2nd ed.) (pp. 2–22). Philadelphia, PA: F. A. Davis.

Ellis, L. B., & Lee, N. (2005). The changing landscape of doctoral education: Introducing the professional doctorate for nurses. *Nurse Education Today, 25*(3), 222–229.

Fink, D. (2006). The professional doctorate: Its relativity to the Ph.D. and relevance for the economy. *International Journal of Doctoral Studies, 3*, 35–44.

Fitzpatrick, J. (2003). The case for the clinical doctorate in nursing. *Reflections on Nursing Leadership*, First Quarter, 8–9, 37, 52.

Fitzpatrick, J. (2008). Doctor of nursing practice programs: History and current status. In J. Fitzpatrick, & M. Wallace (Eds.), *The doctor of nursing practice and clinical nurse leader: Essentials of program development and implementation for clinical practice* (pp. 13–30). New York, NY: Springer.

Flexner, A. (1910). *Medical education in the United States and Canada: A report to the Carnegie Foundation for the Advancement of Teaching*. Bulletin No 4. New York, NY: Carnegie Foundation for the Advancement of Teaching.

Florczak, K. L. (2010). Research and the doctor of nursing practice: A cause for consternation. *Nursing Science Quarterly, 23*(1), 13–17.

Ford, J. (2008). Editorial: DNP a bad idea. Retrieved from http://community.advanceweb.com/blogs/np_1/archive/2008/07/23/editorial-on-dnp.aspx

Fulton, J. S. (2010). Evolution of clinical nurse specialist role and practice in the United States. In J. S. Fulton, B. L. Lyon, & K. A. Goudreau (Eds.), *Foundations of clinical nurse specialist practice* (pp. 3–14). New York, NY: Springer.

Fulton, J., & Lyon, B. (2005). The need for some sense making: Doctor of nursing practice. *Journal of Issues in Nursing, 10*(3), Manuscript 3. Retrieved from www.nursingworld.org/MainMenuCategories/ANAMarketplace/ANAPeriodicals/OJIN/TableofContents/Volume102005/No3Sept05/tpc28_316027.aspx

Gibbons, M., Lomoges, C., Nowotny, H., Schwartzman, S., Scott, P., & Trow, M. (1994). *The new production of knowledge*. London, UK: Sage.

Goodrich, A. A. (1936). Modern trends in nursing education. *American Journal of Public Health, 26*, 764–770.

Gordon, S. (2006). *Nursing against the odds: How health care cost cutting, media stereotypes, and medical hubris undermine nurses and patient care*. Ithaca, NY: Cornell University Press.

Gortner, S. R. (1986). Impact of the division of nursing on nursing research development in the U.S.A. In S. M. Stinson, & J. Kerr (Eds.), *International issues in nursing research* (pp. 113–130). Philadelphia, PA: Charles Press.

Gortner, S. R. (2000). Knowledge development in nursing: Our historical roots and future opportunities. *Nursing Outlook, 48*(2), 60–67.

Grace, H. (1989). Issues in doctoral education in nursing. *Journal of Professional Nursing, 5*(5), 266–270.

Hastings, C. E., Mitchell, S. A., & Loud, J. T. (2010). *Advancing nursing roles in clinical and translational science*. Paper presented at the 2010 Clinical and Translational Research and Education Meeting, ACRT/SCTS Joint Annual Meeting, April 5–7, 2010, Washington, DC.

Hathaway, D., Jacob, S., Stegbauer, C., Thompson, C., & Graff, C. (2006). The practice doctorate: Perspectives of early adopters. *Journal of Nursing Education, 45*(12), 487–496.

Hawkins-Walsh, E. (2004). The "practice doctorate" — What's it all about? *The Pediatric Nurse Practitioner*, July–August 2004, 18.

Hawkins, R., & Nezat, G. (2009). Doctoral education: Which degree to pursue? *American Association of Nurse Anesthetists Journal, 77*(2), 92–96.

Hellerstein, D. (2008). Practice-based evidence rather than evidence-based practice in psychiatry. *Medscape Journal of Medicine, 10*(6), 141.

Hiatt, M. D. (1999). Around the continent in 180 days: The controversial journey of Abraham Flexner. *The Pharos*, Winter 1999, 18–24.

Honig, J., & Smolowitz, J. (2009). Clinical doctorate at Columbia University School of Nursing: Lessons learned. *Clinical Scholars Review, 2*(2), 51–59.

Horrocks, S., Anderson, E., & Salisbury, C. (2002). Systematic review of whether nurse practitioners working in primary care can provide equivalent care to doctors. *British Medical Journal, 324*, 819–823.

Hutchinson, S. A. (2001). The development of qualitative health research: Taking stock. *Qualitative Health Research, 11*, 505–521.

Institute of Medicine. (1999). *To err is human: Building a safer health system*. Washington, DC: National Academies Press.

Institute of Medicine. (2001). *Crossing the quality chasm: A new health system for the 21st century*. Washington, DC: National Academies Press.

Institute of Medicine. (2003). *Health professions education: A bridge to quality*. Washington, DC: National Academies Press.

Jacobson, A., Stern, C., Gaspar, P., Spross, J., Heye, M., France, N., Tibbals, S., Gerard, P., & Sedhorn, L. (2007). *Comparison of National Association of Clinical Nurse Specialist Statement Competencies with DNP Essentials: What is the fit?* Paper presented at the First National Conference on The Doctor of Nursing Practice: Meanings and Models, Annapolis, Maryland, March 28–30, 2007.

Joachim, G. (2008). The practice doctorate: Where do Canadian nursing leaders stand? *Nursing Leadership, 21*(4), 42–51.

Kirkpatrick, M. (1994). The department chair position in academic nursing. *Journal of Professional Nursing, 10*(2), 77–83.

Krugman, P. (2009). The Great Recession versus the Great Depression. *New York Times.com*. Retrieved from http://krugman.blogs.nytimes.com/2009/03/20/the-great-recession-versus-the-great-depression/

Lenz, E. R. (2005). The practice doctorate in nursing: An idea whose time has come. *Online Journal of Issues in Nursing, 10*(3), Manuscript 1. Retrieved from www.nursingworld.org/MainMenu-Categories/ANAMarketplace/ANAPeriodicals/OJIN/TableofContents/Volume102005/No3 sept05/tpc28_116025.aspx

Loomis, J. A., Willard, B., & Cohen, J. (2006). Difficult professional choices: Deciding between the PhD and the DNP in nursing. *Online Journal of Issues in Nursing, 12*(1), 6.

Magyary, D., Whitney, J. D., & Brown, M. A. (2006). Advancing practice inquiry: Research foundations of the practice doctorate in nursing, *Nursing Outlook, 54*(3), 139–151.

Maxwell, T. (2003). From first to second generation professional doctorate. *Studies in Higher Education, 28*(3), 279–291.

McKenna, H. (2005). Doctoral education: Some treasonable thoughts. *International Journal of Nursing Studies, 42,* 245–246.

McKenna, H., & Cutcliffe, J. (2001). Nursing doctoral education in the United Kingdom and Ireland. *Online Journal of Issues in Nursing, 6*(2). Retrieved from www.nursingworld.org//MainMenu-Categories/ANAMarketplace/ANAPeriodicals/OJIN/TableofContents/Volume62001/No2May01/ArticlePreviousTopic/UKandIrelandDoctoralEducation.aspx

McNett, M. (2006). The PhD-prepared nurse in the clinical setting. *Clinical Nurse Specialist, 20*(3), 134–138.

Meleis, A., & Dracup, K. (2005). The case against the DNP: History, timing, substance, and marginalization. *Online Journal of Issues in Nursing, 10*(3), Manuscript 2. Retrieved from www.nursingworld.org/MainMenuCategories/ANAMarketplace/ANAPeriodicals/OJIN/TableofContents/Volume102005/No3Sept05/tpc28_216026.aspx

Melosh, B. (1982). *The physician's hand: Work culture and conflict in American nursing.* Philadelphia, PA: Temple University Press.

Melnyk, B., & Davidson, S. (2009). Creating a culture of innovation in nursing education through shared vision, leadership, interdisciplinary partnerships, and positive deviance. *Nursing Administration Quarterly, 33*(4), 288–295.

Mundinger, M. O. (2005). Who's who in nursing: Bringing clarity to the doctor of nursing practice. *Nursing Outlook, 53,* 173–176.

Mundinger, M. O. (2009). The clinical doctorate 15 years hence. *Clinical Scholars Review, 2*(2), 35–36.

Mundinger, M. O., Kane, R., Lenz, E., Totten, A., Tsai, W., Cleary, P. et al. (2000). Primary care outcomes in patients treated by nurse practitioners or physicians: A randomized trial. *Journal of the American Medical Association, 283,* 59–68.

Murray, B. (2000). The degree that almost wasn't: The PsyD comes of age. *The Monitor, 31*(1), 52.

National Academy of Sciences. (2005). *Advancing the nation's health needs.* Committee for Monitoring the Nation's Changing Needs for Biomedical, Behavioral, and Clinical Personnel. Washington, DC: The National Academies Press.

National Association of Clinical Nurse Specialists. (2009). *Position statement on the nursing practice doctorate.* Retrieved from http://www.nacns.org/LinkClick.aspx?fileticket=TOZlongI258%3D&tabid=116

National Association of Community Health Centers. (2009). America needs more primary care. *Community Health Forum.* Retrieved from http://www.nachc.com/client/documents/200909_Forum_Feature_Doctors.pdf

National Forum on the Practice Doctorate. (2003). *Executive summary.* Washington, DC: Author.

National Institutes of Health. (2009a). *Mentored Patient-Oriented Research Career Development Award (Parent K23), Program Announcement (PA) Number: PA-10-060* Retrieved from http://grants2.nih.gov/grants/guide/pa-files/PA-10-060.html

National Institutes of Health. (2009b). Part II full text of announcement. Section I. Funding opportunity description. 1. Research objectives. In: Institutional Clinical and Translational Science Award (U54), RFA-RM-07-007. Retrieved from: http://grants.nih.gov.ezproxy2.library.drexel.edu/grants/guide/rfa-files/RFA-RM-07-007.html.

National Institutes of Health. (2007). *Reflection & dialogue: Doctor of nursing practice (DNP) April 2007.* Retrieved from http://www.nln.org/aboutnln/reflection_dialogue/refl_dial_1.htm

National League for Nursing. (2010). *Master's education in nursing June 2010.* Retrieved from http://www.nln.org/aboutnln/reflection_dialogue/refl_dial_6.htm

National League for Nursing Accrediting Commission. (2005). *NLNAC Statement on Clinical Practice Doctorates.* Retrieved from http://www.nlnac.org/statementClinPrac.htm

National Organization of Nurse Practitioner Faculties. (2006). *Statement on the practice doctorate in nursing: Response to recommendations on clinical hours & degree title.* Retrieved from http://www.nonpf.com/displaycommon.cfm?an=1&subarticlenbr=16

National Organization of Nurse Practitioner Faculties. (2008). *Practice doctorate nurse practitioner entry-level competencies.* Retrieved from http://www.nonpf.com/associations/10789/files/DNP%20NP%20competenciesApril2006.pdf

Neal, A. (2008). Seeking higher-ed accountability: Ending federal accreditation. *Change: The Magazine of Higher Education Regulation,* Sept-Oct, 25–29.

Nelson, M. (2002). Education for professional nursing practice: Looking backward into the future. *Online Journal of Issues in Nursing, 7*(3), Manuscript 3. Retrieved from www.nursingworld.org/MainMenuCategories/ANAMarketplace/ANAPeriodicals/OJIN/TableofContents/Volume72002/No2May2002/EducationforProfessionalNursingPractice.aspx

Nichols, E. F., & Chitty, K. K. (2005). Educational patterns in nursing. In K. K. Chitty, & B. P. Black (Eds.), *Professional nursing: Concepts and challenges* (3rd ed.) (pp. 31–62). Philadelphia, PA: Saunders.

Nowotny, H., Scott, P., & Gibbons, M. (2001). *Re-thinking science: Knowledge and the public in an age of uncertainty.* Cambridge, UK: Polity Press.

Nurse Practitioner Roundtable. (2008). *Nurse practitioner DNP education, certification and titling: A unified statement.* Washington, DC: Author.

Nutting, M. A. (1912). The educational status of nursing. *U. S. Bureau of Education Bulletin.* No. 7, Washington, U.S. Government: Printing Office.

O'Sullivan, A. L. (2005). The practice doctorate in nursing. *The Mentor: The NONPF Newsletter, 16*(1), 1–2, 12.

Pearson, A., Wiechula, R., Court, A., & Lockwood, C. (2007). A re-consideration of what constitutes "evidence" in the healthcare professions. *Nursing Science Quarterly, 20*(1), 85–88.

Peplau, H. E. (1952). *Interpersonal relations in nursing.* New York, NY: G. P. Putnam and Sons.

Peplau, H. E. (1988). The art and science of nursing: Similarities, differences, and relations. *Nursing Science Quarterly, 1*(1), 8–15.

Peterson, D. R. (1997). *Educating professional psychologists: History and guiding conception.* Washington, DC: American Psychological Association.

Potempa, K. M., Redman, R. W., & Anderson, C. A. (2008). Capacity for the advancement for nursing science: Issues and challenges. *Journal of Professional Nursing, 24,* 329–336.

Reed, P. G. (2006). The practice turn in nursing epistemology. *Nursing Science Quarterly, 19*(1), 36–38.

Reel, S. (2009). *The role of research and rigor in DNP programs: The ongoing debate.* Paper presented at the Second National Conference on the Doctor of Nursing Practice: The Dialogue Continues..., Hilton Head Island, South Carolina, March 24–27, 2009.

Rubenstein, D. (2009). The nurse-crusader goes to Washington. *New York Observe.com,* December 8, 2009. Retrieved from http://www.observer.com/2009/nurse-crusader-goes-washington

Rubio, D. M., Schoenbaum, E. E., Lee, L. S., Schteingart, D. E., Marantz, P. R., Anderson, K. E. et al. (2010). Defining translational research: Implications for training. *Academic Medicine, 85*(3), 470–475.

Rudy, E., & Grady, P. (2005). Biological researchers: Building nursing science. *Nursing Outlook, 53,* 88–94.

Salzman, A. (2010). The DPT degree: Our destiny or a cosmetic change? *Advance for Physical Therapy & PT Assistants, 14*(4), 55.

San Francisco AIDS Foundation. (2008). Confronting the "evidence" in evidence-based HIV prevention: Summary report. *HIV Evidence-Based Prevention,* July 2008, 1–5.

Sayette, M. A., Mayne, T. J., & Norcross, J. C. (2010). *Insiders's guide to graduate programs in clinical and counseling psychology.* New York: NY: Guilford Press.

Schlotfeldt, R. M. (1978). The professional doctorate: Rationale and characteristics. *Nursing Outlook, 26,* 302–311.

Silver, H. K., Ford, L. R., & Day, L. R. (1968). The pediatric nurse–practitioner program: Expanding the role of the nurse to provide increased health care for children. *Journal of the American Medical Association, 204*(4), 298–302.

Smith, M. E., & Dreher, H. M. (2003). Wanted, nursing faculty! If you think the nursing shortage is bad, the nursing faculty shortage is worse. *Advance for Nursing, 5,* 31–32.

Smith Glasgow, M. E., & Dreher, H. M. (2010). The future of oncology nursing science: Who will generate the knowledge? *Oncology Nursing Forum, 37*(4), 393–396.

Sperhac, A. M., & Clinton, P. (2008). Doctorate of nursing practice: Blueprint for excellence. *Journal of Pediatric Health Care, 22*(3), 146–151.

Stew, G. (2009). *The professional/practice nursing doctorate in the United Kingdom.* Paper presented at the Second National Conference on the Doctor of Nursing Practice: The Dialogue Continues. . ., Hilton Head Island, South Carolina, March 24–27, 2009.

Stewart, D. (2009). *Challenges and opportunities for the professional doctorate: A North American perspective.* Paper presented at the European Conference on the Professional Doctorate, London, England, November 5–6, 2009.

Townsend, B. K. (2002). *Rethinking the Ed.D., or what's in a name.* Paper presented at the Annual Meeting of the Association for the Study of Higher Education, Sacramento, California, November 21–24, 2002.

Tri-Council for Nursing. (2010). *Joint statement from the tri-council for nursing on recent registered nurse supply and demand projections.* Retrieved from http://www.nln.org/governmentaffairs/pdf/workforce_supply_statement_final.pdf

Trossman, S. (2009). Nurses discuss economy, DNP degree, care in the ED. *The American Nurse,* March April, pp. 1, 8.

Valian, V. (2005). Beyond gender schemas: Improving the advancement of women in academia. *Hypatia, 20*(3), 198–213.

Valiga, T. (2004). *The nursing faculty shortage: A national perspective.* Congressional briefing presented by the A. N. S. R. Alliance, Hart Senate Office Building, Washington, DC.

Vreeland, E. M. (1964). Nursing research programs of the public health service: Highlights and trends. *Nursing Research, 13*(2), 148–158.

Webber, P. (2008). The doctor of nursing practice degree and research: Are we making an epistemological mistake. *Journal of Nursing Education, 47*(10), 466–472.

Werley, H. H., & Westlake, S. K. (1985). Impact of nursing research on public policy: An examination of ANA research priority statements. *Journal of Professional Nursing, 1*(3), 148–151, 154–156.

Williams, J. C., & Richardson, V. T. (2010). *New millenium, same glass ceiling? The impact on law firm compensation systems on women.* A joint report of the Project for Attorney Retention, Minority Corporate Counsel Association. Retrieved from http://www.pardc.org/Publications/Same-GlassCeiling.pdf

Wilkes, L. M., & Mohan, S. (2008). Nurses in the clinical area: Relevance of a PhD. *Collegian, 15,* 135–141.

Zungolo, E. (2009). *The DNP and the faculty role: Issues and challenges.* Paper presented at the Second National Conference on the Doctor of Nursing Practice: The Dialogue Continues. . ., Hilton Head Island, South Carolina, March 24–27, 2010.

CHAPTER ONE: Reflective Response

Lynne M. Dunphy

This first chapter of this book provides a good anchoring overview for much of the rich discourse which follows throughout the textbook, as references are cited throughout the chapter to later content. Dreher has made a strong choice on the use of the term *political path* in the title, as the convoluted story of the evolution of this role is fraught with political (and social) implications that are difficult to summarize, synthesize, and explain. Here, Dreher succeeds admirably. He also does not attempt to bring premature closure to some of these complex and deep (in the sense of knowledge development and philosophy of science) issues. He challenges the reader to think through the many potential implications of the previous courses of action in *nursing* that have influenced the evolution of doctoral education in nursing in general and the development of the doctorate of nursing practice in particular. I would suggest, this chapter could use additional work—and I would direct the readers of the text to this task—in the further description of nursing in the context of broader historical trends and sociopolitical disciplinary environments in general. Dreher cites the work of labor historian Barbara Melosh, as well as provides the context to ideas about knowledge development by comparing and contrasting the doctorate of nursing practice programs with the evolution of the PysD, for example, in psychology, and similar disciplinary endeavors in pharmacology (the PharmD), physical therapy, and public health, and even occasionally medicine.

However admirable the work of Melosh (which this author by and large endorses), it is only one viewpoint on nursing's rich history. Also, it begs the question of larger issues in the evolution of science, technology, and therapeutics in general across the 20th century, as well as the rise (and fall) of other health professions in the same time frame (medicine comes to mind), and the even broader cultural, political, and social changes that framed the times and these issues. So, I would see the readers of this text being guided to a broader variety of other historical and sociological readings with which to frame the nursing-specific *debates, power plays, and dissension.*

I would also direct the reader to the work of David Allen, critical social theorist in nursing, who was one of the first in nursing to raise the issue (along with Melosh, to be fair) of the limits of advanced education as a "professionalizing strategy" for nursing (Allen, 1986). Historians and sociologists have also pointed out the use of "education" as a pseudonym for class, pointing out that in medicine, requiring the prerequisite of a baccalaureate degree prior to admission to medical school, assured a steady stream of well-educated (read: "well-bred" as in "invariably well-off enough" to be able to AFFORD education) young gentlemen, of a certain class. Equally, any historical and political analysis cannot afford to ignore the gender issue in nursing, as tedious as this discussion may be to some. Ethel Manson Fenwick, organizer of the British Nurses Association and the editor first British journal of nursing (the *Nursing Record*), aptly summed up the situation in 1887 when she said, "The Nurse question is the Women question, pure and simple. We have to run the gauntlet of those historic rotten eggs" (Fenwick, quoted in Baer, 1997, pp. 256–257). Has anything *really* changed?

When one examines the evolution of the nurse practitioner role broadly speaking, within its social context, one gets a sense of the "grass-roots" nature of its development — a response to a social need for primary care (Dunphy & Youngkin, 2008). Nurse Practitioner programs sprung up willy-nilly; certifications and continuing education programs abounded for practicing diploma-prepared nurses to become "nurse practitioners." In contrast, as broadly observed and described in this chapter, the DNP evolved as a much more "top-down" movement, springing from ideas of influential nurse leaders and educators (nurse *professionalizers*) as actualized in various nursing organizations like the American Association of Colleges of Nursing (AACN) and National Organization of Nurse Practitioner Faculties (NONPF). Against the broader backdrop of history, and societal need for health care, debates over titling, splitting hairs over the differentiation of the PhD, DNS, DNSc, and DNP (so well outlined in this chapter!), for example, may fade out.

Although as an academic I applaud the need for "tight" definition and appreciate fully the implications in this endeavor in defining knowledge development, curriculum, and the like, some of these issues emerge as "small" — and possibly petty — when confronted with the magnitude of human need for health care and the subsequent need for nursing *action*. Thus, I posit a broader frame for examining these continually important and compelling issues in nursing.

REFERENCES

Allen, D. (1986). Professionalism, occupational segregation by gender and control of nursing. *Journal of Women, Politics & Policy, 6*(3), 1–24.

Baer, E. (1997). Women and the politics of career development: The case of nursing. In A. M. Rafferty, J. Robinson, & G. Elkan (Eds.), *Nursing history and the politics of welfare* (pp. 242–258). London: Routledge.

Dunphy, L., & Youngkin, E. (2009). Doing what had to be done: Radicals, renegades, and rebels In L. Joel, *Advanced practice nursing: Essentials for role development* (2nd ed., pp. 2–22). Philadelphia, PA: FA Davis.

CRITICAL THINKING QUESTIONS

1. How do you view the state of critical discourse in nursing? Do we debate enough? Do we need more agreement and more consensus? Or should we embrace difference more and be less concerned with conformity?

2. The nursing profession appears to have abandoned the idea of clinical doctorate as an alternative to the PhD and has embraced the title "practice doctorate" to describe the DNP. Discuss whether you think the profession needs a research doctorate (PhD), a practice doctorate (DNP), and a clinical doctorate?

3. Why do you think the EdD in Nursing Education degree model at Teacher's College was never again replicated?

4. What can be done to combat the aging nursing workforce which faces imminent retirements that will not be replaced by the current pool of those entering the profession at all levels?

5. Debate the following: "Resolved, *nursing* is a profession."

6. The ND degree and now the DNP were partly modeled after the doctor of medicine degree (MD). What are your thoughts about this?
7. Discuss whether you think 1,000 total clinical hours should be required for the DNP degree, including practice and clinical executive tracks.
8. Discuss whether original research ought to be part of the formal DNP curriculum.
9. Do you agree that the DNP degree might offer something the PhD degree cannot? Provide your rationale.
10. Discuss why you have chosen the particular doctor of nursing practice program you are currently matriculating in.

CHAPTER TWO

Role Theory and the Evolution of Professional Roles in Nursing

H. Michael Dreher and Jeannine Uribe

INTRODUCTION

In the most explicit sense, the "role" of the registered nurse (RN) *defines* the work of the RN. In other words: What are the job functions of the RN? What are the role boundaries of the RN? How did the evolution of the work of the RN advance to be a professional role (Haase, 1990; Zerwekh & Claborn, 2009)? As one reflects on the history of nursing, one can appreciate the struggles of the profession today.

The very first formal program for nursing in the United States was a 6-month training curriculum established at the Women's Hospital in Philadelphia in 1863 by physician Emmeline Horton Clevelend, MD, an 1855 alumna of the Women's Medical College of Pennsylvania, the world's first medical college for women (Robinson, 1946).[1] The historical and operational creation of the job description of a RN will be discussed in this chapter, because it is only after having some clarity about the role of the RN that one can make assumptions about what the role of the advanced practice nurse should be. Further, with the advent of the relatively new doctor of nursing practice (DNP) degree, the role of the *doctoral advanced practice nurse* then needs to be reflected upon and addressed (Dreher & Montgomery, 2009).[2] Moreover, some serious questions need to be asked and answered: What should the *role* of the doctoral advanced practice nurse be? How is it, or how should it be, different from the roles of the masters-prepared advanced practice nurse? If the roles are not different now and will not differ substantively in the future, then the nursing profession has a problem. *Finally, if a more highly educated advanced practice nurse with a doctorate degree does not improve health, then why bother with the expense and effort of another degree?* This chapter will lay some of the groundwork with which to answer these questions in this text.

This chapter is not meant to be a history of American nursing, which has been excellently provided by Donohue (1996) in *Nursing, the Finest Art: An Illustrated History* (1996), Reverby's (1987) *Ordered to Care: The Dilemma of American Nursing, 1850–1945*, and more recently by Judd, Sitzman, and Davis (2009) in *A History of American Nursing: Trends and Eras*. Robinson (1946) has also written an outstanding text that focuses on the history of nursing globally, but it ends with nurses still active in World War II. This chapter, however, is historical in its approach. What we wish to do differently is to trace the role of nurses (their work) from its early American origins to the emergence of professional nursing roles. Dreher will review the meaning of *role* or *work roles* and discuss how the theoretical aspects of role theory have influenced nursing as a profession. Uribe, a nurse historian, will then trace the evolution of these roles (or work roles) in nursing from Nightingale to just after the turn of the 20th century in the United States, and then through the evolution of the "professional registered nurse" educated at the baccalaureate level in the mid-1960s. As we all know, the American Nurses Association's (ANA) historic 1965 position statement, which called for all RNs to be educated at the baccalaureate level, tragically was never realized (Donley & Flaherty, 2002). Despite the ANA's reaffirmation of that position in 1985, the majority of nurses in the United States are still not educated at the Bachelor of Science in Nursing (BSN) level, with Associate Degree (AD)-level nurses now predominating (Dreher, 2008a; Kraus, 1980). Linda Aiken and colleagues have reported that between 1970 and 1994, of the 1.4 million nurses who entered the workforce, 59% of them earned an AD degree and 41% of them a BSN (Aiken, Cheung, & Olds, 2009).[3] The question is who and what is driving AD nursing education? Is it an issue of economics: A 2-year degree obviously costs less than a 4 or 5-year baccalaureate degree?[4] Does the public not view nursing as a profession and, as a result, potential nurses are steered toward AD programs?

Whether this 45-year-old issue over the entry level for basic nursing practice will ever be fully resolved is unknown. It is therefore not surprising that there is continuing controversy over whether the doctorate will ever fully replace the master's degree for entry-level advanced nursing practice. Do you envision all 50 various state legislatures changing their respective Nurse Practice Acts to eliminate the master's degree requirement in favor of the doctorate? This is an interesting question.

Having defined what the roles of the professional nurse were through the mid-1960s, Chapter 3 will focus on the evolution of what came to be known as "advanced practice nursing" roles. The first iteration of advanced practice nursing began with the certificate pediatric nurse practitioner movement at the University of Colorado in 1965 and culminated in the 1990s with the master's of nursing science as the requirement for all advanced practice nurses (Dreher, 2009; Ford & Silver, 1967). Finally, Chapter 4 builds on these chapters and provides both a contemporary and futuristic analysis of what roles the doctoral advanced practice nurse possesses or should possess. The central thesis of Chapter 4 is: "How do doctoral advanced practice nursing roles differ, or how should they differ, from masters advanced practice nursing roles?" In a real sense, the specific role of doctoral advanced practice nurses, the sphere of influence they will cast, the boundaries of their work, and what they will do with a Doctor of Nursing Practice degree that is explicitly different, are still evolving. In other words, the history of the role of the doctor of nursing practice graduate is being written as you live it!

ROLE AND ROLE THEORY IN THE PROFESSION OF NURSING

Perhaps the seminal book on role theory in the health professions is *Role Theory: Perspectives for Health Professionals*, first published by Hardy and Conway in 1979 followed by a second edition in 1988. Unfortunately, the book did not have a third edition. This chapter extends only some of the work of their contributors and analyzes the content that would specifically pertain to role theory for present-day doctoral advanced practice nurses. The term *role* is largely a sociological one (Biddle, 1986). However, its sociological application has universal meaning for society at both the individual and the group level and for disciplines accorded the status of a profession where roles and role functions are important.

Roles in the Profession

Whereas the early classical professions were divinity, law, and medicine (Klass, 1961), more contemporary definitions of a *profession* include nursing, dentistry, engineering, architecture, social work, accountancy, and others. Professions such as nursing are different from other types of work, as the work of the professional nurse is characterized by the following: professional autonomy; a clearly defined, highly developed, specialized, and theoretical knowledge base; control of training, certification, and licensing of those newly entering the profession; self-governing and self-policing authority; an explicit ethical code especially pertaining to professional ethics; and a commitment to public service (Burbules & Densmore, 1991). A very recent analysis of the word *profession* emphasizes that what makes the work of the professional nurse different from, for example, the work of an engineer is that there is a distinctive reliance on interpersonal skills and on ethical codes of work behavior (Dreher & Dahnke, 2010).

A separate discussion, and not the focus of this chapter, is whether nurses with ADs are also professionals. Many take the position that, while nursing *is* a profession, some practitioners (without a baccalaureate degree) are technically *not professionals* (AACN, 2000; Barter & McFarland, 2001), and the Carnegie Foundation has recently come out strongly in support of a more highly educated nursing workforce (Benner, Sutphen, Leonard, & Day, 2009). Liaschenko and Peter (2004) even declare that nursing is not a profession, but simply "work." Melosh (1982) also flatly writes: ". . . nursing is not and cannot be a profession" (p. 15). Certainly, Melosh was historically correct in her critique in 1982 when she wrote: "Clearly, nurses never gained the large measure of control over their work that defines a profession" (p. 19). She further indicated that, by classical definitions of a profession, "Professionals are their own bosses" (p. 15) and "If professions maintain their authority through controlling the division of labor related to their work . . . then doctors' own professionalization organizes and requires nurses' subordination" (p. 19). Perhaps this was true in 1982 (except where military nurses could outrank their physician colleagues then and now), but in 2010 about 23 states allow completely independent nurse practitioner practices (Ferris, 2001; Pearson, 2010). By contemporary standards, at least by Melosh's definition, some nurses are indeed autonomous and classically "professional." Further, that would mean that the profession of nursing is legitimately partly professional, too. This chapter, however, focuses on the roles of doctoral-educated advanced practice nursing professionals that have evolved from the emergence of professional nursing roles, but the ongoing debate about the nature of the professionalism of nursing continues. Because the health of our citizenry is so important, the roles of nursing professionals are particularly critical to both the development of the profession itself and their impact on society because the highly skilled work they perform.

Role and Its Meaning for New DNP Graduates

At its most basic level, *role* can be defined as "a socially expected behavior pattern usually determined by an individual's status in a particular society" (Merriam-Webster, 2010, p. 1). A more precise sociological view would characterize *role* as occurring within systems (or organizations, or relationships), and therefore a *role* can be considered a "set of systems states and actions of a subsystem, of an organization, including its interactions with other systems of nonsystem elements" (Kuhn, 1974, p. 298). These definitional frameworks lead us to conceptualize an operational definition of the word *role* for nursing. It is suggested that nursing roles are professional, socially constructed, operationalized behaviors that form the boundaries of what a professional nurse does. It is only through a thorough analysis of the work of RNs and the roles they play, enact, or fulfill in the course of their professional work can one ascertain what are *advanced (practice) nursing roles*. Finally, what differs or extends the boundaries of advanced practice to doctoral advanced (practice) nursing roles? In theory, it sounds very simple. In actuality, we believe that it is more complex. Multiple discussions have ensued in our doctor of nursing practice seminars in the last 5 years about nursing roles and the nature of advanced practice nursing. For example, in the scenario of an overweight or obese patient with accompanying negative health conditions that need intervention, how does the 20-minute primary care interaction of an adult nurse practitioner and patient differ operationally from the physician–patient interaction (Dreher, 2008b)? This kind of discussion is particularly germane to doctoral advanced practice nurses, who must now identify how their roles and role functions will be different and *more advanced* than when they had a master's degree. Again, the authors contend that if the skill set is the same, then nursing has a weakened debate calling for a practice nursing doctorate. Meleis' work (1975; Meleis & Trangenstein, 1994) on role transitions is very well applicable to today's doctoral advanced practice graduate, especially one who practiced previously with the master's degree. In her latest work, Meleis suggests, "Role insufficiency may be manifested in assuming any new roles ..." (p. 2), and further indicates that there are "... some losses and gains in their different roles and support systems" (Meleis, 2010, p. 3). Cusson (Cusson & Strange, 2008; Cusson & Viggiano, 2002) has written extensively about nurse practitioner role transitions, especially among neonatal nurse practitioners. The authors are aware that Dr. Cusson is currently extending her work to role transitions among doctoral advanced practice graduates and it is precisely this kind of outcome data that the profession needs.

Sociological Schools of Thought on Roles

There are two very prominent sociological schools of thought on roles and social interactions that serve as frameworks or even paradigms in which individuals, institutions, and systems operate. In Table 2.1, the *functionalist* view, as mostly attributed to the eminent sociologist Emile Durkeim (1964), and the competing *symbolic interaction* perspective best articulated by Mead (1934), Cooley (1964), and Blumer (1969) are summarized.

In a functionalist view, or in structural–functional theory, the roles that individuals play in society evolve out of very organic systems that constantly interact and are somewhat predictable. For example, in the case of the professional nurse, there is a need in society for nurses to perform certain roles (e.g., health educator, caregiver, advocate), and thus most nurses employ those roles in their daily work. Doctoral advanced practice nurses, however, are in a very different place functionally. Society does not yet know exactly what roles they will play (or be required to fill), and the new domain of this *doctoral advanced practice* is being created in real time, even as this text is published.

We therefore propose that the functionalist view of the roles of the professional nurse, where a common socialization of RNs creates stability in the social system, may not theoretically or properly explain the unfolding role of a new type of advanced practice nurse. In a discussion of the roles of professionals, a symbolic interactionist view of doctoral advanced practice nurses would indicate that their emerging roles would evolve from an ongoing examination of their meaning, to a vigorous self-analysis of how satisfying, effective, or well received the exhibition of the role is. In other words, the critical feedback this new practitioner receives, processes, interprets, and reinterprets will ultimately reinforce the role being integrated and assimilated in a new domain of practice. In a study

TABLE 2.1
Two Perspectives on Roles in Social Interactions

Functionalist View (Macro-sociological Analysis)	Symbolic Interactionist View (Micro-sociological Analysis)
Focus of perspective is on the group and its demarcation into smaller sub-groups, units, and systems.	Focus of perspective is on the individual interacting and the symbolic interpretation of both verbal and non-verbal behavior and cures.
Objects and persons are stimuli that act on an individual.	An individual constructs objects on the basis of his ongoing activity. He gives meaning to objects and makes decisions on the basis of his judgments.
Action is a release or response to what the situational norms demand.	The individual decides what he wishes to do and how he will do it. He takes account of external and internal cues, interpreting their significance for his action.
Environmental forces act to 'produce' behavior.	By a process of self-indication, an individual accepts, rejects, or transforms the meaning (impact) of such forces.
Prescriptions for action, or norms, dictate appropriate behaviors. They are social facts.	Others' attitudes are the basis for individual lines of action.
An act is a unitary, bounded phenomenon; that is, it starts and stops.	An act is disclosed over time and what the end of the act will be cannot be foretold at the start.
The act (of an actor) will be followed by the response of another with or without any interpretation taking place on the part of the other.	An act is validated by the response of another.
Persons act on the basis of a generally objective reality; that is, learned responses.	Reality is defined by each actor; one defines a situation as he "sees it" and acts on this perception.
People are socially molded, not forced, to perform societal functions.	Social order is maintained when people share their understanding of everyday behavior.
Group action is the expression of societal demands and shared social values.	Group action is the expression of individuals confronting their life situations.

Adapted from Conway, M. E. (1988). Theoretical approaches to the study of roles. In M. E. Hardy & M. E. Conway (Eds.), *Role theory: Perspectives for health professionals* (2nd ed.) (p. 65).

of "What do people need psychiatric and mental health nurses for?," Jackson and Stevenson (2000) describe the utility of using this critical feedback from patients (which may not be explicit) to answer this question. Similarly, Erving Goffman's (1955) original theory of "face work," which is described by Shattell (2004) as the face of the nurse interacting with the face of the patient in the simplicity or ordinariness of any basic nurse–patient interaction, is an example of how symbolic interaction theory may be highly useful in explaining how two different dyadic doctoral advanced practice nursing roles may evolve.

First, what is the new doctoral advanced practice nurse/patient role? Second, what is the new doctoral advanced practice nursing role in relation to colleagues in other health care disciplinary colleagues? On an operational level, these questions are: (1) How will the individual patient perceive Dr. Jane Smith's role as a nursing primary care provider now using the title "Dr."? (2) How will fellow health profession colleagues perceive the new role of the doctoral advanced practice nurse as *doctoral prepared*, not masters prepared? Will patients have different expectations? Will colleagues have different expectations? Indeed, Goffman in his classic sociological text *A Presentation of Self in Everyday Life* (1959) writes, "When an individual enters the presence of others, they commonly seek to acquire information about him or to bring into play information about him already possessed" (p. 1). Will this new type of advanced practice nurse use the face-to-face feedback to create solutions to any new role conflict or role strain that may occur? While role conflict and role strain in the new doctoral advanced practice nurse will be addressed in Chapter 10 by Smith Glasgow and Zoucha, both sociological concepts are not new to nursing. However, there are likely particular nuances that are different from the role conflict and role strain of the newly educated, master's-prepared advanced practice nurse.

Another important concept in symbolic interaction is that of *role-taking*. Role-taking is a key mechanism of interaction that permits us to take another person's perspective and to see what our actions might mean to the other actors with whom we interact (Schell & Kayser-Jones, 1999). One scholar suggests that the outcome of role-taking is not just the *processing of the influence of the interaction* on behavior, but requires overt behavioral change based on the processing of those interactions (Cast, 2004). In other words, in the new doctoral advanced practice nursing role, the new practitioner is likely to not just think differently, but also to act differently as new face–work interactions with patient and colleagues are experienced. We contend that this change in perspective and change in thinking is more likely to occur as the new practitioner engages in more reflective practice. Johns and Freshwater (2005) are leading scholars supporting the practice of reflection in advanced nursing practice, and in Chapter 20 Stew writes about how reflective practice ought to be even more mature and developed in the DNP/DrNP graduate. With deep reflection about this new role and consideration of what it is or should be (and conversely what it is no longer), the new practitioner is thus likely to experience ambiguity as he or she tries to "figure this new role out." Our view is that the experience of ambiguity is not detrimental, but a sign of progress. As the new practitioner engages in activities that lead to more secure role delineation, we think the ambiguity will lessen. Hopefully, patients will respond differently and positively to the confidence and enhanced skill set of the doctor of nursing practice graduate. Over time, we predict that health profession colleagues will respond similarly.

A vigorous curricular focus on the concept of role is particularly important for the student pursuing a doctor of nursing practice degree. However, it is not likely that the expansion and ultimate role delineation of the DNP/DrNP graduate will be entirely noncontroversial or always well received. There will be resistance from current master's-prepared nurse practitioners, nurse midwives, nurse anesthetists, and clinical nurse specialists who will claim your practice is not different (or better?) than theirs. If their argument prevails, then a given institution, perhaps, may not compensate the doctoral graduate more highly. Thus, in supporting doctoral advanced nursing practice, we are unyielding in our plea that the necessary outcome data must be conducted and disseminated. Nevertheless, there is a bountiful amount of optimism in the profession about your future and this new degree, and as one recent graduate has recently written:

> Since attaining my doctorate, I find myself better equipped to build upon my master's level training. I'm no longer satisfied with doing the "how to," but indeed now relish and crave the "why?" and the "why not?" As a doctoral advanced practice nurse, I am different!
>
> —*Dreher & Montgomery, 2009, p. 530*

We anticipate that in your new role you will also be different.

EMERGENCE OF PROFESSIONAL ROLES IN NURSING: RISING FROM THE TOIL OF PUBLIC HEALTH NURSES

It is with some incredulity that public health nurses are not more duly recognized for their role in the evolution of our discipline. Furthermore, while Nightingale's preeminence still reigns over nursing, her vision for nursing was enacted very differently in the United States. In many ways, the rise of modern nursing has been accomplished despite tension from two equally dogmatic nursing subcultures—the *conservative traditionalists* and the *elite professionalizers* (Melosh, 1982; Reverby, 1987). And as quarrelsome as these two camps have been, progress has indeed been made, and nursing is probably more advanced here than in any other place on the globe.

The Impact of Nightingale

The Nightingale Influence

Florence Nightingale wrote about patients and nursing, beginning a revolution of the roles of nurses, which had been represented up to that point by religious sisters or inmates living in the almshouses where they served. Her ideas on nursing included a reformed vision of employment for women, a profession removing the societal attachment to the idea of womanly work and feminine intuition, and replacing the characterization of a nurse with an educated, highly moral, and stable woman to run the wards. Her nurses required both theoretical and practical training. In Deloughery's (1977) book on the nursing profession, Nightingale changed nursing to "a career and not a last resort" (p. 61) for women in need of employment. Nightingale's ideal plan separated nursing service from education by making student nurses' practical experiences on the hospital wards opportunities for learning with nurse instructors and physicians, rather than just providing service to the hospital.

Scientific progress in medicine, combined with the growing promotion of social reforms in many areas, helped formulate the idea that physicians needed assistants to carry out their complex medical treatments for better results. Recognizing that they were following the physician's orders, Nightingale wanted her nurses to understand the reasons for their actions, and thus promoted the idea of education. She wanted public support for nursing education, which included some medical education—a shift in thinking that was not readily accepted.

In opposition to Nightingale's educational plan for nurses were widely supported ideas such as characterizations of what constituted the natural traditional work of women, and views that too much education would take away the feminine instinct that was related to delivering care. The transfer of the Nightingale tenets to hospitals in the United States altered important educational objectives, which were different from just using student nurses to fulfill the service needs of the hospital.

The Nightingale Nursing Model Becomes "Americanized"

Hospital administrators, physicians, and women in the United States studied Nightingale's ideas and brought them to hospitals that have been established since the late 18th century and staffed with employees providing care without formalized training (Rosenberg, 1987). The first nursing schools formed separate nursing school boards charged with planning and financing the institution. Unfortunately, poor funding removed Nightingale's ideal of student nurses in the hospitals to learn. Instead, students became the sole hospital care providers, in effect paying for their training, which lacked public support (Rosenberg, 1987). Their education became ward service, as theoretical classroom time decreased and practical experience became the teacher. The proliferation of hospitals in the 1870s increased the need for student nurses and the growth of schools of nursing, which led to a diffusion of nursing education and the graduation of a variety of levels of nurses. The reputation of nurses, as well as the quality of the care they provided both in the hospitals and in private duty positions in the home after completing training, varied.

In the late 19th and early 20th centuries, nursing leaders, including a group of women nursing superintendents, shaped nursing education and work and attempted to require prescriptively a level of consistency to nursing care, thus protecting the reputation of the schools and the work done by their graduate nurses. While the superintendent title was mostly associated with the directors of training schools in the profession's early infancy, the "nurse superintendent" was later clarified by Davis (1929) as:

> ... the administrator or executive head of the hospital, *not* the director of the training school. In some of the smaller hospitals (unfortunately) the two positions are combined. The nurse superintendent has her chief field in the non-governmental charitable hospital of less than 100 beds.
>
> —*Davis, 1929, p. 386*

This early cohort of leaders worked together to form committees to evaluate school curricula and the education of specialized tasks performed by nurses. They also promoted heavily the support of alumni groups (and their obvious financial philanthropy) and became a formidable and interested group of active nurses. The American Society of Superintendents of Training Schools, founded in 1894, promoted leadership, higher entrance requirements for potential students, and better schools in an effort to increase the professionalization of nursing and protect trained nurses' legitimate role in society. Renamed the National League of Nursing Education in 1912, members aimed to encourage more women to enter nursing by pushing for progressive reforms, including shorter days, a university education, and a standard curriculum (Dock & Stewart, 1938).

The reputation of hospitals during the 1800s kept many ill people at home to be cared for by their families. With the growth of nursing training schools, those who could afford supplementary care hired a private duty nurse to come to the home to carry out physician treatments and provide skilled nursing care to the sick individual. Demand for private duty nurses increased as female family members increasingly joined the workforce. After the turn of the 20th century, hospitals also arranged for private duty nurses to provide care within the institution, which created employment opportunities for the majority of graduate nurses (Whelan, 2005). These nurse-owned and operated registries were formed to assist nurses with finding work while granting them the freedom to choose the job, although this type of autonomy did not add to the professional image of nurses. When caring for patients in their homes, nurses fought against the image of subservience, especially African-American nurses who had been kept in inferior positions by a White majority of nurses and society alike (Young, 2005). Following Nightingale's promotion of highly moral and educated women, nursing leaders from the first half of the 20th century promoted the ideal nurse to require "the exercise of superior intelligence, a large body of knowledge and skills, sensitiveness, and imagination" (Harmer & Henderson, 1939, p. 4). However, middle- and upper-class women did not join nursing in large numbers, leaving women of the lower class with a high-school diploma to enter training (Dock & Stewart, 1938; Rosenberg, 1987).

The Toil and Contribution of Public Health Nurses to Nursing

Nursing's Role in the Public's Health

On another front, advances in medicine and science during the late 1800s, specifically the wide acceptance of the germ theory, helped change the thinking about infections and debunked the previously held moral aspects of the causes of disease, replacing it with the identifiable and controllable germ as the root cause for illness and disability (Rosen, 1993). A global initiative sprang up asking governments to take responsibility to respond to the public welfare and the need to subsidize improvements in community sanitation, water supplies, and other alterable situations that, if left unattended, could lead to higher morbidity and mortality rates from infectious disease. The federally funded U.S. Public Health Service (USPHS) is one example of the U.S. government's attention to the need for community services to protect the health of citizens. While the USPHS can trace its early history back to 1798 with an Act designed for the relief of sick and disabled seamen, its history was more formally established by legislation in 1889 that formed the USPHS Commissioned Officer program (Williams, 1951). At first, only physicians were admitted to the Commissioned Officer Association, with the first nurses not commissioned as officers until July 1945 (Parascandola, 2007; U.S. Public Health Service Nursing, 2009). Nevertheless, nurses in the 20th century would serve a fundamental role in this agency.

At the turn of the 20th century, the continuing influx of immigrants from around the world and overcrowding in urban areas led to a renewal of social reforms in which nurses participated and started a new role for nurses: caring and educating families in their homes. The settlement house movement, which flourished in many cities beginning in the late 1800s, interested many individuals from all walks of life who subscribed to a belief in social welfare, and who sought to help raise the lives of the poor immigrants (Wade, 1967). Their social activism was intentional and aimed at assisting immigrant families to acculturate to urban life in America by improving their employment, the sanitation of their living arrangements, and their health. Lillian Wald, Mary Brewster, and other nurses formed the famous Henry Street Settlement House in New York in 1893, financed by wealthy patrons who saw the value of improving the health and welfare of the urban working poor (Buhler-Wilkerson, 1991). Living in the neighborhoods they served, nurses visited tenement homes providing nursing care and health education to families, and to educate them about their capacity to care for themselves and to enhance their health. In the new role of the public health nurse another opportunity was provided to increase the professionalism of nurses due to its requirements of higher education, specialized knowledge, and a more autonomous practice (Brainard, 1985).

During the early 1900s, public health initiatives aimed to decrease disease, but the social issues connected with disease remained. Despite great efforts by public health nurses, poverty often limited individual choices. Public awareness of growing health problems created the perfect link between public health and social reforms, forging a place for nurses to address health issues caused by urbanization, poverty, and disease (Porter, 1994). In recognition of this need for more specialized training for this role, Simmons College in Boston in 1904 began an 8-month course for public health nurses (Nutting, 1904). These public health nurses, referred to as *visiting nurses*, worked for two types of agencies, voluntary and official. The privately funded voluntary organizations were funded by communities and philanthropies were run by board members who hired public health nurses.

The National Organization of Public Health Nurses (NOPHN), started in 1912, played a role in shaping public health nursing and attempted to bring this branch of nursing to a higher professional level. The NOPHN promoted standards of education, leadership, supervision, and employment and gave advice to groups looking to employ a public health nurse. Their journal, *Public Health Nurse*, founded in 1912, was a resource for nurses and committees looking for legislation, statistics, health information, and programs. Physicians contributed to the journal, writing about communicable diseases and treatments for illnesses. While NOPHN recommendations were available, there were a very limited number of employable, educated public health nurses who met them. As a result, many organizations overlooked the NOPHN minimum standards and hired unprepared nurses to public health positions, which in many cases did not have supervisors or other nurses to assist the newly hired nurses to fulfill their job requirements (Buhler-Wilkerson, 1987). Although the hiring of public health nurses continued to rise, it was due to the increasing number of agencies hiring only one public health nurse, which ultimately limited the number of people who came into contact with this service (Giacomo, 1953).

With the continued rise of organized nursing and a growing diverse population, philanthropies pushed for national reforms and programs that included positions for public health nurses and helped promote an increase in government support for employing nurses (Magat, 1989). These official agencies were funded by a variety of government levels, and employed public health nurses to address health issues in the hope of decreasing the incidence and prevalence of disease. As public funding increased with the increased incidence of communicable diseases, public health nurses had a choice of employment in official agencies sponsored by the government at the state and federal levels or in voluntary agencies, usually run by a board of community women and men (Beckemeier, 2008).

Public health nurses working in voluntary agencies specialized in caring for families in their homes. They routinely visited many families each day to provide nursing care and to improve public health education practices in the home. These nurses determined the needs of the families and worked in cooperation with local boards and agencies to get services delivered. There were distinct skills required by public health nurses that were not gained from private duty or hospital experience (Dock, 1906). Hospital training did not provide the education to prepare the public health nurse to work with the acute and chronic health care needs in the community. In the early 1900s, public health nurses worked autonomously, caring for patients who could not afford to seek treatment from a physician (Craig, 2003). Their role thus changed with the growing organization of public health and the interest by the federal government in providing services.

Physicians Emerged Dominant Over Nurses in Public Health Role

C.-E. A. Winslow, a Yale professor, physician, and leader in public health, ranked the physician as the head of the team, but he strongly promoted nurses as integral to public health campaigns. Indeed, early on, Winslow (1911) wrote very supportively of visiting nurses, stating:

> Yet it is, I think, more and more clear that the real strategic point is by the bedside of the patient and at the elbow of the convalescent or the carrier. Here the chain of infection can be broken far more surely and more economically than at any point.
>
> —*Winslow, 1911, p. 909*

In his view, however, physicians would still make the diagnosis or program decisions that public health nurses then carried out in the homes, schools, and workplaces in the community. Winslow pushed health education as the change factor for successful public health campaigns, giving the task to nurses to interpret and translate health information to groups, families, and individuals. Attempting to decrease the individual's exposure to communicable diseases, public health nurses broke down scientific health information into doable tasks to be carried out by mothers, workers, children, and teachers. Yet, while he respected their work and realized the necessity of their work in conjunction with public health education, his writings show the continued ambivalent thoughts about the professional role of the nurse. He described a public health nurse as "a community mother but armed with expert knowledge which few mothers can possess" (Winslow, 1923, p. 56).

Supported by administrators in the powerful, pro-medicine Rockefeller Foundation in the 1920s, physicians were formally designated as the public health team leaders in the governmental agencies. Within universities, medical schools and schools of public health joined to educate physicians in bacteriology, statistics, and public health principles and administration (Winslow, 1925). Graduates took positions in health departments and were given the official title of health officer. Public health nurses in official agencies were once again viewed in the position of assisting physicians to carry out public health principles and programs. Public health nurses thus lost some of the autonomy of practice in the homes of their clients and shifted their focus to prevention.

The Public Health Nurse: More Specialized and More Professional?

The public health nurse of the first half of the 20th century had several unique roles described in the textbooks as translator, educator, advocate, and conservator of the public's health (Gardner, 1936). Debate heightened in the 1930s over whether their role should be further specialized into the different services provided, such as child health, maternal health, orthopedics, tuberculosis care, and others (Footner, 1998; Melosh, 1982). With significant medical advances (the first antimicrobial drugs were introduced and new surgical procedures invented), the profession of medicine was becoming more specialized, and of course, physicians needed more specialized nurses *to assist them* (Schulz & Johnson, 2003). However, a generalist role still worked best for most agencies to deliver care efficiently, although nurses debated this issue. Families usually had several problems among various members of the household, and in order to avoid the duplication of services, a public health nurse generalist was able to enter the home and tackle whatever problem the family presented to her. The special tasks of public health nurses, the requirement for additional education, as well as their autonomy in the field outside of the agency, boosted the view of professionalization in nursing.

Indeed, even before the severance of the generalist nurse into the specialist, public health nursing became the first specialty in nursing (Allen, 2007; Alpi & Adams, 2007; Gardner, 1936). Various post-graduate courses educated graduate nurses in public health, sanitation, sociology, ethics, and other subjects to give them a better understanding of the problems as well as approaches to assist different immigrant and impoverished families. Seeing the need for specialized knowledge, nursing leaders promoted the idea of a university education for public health nurses that culminated in 1949 with the Russell Sage Foundation-sponsored Brown Report, which called for nurses to be educated in colleges and universities (Gebbie, 2009; Maraldo, Fagin, & Keenan, 1988). However, nursing continued to be burdened with a label and reputation of "women's work," rather than work that was valued as a "profession." Furthermore, physician control over nursing continued. Group and Roberts (2001) wrote "By the 1930's the American Medical Association (AMA) had established a set of committees on nursing that tightened its control" (p. 148), and the tensions between nursing and medicine would continue for decades.

The Federal Reclassification of Nursing Changes the Profession

The Emergence of the Recognized Professionalism of Nursing

Professionalism for nurses gained momentum just after the turn of the 20th century with endorsements from state and federal legislation. Lusk (1997) points out in her historical study that nursing leaders pushed and promoted the professional classification for nurses based on criteria established in the literature. However, nurses' link to service sometimes placed them in the laborer category, especially students in training whose work hours were limited to 8-hour days. Some nursing leaders fought against these limits to autonomous practice and gained the right for graduate nurses to set their own work hours (Lusk, 1997). Government institutions denied professional status to nurses, which left army nurses during World War I without rank or authority in battlefield hospitals (Donahue, 1985). Nurses fought the federal government classification of nurses as "subprofessionals" in the 1923 legislation (Minnigerode, 1923). However, they did not have enough influence to change the category until 1935, when Harry L. Hopkins of the federal Work Progress Administration (WPA) re-classified nurses from "'skilled non-manual workers" to "Class 4 professional and technical workers" in a simple federal memo (AJN, 1935). Nevertheless, this historic subclassification of nurses' work negatively affected their social standing, but more importantly affected the salaries they earned. And even after this important 1935 regulatory memo, the status of nurses and their work did not substantively change as the ravages of the Great Depression (1929–1940) continued and left nurses with stagnant opportunities for educational advancement (D'Antonio, 2004). However, Byers (1999) views this period as a time of an emerging liberation for women writing:

> Women's roles began to change with World War II as many were forced to find employment and to assume more family responsibilities as a result of the financial devastation of the Great Depression and men being forced to *serve* with the Armed Forces.
>
> —Byers, 1999, p. 12

In reality, nurses utilized expert knowledge, indeed some of the same knowledge utilized by physicians and often taught to them by physicians, but they were not seen as colleagues of the physicians. The public health hierarchy maintained the role of the physician as the head, responsible for making the assessments and the program decisions that directed the care and education to be delivered by the nurse. Therefore, while public health nurses developed a role outside of the hospital and shifted their work from bedside treatment of illness to health promotion and education requiring specialized knowledge, their work was still viewed within the maternal role of women and not considered by society to be "professional level work." The contemporary nursing leadership held a different view and developed education programs to promote the use of scientific knowledge when addressing issues affecting the public. Two pioneers of nursing, Lavinia Lloyd Dock and Isabel M. Stewart, both wrote very provocatively (in almost unheard language of the day by nurses) in 1938 that nursing is not:

> ... a subordinate or 'satellite' vocation ... nursing is as old if not older than medicine and has had an independent existence for hundreds of years. The Nightingale concept of nursing was not that of a sub-caste of medicine or a 'handmaid of medicine'
> —*Dock & Stewart, 1938, pp. 365–366*

They both further stated that:

> The experience of years in many countries tends to show that nursing flourishes best when it is directed and controlled by skilled and experienced nurses and given the largest possible measure of freedom for the exercise of its particular functions
> —*Dock & Stewart, 1938, p. 367*

Earlier, the Rockefeller Foundation, a leader in public health research and education, wanted to evaluate the effectiveness of public health nursing education in order to have workers adequately trained in public health. Nurses effectively bridged the gap between science and home, bringing the ideas to the families in terms they understood in incremental steps they could take to improve their health. The Committee for the Study of Nursing Education, funded by the Rockefeller Foundation in 1919, was charged with studying the education requirements for public health nurses. However, due to the requirement of nurses' training, the committee decided to study hospital training also (Winslow, 1922). Josephine Goldmark subsequently wrote the influential Goldmark Report, published in 1923 (Gebbie, 2009). The study found that the long and difficult hospital training with nursing students used as cheap labor for the hospitals did not attract the interest of middle-class women required for the higher level of knowledge needed to be a public health nurse. The recommendations that came out of the report called for higher entrance standards to nursing school, as well as three years of hospital training plus post-graduate training, which included classroom education as well as public health field work. The committee felt that these steps would encourage more middle-class women to enter nursing, thus bringing more respect to the profession. Ultimately, public health nursing became an expensive endeavor, because their practice remained limited to the poor rather than expanding health education to all levels of society (Buhler-Wilkerson, 1985). Public health nurses' numbers decreased with the draw of nurses to war needs; furthermore, changes in the financial arrangements to pay the public health agencies did not garner public support (Buhler-Wilkerson, 1993).

Nursing's Status Post-World War II—The 1960s

After World War II, the specialized knowledge of the public health nurse became a basic part of nursing education, and the NOPHN blended into the ANA. In pursuing the agenda of professionalization, public health nurses attempted to bring status to all of nursing and to control their nursing work, job qualifications, and education. However, a shortage of educated public health nurses hampered the tremendous need to develop health programs, thus allowing the leaders of the World Health Organization to endorse the utilization of lesser trained workers in public health work (Cueto, 2007).

Post-World War II advancements in medicine and pharmaceuticals, and federal funding of the Hill-Burton Act (which increased the number of hospitals) created changes for the U.S. health care system. The number of nursing homes increased, and the Korean War began in 1950, once again pulling nurses out of hospitals. Nurses experienced innovative programs, such as military flight nurses caring for wounded soldiers on cargo planes and in mobile surgical units close to the battles (Kalisch & Kalisch, 2003). The Truman administration's promotion of the community college system in conjunction with a nursing shortage ultimately made acceptable the idea of a 2-year associate degree for a college-educated nurse. However, community colleges lacked hospital affiliations, raising educational costs due to the needed employment of additional clinical staff (Halloran, 1995). The Nurse Training Act (NTA) of 1964 helped fund nursing education; however, a smaller percentage funded baccalaureate nursing education, while the apprentice system of diploma training schools (still very prevalent, but decreasing in number) and community college ADN programs received a larger share of the money. Incredulously, this inequity still persists some 40-plus years later with the famed researcher, Dr. Linda Aiken, Co-Chair of the Council on Physician and Nurse Supply (2007), reporting:

> However, nurse education is currently balanced toward associate degree nursing (ADN) programs, which receive the bulk of federal funding for nurse education, yet few ADN graduates progress to advanced practice and faculty roles, both of which are needed. The Council urged a national effort to substantially expand BSN training.
>
> —*Aiken, 2007, p. 1*

The ANA's leaders published their stance on nursing education in 1965 promoting the baccalaureate degree as the entry level for professional nurses, but with support for the associate degree for technical nursing practice (ANA, 1965). The intention was to limit the scope of practice of the technical nurse, and develop the leadership aspect of the baccalaureate nurse (Freund, 1990). Ultimately, an increased demand for nurses related to increased health care funding from the Medicare and Medicaid programs added to the persistent nursing shortage in hospitals (Lynaugh, 2007). Despite their best intentions, the nursing leadership had difficulty quantifying the intended levels of care and the lack of differentiation between roles that seemed to blend nurses together. Today, the nursing profession is well aware of its failed efforts to ensure that all nurses have a BSN. However, Donley and Flaherty (2008) write, "If you view the 1965 statement as a call to close hospital schools of nursing and to move all nursing education inside the walls of colleges or universities, then the ANA was successful in implementing its vision" (p. 1). Notwithstanding, they further state, "If, however, you view the 1965 Position Paper as a mandate for a more educated nurse force to enhance patient care, the goal has not been achieved" (Donley & Flaherty, 2008, p. 1).

The sustained progress in medical technology and nursing's emergence as a discipline in the mid to late 1960s again offered nurses specialized knowledge and skill in hospital settings in the newly established cardiac care units (Dreher, 2010). Experiments in 24-hour nursing observation by specialized nurses who learned the skills usually held by physicians gave nurses a larger scope of practice and perhaps a boost to their professionalism (Keeling, 2004). Through skilled observation, these nurses made independent decisions to administer the needed medications based on standing orders and utilized the technology to save patients' lives. Keeling referred to it as "the blurry line" between medicine and nursing, because these nurses gave medications to stop arrhythmias and *then* wrote the verbal orders for physicians to sign at a later time. Increasingly in the 1960s, many nursing tasks involved using new machines and taking new measurements from them, although previously these functions had been limited to the realm of physicians. Physicians, however, embraced the capacity of RNs to manage this ever increasing technology, as they ultimately could not manage and monitor all of this technology themselves.

Was this real progress toward more nursing professional autonomy? Or was it simply acquiescence by physicians that their work depended on the good functioning of nurses and nursing?

SUMMARY

From the origins of American nursing in the 1800s through the 1960s, nursing leaders gradually sought and established higher standards for nurses largely with changes in society. Woods (1996) has also recognized that the rise of professional nursing has been led primarily by nurse educators and public health nurses. Ultimately, however, those "traditionalists" and "professionalizers" (again despite their disagreement on change) did succeed in raising nursing from being simply everyday women's work to a professional career choice for women (and men to a lesser extent), giving women an economic position in the market, albeit undercompensated and still unnecessarily stereotyped. The struggle of nurses to gain true professional status continues today, as their scope of practice and their role in health care expand into the realm of a new doctoral degree, one day possibly to be required for entry into advanced practice nursing. We can only imagine how long that will take! But first, the authors of chapter 3 will characterize the rise of the role of the first advanced practice nurses in the mid-1960s.

NOTES

1. Robinson (1946), who has written a meticulous and gripping history of nursing in *White Caps: The Story of Nursing*, indicates that five separate entities lay claim to the status of the "first nursing school or first training program for nurses," including New York Hospital (1798), Nurse Society of Philadelphia (1828), and the New York Infirmary (1857). However, Robinson favors the authenticity of the more substantial programs established first at the Women's Hospital of Philadelphia in 1863, which was the first 6-month curriculum, and then next a 12-month curriculum founded at New England Hospital in 1872.
2. Is it time for a new acronym to describe this—*DAPN* for the doctoral advanced practice nurse and *DAPRN*—for a description of the practice-doctorate educated traditional APRN who is a nurse practitioner, nurse midwife, nurse anesthetist, or clinical nurse specialist?
3. As diploma nurses only accounted for 5% of all new RNs, they were not analyzed in this calculation (Aiken et al., 2009).
4. Northeastern University founded the first 5-year BSN Co-operative education degree in 1971 and Drexel University followed in 2000.

REFERENCES

Aiken, L. H., Cheung, R. B., & Olds, D. M. (2009). Education policy initiatives to address the nurse shortage in the United States. *Health Affairs, 28*(4), 646–656.

Allen, C. E. (2007). Holistic concepts and the professionalization of public health nursing. *Public Health Nursing, 8*(2), 74–80.

Alpi, K. M., & Adams, M. G. (2007). Mapping the literature of public health and community nursing. *Journal of the Medical Library Association, 95*(1), e6–e9.

American Association of Colleges of Nursing. (2000). *The baccalaureate degree in nursing as minimal preparation for professional practice.* Retrieved from http://www.aacn.nche.edu/Publications/positions/baccmin.htm

American Journal of Nursing. (1935). The WPA and nursing: The nurse's status; projects; state committees [Unsigned Editorial]. *The American Journal of Nursing, 35*(12), 1154–1156.

American Nurses' Association. (ANA). (1965). American Nurses' Association's first position on education for nursing. *The American Journal of Nursing, 65*(12), 106–111.

Barter, M., & McFarland, P. L. (2001). BSN by 2010: A California initiative. *Journal of Nursing Administration, 3*(3), 141–144.

Beckemeier, B. (2008). History of public health and public health nursing. In L. L. Ivanovov, & C. L. Blue (Eds.), *Public health nursing: Leadership, policy, & practice* (pp. 2–26). Clifton Park, NY: Delmar Cengage Learning.

Benner, P., Sutphen, M., Leonard, V., & Day, L. (2009). *Educating nurses: A call for radical transformation.* Hoboken, NJ: Jossey-Bass.

Biddle, B. J. (1986). Recent developments in role theory. *Annual Review of Sociology, 12,* 67–92.

Blumer, H. (1969). *Symbolic interactionism: Perspective and method.* Berkeley, CA: University of California Press.

Brainard, A. M. (1985). *The evolution of public health nursing.* Philadelphia, PA: W. B. Saunders.

Buhler-Wilkerson, K. (1985). Public health nursing: In sickness or in health? *American Journal of Public Health, 75*(10), 1155–1161.

Buhler-Wilkerson, K. (1987). Left carrying the bag: Experiments in visiting nursing, 1877–1909. *Nursing Research, 36*(1), 42–46.

Buhler-Wilkerson, K. (1991). Lillian Wald: Public health pioneer. *Nursing Research, 40*(5), 316.

Buhler-Wilkerson, K. (1993). Guarded by standards and directed by strangers: Charleston, South Carolina's response to a national health care agenda, 1920–1930. *Nursing History Review, 1,* 139–154.

Burbules, N., & Densmore, K. (1991). The limits of making teaching a profession. *Educational Policy, 5*(1), 44–63.

Byers, B. K. (1999). *The lived experience of registered nurses, 1930–1950: A phenomenological study.* A Dissertation in Higher Education submitted to the Graduate Faculty of Texas Tech University. Retrieved from http://etd.lib.ttu.edu/theses/available/etd-07312008-31295013633622/unrestricted/31295013633622.pdf

Cast, A. (2004). Role-taking and interaction. *Social Psychology Quarterly, 67*(3), 296–309.

Cooley, C. (1964). *Human nature and social order.* New York, NY: Schocken Books.

Council on Physician and Nurse Supply. (2007). New council calls for immediate increase in physician and nurse education. *AMN Healthcare.* Retrieved from http://www.physiciannurse-supply.com/Articles/council-meeting-release.pdf

Craig, P. (2003). The development of public health nursing. In S. Cowley (Ed.), *Public health in policy and practice: A sourcebook for health visitors and community nurses* (pp. 25–43). London, UK: Elsevier Science Limited.

Cueto, M. (2007). *The value of health: A history of the Pan American Health Organization.* Washington, DC: Pan American Health Organization.

Cusson, R. M., & Strange, S. N. (2008). Neonatal nurse practitioner role transition: The process of reattaining expert status. *Journal of Perinatal & Neonatal Nursing, 22*(4), 329–337.

Cusson, R. M., & Viggiano, N. M. (2002). Transition to the neonatal nurse practitioner role: Making the change from the side to the head of the bed. *Neonatal Network, 21*(2), 21–28.

D'Antonio, P. (2004). Women, nursing, and baccalaureate education in 20th century America. *Journal of Nursing Scholarship, 36*(4), 379–384.

Davis, M. (1929). The nurse as hospital superintendent. *The American Journal of Nursing, 29*(4), 385–387.

Deloughery, G. (1977). *History and trends of professional nursing.* Saint Louis, MO: Mosby.

Dock, L. L. (1906). Training for visiting nursing. *The American Journal of Nursing, 7*(2), 109–111.

Dock, L. L., & Stewart, I. M. (1938). *A short history of nursing.* New York, London: G.P. Putnam's Sons, The Knickerbocker Press.

Donley, R., & Flaherty, R. (2002). Revisiting the American Nurses Association's first position on education for nurses. *Online Journal of Issues in Nursing, 7*(2). Retrieved from http://www.nursingworld.org/MainMenuCategories/ANAMarketplace/ANAPeriodicals/OJIN/TableofContents/Volume72002/No2May2002/RevisingPostiononEducation.aspx

Donley, R., & Flaherty, M. J. (2008). Revisiting the American Nurses Association's first position on education for nurses: A comparative analysis of the first and second position statements on the education of nurses. *OJIN: The Online Journal of Issues in Nursing, 13*(2). Retrieved from http://www.nursingworld.org/MainMenuCategories/ANAMarketplace/ANAPeriodicals/OJIN/TableofContents/Volume72002/No2May2002/RevisingPostiononEducation.aspx

Donahue, P. (1985). *Nursing, the finest art.* St. Louis, MO: Mosby.

Donohue, P. (1996). *Nursing, the finest art: An illustrated history* (2nd ed.). St. Louis, MO: Mosby.

Dreher, H. M. (2008a). Innovation in nursing education: Preparing for the future of nursing practice. *Holistic Nursing Practice, 22*(2), 77–80.

Dreher, H. M. (2008b). Is poor weight management a failure of primary care? *Holistic Nursing Practice, 22*(6), 312–316.

Dreher, H. M. (2009). Education for advanced practice: The question: Is the PhD or the DNP the right degree model for future advanced practice nurses? L. Joel, *Advanced practice nursing: Essentials for role development* (2nd ed.) (pp. 58–71). Philadelphia, PA: F. A. Davis.

Dreher, H. M. (2010). The path to nursing science today, 1910–2010. In M. D. Dahnke, & H. M. Dreher (Eds.), *Philosophy of science for nursing practice: Concepts and application.* New York, NY: Springer.

Dreher, H. M., & Dahnke, M. D. (2010). Philosophy of science in a practice discipline. In M. D. Dahnke, & H. M. Dreher (Eds.), *Philosophy of science for nursing practice: Concepts and application.* New York, NY: Springer.

Dreher, H. M., & Montgomery, K. (2009). Let's call it "doctoral" advanced practice nursing. *The Journal of Continuing Education in Nursing, 40*(12), 1–2.

Durkeim, E. (1964). *The division of labor in society.* New York, NY: Free Press.

Ferris, D. (2001). Military intelligence. Retrieved from http://www.nurseweek.com/news/features/01-06/military.html

Footner, A. (1998). Nursing specialism or nursing specialization? *Nursing Outlook, 2*(4), 219–223.

Ford, L. C., & Silver, H. K. (1967). Expanded role of the nurse in child care. *Nursing Outlook, 15,* 43–45.

Freund, C. M. (1990). *The unity of education, research, and practice.* Kansas City, MO: American Nurses Association.

Gardner, M. S. (1936). *Public health nursing.* New York, NY: Macmillian.

Gebbie, K. (2009). 20th-century reports on nursing and nursing education: What difference did they make? *Nursing Outlook, 57*(2), 84–92.

Giacomo, R. (1953). The 1953 census of nurses in public health work. *Nursing Outlook, 1*(11), 645–646.

Goffman, E. (1955). On face-work: An analysis of ritual elements in social interaction. *Psychiatry: Journal for the Study of Interpersonal Processes, 18,* 213–231.

Goffman, E. (1959). *The presentation of self in everyday life.* Edinburgh, Scotland: University of Edinburgh, Social Sciences Research Centre.

Group, T. M., & Roberts, J. I. (2001). *Nursing, physician control, and the medical monopoly: Historical perspectives on gendered inequality in roles, rights, and range of practice.* Bloomington, IN: Indiana University Press.

Haase, P. T. (1990). *The origins and rise of associate degree nursing education.* Durham, NC: Duke University Press.

Halloran, E. (1995). *A Virginia Henderson reader: Excellence in nursing.* New York, NY: Springer.

Hardy, M., & Conway, M. (1979). *Role theory: Perspectives for health professionals.* East Norwalk, CT: Appleton & Lange.

Hardy, M., & Conway, M. (1988). *Role theory: Perspectives for health professionals* (2nd ed.). East Norwalk, CT: Appleton & Lange.

Harmer, B., & Henderson, V. (1939). *Textbook of the principles and practice of nursing*. New York, NY: Macmillan.

Jackson, S., & Stevenson, C. (2000). What do people need psychiatric and mental health nurses for? *Journal of Advanced Nursing, 31*(2), 378–388.

Johns, C., & Freshwater, D. (2005). *Transforming nursing through reflective practice* (2nd ed.). Hoboken, NJ: Wiley-Blackwell.

Judd, D., Sitzman, K., & Davis, G. M. (2009). *A history of American nursing: Trends and eras*. Boston, MA: Jones & Bartlett.

Kalisch, P. A., & Kalisch, B. J. (2003). *American nursing: A history* (4th ed.). Philadelphia, PA: Lippincott Williams, & Wilkins.

Keeling, A. (2004). Blurring the boundary between medicine and nursing: Coronary care nursing, circa the 1960s. *Nursing History Review, 12*, 139–165.

Klass, A. A. (1961). What is a profession? *Canadian Medical Association Journal, 85*, 698–701.

Kraus, N. (1980). "The 1985 proposal" for entry into nursing practice: How should the ACNM respond? *Journal of Nurse-Midwifery, 25*(1), 1–3.

Kuhn, A. (1974). *The logic of social systems*. San Francisco, CA: Jossey-Bass.

Liaschenko, J., & Peter, E. (2004). Nursing ethics and conceptualizations of nursing: Profession, practice and work. *Journal of Advanced Nursing, 46*(5), 488–495.

Lusk, B. (1997). Professional classifications of American nurses, 1910 to 1935. *Western Journal of Nursing Research, 19*(2), 227–242.

Lynaugh, J. (2007). Hospitals, nurses, and education—Eternal triangle. In J. Lynaugh, H. Grace, G. Smith, R. Sena, & M. de Villabos (Eds.), *The W.K. Kellogg Foundation and the nursing profession: Shared values, shared legacy*. Indianapolis, IN: Sigma Theta Tau International.

Magat, R. (Ed.). (1989). *Philanthropic giving: Studies in varieties and goals*. New York, NY: Oxford Press.

Maraldo, P. J., Fagin, C., & Keenan, T. (1988). Nursing and private philanthropy. *Health Affairs, 7*(1), 130–136.

Mead, G. (1934). *Mind, self, and society*. Chicago, IL: University of Chicago Press.

Meleis, A. I. (1975). Role insufficiency and role supplementation: A conceptual framework. *Nursing Research, 24*(4), 264–271.

Meleis, A. I. (2010). Transitions from practice to evidence-based. In A. Meleis (Ed.), *Transitions theory: Middle range and situation specific theories in nursing research and practice* (pp. 1–10). New York, NY: Springer.

Meleis, A. I., & Trangenstein, P. A. (1994). Facilitating transitions: Redefinition of the nursing mission. *Nursing Outlook, 42*(6), 255–259.

Melosh, B. (1982). *The physician's hand: Work culture and conflict in American nursing*. Philadelphia, PA: Temple University Press.

Merriam-Webster. (2010). Definition of 'role'. *Merriam-Webster Online Dictionary*. Retrieved from http://www.merriam-webster.com/dictionary/role

Minnigerode, L. (1923). Report of committee on federal legislation. *American Journal of Nursing, 24*(3), 223.

Nutting, A. (1904). A school for social workers. *The American Journal of Nursing, 4*(9), 679–681.

Parascandola, J. (2007). Public health history. *Commissioned Officer Association for the USPHS, Inc.* Retrieved from http://www.coausphs.org/phhistory.cfm

Pearson, L. (2010). The Pearson Report 2010: The annual state-by-state national overview of nurse practitioner legislation and healthcare issues. *The American Journal for Nurse Practitioners, 14*(3). Retrieved from http://www.pearsonreport.com/

Porter, D. (1994). *The history of public health and the modern state*. Atlanta, GA: Clio Medica 26, The Welcome Institute Series in the History of Medicine.

Reverby, S. (1987). *Ordered to care: The dilemma of American nursing, 1850–1945*. Cambridge, MA: Cambridge University Press.

Robinson, V. (1946). *White caps: The story of nursing*. Philadelphia, PA: J. B. Lippincott.

Rosen, J. (1993). *A history of public health*. Baltimore, MD: The Johns Hopkins University Press.

Rosenberg, C. (1987). *The care of strangers: The rise of America's hospital system.* New York, NY: Basic Books.

Schell, E., & Kayser-Jones, J. (1999). The effect of role-taking ability on caregiver–resident mealtime interaction. *Applied Nursing Research, 12*(1), 38–44.

Schulz, R., & Johnson, A. C. (2003). *Management of hospitals and health services: Strategic issues and performance.* Washington, DC: Beard Books.

Shattell, M. (2004). Nurse–patient interaction: A review of the literature. *Journal of Clinical Nursing, 13,* 714–722.

U.S. Public Health Service Nursing. (2009). History of nursing in the USPSH. *Nursing resource manual: USPHS nursing—Mission, responsibilities, and challenge.* Retrieved from http://phs-nurse.org/nurse-resource-manual.html.

Wade, L. C. (1967). The heritage from Chicago's early settlement houses. *Journal of the Illinois State Historical Society (1908–1984), 60*(4), 411–441.

Whelan, J. (2005). "A necessity in the nursing world": The Chicago Nurses Professional Registry, 1913–1950. *Nursing History Review, 13,* 49–75.

Williams, R. C. (1951). *The United States Public Health Service, 1798–1950.* Washington, DC: Commissioned Officers Association of the United States Public Health Service.

Winslow, C.-E. A. (1911). The role of the visiting nurse in the campaign for public health. *American Journal of Nursing, 11*(11), 909–929.

Winslow, C.-E. A. (1922). From the report of the committee on nursing education. *American Journal of Nursing, 22*(11), 882–884.

Winslow, C.-E. A. (1923). *The evolution and significance of the modern public health campaign.* New Haven, CT: Yale University Press.

Winslow, C.-E. A. (1925). The place of public health in a university. *Science, 62*(1607), 335–338.

Woods, C. Q. (1996). Evolution of the American Nurses Association's position on health insurance for the aged: 1933–1965. *Nursing Research, 45*(5), 304–310.

Young, J. (2005). Revisiting the 1925 Johns Report on African-American nurses. *Nursing History Review, 13,* 77–99.

Zerwekh, J., & Claborn, J. (2009). *Nursing today: Transitions and trends* (6th ed.). Philadelphia, PA: Elsevier Health Sciences.

CHAPTER TWO: Reflective Response

Sheila P. Davis

Dreher and Uribe begin the narrative without any hidden punches. They ask, "What should the role of the new doctor of nursing practice graduate be?" (p. 47). This question is answered with the supposition that "if a more highly advanced practice nurse with a doctorate does not improve health, then why bother with the expense and effort of another degree?" (p. 47). Thereafter, one would expect a plethora of arguments and postulates that compare the current and/or emergent new practice doctorate role as either improving health care or not improving health care. However, what is presented in the narrative is a rather extensive and comprehensive history of the evolving role of the nurse. While this history is important, it does not capture the poignant implied thesis of the necessity of the emergent role of the new advanced practice nurse being that of improving health. One reason may be the failure of the profession to adequately document our role in improving health care. Where is the historical body of literature that supports the premise that the value added to the health team by nurses is that of improvement of health for those being cared for? And, perhaps a more important question is, "What impact does the role of the nurse have on the improvement of the nurse's health?" I submit that care of the caregiver is equally as important as care for the recipient.

Permit me to add what I consider to be a blaring omission in mainstream historical texts on the role of nursing. Only if one goes to specialty published nursing history books, can one find substantive information on the role of ethnic minority nurses as it relates to their contributions to nursing. As an example, Dr. Mary Elizabeth Carnegie's book, *The Path We Tread*, methodically and meticulously portrays the roles of nurses of color who endured hardships of entry in the health care profession as professional nurses (Carnegie, 2000). Despite the barriers of being minorities in a majority Caucasian profession, she captures their tenacity in succeeding against the odds and making indomitable strides in nursing. Before African-American nurses were accorded membership in mainstream nursing organizations, Dr. Carnegie, because of her position as president of the Florida Chapter of National Association of Colored Graduate Nurses (FSNA), was made a "courtesy" member of the mainstream Florida Nurses Association. As a courtesy member she did not have a vote, nor was she "supposed" to contribute to the organization's discussions. True to her nature, Dr. Carnegie spoke up in the meeting anyway. And due to the nature of her contributions, the following year in 1949, she was elected to the board of the Florida Nurses Association (Hines, 1993). This is just one of numerous examples of triumphs of ethnic minorities in forging against seemingly insurmountable odds.

As we consider the evolution of nurses' roles and the "placement" of the new advanced practice practitioner, it is imperative to plan for the multicultural smorgasbord of patients, health care professionals, and students. Demographers estimate that by the year 2050, there will no longer be a majority Caucasian population in the United States.[1] What this means is that we will have to incorporate views and truths that we as a profession have not traditionally embraced. To improve care, which Dreher and Uribe pose should be the essence of our role of nurses in general and doctorally advanced practice nurses in particular, I submit that they must also have expert knowledge in multicultural care as a major priority.

Like Dr. Carnegie, at first the new doctorally prepared practitioner may not be understood, and may even face overt ostracism; but, if one perseveres as she did, not only will you be accepted, but your contributions will be valued. Other lessons that can be derived from a study of nurses who have come under the banner of the "minority" nurse, is that when given an opportunity, they often excel: Small wonder that males in the nursing profession advance at a faster pace than women after they have *proven themselves*.[2] Last, consider that unless it is written and published, it is not done. This is akin to giving medications. If it is not charted, it is not considered dispensed. For the role to be known and embraced, new doctorally prepared advanced practice nurses must be *intentional* in informing the nursing profession, the practice community, and the public of their utility. They should *speak up* even if the "rules" dictate otherwise.

In this stage in history, the doctorally prepared advanced practice nurse is a welcome change and critical element to the health care team. Historically, nurses have made a rather gentle and almost apologetic entrance as a member of the health team. We have followed all the rules and remained in our places. It is my opinion that the consequence of this has been that our perceived role has been so marginalized that the public does not know what we do. And, if they do not know what we do, why would they want to pay us more for having the doctorate? Now is the time for radical change. Consider your role as team leaders. Study the past roles of nurses, but embrace the new roles that a doctorate in nursing practice engenders. I wish you every success!

NOTES

1. Website for citation: http://www.census.gov/population/www/projections/usinterimproj/
2. Website for citation: http://www.minoritynurse.com/men-nursing/men-nursing

REFERENCES

Carnegie, M. E. (2000). *The path we tread: Blacks in nursing worldwide*. Ontario, Canada: Jones and Bartlett.
Hines, D. C. (1993). *Black women in America: An historical encyclopedia* (Vols. 1–2). Brooklyn, NY: Carlson Publishing Inc.

CRITICAL THINKING QUESTIONS

1. How do you think the controversy over whether nursing is truly a profession might impact the perception of the doctor of nursing practice graduate by other, more common doctoral-prepared health care professionals?
2. As you read, there are many times in history when nursing roles changed but continued to be limited by internal and external forces. Can you identify any particular forces that might support or work against the proliferation of this new degree?
3. Do you agree the role of the professional nurse is best described using a functionalist perspective, and the role of the doctoral advanced practice nurse is best described

using a symbolic interactionist perspective? What about the role of the master's-prepared advanced practice nurse—is their role more structural–functional or symbolic interactionist?

4. Your new role will interact with two different populations: patients and colleagues. How do you envision your new role evolving with each one?

5. As you are most likely very early in your doctor of nursing practice curriculum, do you already have ideas about how you want your doctoral role to be different from your master's role?

6. As a future nursing leader, how can you utilize historical research for problem solving? In other words, can knowledge of the past prepare one for the future?

7. The information in this chapter points out some of the external influences that affected the nursing profession, leaving nursing leaders with their hands tied. Do you think *nursing leaders* are ably ascertaining the external influences that are affecting nursing today? Discuss.

8. Do you think this chapter points to nurses actively promoting their professionalism or passively accepting the judgment of others? Discuss. How will you advance your role as DNP graduate: active promotion or passive acceptance or maybe somewhere in between?

9. Discuss whether nurses were handed their place in the health care system or did they endeavor to develop roles for nurses in the health care system, placing nurses where they were most effective.

10. Discuss why you are either a *conservative traditionalist* or an *elite professionalizer*.

CHAPTER THREE

The Evolution of Advanced Practice Nursing Roles

Marcia R. Gardner, Bobbie Posmontier, and Michael E. Conti

INTRODUCTION

Nursing, as a discipline, has struggled since the Nightingale era to articulate the unique contribution of its practitioners to health and illness care. This tension comes in part from its own history and in part from its link with, and historical dependence on, other disciplines including medicine for certain types of scientific knowledge, practice skills, and to a large degree, access to patients. Functional skills (e.g., physical examination) and functional knowledge (e.g., pharmacology, pathophysiology of disease, or psychology of illness) are shared with (some might say "borrowed" from) other health disciplines. Mastery of higher level biomedical and pharmacological knowledge, clinical reasoning, and clinical and/or diagnostic skills has emerged as a hallmark of advanced practice nursing as enacted by nurse practitioners, nurse anesthetists, nurse midwives, and clinical nurse specialists. Yet, at the same time, nursing has also labored to establish a distinctive knowledge and practice structure separate from these shared domains.

Nursing's scope in the United States has expanded, contracted, and reexpanded in concert with, and in response to, a variety of social, political, technological, and theoretical forces such as the:

- Influx of poor immigrants into overcrowded tenements at the turn of the century, culminating in Lillian Wald's creation of the Henry Street Settlement (Keeling, 2009);
- Congress's establishment of the Army and Navy Nursing Corps in the early 1900s (Keeling, 2009);
- Advent of World War I and the 1918 influenza epidemic (Buhler-Wilkerson, 2001; Wald, 1922);
- The Great Depression of the 1930s, resultant closing of hospital nursing programs, and movement of graduate nurses into hospitals (Keeling, 2009);
- Nursing shortage during World War II resulting in the Bolton Act, which established funding for basic nursing education and post-graduate education for the preparation of certified nurse anesthetists, educators, and administrators (Spalding, 1943);
- Post World War II development of the acute care hospital system (Fairman & Lynaugh, 1998);

- The Brown Report of 1948 funded by the Carnegie foundation, advocating the transition of nursing education from hospital-based diploma programs into colleges and universities, and recruitment of men and minorities (Donahue, 1996);
- Explosions in scientific, biomedical, and pharmaceutical knowledge, as well as related technologies (Keeling, 2009);
- President Johnson's "Great Society" legislation in 1964 enacting Medicare and Medicaid (Keeling, 2009);
- Growth of the third-party payment system in 1965 (Keeling, 2009);
- Economic pressures and expanding costs of health care and health care coverage (Keeling, 2009); and
- The need to fill the "provider gap" in rural and underserved geographic areas (Keeling, 2009).

In the midst of these social and scientific changes (and possibly in response to them), nursing leaders and innovators in the mid-20th century embraced a growing theoretical and practice focus on individuals and their experiences, rather than on medical diagnoses and treatment (Fairman, 1999). This disciplinary, cognitive shift offered a means to recognize and consolidate nursing's distinctive knowledge and practice methods, to break away from a purely medicalized approach to patient care, and to situate nursing as an independent, collaborative healthcare discipline with a differentiated knowledge base, focus, skill set, and language—particularly differentiated from medicine. Such efforts led to development, articulation, and scientific testing of conceptual models and related descriptive grand theories for the understanding of human responses to health and illness, such as Orem's Self-care Framework, the Roy Adaption Model, or Roger's Science of Unitary Human Beings. Other crucial developments included elucidation of the generally accepted meta-paradigm for nursing practice, research and theory construction: *human/person, environment, health, nursing,* and synthesis and testing of mid-range and other theories to guide practice (Baer, 1987; Fawcett & Alligood, 2005; Phillips, 1996). These efforts were integral to and important in the examination and expansion of nursing's knowledge and practice structures, including its taxonomy, processes, strategies for knowledge generation, scope of practice, and practice strategies (Blegen & Tripp-Reimer, 1997; Fawcett & Alligood, 2005; Moorhead, Head, Johnson, & Maas, 1998; Roy, 2007). Knowledge and clinical practice set the stage for the more recent evolution of, and revolution in, nursing advanced practice roles and scope of practice. The four advanced practice nursing roles, addressed below, include the nurse midwife, nurse anesthetist, nurse practitioner, and clinical nurse specialist, all of whom contributed via their own unique history to shaping advanced practice nursing in the 21st century. We have provided a lengthier analysis of nurse midwifery, as its emergence as an advanced practice role is often minimized in the broader nursing literature.

DEVELOPMENT OF THE NURSE MIDWIFE ROLE

Although records of midwifery practice dates back to the 370–460 BCE at the time of Hippocrates, it was the midwives of the 18th and 19th centuries who shaped the evolution of nurse midwives in the 21st century in the United States (McCool & Simeone, 2002). Midwifery skills among colonial midwives ranged from those formally trained in Europe to illiterate women who became midwives in response to community need. In addition to assisting with childbirth, bathing women after childbirth, and cooking, most midwives also provided primary care to their communities. When the first boat of African slaves arrived from West Africa, the first granny midwives began to practice midwifery on plantations in the rural south for both white and black women, which was based on West African tribal folklore (Graninger, 1996; Morrison & Fee, 2010). The safety and skill of midwives varied widely during the first 250 years in America since there were no educational standards. While some were well educated, others relied on herbs and poultices (Manocchio, 2008). Most midwives were either self-taught or learned by apprenticeship from others.

Dr. William Shippen, a protégé of Dr. William Smellie in England, established the first formal educational program for midwives in Philadelphia in 1765 (Rooks, 1997). Because illiterate women could not qualify for or afford the private education, and midwifery was considered beneath the stature of educated women, Dr. Shippen limited the education to men. By the end of the 18th century, colonial men traveled to England for medical training, and returned to provide obstetric care to upper class women. Morally outraged by men providing care for women, Dr. Samuel Gregory, a graduate of Yale University, established the first formal midwifery education program for women at the Boston Female Medical College in 1848 (Rooks). The 3-month midwifery program graduated 12 midwives between 1848 and 1851, but was forced to close in 1874 due to strong opposition from the Boston Medical Society (Rooks). By the late 19th century, there was massive immigration into the United States from southern and eastern Europe (Dawley, 2003). New immigrants were densely packed into urban areas and suffered poor working conditions, long hours in factories, and overcrowding in tenements (Keeling, 2009). High maternal–infant mortality was blamed on granny and immigrant midwives, who managed 50% of all U.S. births. Public health nursing leaders, including Carolyn Conant van Blarcom, who wrote the first obstetric nursing textbook; Lillian Wald, the founder of the Henry Street Settlement in New York City; Mary Beard, who developed prenatal care; and Mary Breckinridge, who founded the first midwifery service in America, joined with obstetricians to eliminate lay midwives in the United States (Dawley; Stone, 2000). These nursing leaders sought to combine public health nursing and midwifery to create the nurse midwife. Dr. Fred Taussig, a Missouri physician, is credited with coining the term *nurse midwife* in 1925 (Stone).

The 1920s were framed by several pivotal events including:

- Middle and upper class women embracing "twilight sleep" (a combination of morphine and scopolamine for childbirth analgesia and amnesia to decrease and forget labor pain);
- Physicians gaining higher esteem (since upper and middle class women chose them for labor and pain management);
- Physicians becoming more politically organized; and
- The increased use of intervention methods (forceps, episiotomies, scopolamine, and morphine) recommended for all women by obstetrician Joseph Delee (McCool & Simeone, 2002).

Despite the findings in several New York and New Jersey based studies, and the 1925 White House Conference on Child Health and Protection, that midwives had much better maternal–infant outcomes than obstetricians, middle and upper class women felt that the use of midwives should be reserved only for poor women who could not afford the prestigious care of an obstetrician (Keeling, 2009; Rooks, 1997).

The Bellevue School of Midwifery opened in 1911 to train lay midwives, but was forced to close in 1935 by the New York City Commissioner of Hospitals because he considered midwifery superfluous in the current social climate as well as below current medical standards (Varney, Kriebs, & Gegor, 2004). In 1923, the Maternity Center Association's (MCA) Hazel Corbin, RN and obstetrician Ralph Lobenstine, MD sought to open a nurse midwifery educational program in conjunction with Bellevue Hospital in New York City, but they were thwarted by the New York City Commissioner who worried that well-educated nurse midwives would be harder to eliminate than the lay midwives (Dawley, 2003; Dawley & Burst, 2005).

In 1921, Mary Breckinridge conducted a maternal child needs assessment and lay midwifery survey in Leslie County Kentucky while she was studying public health nursing at Columbia Teacher's College (Dawley, 2005; Dawley & Burst, 2005). When Corbin and Lobenstein's nurse midwifery education program failed to open in New York, Mary Breckinridge's friend and colleague Carolyn Conant van Blarcom assisted her with enrolling in an English midwifery school. Upon her graduation in 1925, Breckinridge returned to Hyden, Kentucky to establish the Frontier Nursing Service (FNS). With the help of Louis Dublin, statistician from Metropolitan Life Insurance, Breckinridge compiled statistics which showed positive outcomes among the first 10,000 births assisted by midwives and public health nurses from the FNS (Dawley, 2003; Raisler & Kennedy, 2005).

In 1923, the Preston Retreat Hospital added a midwifery course, which continued to operate despite dwindling enrollment until 1960 (Varney, Kriebs, & Gegor, 2004). In 1927, the FNS and MCA joined forces to draft plans for developing a nurse midwifery educational program and to examine state laws governing midwifery practice. By 1931, the MCA opened its own home birth service (Lobenstein Midwifery Clinic) and by 1932 it opened an educational program, the Lobenstine Midwifery School (Burst & Thompson, 2003; Dawley & Burst 2005; Stone, 2000).

By the late 1930s, after the introduction of penicillin and sulfonamides, improved nutrition, of sanitation use and of improved housing, the maternal death rate dropped dramatically for all women in the United States (Rooks, 1997). Changes in the U.S. healthcare system then influenced midwifery education after World War II (Dawley, 2003). In 1943, the federal government established the Emergency Maternity and Infant Care Program for the wives and children of returning servicemen who could not otherwise afford a hospital birth. In addition, the Hill–Burton Act of 1946 provided funding for the construction of hospitals. Although 9% of all U.S. citizens had health insurance in 1940, by 1950 the percentage had increased to 50%. But despite more widespread health insurance coverage, there was a shortage of obstetricians providing hospital maternity services. In response to the shortage, there was an accelerated increase in midwifery programs from 1940 to 1950. The Medical Mission Sisters of Philadelphia designed and developed a midwifery service and educational program (Catholic Maternity Institute) in New Mexico (Barger, 2005; Dawley). Once established, the New Mexico program provided partial funding for the education of black nurse midwives in Tuskegee, Alabama (1941), as well as in the Flint Goodrich Hospital Nurse Midwifery program (1942) in New Orleans. Racial tensions, however, eventually resulted in closing the programs in 1946 (Burst & Thompson, 2003). By 1947, the Medical Mission Sisters of Philadelphia established the first Masters in Nursing program for nurse midwives at the Catholic University of America to respond to the needs of underserved families in Washington, DC.

Despite the innovations in natural childbirth methods based on Dr. Grantly Dick Read's work developed after World War II, and with increasing public dislike of "twilight sleep," 88% of women chose to deliver in hospitals (Rooks, 1997). During the 1950s, 25 university affiliated hospitals offered graduate nursing programs for maternal–child nursing to provide leaders in teaching, education, and public health. Their socialization was different from the nurse midwife, because they were taught to follow physician standing orders, recognize abnormal labor, and call the physician to the labor room when delivery was imminent. Midwifery was never part of these nursing programs.

In the meantime, MCA recommended moving midwifery education into recognized universities and formulating standard admission requirements and curriculums (Burst & Thompson, 2003; Rooks, 1997). In 1955, Columbia University opened the first graduate nurse midwifery education program with clinical training in an academic medical center. Yale University opened its own program in 1956. By 1958, three of six national midwifery education programs offered a masters degree for nurse midwives.

In 1954, twenty nurse midwives attended the American Nurses Association (ANA) Convention and formed the Committee on Organization because the National League of Nursing (NLN) and ANA would not create a special niche for nurse midwives (Rooks, 1997). In May 1955, the Committee on Organization voted to form the American College of Nurse Midwifery (ACNM) as a separate accrediting body to develop and evaluate nurse midwifery standards, improve nurse midwifery education, sponsor nurse midwifery research, and participate with the International Confederation of Midwives (Burst & Thompson, 2003).

The social changes of the 1960s were marked by the counter-culture activities, rejection of authority, and the enactment of Medicare and Medicaid by President Lyndon Johnson (Keeling, 2009). After Senator Robert Kennedy visited the Mississippi Delta in 1965, federal funding was established for the County Health Improvement Program for Holmes County Mississippi starting in 1969. In addition, the Federal Division of Nursing provided funding for nurse midwifery education in the Department of Obstetrics and Gynecology at the University of Mississippi School of Medicine. Because the requirements for admission initially included a bachelors degree in nursing, most nurses in Mississippi could not participate. In response, the requirements were revised to allow nondegreed nurses to obtain a Certificate in Midwifery (Keeling, 2009).

During the 1970s, the number of infants delivered by nurse midwives doubled, there was a shortage of physicians providing obstetric care to the poor, and the concept of using a nurse midwife for birth moved into the middle class (McCool & Simeone, 2002) Nurse midwifery educational programs increased from 7 in 1960 to 19 in 1979, and nurse midwifery became legal in most states. The National Health Service Corps began to offer scholarships to nurse midwife students willing to work in underserved areas after graduation. In 1973, in response to the increased births and the shortage of physicians, the University of Mississippi began a modular curriculum for nurse midwifery students, based on self-mastery learning that could be completed in less time than traditional education. The modular program included a list of objectives for the entry-level nurse midwife, learning materials in self-contained packages, independent and self-paced learning, and self-assessment measures by which students could decide if they were ready for testing. By 1979, the ACNM established core competencies in nurse midwifery, which specified the body of knowledge, skills, and behaviors expected of nurse midwife graduates (Avery, 2005). The core competencies served as a guide for formulating curricula, accrediting nurse midwifery programs, and setting the standards for the national certification exam.

Because the three branches of military service in the United States had difficulty recruiting and retaining obstetricians, the Air Force started its own nurse midwifery program at Andrews Air Force Base in Maryland in 1973 (Rooks, 1997). The ACNM, however, would not accredit its program. The Air Force affiliated with Georgetown University in 1975 and offered its base as a clinical site. The Army formed its own graduate nurse midwife program in 1974 in affiliation with the University of Kentucky and offered Fort Knox as the clinical site. The Navy chose to send its personnel to already established nurse midwifery programs (Rooks).

By the 1980s there were 21 accredited nurse midwife educational programs ranging from 9- to 18-month certificate programs to 2–3 masters level programs (Burst & Thompson, 2003). In 1980, the Education Program Association opened the first distance learning program for family nurse practitioners and physician assistants desiring to practice midwifery in publically funded clinics in California. This innovation allowed students to continue to live in their own communities, while rapidly completing requirements for graduation. By 1989, the FNS had established its own distance learning by establishing the Community-Based Nurse Midwifery Program (CNEP) in order to increase rural access to nurse midwifery education. CNEP affiliated with Francis Payne Bolton School of Nursing at Case Western Reserve University in order to offer a masters degree in nursing (Burst & Thompson).

Although the number of midwifery programs increased to 28 by 1984, enrollment dropped between 1984 and 1986, largely as a result of the malpractice crisis (Burst & Thompson, 2003; Rooks, 1997). By 1988, however, the Robert Wood Johnson Foundation provided a grant for scholarships to educate and recruit nurse midwifery students to work in West Virginia after graduation (Burst & Thompson). The program increased the number of nurse midwives in West Virginia from 4 in 1989 to 20 in 1992. Between 1991 and 1993, federal financial support provided nurse midwifery education in exchange for working in underserved areas. In 1991, the ACNM task force also identified barriers for nurse midwives and established the goal of 10,000 practicing nurse midwives by 2001. In response to a 50% decrease of practicing obstetricians and 20% increase in births, the Florida Midwifery Resource Center established a call to action in 1993 to educate 600 additional nurse midwives by the year 2000. By 1993, 67–70% of nurse midwives were masters prepared and 4–5% were doctorally prepared (Burst & Thompson; Rooks).

Between 1982 and 1997, ACNM Division of Accreditation (now the Accreditation Commission for Midwifery Education [ACME]) only provided accreditation for nurse midwifery programs (ACNM, 2010). In 1997, however, the ACNM Division of Accreditation recognized the certified (direct entry) midwife credential. The only direct entry midwifery program out of 17, however, recognized by the ACNM is the program in New York City. Graduates of this program must meet the core competencies and may sit for the national certification exam. The ACNM has issued a position statement (Mandatory Degree Requirements for Entry into Midwifery Practice) that a graduate degree will be required for entry into clinical practice by 2010 for both nurse midwife and direct entry midwifery students. However, Certified Nurse Midwives and Certified Midwives educated before 2010 will be permitted to retain licensure to practice. As of 2010, there are currently more than 6,000 nurse midwives and certified midwives, and 38 accredited graduate nurse midwifery programs in the United States (ACNM).

DEVELOPMENT OF THE NURSE ANESTHETIST ROLE

The roots of the certified registered nurse anesthetist (CRNA) emerged during the American Civil War (1861–1865) when surgeons needed the assistance of the Catholic sisters and Lutheran deaconesses trained as nurses to administer chloroform to wounded soldiers during surgery (Wall, 2005). Ten years after the Civil War, Dr. William

Mayo of St. Mary's Hospital in Rochester, MN recognized the value in training nurse anesthetists, because unlike medical students who watched the surgery while administering anesthesia, nurses observed the patient (Keeling, 2007). In 1889, Dr. Mayo trained and hired nurses Edith Granham and Alice Magaw to serve as his anesthetists. By 1913, his six-month program included theoretical education and clinical practice.

Despite the success of the Mayo training program for nurse anesthetists, other physicians began to question the authority of nurses to administer anesthesia (Keeling, 2009). Both the New York State Medical Society and the Ohio State Medical Board tried unsuccessfully to bar nurse anesthetists from practicing medicine without a license. In *Frank vs. Smith* (1917), a landmark case, the Kentucky appellate court ruled in favor of nurse anesthetist Margaret Hatfield, stating that she was not practicing medicine because she was under the supervision of and subordinate to licensed physician Dr. Louis Frank. During World War I, Mayo physicians and Dr. George W. Crile of the Lakeside Hospital anesthesia program in Cleveland Ohio advocated for nurse anesthetists to provide pain relief to wounded soldiers (Keeling, 2009). In addition, nurse anesthetist Agatha Hodgins and Dr. George Crile developed novel anesthetic techniques, including the use of nitrous oxide–oxygen combinations, and scopolamine and morphine as anesthetic adjuncts.

Despite the fact that medicine was laying claim to the specialty of anesthesiology during World War II through its expertise in administering sodium pentathol, endotracheal intubations, and regional blocks, shortages of anesthesiologists on the battlefield necessitated the training of nurse anesthetists (Keeling, 2009). In 1945, certification became a practice requirement for CRNAs (National Board on Certification and Recertification of Nurse Anesthetists, 2010). The Korean War provided yet another opportunity for the expansion of the profession. By the early 1960s, the army established nurse anesthesia programs at Walter Reed Hospital and Letterman General Hospital. Although the number of nurse anesthesia programs decreased during the 1970s due to decreased funding, lack of affiliation with universities, loss of third-party payment, and physician opposition, by the 1980s nurse anesthetists were winning legal battles against physicians and hospitals restricting their practice, and reestablishing third-party payments for anesthesia services (Diers, 1991, Keeling). By the late 1990s, many nurse anesthesia educational programs were offered through graduate schools of nursing at the master's level.

Anesthesia delivery is currently accomplished by three main methods: anesthesiologists working as the sole provider, an anesthesia care team (ACT) or by independent CRNAs. The ACT, where a physician anesthesiologist may supervise one to four CRNAs, is the most common form of delivery. CRNAs work independently, mostly in rural areas, where they deliver approximately 70% of anesthetics in rural hospitals (American Association of Nurse Anesthetists [AANA], 1996).

Nationally, fifteen states have enacted the "opt out," where physician anesthesiologist supervision is no longer required for Medicare and Medicaid patients. This was intended to increase access to care for those patients who resided in primarily rural areas (Agres, 2010). According to 1996 data by the AANA, approximately 39% of CRNAs were employed by hospitals; 36% were employed by anesthesia groups (usually physician employers); 15% were employed by Nurse Anesthesia groups or were self-employed; and 10% were employed by a physician office (dentist, podiatrist), the military, or a university (AANA, 1996). Military CRNAs have had a distinguished history of autonomous practice. On Navy ships and on the battlefield, they have provided and continue to practice without anesthesiologist supervision as the sole provider to the U.S. military (Jenkins, Elliott, & Harris, 2006).

The current scope of practice according to the practice guidelines, published by the AANA include:

- Preoperative assessment;
- Development and implementation of an anesthetic plan;
- Anesthesia delivery (sedation, general anesthesia, regional and neuraxial anesthesia);
- Selection and implementation of noninvasive and invasive monitoring (arterial lines, pulmonary artery [PA] catheters, and central lines);
- Airway management (natural airway, endotracheal intubations, laryngeal mask airway [LMA] placement and implementation of alternative airway techniques, fiber-optic intubations [FOI], needle cricothytotomy);
- Facilitation of emergence from anesthesia; transfer to the post anesthesia care unit (PACU) and PACU management;
- Chronic and acute pain management; and
- The ability to function as a member of emergency response teams (providing cardio-pulmonary support) (AANA, 2010).

It is important to note that the scope of practice for CRNAs is determined by individual state nursing boards and by each facility where the CRNA practices.

Nurse anesthesia has, from its nascence, had to continuously and diligently prove its important contribution to the delivery of anesthetic care within the matrix of the U.S. healthcare system. Two important, recent studies examined the effect of the anesthesia provider on mortality rates (Canadian Coordinating Office for Health Technology Assessment, 2004). First, Pine, Holt, and Lou (2003) examined risk adjusted mortality rates for the following provider models: anesthesiologist as sole provider, CRNAs as sole provider, and the ACT model. Medicare patients undergoing eight surgical procedures were the focus of the study. Results indicate there was no statistically significant difference between provider types. Similar results were found among the sole CRNA provider, anesthesiologists, and ACT personnel (Pine et al., 2003), meaning anesthesia care outcomes were equivalent regardless of provider type. Second, Jordan, Kremer, Crawforth, and Shott (2001) found no statistical difference in adverse outcomes between type of provider and preoperative physical status, patient age, surgical procedure, or method of anesthesia in a study that reviewed 223 closed claims studies from 1989 to 1997. Although only two studies have been cited, it is important to note that CRNAs, who now almost universally have a master's degree, have a long history of providing quality, cost-effective patient care with positive patient outcomes.

DEVELOPMENT OF THE NURSE PRACTITIONER ROLE

The nurse practitioner role has been prominent in terms of controversies, visibility in public and social policy, and scope of practice considerations, particularly in the role's overlap with medical practice. The history of the nurse practitioner movement can be seen as another exemplar for advanced practice nursing's developmental journey. Nurse practitioners step beyond the range of extended health care services, including education, direct care, chronic illness management, and community services that public health nurses had been providing since the 1920s. Formal nurse practitioner practice was "birthed" in 1965 through the joining of primary care pediatrics and public health/family-community nursing. This was the vision of Dr. Henry Silver, a pediatrician associated with the University of Colorado School of Medicine, and Dr. Loretta Ford from the University of Colorado School of Nursing. The nurse practitioner role emerged at a time when pediatric medicine was struggling to extend care to underserved populations during a shortage of health care professionals. At the same time, nursing was also struggling to expand its scope beyond hospital care to develop autonomous practice, to fully embed nursing education in higher education, and to professionalize as a workforce (Bullough, 1976; Ford, 1975; Richmond, 1965).

The new breed of pediatric care providers in the original University of Colorado program were baccalaureate-prepared clinicians with: (i) advanced clinical and diagnostic skills and knowledge; (ii) the ability to monitor child health, growth, and development; and (iii) the ability to provide guidance to families, manage minor acute health problems in pediatric primary care, and function within healthcare teams — particularly for medically underserved populations. The program involved four months of university-based education, followed by clinical training in underserved rural community/primary care pediatric settings. Dr. Ford subsequently argued strongly for embedding nurse practitioner education fully within a graduate nursing education framework; both Ford and Silver were instrumental in communicating the effectiveness of this pediatric nurse practitioner model and in ensuring its replication (Ford, 1975; Mason, Vaccaro, & Fessler, 2000; Silver, Ford, & Day, 1968).

A comparable brief pediatric nurse practitioner program for the care of children from underserved urban families developed soon after at the Massachusetts General Hospital in Boston. In addition, other academic medical care settings also developed nurse practitioner programs that would similarly extend the skills of public health nurses, address access to care for urban underserved children, as well as serve the needs of children in underserved rural areas (Murphy, 1990).

In the following decade, nurse practitioner certificate training programs began to proliferate across the country. Most of these had a particular emphasis on pediatrics and/or family health, and on extending primary care to underserved urban and rural children and families in a time of expanding healthcare needs and growing recognition of disparities in access to care (Davidson et al., 1975; Mason et al., 2000). Most required a short time commitment (less than one year), and not all required a bachelors degree for entry (Mason et al.). The scope of nurse practitioner practice expanded to include family planning and women's health within ten years after Ford and Silver's innovation (Lewis, 2000) and continues to expand in response to current health care needs nationally and globally.

Federal funding through Title VIII of the Nurse Training Act (American Association of Colleges of Nursing [AACN], 2009) provided opportunities for the expansion of nurse practitioner use in family-focused primary care, in women's health, and then in other populations. In addition, regional programs funded by the federal Title X family planning initiative prepared nurse practitioners, therefore significantly expanding the NP workforce in women's health (Bednash, Worthington, & Wysocki, 2009; Manisoff, 1981). By 1978, the Institute of Medicine had taken the stand that state regulations should be revised to accommodate an increased scope of practice and prescription authority for nurse practitioners, albeit under physician supervision (Mason et al., 2000). As the advanced nursing role began to fully take hold, university-based schools of nursing began to integrate nurse practitioner education and training at the graduate level. Title VIII funding was essential in supporting nurses' completion of these programs (AACN, 2009), and thus, expanded the advanced practice nursing workforce. Scope of practice expanded beyond family and pediatric foci, and beyond primary care to include adult health as well as highly specialized and/or system-focused practice (e.g., oncology, cardiology, and psychiatric specialties).

Coincidentally, a variety of forces created opportunities for expansion of the nurse practitioner role. There were regulatory changes for medical education, including pass-through funding adjustments and state-level regulatory restrictions for physician residency training of physicians (hours permitted on-duty). There was also a growing body of evidence supporting cost and treatment outcome effectiveness of nurse practitioners, as well as a growing and better educated nurse practitioner workforce. Along with other forces, these recognized improvements created opportunities for greater incursion of nurse practitioner scope and practice into high acuity patient care. As fewer physician residents were able/available to provide acute patient care coverage, additional opportunities for nurse practitioner employment developed. Adult, pediatric, and neonatal acute care nurse practitioner education was introduced and solidified, as nurse clinicians were poised to fill gaps in the acute care system (Hinch, Murphy, & Lauer, 2005). In the 1990s, the National Council of State Boards of Nursing (NCSBN); American Academy of Nurse Practitioners; American Nurses Credentialing Center; National Certification Board for Pediatric Nurse Practitioners and Nurses, now the Pediatric Nursing Certification Board (PNCB); and National Certification Corporation (NCC) began to jointly consider a cohesive approach to regulation of NP practice (NCSBN, 1998).

The nurse practitioner movement, particularly in its overlap with medicine's functions, created and continues to create controversies both within and outside of its own discipline. Controversies include the overlap into a medically oriented model of practice, educational preparation, and qualifications for practice, role functions, and differentiation from other providers (e.g., physicians, physician assistants, and clinical nurse specialists). There is also controversy about regulation and certification, reimbursement, competition with other providers for a client base, equivalence of health outcomes as compared with physician providers, and costs for equivalent care (Hayes, 1985). NP practice has expanded beyond health professions, shortage areas into the mainstream of primary and acute care. Furthermore, NP clinicians, through their lobbying efforts, have made inroads in reimbursement for the provision of healthcare services. However, professional medical organizations, including the American Medical Association, American College of Physicians, and the American Academy of Pediatrics (AAP), among others, have periodically attempted to limit NP scope of practice, particularly related to autonomous practice, through the creation of policies and standards for physician supervision of nonphysician providers. These are, in some cases, in opposition to state-specific NP practice regulations (AAP, 1999, 2003; Buppert, 2005; Hedger, 2009). In 2010, we now see, at minimum, universal master's preparation for nurse practitioners, and increasingly, NPs-prepared at the doctoral level.

DEVELOPMENT OF THE CLINICAL NURSE SPECIALIST ROLE

Concurrent with expansion of NP practice, programs preparing clinical nurse specialists (CNS) were proliferating. For example, the first CNS program in psychiatric nursing was established in the 1954 at Rutgers University in New Jersey. Subsequently, CNS programs expanded throughout the United States in the 1950s, 1960s, and later (MacDonald, Herbert, & Thibeault, 2006). The clinical nurse specialist role was conceived and then further evolved to an advanced nursing clinician focused on expert practice, improvement of care at the bedside, and intertwining roles as "clinician, consultant, researcher, educator and manager" (Page & Arena, 1994, p. 316). More recent conceptualization of the "research" function of the master's prepared nurse in an advanced role, regardless of specific role, is translation and integration of evidence into clinical practice (AACN, 1996). In its evolution, the CNS scope of practice would include direct patient care services, as well as staff education and macrosystem management of a specialized population, embedded within a nursing or a systems model, rather than the medical model of care.

While the focus of NP practice was conceived as the individual at the direct care level, the focus of CNS practice was to be both individual and macrolevel, incorporating nursing diagnosis and management as well as systems assessment and synthesis of improved approaches to nursing care. Psychiatric mental health CNS practice was a forerunner in extending the focus beyond acute care. In 2000, only about one-third of psychiatric-mental health clinical specialists were practicing in hospital-based settings, while a majority were practicing in other types of settings, providing a variety of mental health therapies (e.g., in clinics; private, or collaborative practices offering counseling and/or psychotherapies; and forensic settings) (Delaney, 2009).

During the 1980s and 1990s, CNS and NP education were similar in some domains—coursework, caseload, practice strategies—although education and scope of practice for both were rapidly evolving (Lindeke, Canady, & Kay, 1997). Some suggested that both CNS and NP clinicians had similar competencies and could overlap in roles and functions. For example, in acute care or psychiatric-mental health care, some graduate programs established joint curricular pathways for both CNS and NP education (Elder & Bullough, 1990; MacDonald et al., 2006; Page & Arena, 1994). However, regulatory authority over clinical nurse specialist titling practice is a relatively recent innovation. Clinicians working as clinical nurse specialists typically were not required by hiring organizations to have specific preparation in the role until late in the 20th century. Many nurses functioned as CNSs based on their clinical experience and expertise, without formal education preparation or certification in the role. In the 1990s, only about half of state nursing boards had statutes or regulations governing CNS scope of practice (Hudspeth, 2009). There remains wide variation at the state level in title protection, regulation, and scope of practice for the CNS. The new consensus model for advanced practice registered nurse (APRN) practice, discussed below, clarifies current and future vision for overlap and differences in education, licensure, regulation, and scope of practice for the CNS and other APRN clinicians, and provides for uniform treatment and regulation of CNS scope of practice at the state level.

UNIFICATION OF APRN EDUCATION, REGULATION, AND PRACTICE

Professional and regulatory organizations continued to move toward a cohesive approach relative to the preparation of advanced practice nurses for entry into practice and toward a unified vision of the scope of advanced practice nursing in general. Lewis (2000) notes that in 1992, both the ANA and the NCSBN took similar positions regarding the need for advanced practice nursing education (with advanced practice nursing defined as nurse practitioner, nurse anesthetist, nurse midwife, and clinical nurse specialist) to be situated only at the graduate level, and made an initial effort to create a regulatory model (NCSBN, 1998). As nursing professional organizations began to take similar positions regarding advanced nursing practice and advanced nursing education, the transition of certificate programs preparing advanced practice nurse clinicians to formal graduate-level programs accelerated.

In the 1990s, the AACN convened a national group representing multiple organizations and specialty stakeholders for the development of consensus guidelines for advanced practice nursing education at the graduate (master's) level: *Essentials of Master's Education for Advanced Practice Nursing* (AACN, 1996). This document recognized only four types of clinicians providing direct, advanced patient care as advanced practice nurses: Nurse Midwives, Nurse Anesthetists, Nurse Practitioners, and Clinical Nurse Specialists. It specified clearly that education for advanced nursing roles should occur at the master's level. The National Task Force for Quality Nurse Practitioner Education, comprised of representatives from a variety of organizations, including the AACN, National Organization of Nurse Practitioner Faculties (NONPF), NP certifying bodies, and a variety of other stakeholder organizations, promulgated targeted educational guidelines for NP preparation. NONPF established a set of specialty-specific educational guidelines outlining competencies for nurse practitioner education in both general and specialty areas of practice (NONPF, 2002, 2003, 2004). In 2008 the National Task Force produced the consensus document—*Criteria for Evaluation of Nurse Practitioner Programs*. Nurse anesthetist, nurse midwife, and clinical nurse specialist education are, in addition, more specifically guided by the respective specialty accrediting organizations. Educational "landmarks" are critical, because they demonstrate the evolution of a cohesive view of advanced nursing practice on the part of those involved in preparing advanced clinicians for practice.

CONSENSUS MODEL AND *LACE*

Advanced practice nursing has continued to grow toward a unified licensure and practice model through the collaboration of a variety of advanced practice nursing stakeholder organizations, including the NCSBN, the APRN Consensus Workgroup, and representatives from multiple professional nursing organizations, building on a framework established in the 1990s. The *Consensus Model for Advanced Practice Registered Nurses* (APRN Consensus Workgroup & NCBSN APRN Advisory Committee, 2008), developed through this collaboration, prescribed the regulatory strategy for advanced practice registered nurses, identified the same four direct care providers as APRNs, and specified that other nurses prepared at the graduate level, whose scope is not direct care, do not fall under the rubric of the APRN as defined by the model. A proposed timeline for implementation of the model has been developed; as it is implemented and state regulations are amended, the title *Advanced Practice Registered Nurse* will be restricted. The model specifies that APRNs will be licensed and will practice in one of the following clinical roles: Certified Nurse Practitioner, Certified Nurse Midwife, Certified Nurse Anesthetist, or Certified Clinical Nurse Specialist. Education for practice will occur within six population foci (adult–geriatric, pediatric, neonatal, women's/gender-related health, psychiatric/mental health, or family/individual lifespan), with certification and licensing within the respective population focus as well. Specialization will involve an additional layer of certification, via professional organizations, beyond the population focus (e.g., adult-gerontology population focus, specialty of oncology) (APRN Consensus Workgroup & NCBSN APRN Advisory Committee, 2008; Partin, 2009; Stanley, Werner, & Apple, 2009).

The model offers a discrete definition of advanced practice nursing and outlines recommendations for uniform regulation of APRN practice via *LACE*: "licensure, accreditation [of APRN educational programs], certification, education" (APRN Consensus

Workgroup and NCSBN APRN Advisory Committee, 2008, p. 7). Characteristics of an APRN as outlined in the consensus statement are that he or she is a clinician:

1. Who has completed an accredited graduate-level education program preparing him/her for one of the four recognized APRN roles.
2. Who has passed a national certification examination that measures APRN, role and population-focused competencies and who maintains continued competence as evidenced by recertification in the role and population through the national certification program.
3. Who has acquired advanced clinical knowledge and skills preparing him/her to provide direct care to patients, as well as a component of indirect care; however, the defining factor for *all* [sic] APRNs is that a significant component of the education and practice focuses on direct care of individuals.
4. Whose practice builds on the competencies of registered nurses (RNs) by demonstrating a greater depth and breadth of knowledge, a greater synthesis of data, increased complexity of skills and interventions, and greater role autonomy.
5. Who is educationally prepared to assume responsibility and accountability for health promotion and/or maintenance as well as the assessment, diagnosis, and management of patient problems, which includes the use and prescription of pharmacologic and nonpharmacologic interventions.
6. Who has clinical experience of sufficient depth and breadth to reflect the intended license; *and* [sic].
7. Who has obtained a license to practice as an APRN in one of the four APRN roles: certified registered nurse anesthetist (CRNA), certified nurse midwife (CNM), clinical nurse specialist (CNS) or certified nurse practitioner (CNP) (APRN Consensus Workgroup & NCSBN APRN Advisory Committee, 2008, pp. 7–8).

UNIQUENESS OF APRN "PRACTICE"

Contemporary views of advanced nursing practice are grounded in the intersection of medical knowledge and skills with nursing's metaparadigm and knowledge base. The unique contribution that APRNs can make in the current health care system can be conceptualized to emerge from a distinctive blend of biomedical and nursing perspectives, skills, and knowledge sets. One crucial challenge for contemporary and future advanced nursing practice is to fully elucidate and articulate the mechanisms by which this fusion occurs (resulting in excellent, cost effective nursing and excellent patient outcomes). Our discipline's appreciation of holism, incorporates an understanding of persons as integrated, continually interacting with their environment, and engaged in the creation of meaning, and our disciplinary attention to the influences of life transitions and health conditions on individuals, families, and communities, form a matrix of underpinnings for advanced nursing practice. Holism, patient/client-centeredness, respect for individual autonomy, respectful communication with active listening, focused preventive care, health education, and integration of services, all of which are combined with clinical knowledge and expertise, are potentially some of the essential components of APRN effectiveness that grow from the nursing meta-paradigm (Donnelly, 2003; Erikson, 2007; Neill, 1999).

Despite an evolving, but still small, evidence base for the uniqueness of APRN practice, many of these disciplinary dimensions of practice need to be systematically examined. For example, Charlton, Dearing, Berry, and Johnson (2008) reported findings of their integrative review of nurse practitioner communication styles. Their review suggested that nurse practitioners' patient-centered communication styles, which they termed "biopsychosocial," compared with "biomedical" styles (2008, p. 383), influenced patient satisfaction, adherence, and health indicators, and was consistent with a specialized model of APRN effectiveness based on nursing's disciplinary perspective. Dunphy and Winland-Brown (2006) proposed a model of APRN practice: the *Circle of Caring*. This model accounts for, and formalizes, the overlapping multidisciplinary perspectives integrated in APRN practice through the standpoint of contextualized understanding in a scientific caring framework. Dunphy and Winland-Brown state that "caring is suggested as one way to bridge the gulf between holistic nursing theories and biomedical nursing praxis" (2006, p. 288). Table 3.1 offers other perspectives by summarizing several

TABLE 3.1
Sample of Studies Examining Influence of Disciplinary Underpinnings on NP Practice Outcomes

First Author	Design	Related Findings
Benkert et al. (2009)	Descriptive-correlational	African-American subjects with moderate cultural mistrust of European-Americans; high satisfaction/moderate trust of NP's
Benkert, Barkauskas, Pohl, Corser, Tanner, and Wells (2002)	Descriptive	Low-income African-American subjects with significantly higher trust scores for NPs vs. MDs; no significant difference in mistrust or satisfaction between providers; significantly higher trust scores for clinicians in nurse-managed vs. jointly managed clinics
Castro (2009)	Descriptive-correlational	Latina (female) subjects seen at least once by an NP clinician. All NP clinicians had either cultural proficiency, competence or awareness; no clinicians with cultural incompetence. Higher NP cultural competence score correlated with higher patient satisfaction scores; higher time spent with provider correlated with higher satisfaction
Donohue (2003)	Descriptive, naturalistic	Middle-aged female subjects described resources expected and received from NP encounters. Resources included services, information, support, time, respect, reassurance, affirmation, reinforcement, trust
Green (2005)	Predictive Modeling	Predictors of patient satisfaction and relationships among NP demographic characteristics, components of Caring Behaviors Inventory, patient satisfaction measures. All NPs with high CBI scores; no differences between male and female; no significant relationships among CBI components and satisfaction

(Continued)

TABLE 3.1
Sample of Studies Examining Influence of Disciplinary Underpinnings on
NP Practice Outcomes (*Continued*)

First Author	Design	Related Findings
Hayes (2007)	Descriptive-mixed method	Patients aged 18–86 receiving NP care; 86% female. High satisfaction with NP communication and style of interaction; high recall of instructions; intention to adhere to treatment plan-very likely. Themes connected with intention to follow treatment plan: trust, expertise, concern for own health
Kotzer (2005)	Descriptive survey	Advanced Practice Nurses in tertiary pediatric setting; 59% in NP role; 21% in combined CNS/NP role. Primary job functions: education/guidance/counseling, care coordination, direct care
Van Leuven (2007)	Descriptive, naturalistic	Interview NPs for perspectives on health promotion activities in practice. Health promotion viewed as implicit in nursing role; differentiates NP from MD; valued by NPs. Obstacles: time, patient care needs, limitations of scope of practice, patient scheduling, practice model (HMO vs other practice)

Source: Benkert et al. (2002); Benkert et al. (2009); Castro and Ruiz (2009); Donohue (2003); Green and Davis (2005); Hayes (2007); Kotzer (2005); Van Leuven and Prion (2007).

studies which examined the influence of a nursing disciplinary perspective as the underpinning for effective patient care by nurse practitioners.

APRN PRACTICE OUTCOMES

Compelling evidence of the effectiveness of APRN-managed care has been in the literature since the 1970s (Lenz, Mundinger, Kane, Hopkins, & Lin, 2004). A variety of patient outcomes of APRN-provided care have been studied, primarily in comparison to that provided by physicians. Patient satisfaction with, and quality outcomes of, APRN care have been studied extensively in the United States across the last three decades, and more recently in Britain and other European countries that have adopted advanced practice/nurse practitioner roles. Satisfaction with quality of NP-provided care in primary care, emergency departments, and specialty-care settings have consistently been found to be high, while researchers acknowledge that various methods, definitions, instruments, data sets, and time frames have been used in the measurement of these outcomes. However, across multiple studies and reviews, findings consistently documented quality of, and patient satisfaction with, APRN-provided care to be equivalent to or higher than physician-provided care (Carter & Chochinov, 2007; Cooper, Lindsay, Kinn, & Swann, 2002; Dierick-van Daele, Metsemakers, Derckx, Spreeuwenberg, & Vrijhoef, 2009; Horrocks, Anderson, & Salisbury, 2002; Jennings, Lee, Chao, & Keating, 2009; Kleinpell,

Ely, & Grabenkort, 2008; Knudtson, 2000; Roblin, Becker, Adams, Howard, & Roberts, 2004). For example, Mundinger and associates' large randomized controlled trial of NP-provided primary care, compared with physician-provided care, with 2 year follow-up, demonstrated no significant differences in patient satisfaction, utilization of services, self-reported health status and physiological measures related to diabetes, hypertension, and asthma outcomes (Lenz et al., 2004; Mundinger et al., 2000). In another large randomized controlled trial of 2957 low-income low-risk women, Jackson and associates (2003) found that birth outcomes of women receiving nurse midwife collaborative care were equivalent to the group of women receiving traditional physician care, but had lower operative intervention, lower use of epidural anesthesia, more spontaneous vaginal deliveries, and less use of medical resources. Pine et al.'s (2003) and Jordan et al.'s (2001) studies of anesthesia morbidity and mortality, noted earlier, demonstrated in a similar fashion the effectiveness, safety, and quality of nurse anesthetist-delivered care.

APRN CURRENT AND FUTURE OUTCOMES

Providers and researchers must, and are, extending the quality focus to a rigorous assessment of the influence of APRN-provided care across the health care system, including primary, acute, and specialty practice. There is evidence, evolving over several decades, that Nurse Anesthetist-provided care has resulted in high-quality patient outcomes that are at least equivalent to those achieved by physicians (AANA, n.d.). In addition, CNM-provided maternity care in the United States has resulted in excellent neonatal and maternal outcomes, including physical health of mothers and infants and satisfaction with care, among others (Davidson, 2002; Oakley et al., 1996; Wilson, 1989). Overall, NP-directed care has achieved excellent outcomes (Lenz et al., 2004). However, these findings should be considered in the context of a changing health care system and rapidly changing population demographics.

Primary care needs of the population are expanding in an era of significant health reform, and many more primary care providers will be required to fill these needs. Management of chronic illness is a growing APRN focus, as the burden of chronic illness grows in our society. This is magnified by an increasingly aged population, by evolutionary technologies that extend life across the developmental continuum, and by health care reform that further pressures the economic bottom line. APRNs are increasingly responsible for caseloads of chronically ill clients who have complex social, behavioral, mental health, and medical needs in primary, acute, and long-term care. Evidence of quality and effectiveness of APRN-provided care in past five decades is strong. The evidence foundation for outcomes of care as provided by NPs, CNMs, CRNAs, and CNSs, including their impact on client health in the short- and long-term, utilization of services, cost, access, quality, and other factors, should, and will, continue to grow in the transformed health care system of the 21st century.

SUMMARY: FROM SILOS TO COMMON VISION

On March 23, 2010 President Barack Obama signed into law the Patient Protection and Affordable Care Act, the first overhaul of the American health care system since Lyndon Johnson signed Medicare and Medicaid into law on July 30, 1965. As the people of the United States stand on the cusp of a new health care system, APRNs wait to see what is in store for their future. During the last decade, several changes have occurred that mesh with this historic healthcare reform. Advanced practice nursing has matured into a powerful force ready to determine its own future. Once separated by practice in separate professional silos, 100,000 APRNs (nurse midwives, nurse anesthetists, nurse practitioners, and clinical nurse specialists) stand ready to join forces under a uniform umbrella to push the profession forward through a common vision (Pearson, 2010).

During the last ten years, APRNs have fought for 100% insurance parity with physicians, universal coverage, and expansion of APRN practice to increase access to care, especially for the underinsured and underserved (Advance for Nurse Practitioners, 2010; Pearson, 2010). Utah and then Iowa adopted the APRN Compact, which allows APRNs in one compact state to practice in other compact states to further increase access to care (NCSBN, 2010). In several states, APRNs have decreased barriers to practice and have won the ability to receive Medicaid reimbursement for health care services. Progressive legislation has resulted in permitting APRNs to write prescriptions for handicap placards for the disabled, order home health care, perform physical exams for drivers and students, sign death certificates, write DNR orders, and become recognized as primary care providers. In many states, APRNs have won the ability to write for Schedule II through V controlled substances, and have their names printed on prescription labels.

Although there have been some losses, APRNs have held their ground in their struggles with Boards of Medicine across the United States to physicians' grip on regulation, supervision, and authority over their profession (Advance for Nurse Practitioners, 2010; Pearson, 2010). In several states, APRNs have managed to change legal language from "physician supervision" to "collaboration" or to "independent practice," and have removed mandatory APRN-to-physician ratios. APRNs have continued to extend their scope with regard to referrals to other healthcare providers, and providing direction to RNs, school nurses, occupational therapists, and respiratory therapists.

APRNs have also increased their numbers in leadership positions on state boards of nursing. In several states, advanced practice nurses have won the protection of the title of APRN (Advance for Nurse Practitioners, 2010; Pearson, 2010). In addition, they have increased their involvement in the business of state legislatures and the federal government. Four nurse practitioners have been elected to powerful positions as state representatives. In several states, APRNs have become major players in malpractice reform, and have been integrally involved in state Medicaid legislation. As the profession has matured, APRNs have hired their own professional lobbyists and formed political action committees. In *Kentucky Association Health Plans v. Miller, Kentucky Commissioner of Insurance*, (2003) the United States Supreme Court upheld *any-willing provider* law where insurers must open their networks to any provider recognized by the state, including APRNs.

In addition to promoting external changes, APRNs have also focused inwardly to improve the quality of practice. APRNs are reexamining the essential degree for entry-level advanced nursing practice (MSN vs. DNP) and moving toward unification through the *Consensus Model for Advanced Practice Registered Nurses* (Advance for Nurse Practitioners, 2010; Pearson, 2010). In addition, APRNs are moving toward uniform regulation of practice through licensing, accreditation, certification, and education. As the nation experiences dynamic changes in its healthcare system, APRNs—both masters and now including those doctorally prepared, stand ready to move the profession forward to provide the highest quality universally accessible healthcare.

REFERENCES

Advance for Nurse Practitioners. (2010). *Annual Legislative updates 2000–2010*. Retrieved from http://nurse-practitioners.advanceweb.com/Editorial/Search/SearchResult.aspx?KW=annual+legislative+update

Agres, T. (2010). California anesthesiologists buck governor over CRNA role. *Anesthesiology News, 36*(1). Retrieved from http://www.anesthesiologynews.com/index.asp?section_id=3&show=dept&issue_id=589&article_id=14427

American Academy of Pediatrics Committee on Hospital Care. (1999). Role of the nurse practitioner and physician assistant in the care of hospitalized children. *Pediatrics, 103*, 1050–1052. Retrieved from http://www.pediatrics.org/cgi/content/full/103/5/1050

American Academy of Pediatrics Committee on Pediatric Workforce. (2003). Scope of practice issues in the delivery of pediatric healthcare. *Pediatrics, 111*, 426–435. Retrieved from http://www.pediatrics.org/cgi/content/full/111/2/426

American Association of Colleges of Nursing. (AACN). (1996). *The essentials of master's education for advanced practice nursing*. Retrieved from http://www.aacn.nche.edu/Education/pdf/MasEssentials96.pdf

American Association of Colleges of Nursing. (AACN). (2009). *Title VIII nursing workforce development programs achieving success: Student recipients report the benefits*. Retrieved from http://www.aacn.nche.edu/government/pdf/FS_StudentSurvey.pdf

American Association of Nurse Anesthetists. (AANA). (n.d.) *Quality of care in anesthesia*. Retrieved from http://www.aana.com/qualityofcare.aspx

American Association of Nurse Anesthetists. (AANA). (2003). *The cost effectiveness of nurse anesthesia practice*. Retrieved from http://www.aana.com/crna/costeffect.asp

American Association of Nurse Anesthetists. (AANA). (2010). *Scope and standards for nurse anesthesia practice*. Retrieved from http://www.aana.com/uploadedFiles/Resources/Practice_Documents/scope_stds_nap07_2007.pdf

American College of Nurse Midwives. (ACNM). (2010). *Accreditation Commission for midwifery education*. Retrieved from http://www.midwife.org/acme.cfm

APRN Consensus Workgroup and NCBSN APRN Advisory Committee. (2008). *Consensus model for advanced practice registered nurses*. Retrieved from http://www.aacn.nche.edu/Education/pdf/APRNReport.pdf

Avery, M. D. (2005). The history and evolution of the Core Competencies for basic midwifery practice. *Journal of Midwifery & Women's Health, 50*(2), 102–107.

Baer, E. (1987). 'A cooperative venture' in pursuit of professional status: A research journal for nursing. *Nursing Research, 36*(1), 18–25.

Barger, M. K. (2005). Midwifery practice: Where have we been and where are we going? *Journal of Midwifery & Women's Health, 50*(2), 87–90.

Bednash, G., Worthington, S., & Wysocki, S. (2009). Nurse practitioner education: Keeping the academic pipeline open to meet family planning needs in the United States. *Contraception, 80*, 409–411.

Benkert, R., Barkauskas, V., Pohl, J., Corser, W., Tanner, C., Wells, M. et al. (2002). Patient satisfaction outcomes in nurse-managed centers. *Outcomes Management, 6*(4), 174–181.

Benkert, R., Hollie, B., Nordstrom, C. K., Wickson, B., & Bins-Emerick, L. (2009). Trust, mistrust, racial identity and patient satisfaction in urban African American primary care patients of nurse practitioners. *Journal of Nursing Scholarship, 41*(2), 211–219.

Blegen, M. A., & Tripp-Reimer, T. (1997). Implications of nursing taxonomies for middle range theory development. *Advances in Nursing Science, 19*(3), 37–49.

Buhler-Wilkerson, K. (2001). *No place like home: A history of nursing and home care in the United States*. Baltimore: Johns Hopkins University Press.

Bullough, B. (1976). Influences on role expansion. *American Journal of Nursing, 76*(9), 1476–1481.

Buppert, C. (2005). Scope of practice. *Journal for Nurse Practitioners, 1*(1), 11–13.

Burst, H., & Thompson, J. (2003). Genealogic origins of nurse midwifery education programs in the United States, Brief report. *Journal of Midwifery & Women's Health, 48*(6), 464–472.

Burst, H. (2004). *Varney's midwifery* (4th ed.). Sudbury: Jones and Bartlett.

Canadian Coordinating Office for Health Technology Assessment. (2004). Surgical anesthesia delivered by nonphysicians. 37. Retrieved from http://www.cadth.ca/media/pdf/273_No37_surgicalanesthesia_preassess_e.pdf

Carter, A. J. E., & Chochinov, A. H. (2007). A systematic review of the impact of nurse practitioners on cost, quality of care, satisfaction and wait times in the emergency department. *CJEM Canadian Journal of Emergency Medical Care, 9*(4), 286–295.

Castro, A., & Ruiz, E. (2009). The effects of nurse practitioner cultural competence on Latina patient satisfaction. *Journal of the American Academy of Nurse Practitioners, 21*(5), 278–286.

Charlton, C. R., Dearing, K. S., Berry, J. A., & Johnson, M. J. (2008). Nurse practitioners' communication styles and their impact on patient outcomes: An integrated literature review. *Journal of the American Academy of Nurse Practitioners, 20*(7), 382–388.

Cooper, M. A., Lindsay, G. M., Kinn, S., & Swann, I. J. (2002). Evaluating Emergency Nurse Practitioner services: A randomized controlled trial. *Journal of Advanced Nursing, 40*(6), 721–730.

Davidson, M. H., Burns, C. E., St., Geme, J. W., Cadman, S. G., Newman, C. G., Bullough, B. et al. (1975). A short term intensive training program for pediatric nurse practitioners. *Journal of Pediatrics, 87*(2), 315–320.

Davidson, M. R. (2002). Outcomes of high risk women cared for by certified nurse midwives. *Journal of Midwifery and Women's Health, 47*(1), 46–49.

Dawley, K. (2003). Origins of nurse-midwifery in the United States and its expansion in the 1940s. *Journal of Midwifery Womens Health, 48*(2), 86–95.

Dawley, K. (2005). Doubling back over roads once traveled: Creating a national organization for nurse-midwifery. *Journal of Midwifery & Women's Health, 50*(2), 71–82.

Dawley, K., & Burst, H. V. (2005). The American College of Nurse-Midwives and its antecedents: A historic time line. *Journal of Midwifery & Women's Health, 50*(1), 16–22.

Delaney, K. R. (2009). Looking 10 years back and 5 years ahead: Framing the clinical nurse specialist debate for our students. *Archives of Psychiatric Nursing, 23*(6), 453–456.

Dierick-van Daele, A. T. M., Metsemakers, J. F. M., Derckx, E. W. C. C., Spreeuwenberg, C., & Vrijhoef, H. J. M. (2009). Nurse practitioners substituting for general practitioners: Randomized controlled trial. *Journal of Advanced Nursing, 65*(2), 391–401.

Diers, D. (1991). Nurse-midwives and nurse anesthetists: The cutting edge in specialist practice. In L. H. Aiken, & C. M. Fagin (Eds.), *Charting nursing's future: Agenda for the '90s* (pp. 159 180). Philadelphia, PA: J. B. Lipincott.

Donnelly, G. (2003). Clinical expertise in advanced practice nursing: A Canadian perspective. *Nurse Education Today, 23*(3), 168–173.

Donahue, P. (1996). *Nursing, the finest art: An illustrated history* (2nd ed.). St. Louis: Mosby.

Donohue, R. K. (2003). Nurse practitioner–client interaction as resource exchange in a women's health clinic: An exploratory study. *Journal of Clinical Nursing, 12*(5), 717–725.

Dunphy, L. M., & Winland-Brown, J. E. (2006). The circle of caring: A transformative model of advanced practice nursing. In W. K. Cody (Ed.), *Philosophical and theoretical perspectives for advanced nursing practice* (4th ed.). Sudbury, MA: Jones & Bartlett.

Elder, R., & Bullough, B. (1990). Nurse practitioner and clinical nurse specialist: Are the roles merging? *Clinical Nurse Specialist, 4*(2), 78–84.

Erikson, H. L. (2007). Philosophy and theory of holism. *Nursing Clinics of North America, 42,* 139–163.

Fairman, J. (1999). Thinking about patients: Nursing science in the 1950's. *Reflections, 23*(3), 30–32.

Fairman, J., & Lynaugh, J. (1998). *Critical care nursing: A history.* Philadelphia, PA: University of Pennsylvania Press.

Fawcett, J., & Alligood, M. R. (2005). Influences on advancement of nursing knowledge. *Nursing Science Quarterly, 18*(3), 227–232.

Ford, L. (1975). An interview with Dr. Loretta Ford. *Nurse Practitioner, 1*(1), 9–12.

Frank vs. South. (1917). 175 Ky 416, 427–428; 194 SW 375, 380.

Graninger, E. (1996). Granny-midwives: Matriarchs of birth in the African-American community 1600–1940. *Birth Gazette, 13*(1), 9–13.

Green, A., & Davis, S. (2005). Toward a predictive model of patient satisfaction with nurse practitioner care. *Journal of the American Academy of Nurse Practitioners, 17*(4), 139–148.

Hayes, E. (1985). The nurse practitioner: History, current conflicts, and future survival. *Journal of American College Health, 34*(3), 144–147.

Hayes, E. (2007). Nurse practitioners and managed care: Patient satisfaction and intention to adhere to nurse practitioner plan of care. *Journal of the American Academy of Nurse Practitioners, 19*(8), 418–426.

Hedger, B. (2009). ACP urges doctors and NPs to work together. *American Medical News*. Retrieved from http://www.ama-assn.org/amednews/2009/03/02/prsa0302.htm

Hinch, B., Murphy, M., & Lauer, M. K. (2005). Preparing students for evolving nurse practitioner roles in healthcare. *MEDSURG Nursing, 14*(4), 240–246.

Horrocks, S., Anderson, E., & Salisbury, C. (2002). Systematic review of whether nurse practitioners working in primary care can provide equivalent care to doctors. *BMJ, 324*(7341), 819–823.

Hudspeth, R. (2009). Understanding clinical nurse specialist regulation by the boards of nursing. *Clinical Nurse Specialist, 23*(5), 270–275.

Jackson, D. J., Lang, J. M., Swartz, W. H., Ganiats, T. G., Fullerton, J., Ecker, J. et al. (2003). Outcomes, safety, and resource utilization in a collaborative care birth center program compared with traditional physician-based perinatal care. *American Journal of Public Health, 93*(6), 999–1006.

Jenkins, C. L., Elliott, A. R., & Harris, J. R. (2006). Identifying ethical issues of the department of the army civilian and army nurse corps certified nurse anesthetists. *Military Medicine, 171*(8), 762.

Jennings, N., Lee, G., Chao, K., & Keating, S. (2009). A survey of patient satisfaction in a metropolitan Emergency Department: Comparing nurse practitioners and emergency physicians. *International Journal of Nursing Practice, 15*(3), 213–218.

Jordan, L. M., Kremer, M., Crawforth, K., & Shott, S. (2001). Data driven practice improvement: The AANA foundation closed malpractice claims study. *AANA Journal, 69*(4), 304–311.

Keeling, A. (2007). *Nursing and the privilege of prescription, 1893–2000.* Columbus, OH: Ohio State University Press.

Keeling, A. (2009). A brief history of advanced practice nursing in the United States. In A. Hamric, J. Spross, & C. Hanson (Eds.), *Advanced practice nurisng: An integrative approach* (4th ed.). Saunders, St. Louis, MO: Elsevier.

Kentucky Association of Health Plans, Inc., et al. (2003). v. Miller, Commissioner, Kentucky Department of Insurance - 538 U.S. 329.

Kleinpell, R. M., Ely, E. W., & Grabenkort, R. (2008). Nurse practitioners and physician assistants in the intensive care unit: An evidence-based review. *Critical Care Medicine, 36*(10), 2888–2897.

Knudtson, N. (2000). Patient satisfaction with nurse practitioner service in a rural setting. *Journal of the American Academy of Nurse Practitioners, 12*(10), 405–412.

Kotzer, A. M. (2005). Characteristics and role functions of advanced practice nurses in a tertiary pediatric setting. *Journal for Specialists in Pediatric Nursing, 10*(1), 20–28.

Lenz, E. R., Mundinger, M. O. N., Kane, R. L., Hopkins, S. C., & Lin, S. X. (2004). Primary care outcomes in patients treated by nurse practitioners or physicians: Two-year follow-up. *Medical Care Research & Review, 61*(3), 332–351.

Lewis, J. A. (2000). Advanced practice in maternal/child nursing: History, current status, and thoughts about the future. *MCN: The American Journal of Maternal Child Nursing, 25*(6), 327–330.

Lindeke, L., Canedy, B., & Kay, M. (1997). A comparison of practice domains of clinical nurse specialists and nurse practitioners. *Journal of Professional Nursing, 13*(5), 281–287.

MacDonald, J., Herbert, R., & Thibeault, C. (2006). Advanced practice nursing: Unification through a common identity. *Journal of Professional Nursing, 22*(3), 172–179.

Manisoff, M. (1981). The nurse practitioner in family planning clinics. *Family Planning Perspectives, 13*(1), 19–22.

Manocchio, R. T. (2008). Tending communities, crossing cultures: Midwives in 19th-century California. *Journal of Midwifery & Women's Health, 53*(1), 75–81.

Mason, D. J., Vaccaro, K., & Fessler, M. B. (2000). Early views of nurse practitioners: A Medline search. *Clinical Excellence for Nurse Practitioners, 4*(3), 175–183.

McCool, W. F., & Simeone, S. A. (2002). Birth in the United States: An overview of trends past and present. *Nursing Clinics of North America, 37*(4), 735–746.

Moorhead, S., Head, B., Johnson, M., & Maas, M. (1998). The nursing outcomes taxonomy: Development and coding. *Journal of Nursing Care Quality, 12*(6), 56–63.

Morrison, S. M., & Fee, E. (2010). Nothing to work with but cleanliness: The training of African American traditional midwives in the South. *American Journal of Public Health, 100*(2), 238–239.

Mundinger, M. O., Kane, R. L., Lenz, E. R., Totten, A. M., Tsai, W. Y., Cleary, P. D. et al. (2000). Primary care outcomes in patients treated by nurse practitioners or physicians: A randomized trial. *JAMA, 283*(1), 59–68.

Murphy, M. A. (1990). A brief history of pediatric nurse practitioners and NAPNAP 1964–1990. *Journal of Pediatric Health Care, 4*(6), 332–337.

National Board of Certification of Nurse Anesthetists. (2010). *Certification.* Retrieved from http://www.nbcrna.com/certification.html

National Council of State Boards of Nursing. (NCSBN). (1998). Using nurse practitioner certification for state nursing regulation: An historical perspective. https://www.ncsbn.org/428.htm

National Council of State Boards of Nursing. (NCSBN). (2010). *APRN compact.* Retrieved from https://www.ncsbn.org/917.htm

National Organization of Nurse Practitioner Faculties. (NONPF). (2002). *Nurse practitioner primary care competencies in specialty care areas: Adult, family, gerontological, pediatric, and women's health.* Retrieved from http://www.aacn.nche.edu/education/pdf/npcompetencies.pdf

National Organization of Nurse Practitioner Faculties. (NONPF). (2003). *Psychiatric-mental health nurse practitioner competencies.* National Panel for Psychiatric Mental Health NP Competencies, Washington, DC: Author.

National Organization of Nurse Practitioner Faculties. (2004). *Acute care nurse practitioner competencies.* Faculties National Panel for Acute Care Nurse Practitioner Competencies, Washington, DC: Author.

National Task Force on Quality Nurse Practitioner Education. (2008). *Criteria for evaluation of nurse practitioner programs.* Washington, DC: AACN. Retrieved from http://www.aacn.nche.edu/education/pdf/evalcriteria2008.pdf

Neill, K. M. (1999). A holistic interdisciplinary health care research model. *Holistic Nursing Practice, 13*(2), 54–60.

Oakley, D., Murray, M. E., Murtland, T., Hayashi, R., Anderson, H. F., Mays, F. et al. (1996). Comparison of outcomes of maternity care by obstetricians and certified nurse midwives. *Obstetrics and Gynecology, 88*(5), 832–829.

Page, N. E., & Arena, D. M. (1994). Rethinking the merger of the clinical nursing specialist and the nurse practitioner roles. *Image: Journal of Nursing Scholarship, 26*(4), 315–318.

Partin, B. (2009). Consensus model for APRN regulation. *The Nurse Practitioner, 34*(6), 8.

Pearson, L. (2010). The Pearson Report 2010. Retrieved from http://www.pearsonreport.com

Phillips, J. R. (1996). What constitutes nursing science? *Nursing Science Quarterly, 9*(2), 48–49.

Pine, M., Holt, K. D., & Lou, Y. B. (2003). Surgical mortality and type of anesthesia provider. *AANA Journal, 71*(2), 109–116.

Raisler, J., & Kennedy, H. (2005). Midwifery care of poor and vulnerable women, 1925–2003. *Journal of Midwifery & Women's Health, 50*(2), 113–121.

Richmond, J. B. (1965). Gaps in the nation's services for children. *Bulletin of the New York Academy of Medicine, 41*(12), 1237–1247.

Roblin, D. W., Becker, E. R., Adams, E. K., Howard, D. H., & Roberts, M. H. (2004). Patient satisfaction with primary care: Does type of practitioner matter? *Medical Care, 42*(6), 579–590.

Rooks, J. (1997). *Midwifery and childbirth in America.* Philadelphia, PA: Temple University Press.

Roy, C. (2007). Advances in nursing knowledge and the challenge for transforming practice. In C. Roy, & D. A. Jones (Eds.), *Nursing knowledge development and clinical practice* (pp. 3–37). New York, NY: Springer Publishing.

Silver, H. K., Ford, L. R., & Day, H. C. (1968). The pediatric nurse practitioner program: Expanding the role of the nurse to provide increased health care for children. *Journal of the American Medical Association, 204,* 298–302.

Spalding, E. (1943). The Bolton Act provides federal funding for postgraduate programs. *American Journal of Nursing, 43,* 833.

Stanley, J. M., Werner, K. E., & Apple, K. (2009). Positioning advanced practice registered nurses for healthcare reform: Consensus on APRN regulation. *Journal of Professional Nursing, 25*(6), 340–348.

Stone, S. E. (2000). The evolving scope of nurse-midwifery practice in the United States. *Journal of Midwifery & Women's Health, 45*(6), 522–531.

Van Leuven, K., & Prion, S. (2007). Health promotion in care directed by nurse practitioners. *Journal for Nurse Practitioners, 3*(7), 456–461.

Varney, H., Kriebs, J., & Gegor, C. (2004). Varney's Midwifery (Fourth ed.). Sudbury, MA: Jones & Bartlett.

Wald, L. (1922). The origin and development of the Henry Street Settlement Text for Broadcasting. [Reel #25 Lillian Wald Papers]. In The Westinghouse Electric Manufacturing Co. (Producer): The New York Public Library.

Wall, B. M. (2005). *Unlikely entrepreneurs: Catholic sisters and the hospital marketplace, 1863–1925.* Columbus, OH: The Ohio State University Press.

Wilson, B. (1989). Delivery outcomes of low risk births: Comparison of certified nurse midwives and obstetricians. *Journal of the American Academy of Nurse Practitioners, 1*(1), 9–13.

CHAPTER THREE: Reflective Response 1

Ann L. O'Sullivan

INTRODUCTION

My first response after reading this succinct history of an Advanced Practice Registered Nurses' (APRNs) growth and development is to say, "It was the best of times, it was the worst of times" (p. 5) from Charles Dickens' (1859/2003) *A Tale of Two Cities*. He was speaking of London and Paris during the time of the French Revolution, just two decades after our own revolution, which certainly had influenced their French Revolution. So, each APRN has had revolutionary behavior to be able to serve people (and society) in the way they need and deserve. In order to have access to care by nurses in any of the four APRN roles, Certified Registered Nurse Anesthetists (CRNAs), Certified Nurse Midwives (CNMs), Clinical Nurse Specialists (CNSs), and/or Certified Nurse Practitioners (CNPs), scopes of practice often overlap with other health care professionals.

Another immediate response is to reflect on a picture from our Barbara Bates Center for the study of the *History of Nursing*,[1] of a young nurse carrying a velvet box holding a thermometer for a physician to use to take a patient's temperature. Today, skill and knowledge, as depicted in this picture that had traditionally been part of medicine, are now part of everyday parenting as we see a revolution in knowledge and skill acquisition by all. Sadly, when reading each profession's response to the American Medical Association's (AMA) 2005 *Scope of Practice Data Series* (which was only recently released in separate modules)[2] that profiles ten nonphysician professions'/professionals' (including audiologists, dentists, naturopaths, nurse anesthetists, nurse practitioners, optometrists, pharmacists, physical therapist, podiatrists, and psychologists) education, accreditation, certification, and licensure, I sense the revolution goes on into the 21st century. The AMA disputes unwarranted scope of practice expansions by nonphysician professionals that they say will threaten the health and safety of patients (Devitt, 2006).

Clearly, the authors of this chapter present data to dispute such claims, as do representatives from each profession in their letters of response to AMA's *Data Series*. On the other hand, if we keep in mind the 2006 collaborative document on *Changes in Healthcare Professions' Scope of Practice: Legislative Considerations* (revised in 2009)[3] developed by: the Federation of State Medical Board (FSMB), National Council of State Boards of Nursing, Inc. (NCSBN), Federation of State Board of Physical Therapy (FSBPT), National Board of Certification on Occupational Therapy (NBCOT), Association of Social Work Boards (ASWB), and National Association of Boards of Pharmacy (NABP), we can be hopeful with their statement "overlapping scopes of practice are a reality in a rapidly changing healthcare environment. The criteria related to who is qualified to perform functions safely without risk of harm to the public are the only justifiable conditions for defining scopes of practice" (National Council of State Boards of Nursing, p. 15, 2009).

ONGOING ISSUES

Therefore, all Doctor of Nursing Practice graduates (DNPs) will need to follow legislation that may influence their practice. Maintaining membership in one's professional nursing organization is essential in order to follow the dialogue on a particular issue, regardless of whether it will negatively or positively influence one's practice. The following are some examples of ongoing issues and organizations that can potentially affect DNP-APRN-CNP practice.

The Scope of Practice Partnership (SOPP) is a coalition of national medical specialty organizations and state medical societies established by the AMA in 2005 to study the qualifications, education, certification, and licensure of nonphysician providers. In addition to nurse practitioners, they are concerned about chiropractors, podiatrists, acupuncturists, naturopathic physicians, and psychologists. They will oppose inappropriate scope of practice expansion or encroachments on physician practice. The AMA staffed the partnership and had allocated $170,000 to pay staff and fund studies that examined the education, accreditation, certification, and licensure of allied health professionals. The partnership had 12 founding members: 6 state medical associations and 6 medical specialty groups (Devitt, 2006).

The Coalition for Healthcare Accountability, Responsibility, and Transparency (CHART) is a new 2006 coalition, introduced bipartisan legislation to increase transparency in the health care system by making it unlawful to misrepresent oneself to one's patients. Members of CHART include the AMA and multiple medical specialty organizations. The coalition believed patients were confused about the qualifications of health care providers. In a telephone survey of 100 adults, they demonstrated that patients were not clear on who was educated and trained as a medical doctor. CHART found that podiatrists, optometrists, psychologists and chiropractors were often considered a medical doctor (Showronek, 2006). They introduced federal legislation (H.R. 5688) to assure that health consumers would not think they were medical doctors just because they used the title *doctor* (govtrack.us, 2006).

DNPs have every right to be called Doctor and are very proud to be nurses and not physicians. They should have no problem being included in such legislation, and like the dental hygienists, their education and training will not be confusing to patients. Currently there is no progress noted on this legislation, but nursing support is crucial since these bills are often introduced two or three times before making headway through the process.

Each year, state legislators are bombarded with bills related to "scope of practice." DNPs need to be aware of ongoing legislation that may infringe on their expanded nursing practice. The publication *Advance for Nurse Practitioners* (http://nurse-practitioners.advanceweb.com/) is one source of such professional information. For example, a July 29, 2009 posting shared the successful end to an NP Restraint-of-Trade Case from Butte, Montana. This case involved two NPs who owned and operated a clinic, whose referrals for imaging beyond routine x-rays were refused by a physician director of radiology and pathology at a nearby hospital, because they did not have physician supervision (which was not required in Montana). After an 8-month delay by the defendants (physician and hospital), the parties settled 4 days into the trial. Advice from these APRNs was "Don't back down, don't allow it, stand up for our rights ..." (Ford, 2009, p. 1).

DNPs should also follow the calls for quick action from professional organizations regarding proposed federal legislation. The NP Roundtable, a coalition of seven national nurse practitioner organizations, works very hard to influence federal legislation (Nurse Practitioner Roundtable, 2008). One hurdle the NP Roundtable is working on is HR2350/S1174 "Preserving Patient Access to Primary Care Act of 2009," in order to remove all physician exclusive language in favor of terms such as clinician, health care provider, or an actual listing by profession in any health care legislation (Sheehan, 2009).

WHAT IS THE COALITION FOR PATIENTS' RIGHTS?

The Coalition for Patients' Rights (CPR) was established in 2006 for the sake of giving patients a choice of providers and fighting barriers to quality care. As of 2010 CPR consisted of more than 35 organizations of a variety of licensed health care professionals who provide safe, effective, and affordable health care to millions of clients each year (CPR, 2010a). CPR was formed to prevent SOPP from implementing unnecessary actions against allied health professionals that "will impede, rather than enhance" (CPR, p. 1, 2006), patient access to evidence-based care by these nonphysician providers. CPR also advocates for "the practice rights of its members for the sake of their patients" (CPR, p. 1, 2010b). CPR seeks to have a balanced study of all health care providers' education, accreditation, certification, and licensure and would like such a study to "assess whether state laws and regulations governing physicians practice contain outdated language that should be eliminated so that the unique skills of licensed healthcare professionals who do not hold a medical license are recognized" (CPR, p. 2, 2006). In addition, such a study would "evaluate the implications of current state laws that allow physicians to practice in any specialty, regardless of the individual qualifications to do so" (CPR, p. 2, 2006). Support statements from over 35 organizations can be found on CPR's website, as well as from media resources. In December 2008, the American Nurses Association (ANA) (a 2006 founding member of CPR) reaffirmed its support for patient access to licensed health care providers of their choice when ANA Chief Executive Officer Linda J. Stierle, MSN, RN, NEA-BC in a press release stated "Patients deserve to have access to the expert care that nurses can give them. Doctors do not have the right to impede nurses merely because we threaten their 'territory.' We can do more to improve patient care by working together rather than at odds with each other" (p. 1). This statement by the ANA was made in concert with the aforementioned 35 other national healthcare organizations to rally toward the "common cause of ensuring that all patients have access to quality care . . ." (CPR, p. 1, 2010b).

Each state's professional society tracks the number of providers that a state has and will need in the next ten years. Sadly, the results of these studies document over and over again the shortage of physician providers to provide primary care to the clients of a particular state. In fact, the American College of Physicians (ACP) released a monograph in 2009 which stated ". . . NPs and physicians have common goals of providing high-quality, patient-centered care and improving the health status of those they serve" (p. 1). Further, the ACP recommended that any demonstration project of the patient-centered medical home model should include one run by an NP (ACP, 2009). This is a perfect position for a DNP-APRN-CNP. AMA still states that DNPs must practice under physician supervision as part of a medical team (PA Nurses Association Update, 2008), but this is much less apt to happen as the physician shortages increase. Clearly the AMA and ACP have different views regarding a pilot of NPs as the leader of a medical home model—one which will in the future hopefully be called a "health home."

One aspect of DNP education, accreditation, certification, and licensure about which the AMA and ACP do agree is that DNP certification should not be obtained through Step 3 of the medical licensing exam of the National Board of Medical Examiners. The discipline of nursing should certify and license the DNP, APRN, and CNP.

CONCLUSION

The challenges of APRN practitioners and their role in the delivery of client-care services to individuals in our society throughout their lifespan will go on for years; but clearly the time has come for better communications, collaboration, and commitment on the part of all health professionals in order to foster health care reform in the 21st century.

NOTES

1. The Center's website at the University of Pennsylvania School of Nursing: http://www.nursing.upenn.edu/history/Pages/default.aspx
2. The AMA Data Series on NPs can be found at: http://www.acnpweb.org/files/public/08-0424_SOP_Nurse_Revised_10_09.pdf
3. The revised 2009 version produced by the NCSBN can be found at: https://www.ncsbn.org/ScopeofPractice.pdf

REFERENCES

American College of Physicians. (2009). *Nurse practitioners in primary care.* Retrieved from http://www.acponline.org/advocacy/where_we_stand/policy/np_pc.pdf

American Nurses Association. (ANA). (2008). *ANA supports patient access to licensed health care providers of their choice.* Retrieved from http://www.patientsrightscoalition.org/About-Us/Statements-of-Support/ANA.aspx

Coalition for Patients' Rights. (CPR). (2006). *Healthcare professionals urge cooperative patient care; oppose SOPP & AMA Resolution 814.* Retrieved from CPRJointStatement.doc

Coalition for Patients' Rights. (CPR). (2010a). Homepage. Retrieved from http://www.patientsrightscoalition.org/default.aspx

Coalition for Patients' Rights. (CPR). (2010b). *Statements of support.* Retrieved from http://www.patientsrightscoalition.org/About

Devitt, M. (2006). American Medical Association creates "partnership" to limit other providers' scope of practice: The next attempt to "contain and eliminate" chiropractic? *Dynamic Chiropractic, 24*(12), 1–7. Retrieved from http://www.dynamicchiropractic.com/mpacms/dc/article.php?id=51219

Dickens, C. (1859/2003). *A tale of two cities.* London, UK: Penguin Classics.

Ford, J. (2009). NP restraint-of-trade case settles. *ADVANCE for Nurse Practitioners.* Retrieved from http://nurse-practitioners.advanceweb.com/Article/Restraint-of-Trade-Case-Settles-2.aspx

govtrack.us. (2006). *H.R. 5688: Healthcare Truth and Transparency Act of 2006.* Retrieved from http://www.govtrack.us/congress/bill.xpd?bill=h109-5688.

National Council of State Boards of Nursing (NCSBN). (2009). *Changes in healthcare professions' scope of practice: Legislative considerations [revised from 2006].* Retrieved from https://www.ncsbn.org/ScopeofPractice.pdf

Nurse Practitioner Roundtable. (2008). *Nurse practitioners: Medical home/coordinated primary care providers.* Washington, DC: American Academy of Nurse Practitioners; American College of Nurse Practitioners; Association of Faculties of Pediatric Nurse Practitioners; National

Association of Nurse Practitioners in Women's Health National Association of Pediatric Nurse Practitioners National Conference of Gerontological; Nurse Practitioners National Organization of Nurse Practitioner Faculties. Retrieved from http://www.acnpweb.org/files/public/2009_ NP_Medical_Home_Coord_Primary_Care_Providers.pdf

PA Nurses Association Update. (2008). *AMA house of delegates considers limits on nursing education and practice.* American Nurses Association response to American Medical Association, House of Delegates Resolution: 214(A-08) "Doctor of Nursing Practice." June 11, 2008. Retrieved from http://allnurses.com/nursing-activism-healthcare/ama-house-delegates-310324.html

Showronek, P. (2006). CHART telephone survey—*Nationwide survey shows widespread consumer confusion over differences among health care providers.* Retrieved from http://www.earnosethroat-associates.com/ent_ news_ archive_0606.html

CHAPTER THREE: Reflective Response 2

Patti Rager Zuzelo

The authors correctly describe the historical "roots" of the Clinical Nurse Specialist, Nurse Practitioner, Nurse Midwife, and Nurse Anesthetist roles. However, it is critical to understand the important contrast between CNS role origins as compared to the genesis of other roles. Midwifery, Anesthetist, and Practitioner roles evolved from unmet public needs often in response to a lack of medical care and, many times, were birthed in practice models informed by medicine or by other non-nursing influences. These origins are in sharp contrast to those of the CNS role, a role *uniquely* grounded in professional nursing.

The term *Clinical Nurse Specialist* was first used in 1938 (Peplau, 1965/2003), and the initial role description of CNS as an advanced practice nurse with expertise in nursing practice in the care of complex patients is credited to Dr. Peplau (NACNS, 2004). These underpinnings contribute to the significant differences found in the subsequent histories, practice barriers, regulatory challenges, and practice domains between advanced practice nursing roles.

Specialization is not unique to the CNS but is a hallmark of this role. The first edition of the Social Policy Statement (American Nurses Association [ANA], 1980) described a CNS as a registered nurse holding a master's degree in nursing with a clinical focus. These clinical foci or areas of specialization often develop along lines of new knowledge, public needs and demands, nurse interests, and available opportunities (Peplau, 1965/2003). Nurse midwife and nurse anesthetist roles are specialized fields but areas of expertise are confined to a particular demographic or a specific type of intervention. CNSs specialize in many practice areas with evidence-based competencies associated with the particular specialty (NACNS, 2004). CNS specialization taxonomy could be organized by population, problem type, setting, care requirement, or disease/pathology/medical specialty (NACNS). Regardless of the specialty area, *nursing* is the center of CNS practice. This observation reinforces the notion that the CNS is "first of all a generalist, so she [sic] can do what is expected of a staff nurse" (Peplau, 2003, p. 7).

The authors note that during the 1980s and 1990s, there was much discussion and published exchange about blending the CNS and NP roles. In part, this discussion was fueled by reduction in workforce decisions made by hospital administrators in response to reduced reimbursements and budget challenges (Barker, 2009). CNS positions were often threatened or lost. There were also educational programs touting blended role programs that typically provided minimal attention to developing the CNS skill set and specialized expertise. Because the CNS role was more vulnerable to workplace reductions and titling protections were often not provided at the state level, nurses interested in the CNS role often gravitated to this role after completing graduate education in a different area of study, including education, administration, or nurse practitioner programs.

The authors point out threats related to CNS title protection, regulation, and scope of practice and these issues are concerning. *The Consensus Model for Advanced Practice Registered Nurses* (APRN Consensus Workgroup and NCSBN APRN Advisory Committee, 2008) offers both opportunities and challenges to CNS practitioners, particularly since specialization is a CNS hallmark of the CNS role and this is an "optional" feature of the model. Limited access to and inadequate availability of necessary certification examinations are also priority CNS issues (Zuzelo, 2010).

A critical aspect of CNS history that is not noted by the authors relates to the conceptualization of the CNS role through efforts of the National Association of Clinical Nurse Specialists (NACNS) and the subsequent opportunities for a CNS "voice" at important national dialogues. This organization was formed in 1995 to represent CNSs, regardless of specialty. Its early work included explicating core competencies for CNS practice (Baldwin, Lyon, Clark, Fulton, Davidson, & Dayhoff, 2007). Prior to this time, the CNS role was typically described in a functional, "laundry list" of sub-roles, including educator, clinician, consultant, researcher, and expert. Notably, other APRNs could reasonably claim to have similar expertise and responsibilities. This list did not provide an encompassing framework to inform CNS practice.

A process that included review of evidence, input and validation of experts, and public comment was used to develop CNS core practice competencies actualized in specialty practice (Baldwin et al., 2007). The essence of CNS practice is recognized as clinical expertise based on advanced nursing science knowledge (NACNS, 2004). Three interacting spheres of influence, guided by specialty knowledge and specialty standards, provide the conceptual framework for CNS practice (Figure 3.1). Recent validation of the 75 core NACNS CNS competencies among practicing CNSs demonstrated that these core competencies remain relevant and useful (Baldwin, Clark, Fulton, & Mayo, 2009). The conceptual framework also provides a meaningful lens through which to explicate clear differences between CNS and NP practice (Zuzelo, 2003).

As a result of the organized leadership provided by NACNS in partnership with other specialty and professional organizations, CNS practice is now viewed in an integrative fashion with expert nursing practice in the patient/client sphere serving as the keystone (Baldwin et al., 2007). The authors have appropriately commented on wide state-level variation in regulation and scope of CNS practice and have observed that there is a history of overlap in roles and functions between CNS and NP. The work of

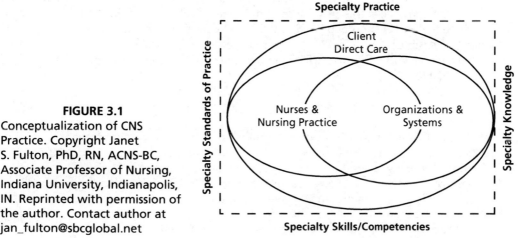

FIGURE 3.1
Conceptualization of CNS Practice. Copyright Janet S. Fulton, PhD, RN, ACNS-BC, Associate Professor of Nursing, Indiana University, Indianapolis, IN. Reprinted with permission of the author. Contact author at jan_fulton@sbcglobal.net

NACNS has provided a vehicle for making a clear case that CNS competencies are unique, built on clinical expertise and specialization, and directly connected to the science of nursing. Efforts currently underway include developing nationally validated education standards for CNS study programs to further ensure that nurses prepared in CNS programs of study are educated to meet CNS core competencies.

REFERENCES

American Nurses Association (ANA). (1980). *Nursing's social policy statement*. Kansas City, MO: Author.

Baldwin, K., Clark, A., Fulton, J., & Mayo, A. (2009). National validation of the NACNS Clinical Nurse Specialist Core Competencies. *Journal of Nursing Scholarship, 2,* 193–201.

Baldwin, K., Lyon, B., Clark, A., Fulton, J., & Dayhoff, N. (2007). Developing clinical nurse specialist practice competencies. *Clinical Nurse Specialist, 6,* 297–303.

Barker, A. (2009). *Advanced practice nursing: Essential knowledge for the profession.* Sudbury, MA: Jones and Bartlett.

National Association of Clinical Nurse Specialists 2004 Statement Revision Task Force. (2004). *Statement on clinical nurse specialist practice and education* (2nd ed.). Harrisburg, PA: Author.

Peplau, H. (1965/2003). Specialization in professional nursing. *Clinical Nurse Specialist, 17*(1), 3–9.

Zuzelo, P. (2003). Clinical nurse specialist practice—Spheres of influence. *AORN Journal, 77*(2), 361–364, 366, 369–372.

Zuzelo, P. (2010). *The clinical nurse specialist handbook* (2nd ed.). Sudbury, MA: Jones and Bartlett.

CRITICAL THINKING QUESTIONS

1. How have social, professional, and economic changes from the 1950s to the present influenced the APRN scope of practice?
2. How can historical factors in the evolution of the APRN shape the role and practice of future APRNs?
3. How is APRN practice different from generalist practice? From medical practice? What accounts for its outcomes in terms of patient satisfaction and health status?
4. APRN practice, particularly NP and CNM practice, may be conceptualized as built on a social justice foundation—to increase access to care for underserved and/or economically vulnerable populations. Current APRN practice has expanded beyond these boundaries, and many APRNs provide health services to clients who have access to adequate health care services, and who have adequate financial resources. How does this fit with nursing's values? How does this fit with the argument that APRNs should provide lower cost care than physicians and care that is more accessible?
5. What factors will influence full implementation of the consensus model for APRN practice? How?
6. What are the barriers to fully autonomous APRN practice?
7. What strategies could be used to increase physician support of autonomous APRN practice?
8. What are the advantages and disadvantages of APRN movement towards the *Consensus Model for Advanced Practice Registered Nurses* and uniform regulation of practice through licensing, accreditation, certification, and education?
9. What are the factors of APRN practice that make it uniquely different than medical practice? How do they enhance or weaken the profession?
10. What are the theoretical factors that set APRNs apart from the discipline of medicine? How does this theory base influence research and practice?

CHAPTER FOUR

How Doctoral-Level Advanced Practice Roles Differ From Masters-Level Advanced Practice Nursing Roles

Kym Montgomery and Sharon K. Byrne

INTRODUCTION

With a new era of health care reform upon us, the doctorate of nursing practice graduate will likely serve as an exemplar of a new form of Advanced Practice Registered Nursing (APRN) excellence (Apold, 2008). According to Burman, Hart, and McCabe (2005), the time is ripe and the nursing profession is ready for innovation in nursing education through this terminal degree. Globally, the ranks of APRNs have exploded over the past 45 years. Despite the number of APRNs in clinical practice, however, there has been a lack of consistency in education that is reflected in poor degree parity compared to other health care professions such as physical therapy, nutrition therapy, occupational therapy, and pharmacy that have successfully developed doctoral programs as entry into their fields of practice. Nursing's first foray into doctoral nursing education began in 1932 at Teacher's College of Columbia University with the awarding of the first Doctor of Education (EdD) degree in Nursing Education (Nichols & Chitty, 2005). Since that time, the profession has been persistently and unsuccessfully seeking a true clinical doctorate degree that showcases the true intellectual triad of the nursing profession. In the past, the profession's support of the PhD, DNSc (Doctor of Nursing Science), DNS (Doctor of Nursing Science), and DSN (Doctor of Science in Nursing), and lukewarm support of the EdD and ND (Doctor of Nursing) degrees, did not yield an appropriate pathway to the "clinical" doctorate. Is it possible that amid this chaos and ongoing scholarly debate about which is the right terminal degree for clinicians, opportunity knocks with the development of the doctor of nursing practice (DNP or DrNP)?[1] The authors of this chapter will hopefully present a thought-provoking discussion regarding the roles of the long-standing and historically MSN-prepared APRN, and contrast it with the newly heralded DNP-prepared APRN, as a new method of achieving a terminal degree that supports superior professional excellence.

THE EMERGENCE OF THE DOCTOR OF NURSING PRACTICE DEGREE

The timeline leading up to the DNP degree for APRNs began with the call of the Institute of Medicine (IOM) (2001) for sweeping redesign of the entire health care system. The IOM outlined basic skills that all health care professionals should have and suggested that new educational options be developed to ensure the safety of patients and close the gap that impedes quality care. The IOM (2001) stated:

> Forced with rapid changes in the healthcare system, the nation's healthcare delivery system has fallen far short in its ability to translate knowledge into practice and to apply new technology safely and appropriately. And if the system can not consistently deliver today's science and technology, it is less prepared to respond to the extraordinary advances that surely will emerge during the coming decades There is a dearth of clinical programs with the multidisciplinary infrastructure required to provide the full complement of services needed by people with common chronic conditions. The healthcare system is poorly organized to meet the challenges at hand.
>
> —*Institute of Medicine, 2001, p. 1*

IOM's challenge ignited a series of responses by a myriad of organizations that called for better-prepared APRNs who could address the complexity of patient care requirements, improve the efficiency of health care environments, and provide for an increased knowledge base for practice and excellence in nursing leadership. Three years later in 2004, the American Association of Colleges of Nursing (AACN) adopted a position to move the level of preparation necessary for advanced practice roles from a master's degree to a doctoral degree. More importantly, the AACN (2004) anticipates that by 2015, the DNP will become the requisite credential for entry into advanced practice nursing.

Similarly, the Commission on Collegiate Nursing Education (CCNE) (2005), the accrediting body of the AACN, decided that only practice doctorate degrees with the credential Doctor of Nursing Practice (DNP) would be considered for accreditation by the CCNE. At the time, this was a controversial stance since the initial 2004 vote was not unanimous (AACN, 2004). Columbia University had proposed an older doctor of nursing practice degree model first, a DrNP, but there were concerns that multiple practice degrees might take the degree model down the path of the DNSc, DSN, DNS alphabet soup path again (AACN). As the first DNP degree founded at the University of Kentucky in 2001 did not prepare practitioners but only clinical executives, it is unclear why the Columbia degree model, which prepared advanced practitioners and clinicians, was not the preferred degree model.

Presently, CCNE continues to accredit Master's in Nursing programs leading to advanced practice (CCNE, 2010). In 2006, The National Organization of Nurse Practitioner Faculties (NONPF) also issued a position statement supporting the practice doctorate in nursing. The NONPF (2006) statement highlighted core competencies expected of entry-level NPs with DNP preparation. This work, along with the *Essentials of Doctoral Education for Advanced Nursing Practice* (AACN, 2006), identified the competencies and outcomes necessary for quality DNP educational programs (Exhibit 4.1).

The DNP Roadmap Task Force stipulates steps to be taken to achieve the 2015 goal relative to educational programs. Having now identified that the DNP will be the terminal clinical practice doctorate supported by the above organizations, the questions still remain—How will the DNP-educated APRN differ from the traditional master's-educated APRN? Can the health care system afford a workforce of exclusively doctoral-prepared APRNs, particularly in this economic climate?

THE MSN ADVANCED PRACTICE NURSE: ONE IS SATISFIED, ONE WANTS *MORE*

The MSN-prepared APRN role has been historically restrictive and prescriptive. According to the American Nurses Association (2004), an APRN is the umbrella term given to a registered nurse who: (a) has met advanced educational and clinical practice requirements,

EXHIBIT 4.1 AACN's *Essentials of Doctoral Education for Advanced Nursing Practice*, **With Commentary**

I. Scientific Underpinnings for Practice

The DNP program prepares the graduate to:

1. Integrate nursing science with knowledge from ethics, the biophysical, psychosocial, analytical, and organizational sciences as the basis for the highest level of nursing practice.
2. Use science-based theories and concepts to:
   ■ Determine the nature and significance of health and health care delivery phenomena;
   ■ Describe the actions and advanced strategies to enhance, alleviate, and ameliorate health and health care delivery phenomena as appropriate; and
   ■ Evaluate outcomes.
3. Develop and evaluate new practice approaches based on nursing theories and theories from other disciplines.

Our View: The MSN graduate should be aware of all current evidence and knowledge to provide quality patient care and remain current in practice.

In Addition: The DNP graduate should design, develop, implement, and publish scientific findings to improve patient care and health care systems; and utilize new scientific evidence to devise protocols and practice plans. Additionally, the DNP graduate should maintain an active professional development plan.

II. Organizational and Systems Leadership for Quality Improvement and Systems Thinking

The DNP program prepares the graduate to:

1. Develop and evaluate care delivery approaches that meet current and future needs of patient populations based on scientific findings in nursing and other clinical sciences, as well as organizational, political, and economic sciences.
2. Ensure accountability for quality of health care and patient safety for populations with whom they work.
   (a) Use advanced communication skills/processes to lead quality improvement and patient safety initiatives in health care systems.
   (b) Employ principles of business, finance, economics, and health policy to develop and implement effective plans for practice-level and/or system-wide practice initiatives that will improve the quality of care delivery.
   (c) Develop and/or monitor budgets for practice initiatives.
   (d) Analyze the cost effectiveness of practice initiatives accounting for risk and improvement of health care outcomes.
   (e) Demonstrate sensitivity to diverse organizational cultures and populations including patients and providers.
3. Develop and/or evaluate effective strategies for managing the ethical dilemmas inherent in patient care, the health care organization, and research.

Our View: The MSN graduate should participate in professional organizations and lobby government officials for access to quality, cost-effective health care.

In Addition: The DNP graduate should represent professional organizations at the table with government officials to ensure health care policy efficacy and quality. The DNP actively and prominently initiates and advances the health care agenda.

III. Clinical Scholarship and Analytical Methods for Evidence-Based Practice

The DNP program prepares the graduate to:

1. Use analytic methods to critically appraise existing literature and other evidence to determine and implement the best evidence for practice.

2. Design and implement processes to evaluate outcomes of practice, practice patterns, and systems of care within a practice setting, health care organization, or community against national benchmarks to determine variances in practice outcomes and population trends.
3. Design, direct, and evaluate quality improvement methodologies to promote safe, timely, effective, efficient, equitable, and patient-centered care.
4. Apply relevant findings to develop practice guidelines and improve practice and the practice environment.
5. Use information technology and research methods appropriately to:
   - Collect appropriate and accurate data to generate evidence for nursing practice
   - Inform and guide the design of databases that generate meaningful evidence for nursing practice
   - Analyze data from practice
   - Design evidence-based interventions
   - Predict and analyze outcomes
   - Examine patterns of behavior and outcomes
   - Identify gaps in evidence for practice
6. Function as a practice specialist/consultant in collaborative knowledge-generating research.
7. Disseminate findings from evidence-based practice and research to improve health care outcomes

Our View: The MSN graduate should understand the need for research to advance nursing science, actively participate in research agendas, and utilize current information to provide quality care.

In Addition: The DNP graduate should design, develop, implement, and evaluate clinical research to improve patient care and outcomes through the development of guidelines, protocols, and informed opinion. The DNP should ensure organizational guidelines are congruent with current evidence-based practice, always with an open eye toward continuous improvement; and maintain a culture of excellence through continued scientific inquiry and personal and professional transformation.

IV. Information Systems/Technology and Patient Care Technology for the Improvement and Transformation of Health Care

The DNP program prepares the graduate to:

1. Design, select, use, and evaluate programs that evaluate and monitor outcomes of care, care systems, and quality improvement including consumer use of health care information systems.
2. Analyze and communicate critical elements necessary to the selection, use and evaluation of health care information systems and patient care technology.
3. Demonstrate the conceptual ability and technical skills to develop and execute an evaluation plan involving data extraction from practice information systems and databases.
4. Provide leadership in the evaluation and resolution of ethical and legal issues within health care systems relating to the use of information, information technology, communication networks, and patient care technology.
5. Evaluate consumer health information sources for accuracy, timeliness, and appropriateness.

Our View: The MSN graduate should have a clear understanding of current technological advances to improve patient care and patient outcomes; and have the ability to evaluate new systems and suggest updates to fulfill the needs of rapidly changing clinical environment.

In Addition: The DNP graduate should participate in the design, development, implementation, and evaluation technology to meet the current and future needs of health care teams nationally and internationally; design, develop, implement, and evaluate databases to improve health care informatics and communications; and lead activist groups to lobby for global electronic medical records to ensure the quality and continuity of patient care.

V. Health Care Policy for Advocacy in Health Care

The DNP program prepares the graduate to:

1. Critically analyze health policy proposals, health policies, and related issues from the perspective of consumers, nursing, other health professions, and other stakeholders in policy and public forums.
2. Demonstrate leadership in the development and implementation of institutional, local, state, federal, and/or international health policy.
3. Influence policy makers through active participation on committees, boards, or task forces at the institutional, local, state, regional, national, and/or international levels to improve health care delivery and outcomes.
4. Educate others, including policy makers at all levels, regarding nursing, health policy, and patient care outcomes.
5. Advocate for the nursing profession within the policy and health care communities.
6. Develop, evaluate, and provide leadership for health care policy that shapes health care financing, regulation, and delivery.
7. Advocate for social justice, equity, and ethical policies within all health care arenas.

Our View: The MSN graduate should have a deep-rooted understanding of financial aspects of quality care, diverse ways to access care, and how to advocate for legislative changes to influence health care delivery systems.

In Addition: The DNP graduate should identify problems within the health care delivery system and actively spearhead legislation to improve and/or change health care policy utilizing advanced negotiating, consensus building, and partnering skills, particularly across other health care disciplines.

VI. Inter-professional Collaboration for Improving Patient and Population Health Outcomes

The DNP program prepares the graduate to:

1. Employ effective communication and collaborative skills in the development and implementation of practice models, peer review, practice guidelines, health policy, standards of care, and/or other scholarly products.
2. Lead inter-professional teams in the analysis of complex practice and organizational issues.
3. Employ consultative and leadership skills with intra-professional and inter-professional teams to create change in health care and complex health care delivery systems.

Our View: The MSN graduate should collaborate and consult with health care providers as well as participate as a member of the health care team to advocate for both quality health care for patients and for the advanced practice role of the nurse.

In Addition: The DNP graduate should create and provide leadership in an interdisciplinary environment to advance health care agendas and improve patient care by utilizing critical and reflective thinking, scientific foundations, and research in all disciplines.

VII. Clinical Prevention and Population Health for Improving the Nation's Health

The DNP program prepares the graduate to:

1. Analyze epidemiological, bio-statistical, environmental, and other appropriate scientific data related to individual, aggregate, and population health.
2. Synthesize concepts, including psychosocial dimensions and cultural diversity, related to clinical prevention and population health in developing, implementing, and evaluating interventions to address health promotion/disease prevention efforts, improve health status/access patterns, and/or address gaps in care of individuals, aggregates, or populations.

3. Evaluate care delivery models and/or strategies using concepts related to community, environmental and occupational health, and cultural and socioeconomic dimensions of health.

Our View: The MSN graduate should provide comprehensive, culturally diverse, and competent care to patients in their scope of practice. The practitioner should investigate all resources to ensure quality care for their population.

In Addition: The DNP graduate should utilize problem solving skills to generate new knowledge that affects patients within and outside their population. The DNP utilizes clinical experience, advanced analytic skills, and leadership abilities to target health care GLOBAL health care issues.

VIII. Advanced Nursing Practice

The DNP program prepares the graduate to:

1. Conduct a comprehensive and systematic assessment of health and illness parameters in complex situations, incorporating diverse and culturally sensitive approaches.
2. Design, implement, and evaluate therapeutic interventions based on nursing science and other sciences.
3. Develop and sustain therapeutic relationships and partnerships with patients (individual, family or group) and other professionals to facilitate optimal care and patient outcomes.
4. Demonstrate advanced levels of clinical judgment, systems thinking, and accountability in designing, delivering, and evaluating evidence-based care to improve patient outcomes.
5. Guide, mentor, and support other nurses to achieve excellence in nursing practice.
6. Educate and guide individuals and groups through complex health and situational transitions.
7. Use conceptual and analytical skills in evaluating the links among practice, organizational, population, fiscal, and policy issues.

Our View: The MSN graduate should practice in a collaborative environment.

However: The DNP graduate should "create" the environment he/she practices in utilizing principles of autonomy and independence, while fostering an interdisciplinary climate. *While some believe this is just a new degree with the same role, we disagree. We encourage more explicit development of doctoral advanced practice nursing competencies.*

Adapted from the 2006 *AACN Essentials of Doctoral Education for Advanced Nursing Practice.*

at a minimum of a master's level, beyond a basic nursing education and licensing required of all RNs; and (b) provides at least some level of direct care to patient populations. As identified in chapter 3, the APRN roles at the master's level are clearly defined. The nurse is educated in and chooses her or his area of specialty and population foci. They then proceed to practice within that particular scope of practice (e.g., Nurse Anesthesia, Nurse Midwifery, Nurse Practitioner, Clinical Nurse Specialist) utilizing expanded skills, experience, and knowledge in assessment, planning, implementation, diagnosis, and evaluation of the care required within their specialized area.

The authors of this chapter acknowledge that well-educated master's-level APRNs provide safe, efficient, comprehensive, high-quality care to the population they serve. Mundinger and colleagues' (2000) classic article in the *Journal of the American Medical Association* reported equivalent master's APRN outcomes compared with physician primary care outcomes; these study findings were replicated 2 years later by Horrocks, Anderson and Salisbury (2002) in the United Kingdom. These studies indicate the DNP degree was certainly not created because MSN APRN care was inferior. Unfortunately, the professional recognition of MSN-prepared APRNs outside of the nursing profession has been stunted because of numerous factors including "cookie cutter" educational training programs (e.g., overly restrictive, lacking innovation, or "designed for the past, not the future") and inaccurate and derogatory perceptions of these providers as being simply *physician extenders* or *mid-level providers*. These are terms that the nursing profession has fiercely tried to negate. As nurse practitioners, what we do is not mid-level anything: We certainly *do not* provide just mid-level care, and we certainly *do not* practice at a mid-level, nor is it mediocral! We suspect you, as well the authors of this chapter, provide high-quality care to the best of your ability all of the time. To us, that is not mid-level. We would prefer to be called by our title or be identified by the role that we hold within the health care domain with an emphasis on maintaining our nursing identity as Advanced Practice Registered Nurses, Advanced Practice Nurses, Doctoral Advanced Practice Registered Nurses, Board Certified Nurses, or the designation provided by respective State Boards of Nursing.

Conversely, the DNP degree is not prescriptive to the clinical specialty areas like master's education. The DNP degree builds upon the MSN level of education, and the student learns to branch out of standard roles in order to assume greater responsibility and accountability for his or her patients, ensuring care continuity that will infiltrate through other disciplines (Mundinger, 2005). If the master's-prepared nurse wants to achieve a practice doctorate simply to earn the respect and the "doctor" title, we urge the matriculating student to stop now or proceed with extreme caution! Doctoral education differs dramatically from MSN education. It commands an overwhelming amount of dedication and an unwavering intellectual curiosity to "pry the lid off" of the road map point of care pathways and to understand the "why"; to think outside the box, to question practice, and to be the conduit to explore causation that might lead to new interventions (Dreher & Montgomery, 2009).

Over 330 master's degree programs that have been accredited by the CCNE or by the National League for Nursing Accrediting Commission (NLNAC) exist with fairly standard and traditional curricula incorporating basic theoretical and conceptual aspects of nursing science, skills performance, research comprehension and application, and leadership proficiency to improve the health care system (AACN, 2006). The graduate APRN is then molded within his/her practice environments to grow and mature in a specialty area. For many master's-prepared clinicians, contentment is found in providing high-quality care to the patients or systems they serve. For others, they may feel they have reached their full potential or the boundary of their practice ability. Their professional contentment slowly dissipates and results in the quest for "more." But just what exactly is *more*?

THE DNP APRN: THE ONE WHO WANTS *MORE*

The DNP is the answer to this resounding question! The emergence of this new title and its associated curricular structure may be just what the *doctor ordered* (no pun intended)[2] to lead APRNs with a progressive thirst for knowledge and armed with the assimilation and integration of new DNP NONPF competencies to merge into a different world of life-long engagement and satisfaction in doctoral advanced practice nursing. In Exhibit 4.1, we have included a very specific commentary where we highlight what the DNP graduate is educated and trained to do beyond the MSN. Both of us having now "lived" the *Essentials* (AACN, 2006) feel our perspective is very valuable as the profession tries to define what exactly is the domain of practice that exists beyond the MSN. The following two scenarios provide cases in-point for readers interested in sharing the journey and personal insight of two DrNP graduates from the start to completion of their terminal degree. We offer our two personal stories openly and hope they may be valuable to current doctor of nursing practice students.

Case I: A Women's Health Nurse Practitioner Who Wanted More

The first author of this chapter is a 40-year-old, well-seasoned practicing APRN. My 15-year practice, specializing in women's health in both clinical and academic arenas, centered on achieving success at providing empathetic, comprehensive care to my patients and was focused on health promotion and disease prevention. Each office day was packed with a full complement of patients with an array of issues ranging from the normal annual well visit to the extremely complex and potentially life threatening disease situations. Booking an appointment with me typically necessitated a 6-month wait. My collaborating physicians' operating room schedules were also booked with referrals stemming from my robust practice. In addition, the number of my pregnant patients delivering with the collaborating physicians greatly contributed to the income of the practice. Needless to say, I successfully cultivated a large and loyal patient volume through hard work, and earned respect from the medical community and my peers through my practice—my ideal clinical APN professional career goal attainment.

However, as the years passed and as each professional milestone was attained, my office hours began to get longer and more mundane. Challenges were fewer and farther between. I did not feel as though I had to put much thought into providing high-quality, effective, and efficient care. I did, however, become more frequently frustrated by existing policies that were incongruent to quality health care options. Somehow, invisible to my patients and initially without my own complete self-awareness, I was intellectually stunted. But what grew out of this discomfiture was a gnawing desire to seek the unknown—to find "more," whatever that was. I thought about taking the LSAT for law school admission, but my unwavering self-identification and dedication as a nurse clinician halted that option. I also explored avenues in forensic nursing, defense law expert for nurses, and even medical school. However, my zest for my specialty and my profession continued to overpower my "wandering eye" into other career areas, until I found the practice doctorate, the DrNP.

In response to another IOM report (2003), *Health Professions Education: A Bridge to Quality*. Many masters-level the AACN interpreted the document's policy recommendations as supportive of more advanced nursing education, and thus the early planning and politicking toward a practice doctorate degree alternative to the PhD was underway. Many master's-level nursing programs had revamped their existing curricula by requiring an expansion of the already challenging and complex credit loads to deal with the IOM's requests. Some thought the MSN degree already conferred this advancement and was almost equal to similar entry-level health profession doctorates. Was nursing about to abandon its history of failed clinical doctorate models in favor of a new practice doctorate degree? The AACN ultimately indicated the new DNP degree was created to meet the demands of the present day fragmentation of services and system failures in health care by preparing nurse clinicians (and later clinical executives) for practice with interdisciplinary, information systems, quality improvement, and patient safety expertise (AACN, 2006). Practically simultaneously, Mary O'Neil Mundinger, Dean of the Columbia School of Nursing, pioneered the first DrNP program to revolutionize the nursing profession and prepare the nurse clinician for more sophisticated and complex advance nursing practices (Yox, 2005). At this juncture, a debate ensued that has really not abated. If the master's degree is still filled with rigor and produces capable and competent APRNs, why are some left asking for "more"? Why go for the DNP?

Before the DNP/DrNP degrees evolved, many passionate APRNs found themselves in PhD programs, not exactly certain what their role would be if they completed the PhD. Typically, APRNs who seek a doctoral nursing terminal academic degree still identify strongly with the clinician role (Bloch, 2005; Chism, 2009). The DNP program "requires competence in translating research in practice, evaluating evidence, applying research in decision-making, and implementing viable clinical innovations to change practice" (AACN, 2006, p. 6). In addition, a strong DNP curriculum should prepare the APRN clinician to become an integral part of a research team. In our program, and perhaps in some DNP programs, the graduate is also prepared to competently spearhead research initiatives, especially those deeply grounded in practice.

The expert APRN's journey into the DNP curricula is definitely not an easy one, Then again, is any doctoral program designed to be navigated effortlessly? For the clinician accustomed to being "on top of her game" in the clinical world, rejoining a very different academic world will often result in frustration. Being a doctoral student mentally means experiencing challenging workloads designed to reprogram the APRN's view of the world, the very same view that was accustomed to confidence and security in both judgment and performance (with a masters degree). In order for the APRN to attain the DNP, an extremely challenging metamorphosis needs to occur. These programs are designed to infuse a deep-rooted understanding of the multifaceted aspects of evidence-based practice and research skills, leadership, administration, and policy into the polished practitioner. The lens from which clinical practice was previously viewed is reinforced, but also changed so that a new broader landscape perspective is seen. The DNP clinician possesses newly acquired skills, which fortify critical thinking about the care provided and empower the nurse to authoritatively and credibly question the standard of care and to participate actively in the revision of current standards to improve patient care.

In my case, my quest to find something "more" and stay true to my clinical roots allowed me to build upon my master's level training. I was truly at the point in my professional career where I was no longer satisfied with doing the "how to," but I craved the "why" and the "why not" in order to *improve* "how to" learning. In this quest, my doctoral education encouraged and challenged me to find novel and creative ways to improve the care I deliver and enabled me to make a greater impact in the lives of not only the patients I encounter, but also the future generations of patients and providers through the dissemination of my clinical scholarship.

Despite an economy in turmoil, the overall number of nursing students enrolled in doctoral programs continues to increase. There are currently 119 nursing schools accepting students into a DNP program with an additional 100 schools contemplating offering a DNP program (AACN, 2010; Fang, Tracy, & Bednash, 2010). Student enrollment in DNP programs has increased a startling 176% ($N = 3,291$), from 1,874 students in 2007 to 5,165 students in 2009 (Raines, 2010). Of particular interest, in research-focused doctoral programs, enrollments increased by only 0.1% or 3 students from 2007 to 2008, but in 2009 there has been a slight increase of 5.1% (AACN, 2009; Fang, Tracy, & Bednash, 2010). As a critical mass of DNP clinicians accrues, their additional education, greater depth and breadth of knowledge, more refined leadership abilities, and enhanced skill set will propel graduates to exert more influence on patient care and demand equivalent input into joint decision-making for their patients. At the same time, the DNP will "profoundly improve the nation's image of nursing" (Mundinger, 2005, p. 174). Mundinger also acknowledges that DNPs, based on their intense advanced education, coupled with their passion for patient care, are raising intriguing questions, offering resolutions, and stepping in with welcome wisdom to improve the care in the systems in which they work. The saga continues.

With the attainment of my DrNP, coupled with my scholarship productivity and expert clinical practice, I am not doing the same thing I was doing when I walked into my first doctoral seminar. I now have a joint appointment in both a prestigious nursing school and medical school, and have published 9 journal articles (3 research related) in respected peer-reviewed journals in my first year of post graduation. My clinical scholarship focuses on helping raise public awareness concerning the issues of HPV in women's health care, both nationally and internationally. I continue to be active in promoting optimal women's health care and I really believe my primary care has improved because of my enhanced abilities at formal clinical inquiry. My doctoral education (and the specific coursework I took) has given me (a clinician!) the tools to evaluate and strengthen woman health nurse practitioner curricula and now educate future "foot soldiers" in women's health advanced practice nursing. I truly believe my doctoral education has enabled me to accept the challenge of the IOM (2001) to help close the gap that impedes the quality of care we give to patients. I also do not see practice on one side of the road and research on the other. Instead, my own degree has helped me professionally build a bridge between the two. I have just finished writing a four-part transdisciplinary education grant that combines diverse expert faculty instruction, multilevel simulation, and collaborative case study learning formats to educate OB/GYN medical students, Women's Health Nurse Practitioner students, Physician Assistant students, and Nurse Anesthesia students *together* in a collaborative setting.

The focus of this degree is to enhance knowledge of roles and responsibilities within the health care system, foster development of team-building skills, improve health care team communication, reduce medical errors, and improve the quality of patient care through simulation in a transdisciplinary environment. Had I kept my head to the grindstone in my clinical practice and never decided to continue on to get my DrNP, I do not believe I would have ever dreamed such issues existed in health care, or that I could be part of a solution. I feel as though the lenses of my clouded glasses were cleaned, and now I can see farther and more clearly than ever before. My doctor of nursing practice education has satiated my quest for "more" and has opened up a new world of endless possibilities that will continue to assist me in my own personal and professional development, as well as help me be a better steward of my profession and discipline.

Case II: One Oncology Nurse's Story: From RN-to-BSN-to-CNS-to-FNP-to-DrNP!

The second author is an APRN who, after 20-plus years of practice evolving from a diploma-prepared registered nurse followed by a BSN degree and master's-level preparation as a Clinical Nurse Specialist, sought and achieved post-master's certification as a Family Nurse Practitioner. After 3 years of competent practice in this role, at both a community-based hospital and university medical center setting, I had the personal drive to "do more." At first this urge was satisfied with supplemental adjunct faculty responsibilities. This role, however, only fueled my desire to be both an expert practitioner and educator. After exploring both PhD and DNP programs for over a year, I knew that my future quest was doctoral education in nursing. As opposed to a PhD in Nursing program, which emphasizes the philosophy of science, nursing science, and research, I chose a hybrid DrNP program as my educational pathway due to the ability to declare a dual track as a scholar in nursing practice and nursing education. Coursework in the program appealed to the practitioner within me, as it included both a clinical and role practicum. In addition, it included core courses in nursing science, advanced practice, research methods, and independent study cognates. A major draw to this program was that attendance at a "DrNP-in-London or -Dublin Program" was required, and this afforded me the opportunity to study abroad and connect with international nursing scholars.

According to Robb (2005), those seeking a DNP option do so because these programs reflect their interests and personalities. The philosophy and tenets of the DrNP program I chose coincided with the ability to achieve subjective satisfaction and purposefulness in my professional role as an APRN. It is highly recommended that every prospective doctor of nursing practice student find a program or curriculum that matches your philosophy and values. I felt that upon completion of my curriculum, I would be prepared at the highest level, practice with the admiration of peers both inside and outside the discipline of nursing, and develop skills that are crucial to becoming a valued nursing faculty member and empowered nurse leader. The latter two skills have been found to be determinative in students' choosing a practice doctorate rather than a research-focused doctorate, and to support those who desire to focus their careers on clinical practice and nursing education (Loomis, Willard, & Cohen, 2007).[3] Likewise, Brar, Boschma, and McCuaig (2010) state the DNP is the most recent credential and source of preparation of new nursing knowledge that has a strong emphasis on advanced leadership in clinical practice.

Following my coursework related to the terminal degree and successful completion of a clinical dissertation, I am pleased to say I was offered a full-time appointment as a Assistant Clinical Professor in a College of Nursing and Health Professions within a large urban university setting, teaching across the curriculum. Most recently, I am to assume the additional role of Track Coordinator for the MSN Family Nurse Practitioner program. Our college is also exploring whether to offer the practice doctorate for entry-level APRN practice as well. My own individual competency and engagement in clinical practice is further fostered by applying the knowledge and skill I gained in my elective cognate coursework to my current role as an Advanced Practice Nurse within a university hospital-based Cancer Institute's Screening Program. I feel strongly that the DrNP degree has contributed to my being able to achieve this perfect balance of teaching and clinical practice.

According to Little and Milliken (2007), there is an "obligation and expectation that nurse educators are experts in clinical practice and education concurrently" (p. 1). By educating future nurse practitioners at the same time as I continue to practice and maintain national certification as a Family Nurse Practitioner by the Academy of Nurse Practitioners (NP-C) and specialty certification as an Advanced Oncology Certified Nurse Practitioner (AOCNP) by the Oncology Nursing Certification Corporation, my commitment to staying current in practice is strengthened. This experience also assists me in translating the work of Benner (1984) related to expert clinical practice as a model of skills acquisition, a model comprised of five stages of development from novice to expert within the classroom and practicum settings. With my practice doctorate, I feel I can serve as an example of a nursing professional that can help lessen the "theory–practice gap" discussed by Little and Milliken. This gap is bridged by remaining current in clinical nursing practice, balancing the demands of holding a academic position, and undertaking other scholarly activities such as research, publishing to disseminate nursing knowledge, providing service to the community and university, and being an active participant as a speaker or poster presenter in a variety of nursing and other inter-disciplinary conferences. I believe I have a responsibility to the profession and discipline to perform these activities; to me, this is what a doctoral-educated clinical nursing scholar does. I also reject any notion that only the PhD graduate can produce empirical evidence for the profession. However, my focus is on the generation of "practice evidence," and I have confidence that my doctoral coursework has equipped me with the basic and prac-tical clinical research skills to accomplish this.

Extending beyond the traditional APRN role and with the support of coursework in my own doctoral program that fostered leadership, I have been able to advocate at both an urban local and county level and to serve as a member on a Cancer Coalition for service improvements to underserved populations in the area of early detection and treatment related to cancer care. As one of two APRNs in an out-patient-based Department of Medicine, Hematology/Oncology practice (and the only one doctorally prepared), I have taken the lead in designing and developing educational outreach pro-jects based on gaming strategies to increase participation of women in breast cancer screening and increase early access to services. This program is the result of funding that was secured through a grant from a nationally recognized organization in the pro-motion of breast health and breast cancer awareness. More recently, I have been assisting in bringing to inception a regionally funded grant for "Lost to Follow-up Participants" in a university hospital-based Breast Cancer Screening Program. This program is based on the National Cancer Institute's Research–Tested Intervention Program script for Breast Cancer Screening among Non-Adherent Women. Leadership skills that match resources to needs, such as those noted above, have been described by Fitzsimmons, Hadley, and Shively (1999) as necessary to generate, guide, and manage change, and to interpret prac-tice outcomes. I believe these skills have been nurtured and supported by my own invol-vement in practice-oriented doctoral education and in my role-development journey from that RN to this Doctoral Advanced Practice Nurse.

SUMMARY

The evolution of APRN education from the master's to the doctorate level appears to be here to stay. As Dreher (2005) stated 5 years ago, "Has this train left the station? If so, just where is it going?" (p. 17). The issues surrounding this transition will most likely continue to be debated for some time, and the ultimate direction of the doctor of nursing practice degree is still unfolding. We think that active, practicing DNP and DrNP graduates can actually shape the future of this degree with our critical mass. We absolutely want more outcome data on what these graduates are accomplishing. We even welcome any constructive criticism, especially if there are DNP programs that proliferate that are not rigorous or that aim to create an easy path to the title "Dr." Weak DNP programs will harm us all and not advance the nation's health. We also call for the doctor of nursing practice graduate to advance "practice knowledge development" as has been recently advocated by Dreher (2010) who also contends the doctor of nursing practice graduate should be the leader in creating practice-based evidence for the discipline. DNP-prepared APRNs have quickly positioned themselves to become an integral part of our discipline's future. They not only carry with them a unique preparation for diverse health care roles, but a plethora of opportunities for advancement in the arenas of practice, leadership, education, and applied research awaits them.

So, exactly how is the MSN different from the DNP? Why take the leap into obtaining a practice doctorate in nursing? The answers to these questions will be different for every nurse practicing in the clinical arena. You will decide if you want *more*. However, one fact is clear . . . *the MSN degree allows you to be part of the change to improve the quality of patient care you provide, while the DNP equips you to collaborate more interprofessionally (and with more confidence) to be the change and advance the discipline.* This degree opens your professional world to a myriad of new lenses, new options, and new agendas with which to advance nursing and make a true impact on the patients you serve *and to the larger aggregate* through your disseminated clinical scholarship. To reiterate our warning at the beginning of the chapter, proceed with caution! When you obtain the DNP, you will be different. Your professional eyes will be open more widely to many more challenges. Your metamorphosis, we attest, will be profound.

NOTES

1. Both initials DNP and DrNP stand for *doctor of nursing practice*, although overwhelmingly, most programs use the DNP initials. Because the DrNP degree is termed a *hybrid professional doctorate* and emphasizes both advanced practice and the conduct of practical clinical research, it uses different initials.
2. On a serious note, however, we *highly discourage* the use of the word *Doctor* to describe one who is actually a physician. There are lots of *doctors* in health care, including DNPs who complete the doctorate. By using the proper title *physician*, we are describing their role and their profession. Even to a patient we recommend saying for example, "What did your physician prescribe for you?"
3. While the educator role may not have been an approved focus of the DNP degree, it has been reported that over 30% of all DNP graduates indeed go in to academia (Zungolo, 2009).

REFERENCES

American Association of Colleges of Nursing. (AACN). (2004). *Position statement on the practice doctorate in nursing.* Retrieved from www.aacn.nche.edu/DNP/DNPPositionStatement.htm

American Association of Colleges of Nursing. (AACN). (2006). *The essentials of doctoral education for advanced nursing practice.* Retrieved from http://www.aacn.nche.edu/DNP/pdf/Essentials.pdf

American Association of Colleges of Nursing. (AACN). (2009). *Despite surge of interest in nursing careers, new AACN data confirm that too few nurses are entering the healthcare workforce.* Retrieved from http://www.aacn.nche.edu/media/NewsReleases/2009/workforcedata.html

American Association of Colleges of Nursing. (AACN). (2010). *Doctor of Nursing Practice (DNP) Programs.* Retrieved from http://www.aacn.nche.edu/DNP/DNPProgramList.htm

American Nurses Association. (2004). *APRNs and FECA.* Retrieved from http://www.nursingworld.org/MainMenuCategories/ANAPoliticalPower/Federal/Issues/APRNsandFECA.aspx

Apold, S. (2008). The doctor of nursing practice: Looking back, moving forward. *Journal for Nurse Practitioners, 4*(2), 101–108.

Benner, P. (1984). *From novice to expert: Excellence and power in clinical nursing practice.* Reading, MA: Addison-Wesley Publishing.

Bloch, J. (2005). Letter to the editor on "Doctor of Nursing Practice. . .". *Online Journal of Nursing Issues, 10*(3). Retrieved from http://www.nursingworld.org/ojin/admin/toc.htm

Brar, K., Boschma, G., & McCuaig, F. (2010). The development of nurse practitioner preparation beyond the masters' level: What is the debate about? *International Journal of Nursing Scholarship*, 7(1), 1–15.

Burman, M. E., Hart, A. M., & McCabe, S. M. (2005). Guest editorial: Doctor of nursing practice: Opportunity amidst chaos. *American Journal of Critical Care*, 14(6), 463–464.

Chism, L. A. (2009). *The doctor of nursing practice: A guidebook for role development and professional issues*. Sudbury, MA: Jones and Bartlett.

Commission on Collegiate Nursing Education. (2005) *Moves to consider for accreditation only practice doctorates with the DNP title*. Retrieved from http://www.aacn.nche.edu/media/NewsReleases/Archives/2005/CCNEDNP.htm

Commission on Collegiate Nursing Education. (2010) *CCNE reaffirms commitment to accrediting all types of master's degrees in nursing programs*. Retrieved from http://www.aacn.nche.edu/accreditation/

Dreher, H. M. (2010). Next steps toward practice knowledge development: An emerging epistemology in nursing. In M. D. Dahnke, & H. M. Dreher, *Philosophy of science for nursing practice: Concepts and application*. New York, NY: Springer.

Dreher, H. M., & Montgomery, K. (2009). Let's call it "Doctoral" advanced practice nursing. *Journal of Continuing Education in Nursing*, 40(12), 530–531.

Fang, D., Tracy, C., & Bednash, G. D. (2010). *2009–2010 Enrollment and graduations in baccalaureate and graduate programs in nursing*. Washington, DC: American Association of Colleges of Nursing.

Fitzsimmons, L., Hadley, S. A., & Shively, M. (1999). The education of advanced practice nurses: A contemporary approach. *Critical Care Nursing Quarterly*, 21(4), 77–86.

Horrocks, S., Anderson, E., & Salisbury, C. (2002). Systematic review of whether nurse practitioners working in primary care can provide equivalent care to doctors. *British Medical Journal*, 324, 819–823.

Institute of Medicine of the Natural Academies. (2001). Crossing *the quality chasm: A new health system for the 21st century*. Retrieved from http://www.iom.edu/reports/2001/crossing-the-quality-chasm-a-new-health-system-for-the-21st-century.aspx

Institute of Medicine of the Natural Academies. (2003). *Health professions education: A bridge to quality*. Washington, DC: National Academies Press.

Little, M. A., & Milliken, P. J. (2007). Practicing what we preach: Balancing teaching and clinical practice competencies. *International Journal of Nursing Education Scholarship*, 4(1), 1–14.

Loomis, J., Willard, B., & Cohen, J. (2007). Difficult professional choices: Deciding between the PhD and the DNP in nursing. *Online Journal Issues in Nursing*, 12(1), 1–16. Retrieved from http://proquest.umi.com.ezproxy2.library.drexel.edu/pqdweb?index=0&did=1737222291&SrchMode=1&sid=1&Fmt=6&VInst=PROD&VType=PQD&RQT=309&VName=PQD&TS=1273105897&clientId=18133

Mundinger, M. (2005). Who's who in nursing: Bringing clarity to the doctor of nursing practice. *Nursing Outlook*, 53, 173–176.

Mundinger, M., Kane, R., Lenz, E., Totten, A., Tsai, W., Cleary, P. et al. (2000). Primary care outcomes in patients treated by nurse practitioners or physicians: A randomized trial. *Journal of the American Medical Association*, 283, 59–68.

National Organization of Nurse Practitioner Faculties. (2006). *Competencies for nurse practitioners: Practice doctorate nurse practitioner entry level competencies*. Retrieved from http://www.nonpf.com/associations/10789/files/DNP%20NP%20competenciesApril2006.pdf

National Research Council of the National Academies. (2005), *Advancing the nation's health needs: NIH research training programs*. Washington, DC: The National Academies Press.

Nichols, E. F., & Chitty, K. K. (2005). Educational patterns in nursing. In K. K. Chitty (ed.), *Professional Nursing: Concepts & Challenges*, (4th ed.) (pp. 31–63). St. Louis, MO: Elsevier Saunders.

Raines, C. F. (2010). *The doctor of nursing practice: A report on progress*. American Association of Colleges of Nursing. Retrieved from http://www.aacn.nche.edu/dnp/pdf/DNPForum3-10.pdf

Robb, W. J. (2005). PhD, DNSc, ND: The ABCs of nursing doctoral degrees. *Dimensions of Critical Care Nursing*, 24, 89–96.

Yox, S. (2005). Clinical doctorate in nursing: A newsmaker interview with Mary O'Neil Mundinger, DrPH. Retrieved from http://70.84.11.146/cmsAdmin/uploads/Yox2005.pdf

Zungolo, E. (2009). *The DNP and the faculty role: Issues and challenges.* Paper presented at the 2nd National Conference on the Doctor of Nursing Practice: The Dialogue Continues..., Hilton Head Island, SC, March 24–27, 2009.

Connie L. Zak

The question of how doctoral-level education versus MS education impacts the role of advanced practice nurses (APNs) is asked by many nursing faculty and APNs nationally. The authors have eloquently presented their own experiences and impetus for pursuing the Doctor of Nursing Practice (DNP). The authors started their discourse with a historical recapitulation of doctoral education in nursing, leading up to the practice doctorate, and going on to give their personal journeys from seasoned practitioner to doctoral student and graduate.

It is important to understand that the inception of a practice doctorate in nursing is not a new concept, but one that has been around for 30 years. Nursing has been debating the need for a practice doctorate for a very long time. Unfortunately, the early practice doctorates, such as the ND (Doctor of Nursing) degree, were not generally accepted. Schools of nursing offering such degrees for nurse practitioners lost students to MS programs and in the end had to phase out such programs.

Subsequently, with the position statement from AACN in 2004 came the era of agreement (for the most part) within the nursing profession of the importance for APNs, and especially nurse practitioners (NPs), to have doctoral education as entry into advanced practice, as noted by the authors (AACN, 2004). This shift in nursing education is timely, given the changes in health care occurring in our nation today, which started with the Institute of Medicine's (IOM) report, outlining the skills needed for improving health care (2001). It is important to highlight that translating research into practice, testing new models of care, and working in transdisciplinary teams, are the essentials of the role of DNP-prepared practitioners. Furthermore, the IOM emphasized the need for all health professions programs to educate students to be able to deliver patient-centered care as members of interdisciplinary teams that emphasize evidence-based practice, quality improvement, and informatics.

It is also important for the reader to understand that the DNP is a degree and not a role. The practice doctorate is not just role oriented, but it is advanced education that gives "added value" to the practitioner to better serve their patients and populations. One must keep in mind the AACN definition of *Advanced Nursing Practice* as conceptualized in the DNP *Essentials* document refers to:

> any form of nursing intervention that influences health care outcomes for individuals or populations, including the direct care of individual patients, management of care for individuals and populations, administration of nursing and health care organizations, and the development and implementation of health policy.
>
> —*AACN, 2006, p. 4*

Although the authors point out that the DNP builds on MSN-level education, it should be understood that the DNP replaces MSN-level education for advanced practice with comprehensive and in-depth knowledge that is necessary to manage the complexities not only for individual patient care, but also for populations and health care systems.

As outlined in Case I, "A Women's Health Nurse Practitioner Who Wanted More," the DNP degree provides the education that practitioners need for responding to the health needs of the nation by being the bridge between research and practice. I would differ in opinion with this author who stated that this degree is for the NP who *wants more*, but I declare it is for the NP who *needs more* to continue to be effective in facing the challenges of taking care of patients in the ever-changing and expanding health care system. This is not to say that MS-prepared APNs are ineffective in their roles, but it is to say that continuing their education to the DNP will allow them to be even more effective, not only in their roles, but also in improving the care they deliver. In doing so, it will be instrumental in changing practice to better serve their patients.

In Case II, "The Oncology Nurse's Story," the author highlights the importance of the DNP-prepared educator. Colleges of Nursing educate practitioners, and what better-prepared faculty is there than the "Practice Expert?" There is a national shortage of qualified nursing faculty that is further contributing to the nursing shortage nationally. The increasing number of DNP programs opening across the nation is one answer to the faculty shortage as it increases the number of faculty who can train nurses at both the entry and advanced levels. I agree with this author that it is very important to choose a DNP program that will fulfill the candidate's future career goals.

Finally, it is important to point out the importance of the DNP-prepared APN as a member of a research team, even as the leader of clinical research endeavors. When it comes to evidence-based practice, it is important to understand that this is not a linear pathway to improving patient care. Rather, it is a circular path that always feeds back into primary research. Without measuring outcomes of evidence-based changes in practice, there is no way to ascertain that such change has actually improved patient care and outcomes. It is imperative that DNP-prepared APNs are able to not only synthesize science, but also to apply it to practice and measure the impact of such change. The question here is, "At what point is the generation of evidence-based practice knowledge considered 'research' and how do they differ?" DNP-prepared practitioners are able to and should be prepared to measure the impact of their practice, whether by measuring the process of a program or practice change or by measuring individual patient outcomes. If this is considered "research," one can comfortably say that it is not primary knowledge generating research, but evidence-based practice that will actually benefit the health care system. Webber (2008) raised an important question regarding the decision of DNP programs not to prepare graduates to be principal investigators of clinical research. She argues that such action "will limit the creation of a broader, more inclusive research environment and thus perpetuates marginalization of research for many faculty, students, and practicing nurses" (p. 466). Webber points out how nurse practitioners rely on medical research to support their practice. She urges the conduct of more practice-focused research based on phenomena unique to the nursing experience which will not happen if DNPs are marginalized from the research enterprise.

In conclusion, the authors have made a very important statement regarding the "added value" that DNP education gives to APNs. With the exciting changes going on in health care today, the road has been paved for DNPs to make their mark by advancing nursing practice, improving health care, and educating the future nursing workforce.

REFERENCES

American Association of Colleges of Nursing (AACN). (2004). *AACN Position Statement on the Practice Doctorate in Nursing October 2004.* Retrieved from http://www.aacn.nche.edu/DNP/pdf/DNP.pdf

American Association of Colleges of Nursing (AACN). (2006). *The essentials of doctoral education for advanced nursing practice.* Washington, DC: Author.

Institute of Medicine. (2001). *Crossing the quality chasm: A new health system for the 21st century.* Washington, DC: National Academies Press.

Webber, P. B. (2008). The doctor of nursing practice degree and research: Are we making an epistemological mistake? *Journal of Nursing Education, 47,* 466–472.

CHAPTER FOUR: Reflective Response 2

David G. O'Dell

INTRODUCTION

Drs. Montgomery and Byrne provided a thoughtful and thought-provoking review of the MSN-prepared Advanced Practice Registered Nurse (APRN) while contrasting it with the DNP-prepared APRN through personal observations, personal experiences, and outcomes they recognize in their respective practices. The history of how we have come to this crossroads of professional development is well articulated, and it must be appreciated in order to advance the discipline of nursing and meet the needs of our patients. It was appropriate and self-reflective to recognize that the MSN-prepared Nurse Practitioner (NP) is content oriented, while the DNP-prepared NP "wants more" in terms of scope and depth of practice. Although some NPs are hesitant to embrace the DNP concept, the time has certainly come for doctorally prepared nurse clinicians to become a larger part of the health care delivery system. The personal experiences and perspectives of both Dr. Montgomery and Dr. Byrne reflect this need for wanting more. Their perspectives are appreciated. I suspect many other DNPs would agree that their paths reflect the personal and professional desires of the DNP-prepared advanced practice nurse.

EDUCATIONAL DISPARITY

These authors also captured a prickly problem that has been the bane of advanced practice nursing, and now doctorally prepared advanced practice nursing. Overly restrictive educational programs designed for the past and not for the future have been a problem, but this is not the essential question to be asked when examining the expectations of doctorally prepared advanced practice nurses. Educational programs have developed and fragmented into many paths to the same degree designation, though the variety of programs is not a reflection of a foundation for doctorally prepared clinical practice. Consider one program that requires 24 semester hours[1] to earn a post-MSN DNP degree, while other post-MSN DNP programs are as high as 54 semester hours.[2] The contrast of rigor and expectations is obvious. Until university deans, department chairs, and the American Association of Colleges of Nurses (AACN) recognize this divergence of requirements, many advanced practice nurses will take the path of least resistance (e.g., seek programs with fewest credit hours) and the general public will have DNPs in practice with a wide range of education and experiences. Is this a safe route for clinicians to take considering the magnitude of our responsibilities? Are we demonstrating true rigor in preparation to take on these roles of advanced practice with the minimum hours or post-master's clinical experiences? All DNPs *are not* alike. It is confusing not only to the consumer and other health care professionals, but to those within our discipline. A DNP designation may not reflect advanced clinical practice. It may demonstrate administrative practice. Also, there are some programs that offer the DNP program in nursing education. I challenge the reader to find a parallel in any other discipline that grants a practice degree as an educator. Is there a Medical Doctor degree in medical education? Is there a Juris Doctorate degree in legal education? I have not found this to be the case. Therefore, are we harming ourselves as a discipline to allow a practice degree to be something other than advanced nursing practice? These are questions that will undoubtedly be debated for many years.

TITLING AND CERTIFICATION

Titling and certification issues also impact how the MSN-prepared NP will be compared to the DNP-prepared advanced practice nurse. Currently, the American Academy of Nurse Practitioners (AANPs) and the American Nurses Credentialing Center (ANCC) are the only nationally recognized certification entities for advanced practice nursing. Will the doctorally prepared NP have a different certification examination in the future? It seems appropriate that this would be the expectation, as the clinical experiences are more advanced than the MSN-prepared nurse clinician. Furthermore, the educational requirements reflect a higher level of practice for all patient populations and systems. Time will tell how certification processes will evolve to reflect a higher expectation of practice to meet the health care needs of our patients. The APRN *Consensus Model for Advanced Practice Registered Nurses* is being debated and aligned to address these very concerns (2008).

The lack of a certification examination reflecting doctorally prepared advanced practice through the AANP and the ANCC bolsters the need and value of the Diplomat in Comprehensive Care certification offered by the American Board of Comprehensive Care. As of this writing, this certification is still controversial, yet does reflect the skills, talents, and expertise of DNP-prepared advanced practice nurses.

RETURN ON INVESTMENT

Perhaps the one key element that has been overlooked in the conversation about doctorally prepared advanced practice is the outcomes and impact on patient care. The information shared by Drs. Montgomery and Byrne reflect a personal perspective of value. This cannot be underestimated, yet how does the consumer appreciate this value? Have we adequately articulated the value of this degree?

I had a fascinating conversation with a retired hospital administrator recently. He was well aware of the DNP degree and what it could be for the discipline of nursing, including the vague definitions of practice that have been the hallmark of nursing practice for decades. His challenging questions were about value. More succinctly he said, "What is the return on investment" of earning this degree? For example, what value can be realized with an MSN-prepared advanced practice nurse over a career in terms of caliber of patient care and quality of lives affected? Compare this to a DNP-prepared advanced practice nurse. Is there an appreciable difference in outcomes? Does the pause in time needed to complete a doctoral degree reflect an increase in productivity or quality? Intuitively, most would say that there is a difference. Is the DNP-prepared advanced practice nurse truly "better?" If so, how is this measured? To date, we are still grappling with this question and are collecting data to demonstrate the value of this degree. A review of DNP conference presentations demonstrates glimpses of doctoral advanced practice scholarship. Have we, as a discipline of professional nurses, articulated to the general public (the consumer of our services) why a DNP-prepared advanced practice nurse is of value? Have our exemplars adequately demonstrated the contributions of DNP-prepared advanced practice nurses? This is a large question that still needs to be answered. I suspect that until the general public recognizes the unique contributions of nurses, at any level of practice, we will not be seen as advanced practice clinicians. Rather, we will continue to be considered extenders of physician practice. That is another discussion—but I encourage the reader to explore the reality of our respective practices as independent, interdependent, and dependent. The doctorally prepared advanced practice nurse brings a higher level of skill and talent to the collective table of clinicians and could (in theory) raise the bar of capabilities for all involved. Can the health care system afford a workforce of exclusively doctorally prepared APRN? I say "How can they afford NOT to afford this level of health care provider?" As discussed by the authors of this and other chapters, restrictive and prescriptive regulations limit the capability of the DNP-prepared advanced practice nurse.

SUMMARY

To paraphrase Dreher (2005), "this train HAS left the station," and it is up to those who have earned the degree to set this locomotive on a productive path. The AACN's *Essentials of Doctoral Education for Advanced Nursing Practice* (2006) provides a description of how to construct this locomotive, yet the path is still to be determined. Doctorally prepared advanced practice nurses have a tremendous challenge ahead of us that includes determining and articulating our contribution to patient care and also, to point out a return on our investment.

NOTES

1. University of Michigan-Flint post-Master's DNP for certified NPs: http://catalog.umflint.edu/preview_program.php?catoid=2&poid=709
2. Baylor University post-master's nurse midwife DNP: http://www.baylor.edu/nursing_grad/index.php?id=56776

REFERENCES

American Association of Colleges of Nursing. (AACN). (2006). *The essentials of doctoral education for advanced nursing practice*. Retrieved from http://www.aacn.nche.edu/DNP/pdf/Essentials.pdf
APRN Consensus Workgroup and NCBSN APRN Advisory Committee. (2008). *Consensus model for Advanced Practice Registered Nurses*. Retrieved from http://www.aacn.nche.edu/Education/pdf/APRNReport.pdf
Dreher, H. M. (2005). The Doctor of Nursing Practice: Has this train left the station? If so, just where is it going? *The Pennsylvania Nurse, 60*, 17, 19.

CHAPTER FOUR: Reflective Response 3

Karen Kaufman

Drs. Montgomery and Byrne provide a thought-provoking analysis of the differences between doctoral-level and master's-level practice roles. The personal stories and experiences they relate are powerful reminders that nurses with practice doctorates, with their advanced knowledge and strong commitment, are making enormous contributions to the nursing field and to health care in general. Most importantly, the authors point to the distinction between the MSN degree, which "allows you to be part of the change," and the Doctor of Nursing Practice (DNP), which equips you "to *be* [sic] the change." In other words, MSNs are qualified to carryout important, necessary changes in the practice of health care, while DNPs are the people with the knowledge and responsibility for actually *driving* that change.

The gulf between these two roles is vast. Our experience working with Drexel DrNP students suggests that no book, seminar, or dissertation is sufficient to transform the DNP/DrNP candidate from a nursing practitioner into a health care *leader*. Indeed, two highly respected Drexel professors, Mary Ellen Smith Glasgow and Vicki D. Lachman (2010) recently documented that at least half of the DrNP candidates in the Drexel DrNP program did not truly see themselves as future leaders, nor did they understand the connection between their unique personality preferences and the role requirements of a leader.

Effecting such a transformation does indeed require advanced knowledge, skills and experiences, and it also requires a significant change in one's self-image—which is the first and most important step in persuading others to see you differently as well. Even the best doctoral programs, because of their academic nature, have difficulty effecting this kind of personal transformation in their students. As a result, most DNPs do graduate with the knowledge to address complex patient care challenges and to improve the efficiency of health care delivery. Where they often have difficulty, though, is in mastering the leadership skills required to enlist others in the effort—to implement real and lasting improvement in the nursing profession and health care in general. In short, to *be* the change—which, after all, is the key reason for obtaining a DNP degree in the first place.

In my years of designing and leading professional development programs, I have noted that doctoral nursing students are not the only ones in need of more comprehensive leadership training, but leadership skills are especially critical in nursing, a field still dominated by women, most of whom have been socialized to cede leadership authority to men. To be sure, male DNPs need leadership skills too, but as more and more women earn DNPs, their ability to lead will have an outsized effect on the profession as a whole—how it is viewed by other health care professionals and by the general public.

I have had the privilege of working with Drexel DrNP students in recent years to enhance their leadership abilities. Like Professors Smith Glasgow and Lachman, I have observed that the typical female student does not see a "disconnect" between her own personality preferences—such as the desire to be liked and avoid confrontation—and the more active role requirements of a leader. Effective leadership depends on a variety of factors, from vision and assembling the right team of people, to the integrity of personal actions and behaviors. However, developing leadership skills has to begin with self-image. We need to think of ourselves as leaders in order to have others see us as leaders.

Impression Management is the term our firm uses to describe the tools for building and expanding the key relationships required to meet complex leadership challenges. It is the art and science of making a favorable, role-appropriate impression on others, both personally and professionally. In our work at Drexel, we discuss and dissect these tools in a classroom setting, but given the relatively small number of students—typically a dozen or so—we are confident that much more could be accomplished one-on-one.

Our preference—and our recommendation for all forward-thinking DNP programs—is to treat DNP candidates as we do our executive coaching clients. To help prepare these students for leadership roles, DNP programs would do well to offer a few individualized sessions in which each candidate is profiled according to his or her unique combination of perceptual, cognitive, behavioral and emotional traits. That analysis can then become the foundation of a customized development plan in which students identify and optimize their strengths while also focusing on areas of weakness.

In other words, DNP programs should adopt a conscious, proactive approach toward transforming nursing practitioners (and other types of DNPs) into health care leaders through detailed analysis and behavioral focus. Such an approach, when consistent with the student's professional goals and advanced knowledge, is the best possible way of transforming nursing practitioners into the leaders that our health care system so urgently needs.

REFERENCE

Smith Glasgow, M. E., & Lachman, V. D. (2010). Impression management: A key leadership skill in DrNP graduates from Drexel University College of Nursing and Health Professions. Poster presentation before the American Association of Colleges of Nursing Doctoral Education Conference, Captiva Island, FL, January 2010.

CRITICAL THINKING QUESTIONS

1. After review of the above chapter, has your individual thoughts or views on the AACN's position to move the level of preparation necessary for advance practice roles from a master's degree to doctoral level as requisite credential for entry into advanced practice nursing changed? Why or why not?
2. If the DNP is mandated by regulatory bodies (Licensure, Accreditation, Certification, and Education), will it be held to the same prescriptive expectations as the masters-prepared ARPN?
3. Is there a need for a standardized, designated title to signify the educational preparation and national credentialing of DNPs? Explain.
4. Do you feel that the DNP degree will support the triad of academia, practice, and research related to the nursing profession? Discuss.
5. Will the DNP degree better prepare nurses to deal with the complexity of patient care environments, expand the knowledge base for practice, initiate and evaluate

evidence-based practice through clinical research, and meet the need for nursing leadership in education and administration beyond that currently found within master's level programs?

6. Can preparation at the DNP level contribute to and sustain the perfect balance between teaching and clinical practice competencies within the nursing profession? In other words, do you feel the DNP may lessen the "theory–practice gap" as discussed by Little and Milliken (2007)?

7. Based on the experience of these two DrNP graduates from the start to the completion of their terminal degree, can you see how the DNP supported a diverse perspective of roles and myriad of opportunities that may have not been otherwise fulfilled with traditional master's-level advanced practice nursing education?

8. Can the health care industry afford a workforce made up of exclusively doctoral-prepared ARPNs (DNPs)? Discuss.

9. The debate on how doctoral level advanced practice nursing roles differ from master's-level advanced practice nursing roles is far from over. What areas of systematic evaluation related to the impact of the DNP on the advanced practice workforce do you see as most pressing?

10. The rationale for the shift in academic preparation of nurses in advanced practice has focused on several issues including how the transition to clinical doctoral preparation for APRNs can be conducted so that master's-prepared APRNs will not be disenfranchised in any way. Based on your knowledge and the information provided within this chapter, can this transition be handled smoothly? How should it proceed?

CHAPTER FIVE

The Role of the Practitioner

Sandra Bellini and Regina M. Cusson

INTRODUCTION

In their 2004 Position Statement, the American Association of Colleges of Nursing (AACN) declared that the future entry-level educational requirement for nurse practitioners (NPs) would be the Doctor of Nursing Practice (DNP) degree. The move has raised many controversies for both currently practicing MS-prepared NPs, as well as NP faculty. Some of the controversies are: (a) whether the DNP is a degree or a role, (b) how DNP-prepared NPs are currently practicing, (c) whether the DNP practice is really different from MS-prepared NP practice, (d) what effect DNP education will have on certification, and (e) whether programs conferring a DNP degree truly are at the doctoral level of scholarship. In this chapter, we explore these issues to date and discuss the potential etiologies for, and resolutions to, many of the issues impacting the future role of the NP.

EVOLVING ACADEMIC PREPARATION FOR THE PRACTITIONER

The academic preparation path for NPs has evolved several times since the initial establishment of the NP role. From early certificate programs, to MS-required preparation, to the more recent 2004 AACN position statement, and elevating future NP entry-level education to the doctoral level, nursing continues to strive for the highest education standards in order to best serve our patients and society. That said, the move to doctoral degree-only preparation for NP education raises many questions, with answers that may remain elusive for some time. As we begin our chapter, we mention as a note to the reader that the term "practitioner" will be used as a broadly inclusive term throughout this chapter, pertaining to traditional APRN roles, not exclusively or specifically to the role of the certified NP.

Among a number of issues to be explored in this chapter, there is one very basic question: What does the DNP degree itself represent? Is it a degree, or is it to be synonymous with a particular advanced nursing role? Since AACN has made this determination, what precisely is different when comparing the current practice of an MS-prepared NP to that of a DNP-prepared NP? What are the potential consequences to our discipline if we move too quickly to close our MS APRN programs? What about the apparent variability in curriculum and foci in DNP programs? Should they all be the same? Do they need to be? Another contentious issue at present is the certification.

When in the educational process should DNPs become certified, in what, and by whom? Does the DNP curriculum prepare graduates to assume full-time academic faculty roles? Finally, this chapter will reexamine the document that got us here: *The Essentials of Doctoral Education for Advanced Nursing Practice* (AACN, 2006); are they fluid enough?

At the present time in our society, with such uncertainty in the economy, an aging population with increasingly diverse health care needs, and the health care system at a breaking point, is this really the moment to undertake such a grand agenda on the part of our profession? Added to these societal issues are other intraprofessional issues that further complicate the picture, such as the nursing shortage, the aging workforce, the nursing faculty shortage, as well as aging faculty soon to retire. Or perhaps at this time in history, with a constellation of such pressing issues, this is exactly the right time.

THE DNP: DEGREE OR ROLE?

Unlike many sweeping changes in education, it is important to remember that the move to the DNP degree for entry into practice for future NPs did not result from poor patient outcomes with NP-managed care. To the contrary, research comparing physician-managed patient outcomes with those of their NP counterparts has demonstrated comparable outcomes (Mundinger et al., 2000; Horrocks, Anderson, & Salisbury, 2002). The decision to elevate the educational requirement for NPs came as a result of a broad consensus among health professions: In order to meet the needs of health care reform, tomorrow's clinicians would need additional skill sets from those currently existing in today's NP programs. Multiple publications by the Institute of Medicine (IOM, 1999, 2001) and the National Research Council of the National Academies (NRCNA) (2005) from earlier this decade highlighted the serious nature of health care quality issues in the United States. These publications also called upon the many health care professions to align their visions and educational processes to produce clinicians with advanced skills and knowledge to address these issues (IOM, 2003). The AACN heeded this call and set about redesigning the role of the NP. This move to DNP education has evidently resonated with many. As of February 2010, a total of 120 DNP programs have been established in 35 states, with reports of an additional 161 programs in the planning stages (AACN, 2010). In fact, in a recent AACN survey of all schools of nursing with APRN programs nationwide, 71.9% are either offering the DNP or plan to do so in the near future (AACN, 2010).

The NP of tomorrow, as articulated by AACN (2006), will need expertise and leadership ability in areas such as quality assessment, outcomes evaluation, evidence-based practice, health policy, systems leadership, and health information technologies—topics identified in the IOM papers—in addition to the current required competencies for NPs. If the goals of health care reform are to be met, the existing research–practice gap, cited as existing for as long as 17 years in some studies, needs to be closed (Balas & Boren, 2000). Important research findings generated at the bench need to be implemented in a far more timely fashion at the bedside. Research findings establish the evidence, upon which clinical practice guidelines are founded. By integrating the most recent research findings into clinical practice and reducing variation in practice, adherence to evidence-based practice guidelines can improve patient outcomes as much as 28% (Heater, Becker, & Olson, 1988). It can be argued that NPs, as frontline care providers, are ideally positioned to contribute toward that goal. Therefore, DNP programs need to have strong emphasis on advancing the evidence base for practice within their curricula.

When discussion of the DNP degree first emerges in conversation, one of the more common controversies that can quickly come to light is whether the DNP is a role or a degree. To be clear, the DNP is a terminal practice degree (AACN, 2006), designated as the required educational level for several advanced nursing practice-registered nurse (APRN) roles as of 2015, including Certified Nurse-Midwife, Certified Registered Nurse Anesthetist, Clinical Nurse Specialist, and Nurse Practitioner (Joint Dialogue Group Report, 2008). That said, the AACN endorses the notion that while all APRNs must be DNPs, not all DNPs will be APRNs. While the DNP will be required for APRN practice, MS-prepared academic nurse educators as well as nurse administrators from practice settings also seek the degree.

The curriculum in DNP programs, as described by the AACN, should focus on advanced nursing practices and issues relevant to advanced nursing practice, and that the process of education should be included only as far as it pertains to patient education. However, the AACN (2006) recommends that DNP programs may offer courses in educational pedagogy beyond the expected courses in the curriculum. This recommendation is also mentioned in the 2006 AACN document for PhD graduates, whose doctoral education focuses on research rather than the process of education. In light of this position by AACN, there has been much debate in academic circles regarding whether the DNP graduate, without additional coursework in education, is prepared to enter the faculty role as an educator.

For NPs prepared with the DNP degree, it would be difficult to argue that they would be unqualified to teach without additional coursework in education, especially if the teaching assignment were to be in corresponding APRN specialty tracks. The rationale for this statement is that, while coursework in educational instruction would undoubtedly be advantageous to the DNP as educator, the reality is that current APRN specialty tracks are frequently taught by MS-prepared APRNs who have not taken such courses. Until this practice changes in the future, it is short sighted to infer that APRNs with the highest educational preparation available are less prepared to teach than their MS-prepared counterparts, who have supported the educational preparation of APRNs with great success for decades.

Conversely, an alternative argument regarding academic preparation and qualifications for teaching various curriculum contents could be raised. Specifically, are DNP graduates who are not APRNs qualified to teach APRN/DNP students? If so, what content is appropriate? What is not? A similar issue may arise in the years to come, as more research-focused faculty obtain BS–PhD degrees that do not include APRN education. Are they qualified to teach APRN/DNP students? Suffice it to say that faculty composition and roles as we know them are likely to change and evolve over the next several years. The allocation of teaching assignments will need to be based on subject matter expertise and the needs of the students. In any event, coursework in the knowledge and process of teaching could benefit all educators, regardless of their specific degree focus, would undoubtedly benefit students, and should therefore be encouraged for all doctoral students.

THE ARRIVAL OF THE DOCTORALLY PREPARED NP: IS IT DIFFERENT FROM THE MS-PREPARED NP?

Now that the first DNP-prepared NPs have arrived in the workforce, who are they, where are they, and what are they doing in these early days? Most importantly, are they practicing any differently than their MS-prepared counterparts? Perhaps, it is too soon to adequately answer this question in light of the small numbers, but we can examine what little evidence is currently available.

In a recent editorial, one new graduate of a DrNP program described ways in which she saw herself as practicing differently than she had as an MS-prepared NP with many years of experience (Dreher & Montgomery, 2009). This "Doctoral Advanced Practice Nurse" articulated a newfound confidence not only in investigating practice issues, but also in the ability to investigate, evaluate, and question the evidence upon which much of clinical practice is founded. Interpreted in another way, these anecdotes speak to larger concepts, such as increased leadership ability and clinical scholarship—concepts articulated in the AACN publications supporting the move to the DNP. These qualities, built upon solid NP education obtained historically at the MS level, combine to give rise to the role and abilities that AACN envisioned for the DNP-prepared NP.

While the literature is quite limited regarding what the first wave of DNP graduates are currently doing in practice, other testimonials from MS-to-DNP graduates have emerged with themes that are remarkably recurrent. In a recent 2010 online article published in the *New England Nursing News* (The DNP: An Emerging Trend), seven DNP graduates and current DNP students relayed similar accomplishments to those cited in the Dreher and Montgomery (2009) article. From the DNP-prepared Chief Nursing Officer to the various NPs from a variety of practice settings, the featured subjects articulated significant perceived benefits from their additional education. The DNPs who were interviewed described increased knowledge regarding evidence-based practice, quality and outcomes evaluation research, systems leadership, the needs of the increasingly complex health care system, and the need to bridge the research–practice gap. Another theme that clearly resonated from the article was that all of the graduates and students felt they now possessed a level of leadership ability to face the challenges of the health care system that they did not previously possess.

To be sure, while the practice setting will certainly be home to the largest numbers of doctorally prepared NPs, the academic setting will also assimilate a portion of these graduates as educators in NP tracks, as members of faculty practice groups, as part of joint appointments bridging the academic and practice settings, and possibly as educators in undergraduate clinical courses. As discussed elsewhere in this chapter, the DNP as educator is a controversial issue because DNP curricula do not include courses in education as part of their core coursework. That said, DNP graduates who obtain elective coursework in educational pedagogy may arguably become quite successful in the academic setting and bring current clinical expertise, advanced educational preparation, and a wealth of experience from the practice setting to the classroom. For those DNP faculty holding joint appointments in order to remain current in the chosen NP specialization area, such an arrangement might be very rewarding. This structure allows the continuation of NP practice and opportunities for involvement in the health care setting at the systems level, as well as the connection to the academic setting. Joint appointments can also provide an opportunity for DNP-prepared NP faculty to make significant contributions to health care organizations in nontraditional ways such as sitting on nursing leadership councils and participating in collaborative translational research studies. Joint appointments can have benefits to the educational setting as well; for example, joint appointments may provide a means to attract experienced NPs with strong devotion to the clinical practice setting to the academic setting, helping alleviate some of the faculty shortage. Perhaps in years to come, joint appointments may become a staple in nursing faculty composition as they have been for decades in medicine.

Perhaps, as time passes and the skill set of DNP graduates becomes clearer, the ability to appreciate the increased leadership skills and clinical scholarship abilities brought to the practice arena by DNP-prepared NPs will erase any lingering resentments toward the degree. After all, the goal for DNP education is to benefit health care institutions and populations of patients by providing NPs with advanced levels of education built upon their core NP education, or to educate the NP of the future—it is not to disenfranchise the NPs of today. The future role of the DNP-prepared NP will likely be oriented toward adding additional areas of expertise to current practice roles and aimed at improving patient outcomes across practice settings. DNPs will also likely lead many organizational-level performance improvement initiatives, take on leadership roles in ensuring best practices based on current evidence, and assume leadership roles in health care legislation and policy at the national level.

The intended scope of practice for DNP-prepared NPs is an issue that needs to be settled, although it is unlikely to be resolved in the near future. A hotly debated topic currently in nursing academic circles is whether the DNP degree will broaden the current scope of practice for NPs, allowing "advanced" NP competencies traditionally held as the purview of physicians, especially in light of calls for "doctoral-level clinical practice." This idea has incited much disagreement and debate among nursing scholars as well as among physicians. In order to lend clarity regarding what is and is not intended regarding scope of practice issues pertaining to the DNP-prepared NP, perhaps the confluence and level of agreement of several documents published by key leading nursing organizations needs to be raised for discussion.

First, there is no evidence put forth by the AACN in any of their documents that the intent of the DNP is to "expand scope of practice" for NPs (AACN, 2004, 2006). In fact, the question is raised and answered unequivocally for all via the AACN website (AACN, 2009a). Aligned with and supported by AACN, neither the APRN Consensus Work Group nor the National Council of State Boards of Nursing APRN Advisory Committee put forth any language supporting expanded scope of practice for NPs in their LACE (licensure, accreditation, certification, and education) document (Joint Dialogue Report, 2008). Finally, there is also no mention of expanding the scope of practice for NPs based on doctoral-level competencies as articulated by the National Organization of Nurse Practitioner Faculties (2006). In contrast, all documents speak to doctoral-level education for APRNs as focusing on the concepts articulated in the *Essentials* documents and aligned with the IOM papers (IOM, 1999, 2001, 2003). These documents seem to identify the need for an APRN provider with a new, unique skill set designed to fill a current need within the health care arena, not necessarily to produce more providers with the skill sets traditionally held by physicians.

Opportunity exists at this time for nursing to say "yes, expand the scope of traditional NP practice," but perhaps not in the manner in which academicians traditionally envision. The notion that "advanced clinical skills" beyond those currently encompassed in NP practice, in light of the content of various relevant publications, although intriguing, seems rather contrary to the intent of the degree and the skill set collectively described by AACN, the National Council of State Boards of Nursing APRN Advisory Committee, and NONPF. For the purposes of clarity, perhaps nursing academics should broaden their application of the word "clinical" to include "things relevant to the practice setting" rather than the single, more traditional use of the term denoting "hands on, individual-level patient management." If the confusion relating to "expanding scope of practice" were to be disavowed, perhaps the lingering resentment of physicians and their opposition to DNP education may also abate. In any case, the domain of DNPs will likely become clearer and less controversial as more DNP-educated practitioners begin to demonstrate their skill set in the health care arena, presenting themselves as credible leaders and collaborative partners with a unique knowledge base rather than as competitors.

CLOSING MS-LEVEL NP PROGRAMS: POTENTIAL PITFALLS

If the 2015 goal cited by AACN (2004, 2006) as the year graduating NPs will be required to have DNP degrees is to be realized, then academic programs currently conferring MS degrees to NP graduates will need to be transitioned prior to that date. In anticipation of this change in degree preparation, many schools of nursing are revising existing curriculum plans, while others have already opened "BS-DNP" programs. While certainly these are positive steps toward reaching the 2015 goal, perhaps it would be prudent to examine some of the potential problems to the nursing workforce and to society if, in fact, all current MS-APRN programs were to close within the next 5 years. Closure of all MS-APRN programs anytime soon, however, seems unlikely in light of the fact that some APRN specialty groups, such as Nurse Anesthetists have opted to delay the 2015 deadline to 2025.

Today, our discipline has its roots firmly established in the academic setting, with nursing now recognized as a scholarly profession rather than as an "apprenticeship" occupation as it was in past decades. This accomplishment was not easily won, however, and this latest move to elevate academic requirements for NPs also will not come easily. Nursing, as a discipline, has a responsibility toward society to care for the sick and to promote wellness in the larger society. In light of current needs, is this really the appropriate time to advance this agenda? What will be the impact to society, to the current nursing workforce, and to the faculty workforce?

It is common knowledge in the United States that there remains a long-standing shortage of registered nurses (RNs). Currently, published reports indicate a lessening in the workforce deficiency, probably influenced by the recession (Buerhaus, Auerbach, & Staiger, 2009). While this is good news, it is unlikely to be sustained. For example, nurses who have traditionally worked part time have increased their work hours in light of the economy; nurses who had retired early have returned to the workforce; and other nurses may now be working more than one job. When the economy eases and financial burdens lessen, these nurses may not continue employment at their current levels.

The recovery from the recession aside, several other factors indicate that the RN shortage will continue to be a pressing issue for many years to come. Considering the aging of the RN workforce, with some estimates placing the average RN's age at 46.8 years (Health Resources Service Administration, 2004), the aging population in the United States will increase the demand for nurses. Other professional issues, such as burnout among nurses resulting from understaffing and perceived unrealistic expectations on the part of employers, may cause them to choose to leave the profession (Buerhaus, 2005). For the foreseeable future, it is likely that the nursing shortage will continue.

At the NP level, shortages exist and are predicted to worsen, especially in certain specialty areas, such as the national shortage of primary care providers (Pho, 2008) increasing the demand for Primary Care Nurse Practitioners (Stanik-Hutt, 2008a), the Acute Care Nurse Practitioner (Howie-Esquivel & Fontaine, 2006), and the Neonatal Nurse Practitioner (Cusson et al., 2008). While some of these shortages result from small numbers of students within and entering existing programs, the larger issue is anticipated increased demand for NPs in these areas.

As a shortage of NPs in these areas exists, what impact will the move to the DNP have on the existing shortage? Will the added time commitment for graduate education, and therefore added expense, combine to act as a deterrent to RNs considering advanced degrees? If so, what impact will this direction have upon schools of nursing if the number of applicants were to fall significantly? What will be the effect of smaller numbers of APRNs to society? For all of these reasons, some would argue that the DNP degree should remain an option rather than a requirement for advanced nursing practice at least for the foreseeable future. With some educators feeling that preparing the post-BS student as an APRN while concurrently attaining the competencies expected of the DNP-prepared NP is perhaps too much, it might give one pause to consider a possible compromise. Perhaps consideration should be given to the possibility of continuing MS-level APRN preparation for initial certification and licensure, with subsequent renewals requiring a DNP degree, which the APRN could earn while practicing and gaining expertise? Would this potential solution meet the needs of all parties? It might, but at least for now it appears that the 2015 plan for DNP entry into APRN practice remains in place despite concerns regarding shortages of NPs.

Another contributing factor to the nursing shortage is the current faculty shortage. Despite the need for more nurses in the workforce and an increased number of qualified applicants to nursing programs, in the 2008 academic year 49,948 qualified applicants were denied admission to baccalaureate and graduate nursing programs due to an insufficient number of faculty and other resources (AACN, 2009b). The underlying reasons for a shortage of faculty include an aging faculty with a significant number retiring within the next decade, the static number of students applying to research-focused degree programs anticipating an academic career, and a lack of competitive salaries offered by academic settings compared to those in the practice setting (AACN, 2009c). Solutions to these problems remain elusive for now, although creative alternatives to classroom teaching—such as increases in online options, especially in specialty-track NP programs requiring specialty-area NP faculty who are not in abundant supply—is one solution currently in use (Bruce, 2007). Another potential suggestion to ameliorate the effects of the faculty shortage would be to encourage post-MS certificates in educational pedagogy, particularly among DNP students and graduates, to ensure a supply of knowledgeable teachers in nursing as articulated by National League for Nursing (2007).

VARIABILITY AMONG DNP PROGRAMS: TO WHAT EXTENT ARE DNP PROGRAMS PRODUCING CLINICIANS WHO ARE DISTINCTLY DIFFERENT FROM MS-PREPARED NPs?

Now that many programs are conferring DNP degrees, what makes them "doctoral-level" rather than "master's-plus?" Undoubtedly, there are programs today that fall into both of these categories. In light of the "credit-creep" rationale mentioned by AACN as part of the reason for the move to the DNP, some programs may have simply added several courses to their current MS-level curriculum to address the DNP *Essentials* and competencies and retitled the degree as a "Doctorate," while philosophically retaining the notion the DNP programs are really "master's-plus" (AACN, 2006). Other programs have embraced the idea that a doctorate degree denotes academic expectations well beyond those expected at the master's level and have designed a truly doctoral-level curriculum. Perhaps this philosophical difference of opinion is more important than we think, and if resolved, might result in programs with more consistent levels of expectation.

The case for and against PhD-style educational rigor in DNP programs has been discussed in the literature (Sheriff & Chaney, 2007), and while both sides of the issue present strong arguments, we would have to make our decision based on a traditional risk–benefit ratio. While the level rigor of DNP programs as perceived by some might not *necessitate* a level consistent with what is expected in a PhD program, the outcomes may offer significant benefits in terms of valuable learning experiences consistent with clinical scholarship and development of leadership abilities, thereby establishing the DNP as a truly learned individual, respected in the academic setting and valuable in the practice setting. Conversely, the question that must be considered is: What is the perceived risk of traditional doctoral-level scholarship if offered to DNP students? It could hardly be argued that DNP students graduating from such rigorous programs would be considered "too scholarly"; therefore, we take the position that expected level of scholarship should be equitable, but with a distinctly different focus.

Important points to consider in this distinction are competencies to be achieved at the DNP level as designated by both AACN (2006) in their *Essentials* document and NONPF (2006). Competencies articulated by both organizations are distinctly different for MS-level programs and for DNP-level programs. Simply stated, MS-level competencies address the expectations for patient care management at the traditional APRN level, while DNP entry-level competencies speak to additional areas of expected expertise having to do with quality assessment, practice inquiry, policy, and leadership (NONPF, 2006). Perhaps going forward, BS-DNP programs might consider various curriculum design schemes whereby mastery of APRN competencies might be attained early in the program, allowing for leadership competencies to be acquired via DNP coursework later in the program. An example of this curricular structure may offer all "traditional," MS-level APRN specialty-focused content within the first two years of the program, while the latter years of study would be devoted to the DNP-level competencies such as systems perspectives, populations and quality focus, the development of clinical scholarship, and leadership skills. True leadership experience may be gained through an immersion experience at the DNP residency level. It is difficult to imagine that mastery of skills at the traditional APRN level could be attained at the same time that leadership expertise within that role is gained. Generally, leadership follows mastery, and to expect concurrent attainment of both sets of skills may be unrealistic.

THE CONCEPT OF SCHOLARSHIP AND THE DNP *ESSENTIALS*

When the AACN issued their Position Statement on the DNP in 2004 and later published the DNP *Essentials* in 2006, the intent was likely to articulate and define their vision of both DNP education, as well as their intent for the DNP role that would follow. Their publications were to serve as a guiding light for nursing programs throughout the nation to establish and refine their DNP programs. In all of the AACN's well-intended and truly inspired documents, however, there may in fact have been a lost opportunity to very clearly state for posterity what the expected level of "scholarship" for DNP programs was intended to be, at least as seen in 2006.

For example, while there are many references to Boyer's model of *Scholarship* (Boyer, 1990) throughout the *Essentials* document (2006) that clearly spoke to research-focused programs such as "Scholarship of Discovery" and practice-focused programs such as "Scholarship of Application," there appears only a brief sentence regarding the final "project" for the DNP degree, which may in fact be at the root of some of the variation in levels of expected scholarship seen today in DNP programs. For the sake of clarity, while there has been much discussion and debate over the last several years regarding the appropriate level of "rigor" for DNP programs, including elsewhere in this chapter, we would like to propose an alternative parameter to evaluate DNP programs, specifically scholarship rather than rigor. As rigor tends to be synonymous with traditional research methodology, scholarship is a broader concept which may actually lend some clarity to our current dilemma.

AACN (2006) says "For practice doctorates, requiring a dissertation or other original research is contrary to the intent of the DNP" (p. 20). The paragraph goes on to offer alternative suggestions that the final project may take. While it can be inferred that the intent was to guide and clarify, it may be that this statement and this entire section of the document have contributed toward much of the resultant confusion. Is it possible that, in an attempt to define and offer guidance, instead conclusions were drawn based on literal interpretation and expected levels of scholarship restricted from further evolution?

While many agree that research dissertations should be the "gold-standard" outcome measure for programs focused on scholarship of discovery, perhaps it was too soon for the AACN to seek to define the gold-standard outcome measure for programs focused on scholarship of application. Perhaps in an attempt to articulate minimum standards, the statements in the *Essentials* document were interpreted as predetermined, confining limits. After all, is there a valid reason that DNP students should be denied the opportunity to demonstrate the level of scholarship traditionally expected at the doctoral level, an original dissertation, with a focus on clinical practice? Is there a drawback to allowing true clinical scholars to develop and emerge from DNP programs? What about the dissemination of scholarly works? Dissertations are indexed in databases, "projects" are not. Therefore, the scholarly contributions of DNP graduates will be invisible, if not accessible from databases.

In other disciplines with practice doctorates, such as psychology, graduates write a dissertation, but again the focus is on clinical practice rather than traditional research. Can nursing, also a practice discipline, consider this as a viable alternative? In this way, DNP students could have the "Clinical Practice Dissertation" (CPD) as their summative, scholarly work. Structural development for a CPD is similar to that of a research dissertation, with the exception of the section on methodology. Methodology for a CPD arguably can and should be different than that of the traditional research-focused dissertation. Appropriate alternative methodologies to consider for the CPD include quality improvement and evidence-based practice change strategies—commonly used in clinical practice settings and intended to "apply" existing, previously "discovered" science to answer the question: "How can I use this body of knowledge to improve patient outcomes?" For faculty still struggling with issues such as defining the expected level of "rigor" for DNP students, perhaps establishing the CPD as the scholarly outcome measure, and then designing a curriculum to support that mission, would lend clarity. Otherwise, the danger to nursing is that DNP graduates may be seen as a certain number of points less scholarly than their PhD counterparts as a matter of course. This would almost ensure that DNP faculty are never truly integrated into the academic setting as equals among scholars of various disciplines, a concern that has been raised in the literature (Dreher, Donnelly, & Naremore, 2005). One could assume that there is little to be gained for nursing in that case.

The other potentially limiting word in the AACN's *Essentials* document (2006) is "original." Again, is there a drawback to allowing, or even requiring DNP students to design, implement, and evaluate an original scholarly work in the form of applied science, again answering the question as to how existing evidence might be implemented in clinical practice to improve patient outcomes? Rather, can it be argued that as the role expectations for DNP-prepared NPs have evolved, and leadership ability as well as clinical acumen have been further emphasized as necessary skills, would it be advantageous to the student to develop these necessary leadership skills as part of their education program, while supported by faculty mentors? Examples of applied-science DNP projects and CPD of recent graduates from one DNP program educated in this manner include: *Implementation of a Skin Cancer Screening Tool in a Primary Care Setting: A Pilot Study; Heparinized vs. Normal Saline for Maintenance of IV Access: An Evidence-Based Practice Change Initiative; and Evidence-Based Sickle Cell Pain Management in the Emergency Department* (University of Connecticut, 2010). Publications have spoken to the need for strong leadership skills for NPs as both care providers and as patient advocates (Edmunds, 2008). If DNP-prepared NPs are expected to embody these skills, they need to be prepared as students to do so. True doctoral-level scholarship expectations will prepare them for that.

DO WE NEED ADDITIONAL CERTIFICATION TO INDICATE "DOCTORAL ADVANCED PRACTICE NURSING"?

Another controversial area concerning NP certification and the DNP degree is certification. When in the educational process should NPs be allowed to sit for initial certification in their specialty area? Historically, NPs have been eligible to sit for certification following successful completion of their APRN programs, having achieved an MS degree. As NP education moves to the doctoral level, assuming the 2015 goal is realized, the APRN Consensus Work Group and the National Council of State Boards of Nursing APRN Joint Dialogue Group Report (2008) will serve as guides for current graduate programs to align their plans for licensure, accreditation, certification, and education. Endorsed by AACN, NONPF, and many other nursing specialty organizations, the Joint Dialogue Group Report stipulates that as of 2015, a DNP will be required to sit for NP certification exams. Further, while all NP programs will produce graduates with DNP competencies, the specialty-specific NP competencies tested in track-specific certification exams will continue to be developed by the specialty-practice organization (APRN Joint Dialogue Report). In other words, while additional competencies will be expected of DNP graduates, the "specialty competencies" will probably remain as they are, with the exams requiring a DNP rather than an MS. In light of the fact that research has demonstrated that outcomes of care delivered by NPs currently holding MS degrees is at least equivalent to those of MDs (Mundinger et al., 2000; Horrocks et al., 2002), this rationale is appropriate.

The approach taken by the APRN Joint Dialogue Report group, the National Council of State Boards of Nursing, AACN, NONPF, and many other nursing organizations seems to indicate a clear path and commonality of purpose. While evidently intended to serve as the collective voice of authority in speaking to the uncertainties of a profession moving forward, not all prominent leaders in nursing agree with the content areas anticipated for future DNP certification exams. For example, some schools of nursing, in conjunction with the Council for the Advancement of Comprehensive Care (CACC), have endorsed the notion that DNP-prepared NPs should sit for certification exams as "Diplomats in Comprehensive Care" (Mundinger, 2008) via an exam prepared and administered by the National Board of Medical Examiners. The CACC has made the argument that the intent of having NPs sit for and successfully pass an exam very similar in content to the exam taken to license MDs is to "assure the public of quality and reliable standards for these new clinical nurse experts" (Mundinger, 2008, p. 4), or the DNP-prepared NP. This position has raised the ire of the American Medical Association, as well as many within nursing. If the underlying assumption for this certification exam is that without it, the "assurance of quality to the public" (Mundinger, 2008, p. 4) would be in question, the idea seems inconsistent with previous research findings (Mundinger et al., 2000; Horrocks et al., 2002), which have shown that NPs (most with MS preparation) and MDs provide equivalent care. While still popular in some circles, the idea that DNP-prepared NPs would be designated by this additional certification has been "debunked" in a 2008 statement from the American Academy of Nurse Practitioners as unnecessary and potentially disenfranchising to the large numbers of MS-prepared NPs in the workforce (Stanik-Hutt, 2008a,b). For the foreseeable future at least, the matter remains unresolved.

THE *ESSENTIALS*: STILL RELEVANT?

The AACN *Essentials* were published following tremendous effort on the part of the DNP Essentials Task Force in 2006. They have served as the foundation upon which all DNP programs have been developed and by whose criteria today's programs are accredited. But are they still current? Are they fluid enough to be adapted in the ever-changing climates of health care and higher education?

What about the decision by the AACN not to recognize ethics as an *Essential* unto itself (it was previously Essential #3 in the last 1996 AACN's *Essentials of Master's Education for Advanced Nursing Practice* which is also currently in revision)? If, in fact, DNP programs include ethical issues at the advanced practice level that are threaded throughout the curriculum and include topics considered nontraditional for clinicians, then this may be a solid decision on their part. While it is imperative to include traditional ethics content for clinicians, such as ethical treatment of patients, it would also be pertinent to include ethics related to participation in research, business ethics, and the role of ethical principles such as "justice" as it relates to health care economics and reform. Topics such as these are important to include, as the DNP graduate is expected to bring a higher, broader level of understanding of the complexity of issues and leadership to the practice setting. If, however, ethics are not truly being incorporated in the light of competing priorities, perhaps the decision not to recognize ethics as a separate *Essential* was not a wise one.

Opinions on these controversies concerning the *Essentials* may vary. What *is* evident, however, is that the content areas addressed in the *Essentials* (e.g., health policy, leadership, quality, advocacy) are still very much relevant. Indeed, they dominate the national news media and inspire national debate. Rather than asking are the *Essentials* fluid enough, perhaps what nursing needs to ask is: "As a discipline, are we creative enough to envision what the *Essentials* do not say?" Myopia is a dangerous condition, regardless of its context.

SUMMARY

The move to require a DNP for entry into NP practice by 2015 has raised many controversies. Among the controversies are: whether the DNP is a degree or a role, how DNP-prepared NPs are currently practicing, whether DNP practice really is different from MS-prepared NP practice, what effect DNP education will have on certification, and whether programs conferring a DNP degree truly are at the doctoral level of scholarship. In this chapter, we have explored these issues to date. As with the rest of the nursing profession, we anxiously await the arrival of large numbers of DNP-NPs (and other DNP-APRNs) for the future. What will be their contribution to health care, to patient outcomes, to faculty roles, and to nursing? While this remains to be seen to a large extent, the potential impact of the DNP-Practitioner role is very promising indeed.

REFERENCES

American Association of Colleges of Nursing. (AACN). (1996). *The Essentials of Master's Education for Advanced Nursing Practice*. Washington, DC: Author.

American Association of Colleges of Nursing. (AACN). (2004). *AACN position statement on the practice doctorate in nursing*. Washington, DC: Author.

American Association of Colleges of Nursing. (AACN). (2006). *The essentials of doctoral education for advanced nursing practice*. Washington, DC: Author.

American Association of Colleges of Nursing. (AACN). (2009a). *DNP frequently asked questions*. Retrieved from: http://www.aacn.nche.edu/DNP/pdf/faq

American Association of Colleges of Nursing. (AACN). (2009b). *2008–2009 Enrollment and graduations in baccalaureate and graduate programs in nursing*. Washington, DC: Author.

American Association of Colleges of Nursing. (AACN). (2009c). *Special survey on vacant faculty positions*. Washington, DC: Author.

American Association of Colleges of Nursing. (AACN). (2010). *Amid calls for more highly educated nurses, new AACN data show impressive growth in doctoral nursing programs*. Washington, DC: Author.

APRN Joint Dialogue Group Report. (2008). *Consensus model for APRN regulation: Licensure, accreditation, certification & education*. Consensus Work Group & the National Council of State Boards of Nursing APRN Advisory Committee.

Balas, E. A., & Boren, S. A. (2000). *Managing clinical knowledge for health care improvement*. Yearbook of Medical Informatics, 65–70.

Boyer, E. L. (1990). *Scholarship reconsidered: Priorities of the professoriate*. Princeton, NJ: Carnegie Foundation for the Advancement of Teaching.

Bruce, T. J. (2007). Online tutors as a solution to the shortage of nurse practitioner educators. *Nurse Educator, 32*(3), 122–125.

Buerhaus, P. (2005). Six-part series on the state of the RN workforce in the United States. *Nursing Economics, 23*(2), 58–61.

Buerhaus, P., Auerbach, D. I., & Staiger, D. O. (2009). The recent surge in nurse employment: Causes and implications. *Health Affairs ~ Web Exclusive, 28*(4), w657–w668. Doi:10.1377/hlthaff.28.4.w657.

Cusson, R. M., Buus-Frank, M. E., Flanagan, V. A., Miller, S., Zukowsky, K., & Rasmusssen, L. (2008). A survey of the current neonatal nurse practitioner workforce. *Journal of Perinatology, 28*, 830–836.

Dreher, H. M., Donnelly, G., & Naremore, R. (2005). Reflections on the DNP and an alternate practice doctorate model: The Drexel DrNP. *Online Journal of Issues in Nursing, 11*(1). Retrieved from: http://nursingworld.org/MainMenuCategories/ANAMarketplace/ANAPeriodicals/OJIN/TableofContents/Volume112006/No1Jan06/ArticlePreviousTopic/tpc28_716031.aspx

Dreher, H. M., & Montgomery, K. (2009). Let's call it "Doctoral" advanced practice nursing. *The Journal of Continuing Education in Nursing, 40*(12), 530–531.

Edmunds, M. (2008). Nurse practitioners' responsibility to resolve health disparity. *The Journal for Nurse Practitioners, 4*(10), 738. Doi:10.1016/j.nurpra.2008.09.010.

Heater, B., Becker, A., & Olson, R. (1988). Nursing interventions and patients outcomes: A meta-analysis of studies. *Nursing Research, 37*, 303–307.

Horrocks, S., Anderson, E., & Salisbury, C. (2002). Systematic review of whether nurse practitioners working in primary care can provide equivalent care to doctors. *British Medical Journal, 324,* 819–823.

Howie-Esquivel, J., & Fontaine, D. (2006). The evolving role of the acute care nurse practitioner in critical care. *Current Opinion in Critical Care, 12,* 609–613.

Health Resources and Services Administration. (2004). *The registered nurse population: Findings from the March 2004 National Sample Survey of Registered Nurses.* Washington, DC: Department of Health and Human Services.

Institute of Medicine. (1999). *To err is human: Building a safer health system.* Washington, DC: National Academies Press.

Institute of Medicine. (2001). *Crossing the quality chasm: A new health system for the 21st century.* Washington, DC: National Academies Press.

Institute of Medicine. (2003). *Health professions education: A bridge to quality.* Washington, DC: National Academies Press.

Mundinger, M. (2008). Certification is the answer: What is the question? *Clinical Scholars Review, 1*(1), 3–4.

Mundinger, M., Kane, R., Lenz, E., Totten, A., Tsai, W.-Y, Cleary, P. et al. (2000). Primary care outcomes in patients treated by nurse practitioners or physicians: A randomized controlled trial. *Journal of the American Medical Association, 283*(1), 59–68.

National League for Nursing. (2007). Reflection and dialogue: Doctor of nursing practice. Retrieved from: http://www.nln.org/aboutnln/reflection_dialogue/refl_dial_1.htm

National Organization of Nurse Practitioner Faculties. (2006). *Practice doctorate nurse practitioner entry-level competencies.* Washington, DC: Author.

National Research Council of the National Academies. (2005). *Advancing the nation's health needs: NIH research training programs.* Washington, DC: National Academies Press.

Pho, K. (2008, March 13). Shortage of primary care threatens health system. *USA Today,* pp. A.11.

Sheriff, S., & Chaney, S. (2007). Should DNP programs follow the same rigorous coursework as PhD programs? *The Journal for Nurse Practitioners, 3*(10), 704–705.

Stanik-Hutt, J. (2008a). Who will provide primary health care? Nurse practitioners. *USA Today Forum.* March 27. Retrieved from http://www.acnpweb.org/files/public/USA_Today_Primary_Care_03-27-08.pdf

Stanik-Hutt, J. (2008b). Debunking the need to certify the DNP degree. *The Journal for Nurse Practitioners, 4*(10), 739.

New England Nursing News. (2010). *The DNP: An emerging trend: Doctor of Nursing Practice graduates and students share why they chose to pursue a DNP and how it has influenced their careers.* Retrieved from: http://news.nurse.com/article/20100111/NE01/101110008

University of Connecticut. (2010). DNP Abstract Titles. Retrieved from http://nursing.uconn.edu/index.php?option=com_content&task=view&id=307&Itemid=562

CHAPTER FIVE: Reflective Response

Lucy N. Marion

In Chapter 5, *The Role of the Practitioner*, the authors presented a lively and interesting discussion primarily concerning the debate within the profession about Doctorate of Nursing Practice (DNP) educational issues. These issues include the DNP role versus the degree, the future of the Master of Science (MS) versus DNP practice degrees and respective levels of practice, the level of rigor versus scholarship also related to the DNP practice project versus the DNP dissertation, and traditional certification within the DNP and certification at the end of the program. The authors also addressed the scope of practice changes and qualifications to teach in nursing education programs.

After reading the chapter, I revisited three publications describing the new DNP and the issues we faced or expected to face over the next few years (Marion et al., 2003; Marion, O'Sullivan, Crabtree, Price, & Fontana, 2005; O'Sullivan, Carter, Marion, Pohl, & Werner, 2005). These publications were written by National Organization of Nurse Practitioner Faculties (NONPF) Board members during very exciting times when NONPF, along with other organizations, took much of the early leadership in defining DNP/NP parameters (NONPF, 2004). Later, serving on the NONPF DNP Task Force, we provided leadership of national forums, creation and implementation of DNP teleweb conferences, and early writing of DNP/NP competencies. I was honored to represent NONPF on the first American Association of Colleges of Nursing (AACN) DNP Task Force, with Dr. Elizabeth Lenz as Chair, and on the Council for the Advancement of Comprehensive Care (CACC), with Dr. Mary Mundinger as Chair (AACN, 2004). In 2005, I shepherded the development of the first DNP program in Georgia at the Medical College of Georgia and over time served as consultant to several DNP planning committees across the nation. Reading Chapter 5 reminded me of those "all-day" and "late-night" discussions. Indeed, Chapter 5 validated our vision for anticipated struggles and our trust in future leadership to tackle issues as they arose.

Although the authors cited the AACN as being largely responsible for decisions and troubling unresolved issues, a much larger group of organizational and individual participants were active in causing the DNP to become a mainstream rather than a "fringe" degree. Societal forces such as complexity of health care, changing demographics, increased education and degrees in other health professions, and the rapidly emerging need for nurse practitioners (NPs) to provide much of the nation's primary care, set the stage for change in advance practice nursing education. Many forces came together to cause the stampede to create DNP programs, growing in number from 4 in 2000 to 120 in 2010 and 161 more in progress (AACN, 2010). In spite of the cries of folly (Dracup, Cronenwett, Melies, & Benner, 2005) and worries caused by the DNP, many issues have been resolved: the accreditation process is complete, the number of

PhD students has increased instead of the feared decrease, and DNP graduates do get jobs or advance in their current positions. We may have reached the tipping point after just 10 years, with more doctoral-level nursing programs initiating DNP programs and exploring how to maximize the DNP contribution to health care improvement through practice, research, and education (AACN, 2009). Of the several important and well-documented DNP issues addressed, I will target methodological rigor, differences in practice capability with MS and DNP programs, the potential of DNPs as educators, and the closing of MS APRN programs.

In my opinion, the appropriate level of methodological rigor is the most challenging question in DNP education today. If we were using other health care professions (other than psychology) as the model, there would be little debate. Medicine, dentistry, pharmacy, and others do not debate this issue. Their faculty includes applied research methodologies in the curricula as a foundation for evidence-based health care, and many require a scholarly project. Many disciplines have the option of a dual practice/research (PhD) degree for more basic research with a dissertation. Nursing, on the other hand, has had challenges with its practice doctorates. Early efforts in creating a Doctorate of Nursing Science and other such non-PhD nursing degrees resulted in PhD look-alikes (AACN, 2009). The Nursing Doctorate (ND) did not flourish. Could this reticence to embrace a nursing practice doctorate result from the strength of the PhD in Nursing Science and perceived lack of prestige or usefulness of scholarship of other doctorates? Do we impose the PhD model on every ND, regardless of intent? The authors of Chapter 5 suggested a "Clinical Practice Dissertation." They make good points, that is, dissertations are disseminated through official channels and DNP projects are not; so many excellent projects are not available to the public. Another interesting facet of this issue is the NIH (National Institutes of Health) goal of advancing translational, implementation, and dissemination science. Can our DNP programs prepare the learner to conduct these types of research? Write the grants? Time will tell, but DNP students and graduates can further develop their expertise in research through joint and dual degrees, post-doctoral research fellowships, and research team membership. In my opinion, the DNP is the degree for improving practice and patient outcomes through evidence-based practice change, and a dissertation with PhD-level methodological rigor will detract from the primary purpose.

In the early years of the previous decade, open forums with advanced practice nurses and faculty about the viability and usefulness of the DNP revealed participant themes (Fontaine, Stotts, Saxe, & Scott, 2008). We heard the need for synthesis of content, more evidence-based practice, and more genomics, ethics, informatics, cutting-edge pharmacology, systems leadership, and so on. Strong themes were later incorporated in AACN *Essentials* (2006) and NONPF competencies. The few indicators we have suggested are that DNP practice is different from the MS, as would be expected— albeit mostly in the systems arena. However, the authors use the Mundinger study comparing NP and physician care as the evidence for quality of MS-educated nurses (Mundinger et al., 2000). I wonder about the validity of this finding of equivalent care of MD and MS NP, and the more recent study of veteran satisfaction with NPs more than with MDs (Budzi, Singh, & Hooker, 2010) in light of the question: Is DNP practice better than/different from MS practice? Specifying this comparative effectiveness issue and determining the questions and analyses to answer the effectiveness questions will require a complex design and methods.

Doctorally prepared nurses are relatively rare, and with the current faculty shortage, they are welcome in most educational settings (AACN, 2006). The question of whether the DNP graduate is qualified to teach is argued relative to the quality teaching by MS clinicians, but the real argument is whether anyone can or should teach without meeting minimal expectations in formal learning to be an educator. The authors describe how DNP programs could add education courses to the curriculum. Most often, the clinician is employed without preparation in pedagogy and curriculum, and the nursing program then is held accountable for extensive faculty orientation and development to ensure quality teaching. This is a monumental problem in nursing education—especially in that clinical faculty members may decide that the educational work environment is not a match for them and return to the clinical setting after extensive faculty development efforts. The question of *WHO* is qualified to teach DNP students is interesting. Overall, many nursing programs generally accept that credentialed professionals with requisite skills and teaching ability can teach selected components of the curriculum to any level of nursing students. Interprofessional learning is a goal for many health science centers if not already there. For example, a physician's assistant who performs a screening test or treatment proficiently several times each day should be considered qualified to teach that skill to an NP student. Similarly, a DNP/NP faculty member should be able to teach health assessment to medical students. On the other hand, a DNP faculty member is not usually expected to teach all components of the entire DNP curriculum because of the wide range of topics. Of course, nursing programs must stay within the limits of accreditation standards, most of which are not yet evidence based, but are the product of collective wisdom of educators and will likely change as we gather more data on process and outcomes.

Finally, the authors discussed the closing of MS APRN programs by the AACN sanctioned date of 2015. This aspiration will not be reached because there is a growing demand for primary care APRNs in the face of health care reform; nursing anesthesia programs have a different time frame for closure, and many smaller programs cannot accommodate this time frame and are not sure they want to. It will take years to mandate this requirement in state law, and accreditation and certification bodies are not obligated to follow the AACN membership vote. With the serious budget shortfalls for many nursing programs in the current financial climate, nursing administrators are fearful that closing traditional MS APRN programs will cause further loss of income (AACN, 2009). However, sufficient numbers of programs will achieve the goal of DNP as entry to APRN practice to guide others in the transition. Some creative partnership models have already emerged and more will follow (AACN, 2006). The unintended negative consequence of program conversion from MS to DNP is that the students may not have access to a fully qualified, doctorally prepared faculty to teach at the DNP level. An unintended positive consequence could be that large, efficient interprofessional coalitions are created to teach more students with better-prepared faculty. The authors of Chapter 5 have courageously undertaken topics that are still controversial and have provided reasonable questions or solutions. My comments are a reflection of my perspectives and are intended to complement the work to date.

REFERENCES

American Association of Colleges of Nursing (AACN). (2004). *AACN position statement on the practice doctorate in nursing.* Retrieved from http://www.aacn.nche.edu/dnp/pdf/dnp.pdf
American Association of Colleges of Nursing (AACN). (2006). *The essentials of doctoral education for advanced nursing practice.* Retrieved from http://www.aacn.nche.edu/dnp/pdf/essentials.pdf

American Association of Colleges of Nursing (AACN). (2009). *Annual report: Advancing higher education in nursing*. Washington, DC. Retrieved from http://www.aacn.nche.edu/media/pdf/AnnualReport09.pdf

American Association of Colleges of Nursing (AACN). (2010). *Fact Sheet: The Doctor of Nursing Practice (DNP)*. Retrieved from http://www.aacn.nche.edu/Media/FactSheets/dnp.htm

Budzi, D., Singh, K., & Hooker, R. (2010). Veterans' perceptions of care by nurse practitioners, physician assistants, and physicians: A comparison from satisfaction surveys. *Journal of the American Academy of Nurse Practitioners, 22*, 170–176.

Dracup, K., Cronenwett, L., Meleis, A., & Benner, P. (2005). Reflections on the doctorate of nursing practice. *Nursing Outlook, 53*(4), 177–182.

Fontaine, D., Stotts, N., Saxe, J., & Scott, M. (2008). Shared faculty governance: A decision-making framework for evaluating the DNP. *Nursing Outlook, 56*, 167–173.

Marion, L., O'Sullivan, A., Crabtree, K., Price, M., & Fontana, S. (2005). Curriculum models for the practice doctorate in nursing. *Topics in Advanced Practice Nursing eJournal, 5*(1). Retrieved from http://www.medscape.com/viewarticle/500742

Marion, L, Viens, D., O'Sullivan, A. L., Crabtree, K., Fontana, S., & Price, M. M. (2003). The practice doctorate in nursing: Future or fringe? *Topics in Advanced Practice Nursing eJournal, 3*(2). Retrieved from http://www.medscape.com/viewarticle/453247

Mundinger, M., Kane, R., Lenz, E., Totten, A., Wei-Yann, T., Cleary, P. et al. (2000). Primary care outcomes in patients treated by nurse practitioners or physicians. *Journal of the American Medical Association, 283*(1), 59–68.

National Organization of Nurse Practitioner Faculties (NONPF). (2004). *Updated statement from the NONPF board of directors on the practice doctorate*. Retrieved from http://www.nonpf.com/displaycommon.cfm?an = 1&subarticlenbr = 16

O'Sullivan, A., Carter, M., Marion, L., Pohl, J., & Werner, K. (2005). Moving forward together: The practice doctorate in nursing. *Online Journal of Issues in Nursing, 10*(3), Manuscript 4. Retrieved from www.nursingworld.org/ojin/topic28/tpc28_4.htm

CRITICAL THINKING QUESTIONS

1. What strengths does preparation as a DNP bring to the advanced practice practitioner role? In what ways do you think NP practice will change once the majority of NPs are prepared at the DNP level?
2. What is the role of teachers of various educational backgrounds in the education of the DNP practitioner? Should the majority of DNP educators be practicing clinicians? Explain.
3. Do you anticipate that outcomes should be different from MS-prepared practitioners? What outcomes can be expected from DNP-prepared practitioners?
4. Do you think that attaining competency as an NP is necessary before becoming a change agent? How will DNP student practitioners gain the skills to become change agents in clinical practice if they cannot practice as NPs until they complete their DNP education?
5. Should DNP students be encouraged to develop original scholarly work through the scholarship of application? Would this approach better prepare NPs with the skills to demonstrate enhanced patient outcomes resulting from their care? In what way?
6. Should NPs and MDs take the same certification exams? What are the advantages and drawbacks of this approach to determining competencies?

7. Are AACN's *Essentials* relevant and futuristic enough to provide guidance in the development of the practitioner going forward? Should an *Essentials* document be futuristic?
8. Should ethics be added as an essential? Discuss ways to incorporate ethics appropriately throughout the curriculum.
9. Should PhD and DNP students be educated together? Are there areas where each should be educated separately? What areas should be shared?
10. What level of rigor should exist in a DNP program? Should it be similar to the PhD program?

CHAPTER SIX

The Role of the Clinical Executive

Tukea L. Talbert and Robin Donohoe Dennison

INTRODUCTION: SUPPLY, DEMAND, AND PREPARATION OF A CLINICAL EXECUTIVE—WHY IS IT IMPORTANT?

Over the last decade, there has been emerging evidence of the connection between organizational performance and leadership (Frearson, 2002; Hallinger & Heck, 1996; Muijs, Harris, Lumby, Morrison, & Sood, 2006). The Institute of Medicine (IOM) Committee on the Quality of Health Care in America has issued a mandate to the American health care community to bring "state-of-the-art" health care to all Americans (Fasoli, 2010, p. 25). Fasoli indicates that nursing has reached a point of inflection, a tipping point, and the nursing role must evolve in order to remain fully engaged in health care. Of even greater importance, the nurse leader must be prepared to change and create health care policies, create and implement evidence-based practice guidelines, and embrace and represent quality nursing practice at every level of the organization and of society. Now is the time to ensure that the right people are in key leadership positions, and that those individuals are well prepared to face the dynamic environment and challenges of the health care milieu. Organizational performance during this turbulent time in health care will be contingent on the effectiveness of the leadership team.

The American Association of Colleges of Nursing (AACN) in their position statement (2004) puts forth that the transformation in the health care delivery system will require clinicians to design, evaluate, and constantly improve the context in which care is delivered. The AACN strongly believes that nurses with doctoral preparation that encompasses clinical, organizational, economic, and leadership skills are most likely capable of critiquing scientific findings and subsequently developing programs of care that significantly impact health care and that are economically feasible. The AACN adopted the Doctorate of Nursing Practice (DNP) Position Statement in October of 2004 calling for a transformational change in the education necessary for professional nurses who will practice at an advanced level of nursing practice (*Essentials of Doctoral Education for Advanced Nursing Practice* Document, 2005). The AACN recognizes the practice demands affiliated with an increasingly complex health care system amid a major health care reform that has gotten new momentum from the President Obama administration. One can conclude that these demands comprise a new strain with a different genotype that is placing new pressure on the preparation of those nurses in senior leadership positions and on their level of preparation.

In this chapter, the following areas will be discussed: an operational definition of the clinical executive; the AACN's *Essentials of Doctoral Education for Advanced Nursing*

Practice; a comparison of the AACNs *Essentials for Master's Education* with the *Essentials of Doctoral Education for Advanced Nursing Practice*; a comparison of the DNP degree with the MSN and MBA; and the position of the American Organization of Nurse Executives (AONE) regarding the DNP degree requirement for nurse executives. The objectives of this chapter are to give readers the opportunity to have a more in-depth view of the demand for a different level and type of education beyond the master's degree for clinical executive leadership; the results of a DNP education; and the potential challenges of making the DNP a requirement for nurse executives.

DEFINITION OF A CLINICAL EXECUTIVE

Webster (2000) defines an executive as, "capable of, or concerned with, carrying out duties, functions . . . or managing affairs in a business or organization; empowered and required to administer" (p. 497). One cannot fully respect the role of the clinical executive without acknowledging the context in which it occurs. The clinical executive must oversee all aspects of clinical practice in health care organizations. The nursing practice within any organization is a "24/7" accountability for processes, structures, and outcomes of care delivery (Fasoli, 2010). The responsibility of the clinical executive is ever changing and growing, and the expectations upon those in the role are greater. For the purposes of this chapter, both authors agree that senior-level nursing leadership (Chief Nursing Officer, Chief Nursing Executive, and VP of Nursing) in a health care setting is a form of advanced nursing practice as evidenced by the differentiation option offered by the DNP degree, which is the eighth option beyond the seven core essentials.

AACN *ESSENTIALS OF DOCTORAL EDUCATION FOR ADVANCED NURSING PRACTICE*

The AACN (2006) identified seven core competencies for the DNP along with two additional differentiated competencies for nurses who choose to focus more on an advanced practice administrative role (i.e., clinical executive role) or an advanced practice-focused role (nurse anesthetist, nurse practitioner, midwife, clinical nurse specialist). The seven core essentials are: (1) scientific underpinnings for practice; (2) organizational and systems leadership for quality improvement and systems thinking; (3) clinical scholarship and analytical methods for evidence-based practice; (4) information systems/technology and patient care technology for the improvement and transformation of health care; (5) health care policy for advocacy in health care; (6) inter professional collaboration for improving patient and population health outcomes; (7) clinical prevention and populations health for improving the nation's health; (8a—practice-focused) individual, family, and population-focused advanced nursing practice competencies for improving patient care processes and outcomes; and (8b—executive/administrative) systems or organization-focused advanced nursing practice competencies for improving patient care processes and outcomes.

Both authors of this chapter strongly believe that the DNP degree offers an expansive educational experience very different from that of the administrative tract of the Master's of Science degree. This belief hinges on some of the following benefits from the DNP degree that includes extensive literature on leadership theory that encompasses the process of leadership and more specifically leadership in health care; mentoring opportunities with other leaders in advanced practice roles as part of residency/practicum; the differentiated option to focus more on students' desired specialization in the program; and the capstone project, which is a work in progress throughout the program. The capstone project serves as the student's population focus. Throughout the program, the chosen population focus will undergo several analyses that include cost–benefit analyses/return on investment, statistical analyses, utilization focused evaluations, and extensive literature reviews, especially if students have interventional studies as part of their capstone projects.

THE DNP CLINICAL EXECUTIVE PRACTICA: A CRITICAL ELEMENT

Although all aspects of the DNP educational experience are important, additional focus will be spent on the practicum experience and the capstone project. The practicum experiences for each student are designed around the student's choice for specialization (administrative/executive or practice focused). The first author's (TT) practicum took place at Dartmouth Hitchcock Medical Center in Lebanon, New Hampshire, with the VP of Nursing. During the experience, the VP of Nursing along with other members of the senior leadership team undertook a restructuring of the organizational chart. The change, as you can imagine, was enormous. It not only was going to impact the hospital, but also had implications for change for other hospitals that were part of an alliance with Dartmouth. The VP of Nursing was able to articulate the communication plan at every level of the facility and to those hospitals outside the physical boundaries of Dartmouth. The ability to participate in this monumental event at that hospital was vastly different from any of the clinical experiences in the Master's of Science in Nursing (MSN) program experienced by this author 10 years prior to the DNP program.

During the practicum at Dartmouth, as a doctoral student I functioned as a consultant and generated questions that might be posed by stakeholders and various team members within and outside the organization. During the residency, students are expected to exhibit critical thinking and participate in scholarly discussions. The key objective during the residency hours (practicum) is that the students drive the learning experience by being active participants who are not simply in an organization solely to shadow their mentors. Each course has course objectives that provide guidelines for students' practicum experiences; however, the students also create unique objectives for each practicum experience, which results in ownership of the process and outcome of the residency. Although there were other practicum experiences (see Table 6.1.), the Dartmouth experience demonstrated the practice of an effective leader dealing with a very toxic change in a major health care organization. The overall focus of this practicum therefore was on the process of leadership and leadership style, and its effect on organizational culture.

A second practicum occurred at The University of Texas MD Anderson Cancer Center in Houston, Texas, one of the top oncology health care facilities in the nation. The focus of this residency revolved around my (TT) capstone project, which actually was a quasi-experimental pre- and post-test design study that investigated psychological distress among patients undergoing hematopoietic stem cell transplants. During this time, I was able to examine protocols and isolation practices used by experts in hematopoietic stem cell transplants. This practicum provided insight on current versus traditional practices for isolation and outcomes associated with various isolation interventions. The overall focus of this practicum was to evaluate the impact of leadership on the development of practice policies, standards, processes, and patient outcomes.

TABLE 6.1
Student's (TT) Practica Experiences

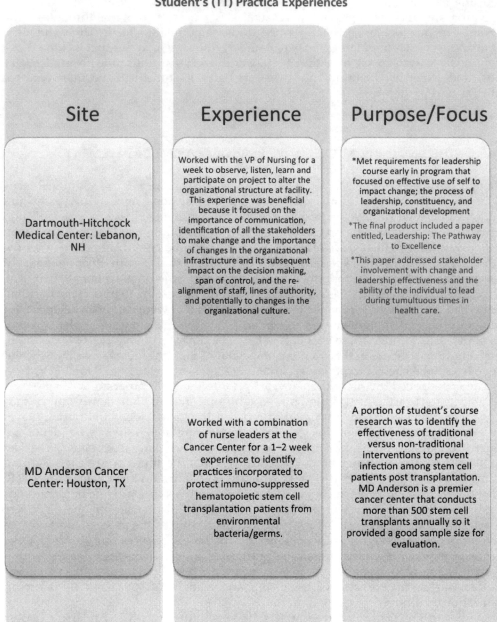

Site	Experience	Purpose/Focus
Dartmouth-Hitchcock Medical Center: Lebanon, NH	Worked with the VP of Nursing for a week to observe, listen, learn and participate on project to alter the organizational structure at facility. This experience was beneficial because it focused on the importance of communication, identification of all the stakeholders to make change and the importance of changes In the organizational infrastructure and its subsequent impact on the decision making, span of control, and the re-alignment of staff, lines of authority, and potentially to changes in the organizational culture.	*Met requirements for leadership course early in program that focused on effective use of self to impact change; the process of leadership, constituency, and organizational development *The final product included a paper entitled, Leadership: The Pathway to Excellence *This paper addressed stakeholder involvement with change and leadership effectiveness and the ability of the individual to lead during tumultuous times in health care.
MD Anderson Cancer Center: Houston, TX	Worked with a combination of nurse leaders at the Cancer Center for a 1–2 week experience to identify practices incorporated to protect immuno-suppressed hematopoietic stem cell transplantation patients from environmental bacteria/germs.	A portion of student's course research was to identify the effectiveness of traditional versus non-traditional interventions to prevent infection among stem cell patients post transplantation. MD Anderson is a premier cancer center that conducts more than 500 stem cell transplants annually so it provided a good sample size for evaluation.

Throughout the DNP program, each student works with a patient population for which she must identify an evidence-based health care intervention to implement. Other critical components associated with the intervention and/or practice change includes cost-effective analyses, program evaluation, literature review in search of best practices, and identification of stakeholders that may influence the practice change and/or be affected by the change.

Another key focus of the DNP program is program evaluation. Several options for evaluation are introduced to students that include utilization-focused evaluation, and formative and summative evaluations. In comparison to the MSN administrative track, the detail with evaluation, research, evidence-based interventions, cost-effectiveness analysis, and policy development associated with health care initiatives, interventions, and outcomes was significantly different. Each of the authors believes that with the completion of the DNP program, we acquired a new level of thinking about program development and evaluation; identification and placement of best practices into practice settings; advanced practice in health care; interpretation of patterns from large data sets; and, most importantly, leadership in health care. Overall, the DNP practicum (residency) experiences greatly enhance the learning experience of students and it enables them to view advanced practice from a macroscopic perspective, which is vastly different from the more microscopic approach experienced in the MSN administrative track.

COMPARISON OF THE *ESSENTIALS OF MASTER'S EDUCATION* AND *ESSENTIALS OF DOCTORAL EDUCATION FOR ADVANCED NURSING PRACTICE*

This section highlights some of the key areas of difference between the 1996 *Essentials of Master's Education for Advanced Practice Nursing* document (which is currently under revision) from AACN and the 2006 *Essentials of Doctoral Education for Advanced Nursing Practice* (see Table 6.2). Table 6.2 demonstrates some of the key differences noted between the traditional MSN educational preparation and DNP competences as defined by AACN. There are four critical differences noted: (1) The DNP competencies are more system wide and provide a macroscopic view of health care that combines all the sciences and better prepares graduates to engage in partnerships that will impact change in health care at a higher level. The student's focus reaches beyond the traditional patient setting within the organization. (2) DNP competencies are geared toward creating graduates who lead to change as opposed to assisting with change, which seems to be more the case with the MSN competencies. This competency is evident through the residency hours and the capstone projects. Students through their residency hours and capstones potentially generate new knowledge, and, in most cases, focus on adapting best practices to the clinical setting. (3) The DNP graduate demonstrates the nursing role to the community at large (even nationally) through both performance and communication, while the MSN graduate competencies focus more on communication of the nursing role on a more narrow scope. (4) The DNP competencies are more population based and prepare a graduate to make change globally, while the MSN competencies are more population and community specific, thus limiting one's impact on health care to a smaller scale. Table 6.2 illustrates a juxtaposed comparison of each set of competencies, pointing out key differences, which are bolded. Although there is a small amount of overlap with a few of the competencies, the differences stated above clearly indicate the variation in the level of preparation among graduates from the two programs.

Many authors conclude that success at the executive level hinges on being visionary and making decisions on a macroscopic level. Hader (2010a), Senior VP and Chief Nursing Officer (CNO) of Meridian Health System in New Jersey, states that the CNO's strategic plan must reach beyond the traditional scope of nursing practice. He notes that the CNO's influence will likely extend to areas outside of nursing. The CNO must engage in

TABLE 6.2
Comparison of Essentials of Masters Education and Doctorate of Nursing Practice

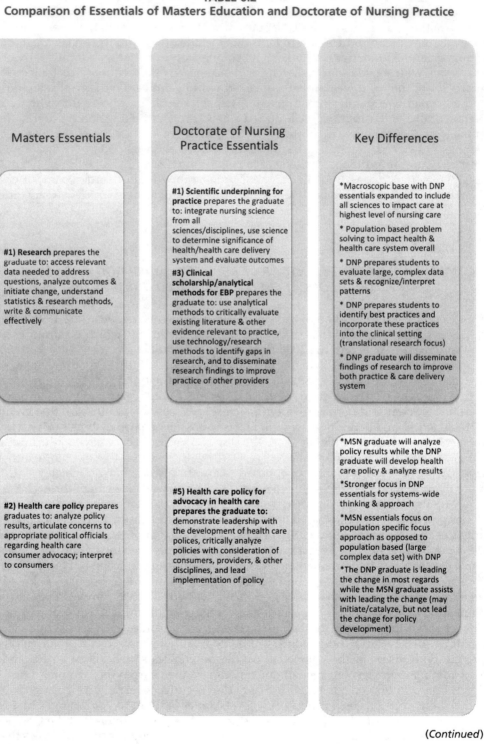

Masters Essentials	Doctorate of Nursing Practice Essentials	Key Differences
#1) Research prepares the graduate to: access relevant data needed to address questions, analyze outcomes & initiate change, understand statistics & research methods, write & communicate effectively	**#1) Scientific underpinning for practice** prepares the graduate to: integrate nursing science from all sciences/disciplines, use science to determine significance of health/health care delivery system and evaluate outcomes **#3) Clinical scholarship/analytical methods for EBP** prepares the graduate to: use analytical methods to critically evaluate existing literature & other evidence relevant to practice, use technology/research methods to identify gaps in research, and to disseminate research findings to improve practice of other providers	*Macroscopic base with DNP essentials expanded to include all sciences to impact care at highest level of nursing care * Population based problem solving to impact health & health care system overall * DNP prepares students to evaluate large, complex data sets & recognize/interpret patterns * DNP prepares students to identify best practices and incorporate these practices into the clinical setting (translational research focus) * DNP graduate will disseminate findings of research to improve both practice & care delivery system
#2) Health care policy prepares graduates to: analyze policy results, articulate concerns to appropriate political officials regarding health care consumer advocacy; interpret to consumers	**#5) Health care policy for advocacy in health care prepares the graduate to:** demonstrate leadership with the development of health care polices, critically analyze policies with consideration of consumers, providers, & other disciplines, and lead implementation of policy	*MSN graduate will analyze policy results while the DNP graduate will develop health care policy & analyze results *Stronger focus in DNP essentials for systems-wide thinking & approach *MSN essentials focus on population specific focus approach as opposed to population based (large complex data set) with DNP *The DNP graduate is leading the change in most regards while the MSN graduate assists with leading the change (may initiate/catalyze, but not lead the change for policy development)

(Continued)

TABLE 6.2
Comparison of Essentials of Masters Education and Doctorate of Nursing Practice
(Continued)

Masters Essentials	Doctorate of Nursing Practice Essentials	Key Differences
#3)Ethics prepares the graduate to: identify & analyze common ethical dilemmas; evaluate ethical methods of decision-making; understand the role of ethics in the health care system	* **No specific essential for ethics**	*No specific essential for ethics
#4)Professional role development prepares the graduate to communicate, advocate about the nursing profession including advanced practice role; functions as change agent;	**#6) Interprofessional collaboration for improving patient and population health outcomes** prepares the graduate to: partner with other professionals to analyze complex clinical issues; assume leadership roles in interprofessional team to develop practice models, guidelines & health policy	*DNP focuses on development of partnerships & is more actively involved in defining the role of the DNP prepared nurse

*DNP graduate better able to effectively develop the partnerships based on system-wide approach, ability to be involved in collaborative relationships with others beyond the traditional organizational boundaries

*DNP graduate has a greater self knowledge & self mastery from extensive study of leadership theory & leadership development exposure-this creates a strong foundation for effectiveness with leadership |

(Continued)

TABLE 6.2
Comparison of Essentials of Masters Education and Doctorate of Nursing Practice
(*Continued*)

Masters Essentials	Doctorate of Nursing Practice Essentials	Key Differences
#5) Theoretical foundations of nursing practice prepares the graduate to: critique & evaluate a variety of theories, apply & use appropriate theories to improve health care	**#2) Organizational & systems leadership for QI and systems thinking** prepares the graduate to: use advanced communication skills/processes to **lead change,** employ principles of business, finance, health law **to develop plans** for practice level and/or system-wide improvement	*Key differences again continues to be the scope of practice (macroscopic-DNP versus microscopic-MSN) *DNP graduate will exhibit the ability to incorporate leadership, organizational, & systems theories to impact change with large data sets over many organizational boundaries/nationally *MSN focuses on application of principles while the DNP will develop organizational-wide improvements for application *The MSN continues to have a limited focus on population and/or community focused/specific issues while the DNP focuses on national trends to address health care issues across several boundaries and geographic areas
#6 Human diversity/social issues prepares the graduate to confront subcultural influences on human behavior, including ethnic, racial, gender, and age differences; deliver multicultural competent advanced nursing care	**No specific essential**	No specific essential – although these concepts are embedded in the DNP *Essentials*

(*Continued*)

TABLE 6.2
Comparison of Essentials of Masters Education and Doctorate of Nursing Practice
(Continued)

Masters Essentials	Doctorate of Nursing Practice Essentials	Key Differences
#7) Health promotion/disease prevention: prepares students to: *use epidemiological, social, & environmental data to draw conclusions regarding health status of client populations (i.e. families, individuals, groups, & communities) *Develop & monitor comprehensive, holistic plans of care that address the health promotion & disease prevention of client populations	**#7) Clinical prevention & population health for improving the nation's health** prepares student to: *analyze epidemiological, biostatistical, environmental & other appropriate data related to population health *Develop, implement & evaluate interventions to improve health status/access patterns and/or address gaps in care within a community	*DNP clearly has a broader scope of practice *Continues to analyze health endpoints of large data sets/make changes that reach beyond traditional boundaries *MSN impact much more limited *Both the DNP & MSN essentials incorporate principles of epidemiology while the DNP does also integrate biostatistics as a means to analyze and interpret data & identify trends
No specific competency	**#4) Information systems/technology and patient care technology for the improvement and transformation of health care** prepares the graduate to: access, use, & evaluate data to alter health care system	No specific MSN competency for this essential

(Continued)

TABLE 6.2
Comparison of Essentials of Masters Education and Doctorate of Nursing Practice
(Continued)

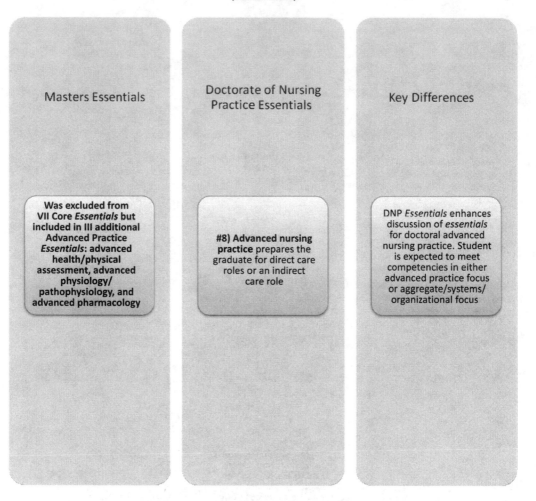

Masters Essentials	Doctorate of Nursing Practice Essentials	Key Differences
Was excluded from VII Core *Essentials* but included in III additional Advanced Practice *Essentials*: advanced health/physical assessment, advanced physiology/pathophysiology, and advanced pharmacology	#8) Advanced nursing practice prepares the graduate for direct care roles or an indirect care role	DNP *Essentials* enhances discussion of *essentials* for doctoral advanced nursing practice. Student is expected to meet competencies in either advanced practice focus or aggregate/systems/organizational focus

collaborative professional relationships with other key stakeholders in the health care organization that include the Chief Medical Officer (CMO), Chief Financial Officer (CFO), Chief Executive Officer (CEO), and Board of Trustee Members. The inability to think and function on a macroscopic level will greatly limit the level of effectiveness of decision making and subsequently the organizational success. Nurse executives exert a great deal of power from the perspective of title and capacity to influence. Nurse executives generally have the majority of the workforce under their span of control, due to their position and the fact that nurses generally are one of the largest sectors of the health care workforce within health care organizations. This opportunity to influence many people who ultimately provide the delivery of care at the bedside is not a position to be understated. It is critical that the individuals in these roles are well prepared for the challenge and are capable of making a difference in health care outcomes.

Our view is that the DNP clinical executive tract is unique in that this degree prepares nurses to be better leaders in a very challenging, dynamic health care arena. Nurses in the role of the clinical executive are no longer invited to the table solely based on their clinical insight, but more so for their ability and capacity to lead organizations based on their leadership competencies. Many of these key competencies are outlined in the AACN *Essentials for Doctoral Education for Advanced Nursing Practice* document and they include organizational and systems leadership, health care policy for advocacy in health care, and inter professional partnerships for improving patient and population health outcomes.

NURSE EXECUTIVE PREPARATION: THE DNP VERSUS OTHER DEGREE OPTIONS

In terms of reviewing options to prepare the contemporary nurse executive (aside from the DNP or DrNP at one school), the options include: a Masters of Science in Nursing (MSN) degree with an administrative focus and a Masters of Business Administration (MBA); some colleges offer a combination of the MSN/MBA as a concurrent option.

Curriculum and course descriptions were obtained and reviewed from an online search of the following institutions: Indiana Wesleyan University (MBA); University of Texas Tyler (MSN/MBA); and hard copies were obtained from the University of Kentucky (DNP) and Eastern Kentucky University (MSN).[1] Through a juxtaposed comparison, some of the following initial conclusions can be made: The MSN with an administrative focus appears to be more focused on a microperspective of leadership development, preparing a novice leader or someone with leadership aspirations; the MBA seems to offer a broader base of courses to better equip the nurse executive, because it includes management concepts, managerial economics, ethics, law, and some leadership courses as well; the MSN/MBA option seems to be the most broad in that it has a good blend of the financial competencies along with some basic entry-level leadership development courses. Overall, any of these three options would be feasible pathways to prepare novice leaders or individuals pursuing a leadership career. In comparison, the post-masters DNP degree with a clinical executive option offers a much more in-depth preparation for advanced leadership roles such as the clinical executive who may serve as the VP of Nursing, Chief Nursing Officer, Chief Operating Officer, and/or the Chief Nurse Executive. With the DNP, one satisfies the requirements of a doctorate, which prepares the individual on a different graduate level (a doctorate) in comparison to the MBA and the MSN options (i.e., a master's degree). Although being a doctorally prepared nurse executive does not always confer credibility, it does confer the unique competence of the individual who holds the degree (Gerrish, McManus, & Ashworth, 2003).

When further comparing these different degree programs, the DNP degree appears to offer a more in-depth overview of leadership and focus on reaching leadership capacity through self-knowledge and self-mastery. The key benefits revolve around the well-designed, focused residency hours; the extensive overview of leadership literature from diversified author-based sources; the initiation of the capstone project at the inception of the DNP program; the liberty to take elective courses outside the College of Nursing, which included Geriatric Policy and the College of Business courses for this chapter's first author; research principles and courses required for a doctoral degree; and the exposure to theory on health policy development. In concert with the above benefits, the student is prepared to constantly ask why, always seek new knowledge through research and evidence-based practice, and to design programs and policy with the ability to evaluate these initiatives clinically and financially. DNP graduates demonstrate the importance of always asking the best next question(s). They recognize that while one may not always have the answers, it is the question that may be more important because it highlights an aspect of a complex situation that may have been missed. Students have a sharpened sense of critical thinking outside the scope of nursing which forces the doctoral clinical executive scholar to examine how health care is truly integrated both horizontally and vertically.

The DNP degree is an option that prepares nurse executives to perform at a higher level. We are not suggesting that the other degree options reviewed are inferior, because they are not. The authors believe that they offer a very sound preparation for one interested in leadership, while the DNP offers an advanced level of preparation for someone who desires more knowledge and preparation. The DNP is not more of the same, but a newer version or model of preparation for the nurse executive who functions as the senior nurse leader in organizations with other members of the executive team. The primary difference in the DNP is best described by Hader who states "The curriculum and expectations of academic performance in the clinical doctorate programs are far more extensive than those in a traditional graduate program" (2010b, p. 6). The focus of the DNP program is uniquely different and, in theory, does create a different type of graduate with the ability to think outside traditional boundaries and develop collaborative partnerships to move organizations forward successfully.

AMERICAN ORGANIZATION OF NURSE EXECUTIVES NURSE EXECUTIVE COMPETENCIES

At this time, the American Organization of Nurse Executives (AONE) has not endorsed the proposal that the DNP should be a requirement for either the clinical nurse executive or practiced-focused nurse in advanced nursing practice roles. In their position statement, AONE (2007) supports the DNP as a terminal degree option for practice-focused nursing. They believe, however, that master's nursing degree programs in both generalist and specialty courses of study should remain intact. The Professional Practice Policy Committee of AONE concludes that questions and concerns that have been voiced regarding patient outcomes, salary compensation, and financial impact on organizations have not been fully identified, investigated, or addressed as they relate to the DNP requirement.

Having said the above, AONE considers nurse leadership a subspecialty within nursing practice that requires competence and proficiency unique to the executive role. They believe that there are five core competencies that are common to nurses in executive practice regardless of their educational level or title (AONE Nurse Executive Competencies, 2005). These five competencies are: (1) communication and relationship building; (2) knowledge of the health care environment; (3) leadership; (4) professionalism; and (5) business skills. These core leadership competencies align with specific core essentials of the AACN *Essentials of Doctoral Education for Advanced Nursing Practice*, such as interprofessional collaboration, organizational and systems leadership, and clinical scholarship. AONE recognizes that their competencies are core competencies and are not exhaustive of all areas of expertise for the nurse executive. They believe that the core competencies establish the standard for executive practice and can be used as a guideline for educational preparation of nurses seeking knowledge in executive practice.

The authors agree with the position of AONE in that there needs to be more evidence to support making the DNP a requirement for those nurses functioning in clinical leadership advanced nursing practice roles. The authors, DNP graduates themselves, aver that this degree is scholarly, uniquely different from a graduate-level preparation for leadership, and is an educational process that prepares the nurse executive to think and function at an advanced level as evidenced by the positions held by these individuals and their accomplishments in these roles. Having said this, it is necessary to address some key questions before concluding that the DNP must be a requirement for any nursing leadership roles. In addition to the questions posed by AONE, other questions need to be addressed as well. First, one must determine for what level of nurse leadership should the doctorate be required. It is the belief of both authors that it would be illogical to require all nurses in leadership to be doctorally prepared. As stated by Jones (2010), this becomes a scope of practice and level of accountability issue. It connects back to the level of preparation offered by the DNP that has been highlighted as producing graduates able to function at a macroscopic level. The nurse executive at the most senior level in the organization needs to see the big picture that often times transcends traditional organizational boundaries. Second, what impact, if any, would such a requirement have on MSN programs? This issue is also raised by AONE in their position statement. Some colleges have or are moving in the direction to eliminate MSN tracks as they create DNP degree options as part of their academic offerings. Third, what impact would the potential elimination of MSN programs have on the supply of nurses? AONE recognizes that nurses may choose other disciplines to acquire a master's degree, which may result in outward migration from the nursing profession. Overall, the reduction of the number of MSN programs or their elimination may result in some unintended consequences that may have long-term effects on the nursing profession and particularly on providing a steady pool of highly educated clinical nurse executives at a variety of levels.

FUTURE PERSPECTIVES

Future considerations regarding the DNP degree need to include three key components. (1) The profession must find a way to ensure that the degree can withstand the test of time through evidence to support its benefits. Since the inception of the DNP degree, there is growing evidence of its impact as demonstrated by successful graduates of the program functioning as effective clinical executives. Key indicators, as highlighted by AONE, that need to be further investigated include the financial impact of increasing salary expectations of doctorally prepared executives and the corresponding financial impact on organizations, patient satisfaction with holders of this degree, and specific degree-related patient outcomes as evidenced by organizations' performance with core measures established by the Centers for Medicare and Medicaid (CMS) and Hospital Consumer Assessment of Health-care Providers and Systems (HCAHPS) scores. (2) The profession must carefully examine the scope of practice and level of accountability of nurses who would benefit most from a DNP degree. Jones (2010) indicates that executives at the top level of nursing administration are accountable for the executive level of patient services. She further states that executives will be expected to function at a macrolevel with decision making and actions that impact patients and others within the organization. Mid-level managers have a narrower focus and span of control within organizations and are more likely to function at a microlevel by virtue of the organizational chart and structure of organizations. The nurse executive will work across both microsystem and macrosystem levels that include groups both internal and external to the organization. As stated earlier, one of the unique qualities of the DNP degree is its preparation of the nurse executive to think and function on a macrosystem level. (3) Investigators must continue to monitor the market and demand for DNP graduates. Many authors have noted the turbulence, variability, and increasing complexity of the health care environment (AACN Fact Sheet, 2010; Fasoli, 2010; New, 2010; Schaffner & Shcaffner, 2009). All of these factors continue to add momentum to the demand for preparation beyond a graduate level. The AACN (2010) provides the following statistics with regard to DNP programs: 120 programs are enrolling students nationwide, and an additional 161 DNP programs are in planning stages; DNP programs are present in 36 states and the District of Columbia; from 2008 to 2009, the number of DNP enrollees increased from 3,415 to 5,165; and to date, 18 DNP programs are accredited by the Commission on Collegiate Nursing Education (CCNE) with an additional 70 DNP programs pursuing CCNE accreditation. Coupled with the above, one other significant finding is that employers have quickly recognized the contributions DNP graduates are making in the practice setting (Waxman & Maxworthy, 2010). This last point is further supported by early studies that show the DNP is perceived as a viable advanced education option and enables students to make viable contributions to the nursing profession (Loomis, Willard, & Cohen, 2006). In closing, the supply is present and the demand continues to create a need for clinical executives who are prepared beyond a master's level. Based on the data above, the DNP is necessary and should continue to be an option for nurses seeking a clinical executive specialty in advanced nursing practice.

A PIONEER'S PERSPECTIVE: A GRADUATE FROM
THE NATION'S FIRST DNP PROGRAM

As the first author of this chapter (TT) and a member of the first DNP graduating class in the United States (at the University of Kentucky), I recall a moment in time that I shall not forget. One of the members of my Doctoral Capstone Committee asked me what was most beneficial about the DNP program. My response at that time was that I had a better understanding of myself and my personal leadership style. Although this may sound somewhat trivial, it was and continues to be, for me, a profound realization. This realization continues to facilitate my personal leadership journey and development, because I better understand what makes me successful as a leader. It also illuminates and highlights what skill sets are necessary to improve my leadership. Through reflection and my current practice, other responses to that question would include the increased confidence and competence to create a culture of collaboration by navigating through departmental and organizational borders by using focused evaluations, evidence-based practice, and influencing others beyond the traditional boundaries of the nursing component of health care. One could also say that health care today has an entirely different look; it is something that stretches beyond the physical and sometimes human boundaries of the health care facility. Successful clinical executives must be willing and equipped to see the new paradigm and context in which health care is practiced. As a graduate of a DNP program (TT), I am able to see the difference and the shift in the health care paradigm, and understand that it requires one to think and function at a different, more advanced level.

SUMMARY

Nurses in the clinical executive role are no longer invited to the table solely based on their clinical insight but more so for their ability and capacity to lead organizations based on their leadership competencies. The nursing profession can lead the "way to knowing" and the capacity to lead by continuing to offer the DNP as a credible degree option for nurses seeking to expand their leadership skill set and knowledge to be better prepared to function in the increasingly turbulent health care environment.

In summary, because there are other strategies necessary to prepare nurses for clinical executive roles, the nursing profession cannot solely depend upon a new degree. They must be proactive in developing a framework that ensures ongoing development of leaders in executive roles that can be incorporated in the context in which they practice. These frameworks must include organizational charts that are aligned with the corporate strategic plan and that create the propensity for nurse leaders to have the capacity to lead and be involved in decision making at every level. The frameworks must provide ongoing opportunities for professional development, mentoring opportunities, and, last but not least, succession planning. Leadership development should not be by default or a second thought, but by design. It must be part of the culture established and supported by the nurse executive in collaboration with the other executive team members. It is too soon to say that a DNP should be required for individuals in clinical executive advanced nursing practice roles. However, it is not too soon to reexamine the process in which nurse executives are prepared for their leadership roles. Because leadership development is a process, it cannot be learned in a day or by completing another degree. The DNP degree offers an innovative educational experience that superbly prepares the nurse executive, but it is only the beginning of the process of leadership development. Nurse executives must be proactive and create organizational cultures that cultivate empowerment, ongoing professional development, and succession planning so that no leader is left behind and organizations advance from good to great.

NOTE

1. Websites for each program are as follows: a) Indiana Wesleyan University MBA: http://www.indwes.edu/Adult-Graduate/MBA/; b) University of Texas Tyler MSN/MBA: http://www.uttyler.edu/nursing/graduate/MSNMBA.html; c) University of Kentucky DNP Clinical Leadership: http://www.mc.uky.edu/Nursing/academic/dnp/default.html; and d) Eastern Kentucky University MSN in Advanced Rural Public Health Nursing with a concentration in Administration: http://www.bsn-gn.eku.edu/docs/PublicHealthNursingCurriculum.pdf

REFERENCES

American Association of Colleges of Nursing. (AACN). (1996) *The essentials of master's education.* Retrieved from http://www.aacn.nche.edu/education/pdf/MasEssentials96pdf

American Association of Colleges of Nursing (AACN). (2004). *AACN position statement on the practice doctorate in nursing October 2004.* Retrieved from http://www.aacn.nche.edu/DNP/pdf/DNP.pdf

American Association of Colleges of Nursing (AACN). (2006). *The essentials of doctoral education for advanced nursing practice.* Retrieved from http://www.aacn.nche.edu/DNP/pdf/Essentials.pdf

American Association of Colleges of Nursing (AACN). (2010, March). *Fact sheet: The doctor of nursing practice (DNP).* Retrieved from http://www.aacn.nche.edu/Media/FactSheets/dnp.htm

American Organization of Nurse Executives (AONE). (2005). Nurse executive competencies. *Nurse Leader, 3*(1), 50–56.

American Organization of Nurse Executives (AONE). (2007). *Consideration of the doctorate of nursing practice.* Retrieved from http://www.aone.org/aone/docs/PositionStatement060607.doc

Fasoli, D. R. (2010). The culture of nursing engagement: A historical perspective. *Nursing Administration Quarterly, 34*(1), 18–29.

Frearson, M. (2002). *Tomorrow's learning leaders: Developing leadership and management for postcompulsory learning. 2002 Survey Report.* London, UK: LSDA.

Gerrish, K., McManus, M., & Ashworth, P. (2003). Creating what sort of professional? Master's level nurse education as a professionalizing strategy. *Nursing Inquiry, 10*(2), 103–112.

Hader, R. (2010a). Success in the "C-Suite." *Nursing Management, 41*(3), 51–53.

Hader, R. (2010b). Who's the doctor, anyway? *Nursing Management, 41*(5), 6.

Hallinger, P., & Heck, R. H. (1996). Reassessing the principal's role in school effectiveness: A review of the empirical research. *Educational Administration Quarterly, 32*(1), 27–31.

Indiana Wesleyan University College of Adult & Professional Studies—CAPS. (2009). Retrieved from http://www.indwes.edu/Adul-tGraduate/MBA/

Jones, R. A. (2010). Preparing tomorrow's leaders: A review of the issues. *The Journal of Nursing Administration, 40*(4), 154–157.

Loomis, J. A., Willard, B., & Cohen, J. (2006). Difficult professional choices: Deciding between the PhD and the DNP in nursing. *Online Journal of Issues in Nursing, 12*(1), 6.

Muijs, D., Harris, A., Lumby, J., Morrison, M., & Sood, K. (2006). Leadership and leadership development in highly effective further education providers: Is there a relationship? *Journal of Further and Higher Education, 30*(1), 87–106.

New, N. (2010). Optimizing nurse manager span of control. *Nurse Leader, 7*(6), 46–48, 56.

Schaffner, M., & Schaffner, J. (2009). Leadership amid times of economic challenge. *Gastroenterology Nursing, 32*(1), 50–51.

Waxman, K. T., & Maxworthy, J. (2010). Doctorate of nursing practice and the nurse executive: The perfect combination. *Nurse Leader, 8*(2), 31–33.

Webster's New World College Dictionary. (2000). *Defining the English language for the 21st century* (4th ed.). Foster City, CA: IDG Books Worldwide, Inc.

CHAPTER SIX: Reflective Response

Patricia S. Yoder-Wise

Talbert and Dennison pose some questions and insights related to the DNP preparation for clinical nurse executives. They compare master's preparation (in nursing and in business administration) with the DNP. However, they omit comparison of the DNP with the PhD and how each of those degrees might contribute to the excellence of clinical nurse executives. They also discuss briefly the position of the American Organization of Nurse Executives and address its core competencies for clinical nurse executives. However, they omit addressing the position of the American Nurses Association and its scope and standards document governing nursing administration. Finally, they are clearly enthusiastic supporters of this degree that seems to be so relevant to leading clinical work. Yet, no mention is made of the huge numbers of nurses in administrative positions who are not even prepared with a baccalaureate degree in nursing. This diversity in the educational qualifications for someone who has the ultimate accountability for the nursing care of patients creates an overwhelming challenge to address before the refinement of the question (master's or doctorate?) can be resolved.

Talbert and Dennison make an excellent case for why clinical executives need solid educational preparation. The idea that nurses in those positions have "24/7 accountability for processes, structures and outcomes" (p. 142) and that these positions often encompass multiple professional groups is an important consideration. The authors point out the value of the *practica* and the *capstone* in shaping the contributions the graduate can make. Although these two experiences are similar to clinical intensives and capstone work at the undergraduate level and the practica and thesis options at the master's level, the richness of the backgrounds learners bring to doctoral level study provides a higher-level experience. In short, every nurse learns through clinical experiences and focused work. If an individual is learning to be a nurse, that level of insight differs greatly from what a nurse, often with multiple years of experience, brings to doctoral-level study.

But what about the difference between the PhD and the DNP? Because I am teaching in both programs, although different courses, I appreciate the distinction in why nurse leaders choose different programs. While I personally tend toward the execution side of leadership, I value those who select a research path. If they did not continue to contribute to our ongoing body of knowledge, we would have less substantive backing in the application of that knowledge. Both of these graduates (the DNP and the PhD) see the macroscopic perspective, but they see it through a different lens.

From my perspective, PhD programs tend to be more similar than varied. The same is not true for DNP programs. The range of what comprises the DNP programs is between high-level application and capstone projects consisting of work we might call intense quality improvement and, at the other end, considerable theoretical perspectives and capstone projects that would be difficult to differentiate from dissertations. As is always true in nursing, our diversity is one of our greatest benefits and one of our greatest liabilities. Until we have some better description of what best comprises a DNP program, it is difficult to compare that type of programming with other degree programs.

One final point about the value or preference for a PhD or a DNP, or for that matter between the DNP and one of the master's programs: The numbers of nurses prepared at the master's and doctoral levels continue to be relatively small in comparison to the 3.1 million registered nurses. Rather than worrying about which is better, we should worry about how we move nurses toward graduate education more quickly and consistently. As Talbert and Dennison point out, "Organizational performance during this turbulent time in health care will be contingent on the effectiveness of the leadership team" (p. 141).

Talbert and Dennison pose several excellent questions related to DNP education for nurse leaders. As more DNP graduates emerge from the expanding number of programs, major medical centers and systems will likely expect that the chief nurse executive hold a doctoral degree. In those organizations, many others will likely be prepared at that level. However, we know from past studies about the profile of nurses in clinical leadership positions; they are often prepared at the baccalaureate, or less, level. This fact suggests that we are unlikely to quickly advance a new educational expectation for nurse leaders. That said, we would be remiss if we did not strongly encourage increased education for nurses at every level.

Two key points resonate for me. One is that nurses are not invited to the table based solely on clinical insight; those extending invitations today look for those who are capable leaders. The second point is that ongoing development is critical for anyone in a leadership position. Whether a nurse is prepared with an MSN or a DNP is not the critical question. The question is, "What is the plan for ongoing professional development to remain relevant to the rapidly changing world?" Thus, if we are not learning and improving, we no longer are standing still. We are falling behind.

Programs that produce clinical leaders through strengthening their leadership abilities and through inculcating the skill of continued professional development have the best opportunity to create key leaders for tomorrow's big challenges.

CRITICAL THINKING QUESTIONS

1. Because leadership can be developed through learning and practice, what do you believe would be the essential content and experiences in a DNP program for a nurse either in or desiring to be in a clinical executive position?
2. As it is the opinion of some that DNP programs should be for advanced practice nurses only, do you believe that the clinical executive's indirect role in influencing patient outcomes falls within the role of the DNP?
3. Do you believe that having a doctoral degree would positively affect a clinical executive's authority and influence with physicians? With other administrators? With other nurses?
4. Many clinical executives have earned a PhD but are not actively engaged in research. Considering the differences in coursework and focus between PhD and DNP programs, which do you believe would be the most appropriate in development of the required skill set of a clinical executive?
5. Considering the health care environment where you live and/or are employed, do you feel that it is desirable and/or possible to require nurses in clinical executive positions to hold a DNP?

6. What do you see as the advantage and disadvantages of MSN, MBA, and DNP preparation of clinical executives?
7. What would be the appropriate criteria to evaluate the effect of a DNP for clinical executives?
8. In your opinion, should the nursing profession address the issue of doctoral preparation for nurse executives and possibly establish a precedent and/or standard of preparation for other executives in top leadership roles? Why or why not?
9. What were your personal reasons for choosing a DNP program, and what track do you believe best meets your rationale for choosing a DNP program?
10. What do you believe are some of the current pitfalls with the preparation of nurse executives and how do you believe the DNP clinical track could address these issues/concerns?

CHAPTER SEVEN

The Role of the Educator

Ruth Wittmann-Price, Roberta Waite, and Debra H. Woda

INTRODUCTION

Despite the initial intent of the American Association of Colleges of Nursing (AACN), DNP (Doctorate of Nursing Practice)[1] graduates are entering academia in substantial numbers. Therefore, it would be professionally negligent *not* to seek further clarification about the role of the DNP-prepared nurse as a nurse educator or *not* to facilitate their successful movement into academic roles. A paradigm shift is upon us and the DNP is becoming an appropriate "terminal degree" for a nurse educator in many institutions. This shift is not only logical, but also practical, because nurse educators are sorely needed. Nursing education should no longer be upheld as a distinct and different entity from other nursing practices. Is it not obvious that nurses today do engage in "the practice of nursing education?" Further, nursing education practice does not exist solely for the purpose of pure knowledge generation in a static format, but also actively involves using innovative classroom and clinical evidence. The universal context in which nursing education takes place reflects its practice-orientation, and the goal of nursing education includes knowledge generation as well as knowledge application or practice. Today's nurse educators are facilitating the development of tomorrow's nursing professionals as practicing professionals, be it at the bedside, in the classroom, in research capacities, in the community, or in administrative offices. The nursing profession needs to expand and redefine the word "practice" in order to encompass and recognize the practice of nurse educators.

In order to facilitate the discussion about the role of the DNP-prepared nurse in relation to the nurse educator role, this chapter is divided into three distinct, but related sections. First, we will provide a case study of a DNP graduate who entered academia. Next, the role of the DNP in relation to nursing education, theoretically and practically will be discussed. In addition, the practice of education, accrediting agencies' stance on nurse educator preparation on certification and education for nurse educators, and a discussion of tenure issues will be emphasized. Finally, we will analyze the educational preparation being received by DNP students in various schools in relation to nurse educator courses, and then conclude with some recommendations for the future.

The following case study is the personal experience of a DNP graduate who is functioning in a nurse educator role in an academic setting. It is just one perspective. Nevertheless, it is an important one because it discusses the rationales for accepting DNP-prepared nurses as educators and professors, and identifies real barriers that we as a profession are creating within the academic realm for DNP-prepared faculty.

Case Study: A DNP-Prepared Nurse Midwife Goes into Academia

As a DNP graduate who went into academia immediately upon graduation, there are indeed challenges to being a DNP-prepared nurse in an educator role. My short experience has already taught me that there are a number of barriers for DNP faculty, as well. The nature of academia is often a treacherous place for practice-focused, doctorally prepared faculty. The issue is not competence, but the definition of scholarship by the larger academic community. The roles of the PhD and DNP have been adequately defined by the DNP *Essentials* (AACN, 2006) in terms of their respective roles in the generation and use of nursing knowledge and evidence, but in academia these differing roles are often more ubiquitous. The traditional perspective of original research is very linear and limited in that it is seen as the one true avenue of scholarship; this viewpoint persists whether it is verbalized or not. This is a contradiction to the more contemporary concept of evidence-based practice, which is being demanded of nurses in all realms, even education. Differing approaches to DNP education as is noted in this text do not make this easier, since curricula vary greatly from program to program. In other words, there are likely DNP degree programs that are rigorous and others that are not. If research is being conducted within the academic realm using varied approaches to prepare nurse educators,[2] a tug of war over who owns (or controls) the research enterprise can occur; this can accentuate problems and cause additional havoc.

Participating in evidence-based research programs that change practice in clinical or educational settings ultimately improves nursing practice and patient outcomes. The generation of this evidence promotes scholarly practice among the faculty and often incorporates the best of the DNP skill sets. However, many research endeavors cannot be accomplished without external funding for salary, as this type of scholarship cannot simply be compounded upon a normal teaching load. Often it is the perception in a respective nursing research department that implementing a new research project, or that creating new evidence, cannot be done without a research partner with a PhD. This can also be a limiting factor to the DNP faculty member when no PhD faculty have an interest in the project, and the department does not afford the resources to support grant writing (even for program grants) to the DNP-prepared nurse.

My experience is that scholarship seems mostly defined by the written or spoken word. The presentation of clinical papers and evidence-based guidelines are good avenues for DNP faculty. However, with the current faculty shortage (and the resulting need for more teaching) there is little time to undertake this avenue of scholarship, and it is difficult, at best, to carry it out consistently. This places the DNP-prepared faculty at a disadvantage because good writing skills need to be developed, and used often, in order for one to become proficient in publishing. Presentations require time and travel support in order to move toward enhancing one's reputation (and thus the department or college's reputation, as well) as a clinical scholar at the national level. Such protected time is often not possible (or perhaps not valued?) for DNP faculty who are deemed "clinical faculty" and who are required to carry very heavy course loads and spend long hours in the clinical area, particularly in undergraduate nursing programs.

Scholarship for the DNP should also be defined by excellence in clinical practice — the goal of the clinically focused DNP is more proficient and expert advanced practice. However, not every School or College of Nursing recognizes this as an important aspect of scholarship. Specific and current skills in clinical practice are necessary for effective clinical teaching at both the undergraduate and graduate level. Yet, academic appointments for DNP-prepared advanced practice faculty teaching at the graduate level are particularly challenging when accrediting bodies require significant practice hours for recertification, but nursing departments do not typically allot time for practice and practice is not considered a scholarly endeavor. This issue has been largely ignored by schools that are actively seeking DNP graduates to teach in their respective DNP programs.

While tenure and promotion of doctorally prepared faculty should not be an issue, those disciplines that have practice-focused doctorates still lag behind in having access to tenure track positions, because the current system does not look favorably upon the type of scholarship these faculty produce. This barrier makes academia less attractive to DNP graduates. Until major research universities address these issues, there is little hope for parity for faculty who are doctorally prepared and active in practice. Mixed messages of valuing researchers (who don't practice), but taking for granted the immense time commitment *to practice* that advanced practice faculty require to teach competently and expertly, is not a prescription to attract faculty in a shortage.

Another issue is the leveling of doctorally prepared faculty in academia. The DNP-prepared nurse educator is often viewed as a second-class citizen, one who is not eligible for full faculty privileges. Unfortunately, this is not only propagated by the larger academic system, but it is propagated by nurse educators and leaders who view their role as PhD-prepared nurses as the true terminal degree. This sets up an oppressive system ripe for horizontal violence (DalPezzo & Jett, 2010). Therefore, consideration of the aforementioned concerns is not only a professional mandate, but it is also an ethical imperative that the profession of nursing must address to enable uplifting of all our doctorally prepared nursing colleagues.

As a DNP-prepared nurse educator, I have experienced both career development benefits and liabilities. My chosen path has afforded me an opportunity to accomplish my passion to help educate the next generation of nurses, the individuals who will positively affect patient care. It has allowed me to use my clinical expertise in an educational setting and provide mentorship and role modeling to graduate and undergraduate students. The liabilities of being in the role include the lack of time in academia to pursue scholarly activity, and experiencing the rigidity of the system in relation to promotion and tenure. Overall, I choose to continue in this role because of the fulfillment I receive from witnessing the students' growth as they develop into the professional nurses and doctoral advanced practice nurses (whatever their role) so desperately needed in today's health care environment.

THE PRACTICE OF "THE NURSE EDUCATOR"

To expand on this concept further, nursing practice is not bound by hospital walls, outpatient clinics, community centers, or homes of the ill. A nursing practice environment is any environment in which nurses can affect health care outcomes. Leadership, role modeling, and research endeavors each facilitate change, as does the practice of nurse educators in affecting the nursing care of individuals and aggregate populations.

Nurse educators are in demand (DalPezzo & Jett, 2010)! Currently, the only deficit in the nursing profession larger than the nursing shortage itself is the declining number of nurse educators who teach students to become nurses (Joint Commission, 2003). In the 1960s, many nursing programs moved from diploma schools to college and university settings, and rightfully so. Other schools chose to remain as two- or three-year programs, in spite of the baccalaureate-level entry debate which surfaced intensely at the time. In the collegiate setting, the PhD or its equivalent (DNS, DSN, or DNSc—hereby referred to as research doctorates) became the accepted credential for a nurse educator. The EdD will not be addressed separately throughout this chapter because it is well recognized as an educational degree, and it was indeed the first nursing doctorate awarded in 1932 at Teacher's College, Columbia University, New York (Nichols & Chitty, 2005).

Although the "entry-into-practice" debate still looms over the nursing profession on one end of the educational spectrum, the DNP has most recently threatened the educational stability of the profession on the other end of the educational continuum, "the terminal degree" side. Now that the DNP is well accepted as the degree for advanced practice nurses in the realms of practice, administration, and in some programs, clinical trials research (Donnelly, 2007), the nurse educator role also needs to be reexamined in the current context of declining numbers of faculty. Also notable in this discussion is that the majority of faculty in associate and diploma schools (>90%) hold a Masters of Science (MSN) degree (National League for Nursing News, 2006).

The authors of this chapter are aware that the AACN/CCNE (Commission on Collegiate Nursing Education) does not recognize DNP programs that formally prepare the DNP-prepared nurse for the "educator role" as part of the standard. DNP curriculum, the National League for Nursing, National League for Nursing Accrediting Commission (NLN/NLNAC) has no such prohibition. The NLN's position statement on the "Preparation of Nurse Educators" (NLN, May 18, 2002) has stated, "schools of nursing can demonstrate their commitment to excellence in nursing education by offering master's, post-master's, or doctoral programs that prepare nurse educators. Schools that offer such options are to be commended, supported, and rewarded" (p. 4). The NLN position statement further elaborated in the recommendation section for program development that:

> some doctoral programs should offer an option that allows students to specialize in nursing education and conduct pedagogical research, thereby contributing significantly to the development of a strong cadre of expert faculty-scholars who will assume leadership roles in nursing education and contribute to the ongoing development of the science of nursing education.
>
> —*NLN, 2002, p. 4*

Thus, with the two major nursing organizations and therefore the two nursing education accrediting agencies, the CCNE and the NLNAC, taking very divergent positions on this issue, we view it as unsettled and requiring more study.

NURSING ACCREDITING BODIES' VIEW OF THE DNP/EDUCATOR ROLE

The NLNAC (2008) has developed standards in order to evaluate and certify clinical doctorate degree programs (they prefer to use the term 'clinical doctorate' rather than 'practice doctorate'), such as the DNP. The six evaluative standards do not specifically exclude nurse educator tracks. Standard 4 states, "The curriculum is designed to prepare graduates to practice from an evidence-based research perspective in their advanced practice role through effective use and collaborative production of clinically based evidence" (2008, p. 3). Our interpretation is that if nursing expands its vision of practice from just clinical, to education in both the classroom and clinical realms, then this standard is suitable for education tracks in DNP programs.

In response to the urgent need for more nurse educators, there are some DNP programs that have either ignored the AACN and implemented educator tracks, or that have developed educator role opportunities within the standard DNP curriculum (in the form of additional credits or cognates). Admittedly, this is an emotionally charged debate on the issue of the proper terminal degree for nurse educators and we believe it is futile and unproductive to uphold the academic façade that only faculty with research doctorates can teach. However, the current context of 'who is going into nursing education' contains counter evidence. Over 30% of all DNP-prepared nurses are now teaching in academia, despite the original intent of the degree to prepare only practitioners and administrators (Zungolo, 2009).

DNP STUDENTS: ESSENTIALS AND COMPETENCIES

The acceptance of the DNP role has been a fairly smooth transition in relation to idealism, time, and resources within the nursing profession. Schools initially responded by taking risks and developing innovative programs (Cartwright & Reed, 2005). Subsequently, after the first cohort of programs were established mostly in 2005, schools of higher education used *The Essentials for Doctoral Education for Advanced Nursing Practice* developed by the AACN (2006). As educators know, essentials and related competencies are expected outcomes developed by established nursing organizations who govern and accredit nursing education programs that define educational missions, program development, and evaluation (Rogan, Crooks, & Durrant, 2008). The eight essentials put forth by the AACN (2006) for the DNP, however, are only guidelines for development of the role. However, the issue is now raised as to whether the 2006 essential standards are already becoming outdated.

The DNP was developed as a clinical degree with an emphasis on practice to further legitimize the advanced practice nurse's role. Some might even argue that the addition of the clinical executive role in the second year of the DNP roll-out by the AACN was somehow confusing to the original intent of the DNP degree, which was to prepare clinicians or practitioners. Nevertheless, this forward progression of role development has assisted the nursing profession to recognize varying expertise. Specifically, the AACN (2006) defines advanced nursing practice as:

> any form of nursing intervention that influences health care outcomes for individuals or populations, including the direct care of individual patients, management of care for individuals and populations, administration of nursing and health care organizations, and the development and implementation of health policy.
>
> —*AACN, 2006, p. 2*

Furthermore, the DNP role is justified by the AACN (2004) by some of the following benefits:

- Development of needed advanced competencies for increasingly complex practice, faculty, and leadership roles;
- Enhanced knowledge to improve nursing practice and patient outcomes;
- Enhanced leadership skills to strengthen practice and health care delivery;
- Better match of program requirements and credits with the credential earned;
- Provision of an advanced educational credential for those who require advanced practice knowledge, but do not need or want a strong research focus (e.g., practice [sic] faculty);
- Enhanced ability to attract individuals to nursing from non-nursing backgrounds; and
- Increased supply of faculty for practice [sic] instruction (adapted from p. 7–8).

Clearly, the AACN mutates the role of educator within the DNP to that of clinical faculty, although the role of clinical faculty is no less important or grounded in educational theory than classroom teaching (McKinley, 2009). In addition, it assumes that clinical expertise equates to educational expertise, and in some instances this may be detrimental to the overall development of undergraduate curriculum (Zungolo, 2004). Being an expert clinician does not automatically assure expertise in clinical teaching.

The rationale for not including educator in the role of the DNP may have been to hold the research doctorate as the most esteemed degree for the educational role and may have been intentional. Most of the DNP developers were and are faculty with research degrees. This possible attempt to "hold sacred" one terminal degree for the nursing profession as the only one capable of the educator role is contradictory to the literature which speaks to the underutilization of advanced practice nurses in nonclinical domains (Bryant-Lukosius, DiCenso, Browne, & Pinelli, 2004). It also establishes an environment that has a layered system ripe for oppression when one terminal degree is held in more esteem than another, particularly when one cohort of doctoral teaching faculty are tenurable and one are largely not.

REDEFINING "PRACTICE" TO INCLUDE THE DOMAIN OF THE NURSE EDUCATOR

Several areas of concern will be raised regarding the concept of "practice." The first is that practice is narrowly and obliquely defined by the AACN as being a place in which there are patients, yet they make exceptions in the case of health care policy makers and administrators. Health care policy makers and administrators are indeed affecting patient care. Are not nurse educators affecters of patient care? Cannot the classroom be the place of their "practice" just as logically as the offices are for administrators and health care policy makers?

Second, the role of clinical educator is an acceptable DNP role, yet the clinical education of nurses is no less important and should be no less grounded in educational theory and research than didactic instruction. There has been much written on the trials and tribulations of clinicians transitioning into education (Penn, Wilson, & Rossiter, 2008; Wetherbee, Nordrum, & Giles, 2008; Zungolo, 2004). Today, clinical education in nursing is amidst another shifting paradigm. The lack of traditional clinical sites as well as legal liability issues has moved more and more of student psychomotor learning from the clinical to a laboratory situation. Therefore, this "new clinical" elicits different teaching skills and practice. It is important to ask the leaders in the AACN if simulation and laboratory were envisioned as appropriate or inappropriate practice sites for the DNP educator, because they creatively combine traditional practice and educational expertise.

Third, to what extent did members of the AACN (composed of research qualified college and nursing school Deans) fully vet the implications for including the executive role as "advanced practice" but excluding the educator role as "advanced practice"? It is confusing that it is now considered visionary (by some, perhaps many) for nurse educators themselves to have excluded the nurse educator role from the DNP degree model. *Who did they foretell would ultimately teach other DNPs?* With the AACN not endorsing DNP programs that have the components needed to produce knowledgeable advanced practitioners in the field of nursing education, they have attempted to cling to and uphold the existing hierarchical academic system. By taking this stance on the role of the DNP-prepared nurse in nursing education, leaders have by default set up a tiered academic system that is already being reported as oppressive to nurse educators who are DNP-prepared. This is an unacceptable consequence in the evolution of DNP role development and should be morally distressing for all nurse educators and leaders. Furthermore, the aims and benefits of the DNP put forth by the AACN are contextually poor in the sense that the profession of nursing has had a protracted and long-standing severe need for doctoral level nurse educators who have expertise in education and this degree model did not address this. Indeed, the Joint Commission (2003) places nurse educators on the endangered list for reasons that are obvious to those in the profession.

For the reasons provided, the DNP in the nurse educator role must be reconsidered. A closer examination of the AACN (2006) *Essentials for the Doctorate of Nursing Practice*, which does not promote the DNP in the nurse educator role, and the NLN (2005) *Competencies of the Nurse Educator*, which does not prohibit DNPs from the role, reveals professional outcomes that are actually more conceptually congruent than different.

TABLE 7.1
Comparison of DNP Nurse Educator Capabilities

AACN (2006) Selections from the *Essentials of Doctoral Education for Advanced Nursing Practice*	NLN (2005) Selections from the *Competencies of the Nurse Educator*
Essential II: Organizational and Systems Leadership for Quality Improvement and Systems Thinking DNP graduates' practice includes not only direct care but also a focus on the needs of a panel of patients, a target population, a set of populations, or a broad community (p. 10)	*Competency 2: Facilitate Learner Development and Socialization* Recognizes responsibility for helping students develop as nurses and integrate the values and behaviors expected of those who fulfill that role (p. 2)
Commentary: Nursing educators, although not providing direct care, are focused on a broad community, nursing students who will deliver direct care.	
Essential III: Clinical Scholarship and Analytical Methods for Evidence-Based Practice Scholarship and research are the hallmarks of doctoral education. Although basic research has been viewed as the first and most essential form of scholarly activity, an enlarged perspective of scholarship has emerged through alternative paradigms that involve more than discovery of new knowledge (Boyer, 1990, p. 11)	*Competency 7: Engage in Scholarship* Nurse educators acknowledge that scholarship is an integral component of the faculty role, and that teaching itself is a scholarly activity. To engage effectively in scholarship, the nurse educator draws on extant literature to design evidence-based teaching and evaluation practices (p. 7)
Commentary: The role of research into all graduate nursing education is needed to advance the science and produce evidence for practice (Nolan et al., 2008). The role of using evidence-based practice is a clear outcome for DNPs and nurse educators. The AACN recognizes alternative forms of scholarship, for example, teaching.	
Essential IV: Information Systems/ Technology and Patient Care Technology for the Improvement and Transformation of Health Care DNP graduates are distinguished by their abilities to use information systems/ technology to support and improve patient care and health care systems, and provide leadership within health care systems and/or academic settings (p. 12)	*NLN Competency IV: Participation in Curriculum Design and Evaluation of Program Outcomes* Nurse educators are responsible for formulating program outcomes and designing curricula that reflect contemporary health care trends and prepare graduates to function effectively in the health-care environment (p. 4)
Commentary: The nurse educator uses technologically advanced methods to facilitate learning for application in the current health care environment. Informatics in all aspects of nursing needs to be strongly and consistently integrated (Jenkins, Wilson, & Osbalt, 2007).	

(*Continued*)

TABLE 7.1
Comparison of DNP Nurse Educator Capabilities *(Continued)*

AACN (2006) Selections from the *Essentials of Doctoral Education for Advanced Nursing Practice*	NLN (2005) Selections from the *Competencies of the Nurse Educator*
Essential V: Health Care Policy for Advocacy in Health Care Health care policy—whether it is created through governmental actions, institutional decision making, or organizational standards creates a framework that can facilitate or impede the delivery of health care services or the ability of the provider to engage in practice to address health care needs. Thus, engagement in the process of policy development is central to creating a health care system that meets the needs of its constituents (p. 13)	*Competency 5—Function as a Change Agent and Leader* Nurse educators function as change agents and leaders to create a preferred future for nursing education and nursing practice (p. 5)

Commentary: By educating students effectively, nurse educators are meeting the need of their constituents, and by examining organizational standards or curriculum address health care needs.

Essential VIII: Advanced Nursing Practice The increased knowledge and sophistication of health care has resulted in the growth of specialization in nursing in order to ensure competence in these highly complex areas of practice. The reality of the growth of specialization in nursing practice is that no individual can master all advanced roles and the requisite knowledge for enacting these roles. DNP programs provide preparation within distinct specialties that require expertise, advanced knowledge, and mastery in one area of nursing practice. A DNP graduate is prepared to practice in an area of specialization within the larger domain of nursing (p. 16)	*Competency 6: Pursue Continuous Quality Improvement in the Nurse Educator Role* Calls for continuous quality improvement in the role of education as a multidimensional function, while as providing an educational environment that facilitates learning (p. 4)

Commentary: Nursing education is *indeed* an area of specialized nursing practice, because it affects the health of the population through the educational preparation of nurses.

Table 7.1 provides comparisons of selected items from AACN's (2006) *Essentials for the Doctorate of Nursing Practice* and several from the NLN's (2005) *Competencies of the Nurse Educator* as examples. After each comparison, a short commentary is provided.

CERTIFICATION FOR NURSE EDUCATORS

The American Nurses Association (ANA) attempted to remove the nurse educator from the certification realm of the advanced practice nurse model with the following statement (ANA, 2008):

> Many nurses with advanced graduate nursing preparation practice in roles and specialties (e.g., informatics, public health, education, or administration) that are essential to advance

the health of the public but do not focus on direct care to individuals and, therefore, their practice does not require regulatory recognition beyond the Registered Nurse license granted by state boards of nursing.

—ANA, 2008, p. 5

Although the ANA does state that practitioners of the specialty roles should be educated on the graduate level, their short sightedness does not acknowledge the value of certification for these roles, even though they affect the aggregate health of populations. Again the term *direct patient* care is used to confine rather than to expand care that is inclusive of many venues.

The AACN (2006) also states that, "All DNP graduates, prepared as APNs, must be prepared to sit for national specialty APN certification" (AACN, 2006, p. 17). The NLN's CNE (Certified Nurse Educator) examination is the advanced specialty certification for nurse educators (Wittmann-Price & Godshall, 2009). Even though many DNP-prepared nurses are CNEs, unfortunately, the NLN has not differentiated between types of doctorates in the demographic calculations of those nurse educators who have successfully completed the certification exam (National League for Nursing, personal communication November 2, 2009).

In order for nurse educators to be eligible to take the CNE examination, they must meet the requirements of one of two options. Option one calls for the nurse educator to have nine credits in graduate nursing education. Knowing that many nurse educators do not have educational courses, there is a second option that calls for four years of teaching. However, unfortunately this again is likened to an apprenticeship model, rather than a scholarly model of professional growth. As the role of the nurse educator evolves, and is respected as an advanced practice role equivalent to the other roles in the realms of practice, administration, and research, the criterion developers of the NLN for the specialization examination will hopefully distance themselves from the apprenticeship model.

PEDAGOGICAL EDUCATION FOR NURSE EDUCATORS

A closer look at the varying degrees held by nurse educators reveals that they are comprised of varying amounts of actual educational courses, and this will be further explored in the third part of this chapter. Many nursing research doctorates have virtually no courses related to the discipline of education, yet that degree is required to apply for tenure as "teaching faculty" at many institutions. This terminal degree is primarily a research doctorate, and the research that is sought is often clinical, not educational, although educational research is greatly needed. There are schools that intertwine educational courses within their research-oriented doctoral nursing programs, and some actually offer a post-masters certificate in education when a specific number of educational courses are successfully completed. Most nurse educators would agree that courses basic to education are those that contain content about:

- Educational philosophies;
- Teaching/learning theories;
- Curriculum development;
- Instructional design and methodologies;
- Technological utilization in education;
- Nurse education's role of scholarship, discovery, teaching, and integration; and
- Evaluative approaches.

The AACN in a white paper dated August 6, 2007 states that educators of nursing students at the baccalaureate and doctorate level should possess a doctorate as well as advanced degrees in their specialty area. It explicitly states that "nursing courses will be taught by faculty with graduate-level specialty educational preparation and advanced expertise in the areas of content they teach. Doctorally prepared faculty have overall responsibility for all nursing courses" (p. 1). Yet the AACN white paper does not define "doctorally prepared" as practice or research-based and does not recognize that many faculty with research-based doctorates are ill-prepared to teach a multitude of clinically based courses.

Nurse educator programs are abundant in MSN programs and these programs are specifically designed with an objective: to produce nurse educators on the graduate level. Although these graduates are well prepared in the practice of education, normally they are not prepared in traditional educational research methods. Therefore, they need further education on the doctoral level, as do other practitioners, but they can contribute to evidence-based educational practice. The best scenario for nurse educator preparation is to have pedagogical courses as well as a doctoral degree—either practice, to contribute to the evidence-base, or research to contribute to original knowledge. Both are needed and should be equally valued in academia.

Therefore, DNPs are currently at no disadvantage in courses about educational content when compared to graduates of most other nursing doctorates. It is the educational courses in pedagogy, curriculum, and evaluation that set nurse educators apart as practice experts in the classroom and clinical areas. The nursing profession needs to reconsider how it evaluates the role of nurse educator. It does not make sense *not* to think of education as an advanced practice, especially if the work of the clinical executive is considered advanced practice.

THE DNP DEGREE AND TENURE

Tenure is another formidable issue that surfaces with the discussion of the DNP's role in nursing education. A brief discussion will be presented related to tenure and the current educational culture that is increasingly questioning the advantages of tenure. Institutional criteria for tenure and promotion have been, and will continue to be, a topic of conversation among nurse educators. Many nursing departments use the Boyer (1996) model of scholarship. The weight an academic institution places on each of the four components of Boyer's model differs according to their educational mission. Many DNP-prepared nurses in nurse educator roles are thoroughly fulfilling the tenure criteria of their institutions, despite, more likely than not, not being permitted to be on the tenure track. They are publishing, presenting, appraising and utilizing evidence and integrated knowledge across disciplines, and are demonstrating teaching excellence. Further, outside of research-extensive or research-intensive institutions, there is no expectation that faculty (any faculty) obtain external research funding. Therefore, at least in teaching institutions, the prohibition of DNPs from tenure track positions seems almost unethical. DNPs hold a terminal degree in nursing and therefore should not be excluded from tenure track positions. Alternatively, tenure guidelines in research-intensive institutions that are based on a track record of original research also do not necessarily exclude DNPs. DNPs should be eligible for tenure in these institutions if they have had course work that provides them with a research background and have chosen to continue on a research career path. Indeed, in this text there are many chapters where the authors have identified programs where the DNP or DrNP graduate has conducted empirical clinical research.

Tenure guidelines are being questioned in today's academic context and have long been a detriment in retention of nurse educators (Holland, 1992; Trower, 2009). The tenure system in academia also needs to be reexamined, given that it was a system that arose in the 1930–1940s developed by white males with stay-at-home wives (Trower, 2009). Tenure's applicability to today's economic system and female gender-based professions desperately needs fair and unbiased appraisal. The tenure system itself still oppresses the nursing profession's position within academic institutions, and without evaluating the actual coursework and scholarship of the individual doctoral degree recipient (rather than just the type of doctorate), the oppression will continue.

DOCTOR OF NURSING PRACTICE CURRICULA TODAY

Most of the new DNP programs do not include preparation for being an educator, because the focus of the DNP program for many institutions is to prepare APNs to function in an advanced practice role that includes leadership and health policy skills (Siela, Twibell, & Keller, 2009). However, the DNP-prepared nurse may still be hired in an academic role and literature indicates that many nurses do become academicians who are responsible for clinical program delivery and clinical teaching. Fitzpatrick (2002) reports that clinical doctorate graduates have a firm foundation in practice and high levels of clinical knowledge and skill which are foremost when considering requirements for nursing faculty. DNP graduates may therefore comprise the majority of nursing faculty in the future (Wall, Novak, & Wilkerson, 2005). In the *Essentials of Doctoral Education for Advanced Nursing Practice*, the AACN (2006) also acknowledges that many DNP graduates desire and will accept faculty positions upon completion of their program. However, the AACN reports that DNPs are not expected to assume a faculty role without additional education.

By preparing graduates whose credentials will not prepare them for full participation in the academic community, the DNP disrupts the flow of graduates to a single terminal degree (AACN, 2004). It is therefore critical to examine how DNP programs are serving as a catalyst in valuing the teaching role and in preparing future leaders in the academic arena. There is a need for formal pedagogical programs to enhance their ability to teach the science of the profession they practice. This formal coursework could be integrated within the context of the DNP program. To examine how some schools are addressing this concern, a random review of course requirements was conducted via website for ten nursing doctor of nursing practice programs within the United States.

Doctor of Nursing Practice curricula for the following programs were examined (noted in alphabetical order): Columbia University, Case Western University, Drexel University, Duke University, New York University, Northeastern University, Old Dominion University, University of Kentucky, University of Medicine and Dentistry in New Jersey, and the University of Minnesota. A brief description of the curriculum and credits required for graduation will be noted with specific emphasis on post-master's DNP students.

- Columbia University (60 credits, post-master's entry) has seven core support courses and nine clinical core courses. The curriculum includes content on: (i) complex diagnostic and treatment modalities, (ii) sophisticated informatics and decision-making technology, and (iii) in-depth knowledge of biophysical, psychosocial, behavioral and clinical sciences. In addition, students complete a residency and portfolio which aim to provide mastery and evidence of competency achievement.

- Case Western University (34 credits, post-master's entry) has ten required core courses and four elective courses. Core curriculum includes content on: (i) applied statistics and research methods, (ii) leadership and health policy, and (iii) nursing theory and translating evidence into nursing practice. In addition, two educational leadership and two practice leadership electives courses are offered. Students also complete a practicum, scholarly project, and proposal.

- Drexel University (DrNP) (48 quarter credits, primarily post-master's entry) has five core fields: nursing science (four courses), nursing practice (four courses), research methods (three courses), cognate (two courses), and dissertation (five sections). The curriculum includes content on: (i) politics in health and ethics in nursing practice; (ii) epidemiology and biostatistics, quantitative methods for clinical nursing inquiry, and qualitative methods for clinical nursing inquiry; and (iii) two cognates that must support the students identified track. Students have four tracks from which they can select as their primary and secondary focus—The Practitioner, The Educator, The Clinical Scientist, and The Clinical Executive. Students also complete a residency, role and clinical practicum, and a clinical dissertation.

- Duke University (34 credits, post-master's entry) has five required core courses, two electives, and a DNP capstone. Students' program of study includes content on: (i) evidence-based practice and applied statistics, (ii) data-driven health care improvement, (iii) financial management and budget planning, (iv) effective leadership, and (v) health systems transformation.

- New York University (40 credits, post-master's entry) requires eight didactic courses, a capstone project, and an internship. Student's course of study includes content on: (i) genomics across the life span, (ii) health care economics and finance for advanced nursing practice, (iii) evidence-based practice, and (iv) issues in health policy and improving health outcomes through quality.

- Northeastern University (30 credits, post-master's entry) requires six core courses, one elective, and a capstone project. Content covered in the student's course plan include: (i) leadership in advance practice nursing, (ii) health informatics, (iii) epidemiology and population-based health, (iv) health care finance and marketing, (v) health care policy, and (vi) translating evidence into practice.

- Old Dominion University (30 credits, post-master's entry) requires eight core courses, a clinical residency, and a capstone project. The students' program of study emphasizes content on health disparities, barriers to care, and culture (two classes); along with practice focused research (two classes); systems leadership (two classes); and advanced clinical training (four classes).

- The University of Kentucky (40 credits, post-master's entry) calls for eleven courses and a residency. Content studied during the students' program of study include: (i) development of advanced competencies for complex practice, and (ii) research utilization for the improvement of clinical care delivery, patient outcomes, and system management. Each student must complete a research utilization project.

- The University of Medicine and Dentistry in New Jersey (40 credits, post-master's entry) requires two foundational courses, ten universal core courses, two cognate courses, a residency, and a capstone project. The students' program of study includes content on: (i) information technology and health care ethics; (ii) evidence-based advance practice nursing and health policy; (iii) epidemiology and statistics;

(iv) health promotion across diverse cultures; and (v) leadership, health care economics, and the business of practice. A selected practice cognate for the DNP role development includes an option for education, health policy, administration, leadership, advanced practice, or clinical informatics.

▓ The University of Minnesota (36 credits, post-master's entry) requires core courses in science and philosophy, leadership, and practice. The students' program of study emphasizes content on (i) program evaluation and epidemiology, (ii) interprofessional health care ethics, (iii) science of nursing intervention, (iv) science of teaching and learning in nursing, (v) health care and health policy leadership, and (vi) evidence-based practice and economics of health care. A leadership project is completed as a core outcome of the program.

Despite the fact that there is no national agreement on the need for pedagogical courses or experiential courses on education for DNP students, several programs have moved ahead to integrate these skills. Of the 10 schools, 4 programs had curricula that identified content regarding an educational track or cognate where students could gain skills in measuring learner outcomes, teaching basics, educational theory, and/or through experiential practice. Only two programs explicitly identified an educator track as a central focus of their doctor of nursing program—Drexel University's Educator Track and Case Western Reserve's Educational Leadership Track. There may, however, be programs where the education of DNPs into the educator role is also taking place, but at least less visibly on their websites.

The authors of this chapter propose that on-the-job training alone may not promote quality outcomes when preparing DNP students who may teach in academic settings. While thriving to gain parity with other professional groups whose graduates earn a practice doctorate, DNP programs have been strong in orchestrating courses that: (i) enhance knowledge to improve nursing practice and patient outcomes and (ii) increase knowledge in leadership skills and roles. Given the significant faculty shortage, the role of DNP educators needs to be recognized and emphasized as fully as other roles in these programs.

It is requisite that DNP programs that use multiple levels of preparation for their graduates appropriately assess how faculty ranks are determined to support clinical tracks that will enable these future nursing leaders to thrive in university settings. Programs must look for ways to provide support for DNP students who want or need pedagogical skills to enhance their ability to teach the science of the profession they practice. The profession of nursing can also be influenced and strengthened if *both* research-focused and practice-focused doctorate programs receive preparation in teaching methodologies, curriculum design and development, and program evaluation methodologies.

To promote this paradigm shift, it is important to think outside the box about those who may be able to fulfill faculty roles and obligations (e.g., DNP graduates). If change is to occur that mitigates the faculty shortage and enables our fellow colleagues to flourish in this new found role, DNP graduates who may guide students in clinical arenas at all levels must be better equipped (didactically and experientially) to lead the next generation of students. Having diversely prepared faculty members may serve us well, especially when the strengths of the individual and his or her educational preparation can be capitalized upon. Some programs have done just that. To this end, this section of the chapter will conclude with a quote by Ralph Waldo Emerson, which is quite fitting for programs taking the lead with this initiative: "Do not go where the path may lead, go instead where there is no path and leave a trail."

WHERE WE STAND NOW

A shortage of doctorally prepared faculty is now a reality as the baby boomers in great numbers have begun to retire. These factors make the DNP an attractive option for faculty who would like to continue their education and obtain a terminal degree. But academia may truly not be ready for clinically focused, doctorally prepared faculty.

There are a number of important reasons why it is important for the DNP graduate to assume a faculty role. The DNP-prepared nurse has a true passion for health care and client interaction. The clinical skill and enthusiasm possessed by this group of faculty is infectious and is an asset for both clinical and classroom teachers, as well as being role models and mentors at both the graduate and undergraduate levels. Again, we strongly emphasize that it is the highly competent, practicing practitioner who is best positioned to teach and best mentor the large cadre of current DNP students—especially in clinical courses.

The ANA (2008) believes strongly that, "Advanced Practice Registered Nurses are one of the keys to solving America's health care crisis" (p. 1). Furthermore, part of that crisis is being produced by a lack of nurse educators to teach the next generation of nurses. The current shortage of nurse educators has prompted over 30% of DNP graduates (Zungolo, 2009) to fill the much needed role of nurse educator. It is thus confusing to us that the AACN admits the PhD and DNP degrees both do not necessarily prepare the graduate for teaching, and yet the PhD is still the preferred degree for the teaching mission (AACN, 2006). However, if PhD graduates have less emphasis on practice, then who is best prepared to teach future DNPs? Retrospectively, this exclusion of the educator role seems inappropriate and poorly planned.

Therefore, here is the summation of the presented dilemma. The research doctorate is the degree which is considered appropriate for a nurse educator, yet it may be conferred with no pedagogical or educational course requirements. The same is true for the DNP. Both education and practice are mandated by virtue of national patient safety goals to use best evidence in both teaching and practice. Our interpretation of the *Essentials* document (AACN, 2006) indicates only graduates with research doctorates are educated to "create" evidence. The DNP graduate is positioned to appraise and use evidence, except in the rare instance in which the generation of clinical research has been built into the curriculum, such as the DrNP degree (Dreher, Donnelly, & Naremore, 2005) or within a few other DNP programs that indeed do include an empirical research project. The master's level graduate may be fully prepared in education, but does not hold a terminal degree. Therefore, the recommendation is to recognize the nurse educator role as an advance practice nursing role and that their "practice" is education; then develop that role with the appropriate courses as a track within the DNP degree. According to the NLN (2002),

> The nurse educator role is essential to the ongoing development of the profession and the ability of the discipline to meet society's needs for quality nursing care. There is specialized knowledge and preparation that is essential for practice as a nurse educator, and that knowledge and skill must be recognized and rewarded by the nursing and higher education communities. Competence as an educator can be established, recognized, and expanded through master's and/or doctoral education, post-master's certificate programs, continuing professional development, mentoring activities, and professional certification as a faculty member.
>
> —*NLN, 2002, p. 1*

SUMMARY

DNP graduates entering the academic realm of nursing are needed to decrease the faculty shortage gap. Other nursing DNP roles that are not direct patient practice, such as administration, are accepted, yet DNPs in the education role are not. PhDs, who are accepted as nurse educators, may have no more educational courses than DNP graduates. DNP graduates are exposed to varying curricula, many with educational courses. DNP as well as PhD curricula vary greatly with respect to educational courses. The NLN certifies nurse educators with pedagogical courses but also with experience, which translates into the apprenticeship model. DNP graduates who are excellent educators and bring up-to-date evidence-based practice issues into the classroom and clinical educational environment are being devalued by a patriarchical, traditional educational system that has long-standing, overly traditional tenure expectations, which do not recognize the worth of DNP's practice scholarship.

Much more dialogue is needed about the role of the DNP graduate as a nurse educator. Nurses also must address the curricula for all doctorally prepared nurse educators to ensure doctoral nursing curricula (PhD or DNP) have the tools to competently teach, should that be their career goal. More importantly, nursing scholars need to be open-minded enough to examine and revisit the current definition of "practice." Most importantly, we must envision the development of the practice doctorate as a step in the journey to define the many aspects of our nursing realm. We must remember that there are many ways, as nurses, to affect the health care change nationally and globally, and we should applaud DNP-prepared nurses for using their expert practice, be it clinical, educational, or administrative, to help the nursing profession reach its goal.

NOTE

1. For the purposes of this chapter, when we refer to the Doctor of Nursing Practice degree, we include both DNP and DrNP degrees, but will use the DNP initials for simplicity.
2. In other words today's doctorally prepared nurse educator can have a PhD, EdD, DNP, and other degrees.

REFERENCES

American Association of Colleges of Nursing (AACN). (2004). *Position statement on the practice doctorate in nursing*. Retrieved from http://www.aacn.nche.edu/DNP/DNPPositionStatement. htm

American Association of Colleges of Nursing (AACN). (2006). *The essentials of doctoral education for advanced nursing practice*. Retrieved from http://www.AACN.nche.edu/DNP/pdf/Essentials. pdf

American Association of Colleges of Nursing (AACN). (2007). *Draft position statement AACN guidelines regarding faculty teaching in baccalaureate and graduate nursing programs*. Retrieved from http://www.aacn.nche.edu/Education/pdf/Facexpect.pdf

American Nurses Association (ANA). (2008). *Advanced practice nurses, key to a reformed U.S. Health Care System*. Retrieved from http://www.nursingworld.org/EspeciallyForYou/Advanced-PracticeNurses.aspx

Boyer, E. (1996). *Scholarship reconsidered: Priorities of the professoriate*. San Francisco, CA: Jossey-Bass.

Bryant-Lukosius, D., DiCenso, A., Browne, G., & Pinelli, J. (2004). Advanced practice nursing roles: Development, implementation and evaluation. *Journal of Advanced Nursing, 48*(5), 519–529.

Cartwright, C. A., & Reed, C. K. (2005). Policy and planning perspectives for the doctorate in nursing practice: An educational perspective. *Online Journal of Issues in Nursing, 30,* 1–10.

DalPezzo, N. K., & Jett, K. T. (2010). Nursing faculty: A vulnerable population. *Journal of Nursing Education, 49*(3), 132–136.

Donnelly, G. (2007). Doctor of Nursing Practice Program (DrNP): About the program. Retrieved from http://www.drexel.edu/cnhp/drnp_program/about.asp

Dreher, H. M., Donnelly, G., & Naremore, R. (2005). Reflections on the DNP and an alternate practice doctorate model: The Drexel DrNP. *Online Journal of Issues in Nursing, 11*(1), Retrieved from www.nursingworld.org/ojin/topic28/tpc28_7.htm

Fitzpatrick, J. J. (2002). The balance in nursing: Clinical and scientific ways of knowing and being. *Nursing Education Perspectives, 23,* 57.

Holland, C. B. (1992). The influence and organizational commitment on intention to leave of nurse educators (Doctoral dissertation, Louisiana State University, 1992). *Dissertation Abstracts International, 53,* 09A.

Joint Commission on Accreditation of Healthcare Organizations. (2003). *Health care at the crossroads: Health strategies for addressing the evolving nursing crises.* Retrieved from http://www.jointcommission.org/NR/rdonlyres/5C138711-ED76-4D6F-909F-B06E0309F36D/0/health_care_at_the_crossroads.pdf

McKinley, M. G. (2009). Go to the head of the class: Clinical educator role transition. *Advanced Critical Care, 20*(1), 91–101.

National League for Nursing. (2002). *Position statement on preparation of nurse educators.* Retrieved from http://www.nln.org/aboutnln/PositionStatements/prepofnursed02.htm

National League for Nursing. (2005). *Core competencies of nurse educators with task statements.* Retrieved from http://www.nln.org/facultydevelopment/pdf/corecompetencies.pdf

National League for Nursing. (2006). Nurse faculty support continues to fall short, July 24, 2006. *National League for Nursing News.* Retrieved from http://www.nln.org/newsreleases/nurseeducators2006.htm

National League for Nursing Accrediting Commission. (2008). *Standards and criteria: Clinical doctorate degree programs in nursing.* Retrieved from http://www.nlnac.org/manuals/SC2008_DOCTORATE.htm

Nichols, E. F., & Chitty, K. K. (2005). Educational patterns in nursing. In K. K. Chitty (Ed.), *Professional Nursing: Concepts & Challenges* (4th ed.) (pp. 31–63). St. Louis, MO: Elsevier Saunders.

Penn, B. K., Wilson, L. D., & Rossiter, R. (2008). Transitioning from nursing practice to a teaching role. *Journal of Issues in Nursing, 13*(3), 1–16.

Rogan, M. K., Crooks, D., & Durrant, M. (2008). Innovations in nursing education standard development for nurse educator practice. *Journal of Nursing and Staff Development, 24*(3), 119–123.

Siela, D., Twibell, K., & Keller, V. (2009). The shortage of nurses and nursing faculty: What critical care nurses can do. *AACN Advances in Critical Care, 19*(1), 66–77.

Trower, C. A. (2009). Rethinking tenure for the next generation. *The Chronicle of Higher Education, Sept. 7.* Retrieved from http://chronicle.com/article/Rethinkin-Tenure-for-the-N/48262/

Wall, B. M., Novak, J. C., & Wilkerson, S. A. (2005). Doctor of nursing practice program development: Reengineering health care. *Journal of Nursing Education, 44*(9), s396–s403.

Wetherbee, E., Nordrum, J. T., & Giles, S. (2008). Effective teaching behaviors of APTA-credentialed versus noncredentialed clinical instructors. *Journal of Physical Therapy Education, 22*(1), 65–74.

Wittmann-Price, R. A., & Godshall, M. (2009). *Certified nurse educator (CNE) review manual.* New York, NY: Springer.

Zungolo, E. (2004). Faculty preparation: Is clinical specialization a benefit or a deterrent to quality nursing education? *The Journal of Continuing Education in Nursing, 35*(1), 19–23.

Zungolo, E. (2009). *The DNP and the faculty role: Issues and challenges.* Paper presented at the Second National Conference on the Doctor of Nursing Practice: The Dialogue Continues..., Hilton Head Island, South Carolina, March 24–27, 2010.

CHAPTER SEVEN: Reflective Response

Eileen H. Zungolo

INTRODUCTION

At the outset, I want to congratulate the authors of this chapter on a thought provoking and timely discussion of the role of the DNP-prepared nurse as an educator. Many of the issues they address have been on my radar screen for a number of years, and writ large in the last few years as the DNP "movement" has evolved. Furthermore, the authors used some interesting approaches to explicate their viewpoint—like good educators—and provided a number of excellent examples.

EXPERIENCE OF ONE DNP-PREPARED FACULTY

First they described, through the experience of one DNP-prepared person, those aspects of the faculty position that she found especially challenging as she moved into a faculty role. On the one hand, this personal narrative brought the feelings and viewpoints into focus, and at the same time, the narrator described elements of higher education that are far outside the direct control of one discipline. For example, the dimensions of scholarship that a DNP-prepared faculty member may develop is laudable, but most institutions of higher education have criteria for scholarship and advancement in rank that are more traditional. These disparate interpretations of scholarship do not only affect DNP-prepared faculty, they often impact all faculty members who function in applied areas of study—lawyers, pharmacists, allied health professionals, and so on, regardless of the academic credential they hold.

An element brought home to me in this piece is the extent to which successfully funded scholarship is equated with strong faculty performance. Are these dimensions really well correlated or do we assume that researchers are good educators?

I was also disappointed that this narrative did not describe the educational preparation of the DNP-prepared faculty member. The acquisition of the credential is only half the story. What did the educational program leading to that degree prepare the individual to accomplish? All too often in explicating what the DNP graduate does not have—credibility as a researcher—detracts from what he/she does have—excellence in practice. Focusing on the scholarship inherent in the role, whether that be in clinical practice, administrative practice, or educational practice, seems a stronger argument to support the integrity of the credential than comparing applied investigations to original research. Since this is the area in which there is more consensus—DNP-prepared individuals are not researchers—it seems a moot point to aim for parity in an area where the incumbents *should* be different. It seems a much more profitable route for the

DNP-prepared faculty member to find a niche within the domain of scholarship that is a better reflection of the preparation the individual is presumed to have had. I encourage learning about the Scholarship of Teaching and Learning, an approach to the faculty role which fosters the development of expertise in pedagogy (McKinney, 2007).

At the same time, if the DNP-prepared faculty member focused the entire study at the DNP level on the acquisition of knowledge and experience in clinical practice, the preparation for the faculty role may be absent. All new faculty members suffer some trauma in a new position with new expectations, and like all new kids on the block, they will need to learn the ropes. The entry into higher education is fraught with new challenges for which new faculty members will be poorly prepared if they have not been afforded learning opportunities about the faulty role and teaching. So, I wish that the description of the DNP-prepared faculty would have focused more on challenges in the classroom and clinical setting with students as the focus, not patients.

To complicate this comparison further, the personal experience description was supplied by a nurse midwife. We assume this individual is teaching students in a midwifery program. As such, this faculty member is fulfilling a role in graduate education for which doctoral level preparation has long been the goal. Thus, while there is no "elevation" in faculty credential with this individual (lessened in this faculty member's view since she cannot be on the tenure track at this institution), what *decreases* is the probability that the DNP-prepared faculty will be viewed as "lesser" than previously established faculty prepared at the masters level in an advanced practice program.

I am increasingly concerned about the management of DNP-prepared faculty in their employment settings. While I sympathize with the concerns about advancement and equity in the distribution of resources, are these not part of the initial employment discussions? If DNP-prepared individuals accept a faculty appointment, they should know at the outset what they can expect. If informed that tenure is not an option at the institution for those who do not hold a PhD or comparable credential, the DNP-prepared person needs to decide whether or not to take the position. Complaining about existing conditions that were clearly explained during the recruitment process is just not good business. I urge all prospective faculty, regardless of their preparation, to explore the opportunities for growth and personal satisfaction in a position before they commit to the offer. Once employed, the faculty member's only recourse is to identify some failure of promises at hire.

THE PRACTICE OF "THE NURSE EDUCATOR"

I am a very strong supporter of the basic tenet of this chapter, which is that *educational practice* is as important and central to the provision of safe, high-quality patient care, as clinical practice or administrative practice. Somehow, over the last 20 years or so, we have diminished the role of the educator to one which appears to require no preparation. As the authors very clearly identify throughout their paper, it seems as if the profession of nursing believes that if you possess content knowledge, you will automatically have the talent to transmit that knowledge to others. As an occupational group we have gone from having a strong, theory based workforce in education, to a group that dismisses educational preparation for higher education as a suitable faculty development enterprise. While faculty development is very important to foster quality educational programs, it is not a substitute for basic preparation for the role.

It is a constant source of amazement to me to have discussions with experts in clinical practice and hear their emphasis on the need for both neophyte nurses and those with advanced practice to possess knowledge of the health care system, and institutional organization priorities. *Yet, these same individuals do not see the need to have candidates for faculty positions who possess these knowledge points about higher education.*

This transition in the value of nurse educator preparation has occurred at a time when the teaching of nursing has become painfully complex, and the world of practice in which our graduates will work has become highly demanding, technological and fraught with an extraordinary array of problems. Yet, as the authors make clear in this manuscript, and years of personal experience has well documented, individuals who hold a credential approved by the local state board of nursing will be hired into faculty positions with no experience or education in the faculty role.

The last year has witnessed the publication of the much awaited study on nursing education from the Carnegie Foundation for the Advancement of Teaching. *Educating Nurses: A Call for Radical Transformation* (Benner, Sutphen, Leonard, & Day, 2009) outlines many issues and weaknesses of our national system of nursing education. Many of these observations and the recommendations derived from them have received considerable national attention. However, very limited debate or discussion has occurred with respect to the preparation of faculty. Yet, Benner and colleagues note:

> We found that many teachers and students are dissatisfied with the teaching preparation of current nursing faculty... we note that current graduate nursing programs do not systematically offer opportunities for learning how to teach . . . .
> —*Benner, Sutphen, Leonard, & Day, 2009, p. 32*

> To be responsible stewards of the discipline all graduate nursing programs need to support the study of pedagogies designed and evaluated for nursing education.
> —*Benner, 2009, p. 224*

Hence, it is clear that a national study of nursing education found the preparation of faculty to be limited and not successfully producing well-prepared educators.

SUMMARY: TRENDS AND NURSING ORGANIZATIONS

The review of the relative positions of the AACN and the NLN related to the DNP and roles in the manuscript is informative, as is the summary of some of the educational programs leading to the DNP degree. Nonetheless, I think the major questions related to the issue of the DNP and the role of educator have not been raised. These are:

1. What is the appropriate preparation for nurse educators in pre-licensure programs?
2. What is the appropriate preparation for nurse educators in advanced practice programs?

Over the years, the National League for Nursing has focused intensely on the needs of faculty as they advance in the academy and has developed many documents to assist in that process (Halstead, 2007). Among the most directive, helpful, and germane to this discussion is the *Core Competencies of Nurse Educators* (2005).[1] This document delineates all of the competencies that faculty need to possess across the spectrum of roles a nurse educator must fulfill. *In my judgment, the actual degree a faculty member holds is less important to their success in the academic community than the degree to which they possess these competencies.* Unfortunately, at the present time, DNP programs *are not* addressing these competencies, nor endeavoring to assist students in developing the knowledge and skills that support such abilities. The result is found in work such as Benner's. I believe, as a profession we need to identify the preparation of future nurses as work, important enough to be deemed advanced practice.

NOTE

1. The website to retrieve this document: www.nln.org/facultydevelopment/pdf/corcompeten-cies.pdf

REFERENCES

Benner, P., Sutphen, M., Leonard, V., & Day, L. (2009). *Educating nurses: A call for radical transform-ation.* San Francisco, CA: Jossey-Bass.

Halstead, J. A. (2007). *Nurse educator competencies: Creating an evidence-based practice for nurse educa-tors.* New York, NY: National League for Nursing.

McKinney, K. (2007). *Enhancing learning through the scholarship of teaching and learning.* San Francisco, CA: Anker Publishing.

National League for Nursing. (2005). *Core competencies of nurse educators with task statements.* Retrieved from http://www.nln.org/facultydevelopment/pdf/corecompetencies.pdf

Nolan, M. T., Wenzel, J., Han, H., Allen, J. K., Paez, K. A., & Mock, V. (2008). Advancing a program of research within a nursing faculty role. *Journal of Professional Nursing, 24*(6), 364–370.

CRITICAL THINKING QUESTIONS

1. What methods of evaluation can nurse leaders use to study the effectiveness of DNP graduates in the role of nurse educator?
2. When assessing a DNP candidate for an educational role in nursing, what criteria of assessment should be used?
3. Your nursing program is preparing for an accreditation visit; what role should your faculty member (e.g., a DNP teaching critical care) play in developing the accredita-tion report?
4. A faculty member with a DNP degree is being evaluated for tenure. The faculty handbook states under degree criteria .... "a terminal degree in your discipline." How would you compose a letter of support for the tenure candidate?
5. You are a DNP faculty member on the curriculum revision team for the baccalaureate program. One of the team members has a PhD in public health and is being uncivil because you do not have a PhD. How would you educate that person in relation to your role, education, and preparation as a nurse educator?
6. What are some of the major differences in preparation between the DNP and PhD in preparing students for an educator role?
7. How do key features of the "practice environment" affect curriculum within the paradigm of nursing education?
8. What are some of the definitions of scholarship that are attainable in the DNP role and should be valued as tenurable?
9. Can you foresee that two different doctoral degrees in academia may lend themselves to establishing an environment that enhances or detracts academic collegiality?
10. Can you think of positive collaborations that could take place in the academic environment between nurse educators with a practice and research doctorate?

CHAPTER EIGHT

The Role of the Clinical Scientist

H. Michael Dreher, Sandra N. Jones, and Cynthia Gifford-Hollingsworth

INTRODUCTION

The doctoral advanced practice role of the Clinical Scientist is a role that is unique to Drexel University's doctor of nursing practice program. However, there are certainly many advanced practice nurses across the country who are working in the clinical trials/pharmaceutical industry who are pursuing various doctor of nursing practice degree programs. This role was created in 2005 at Drexel University as one of the four tracks in our new DrNP program. At the program's inception, we offered two primary tracks: the *Practitioner Track* and the *Educator Track*. The former is recognized by the American Association of Colleges of Nursing (AACN) as a DNP track that the Collegiate Commission on Nursing Education (CCNE) will accredit. And while the CCNE will not accredit DNP Educator Tracks, the National League for Nursing Accrediting Commission (NLNAC) will.[1] We also offered two secondary tracks: the Clinical Executive Track and the Clinical Scientist Track. Again, the CCNE will accredit the former (Clinical Executive), but not the latter. Our assumption is that the progressive stance of the NLNAC toward the titling of the clinical doctorate would make it eligible for accreditation, too (NLNAC, 2005). Because Philadelphia is an international hub of the pharmaceutical research industry and has a large pool of master's-prepared nurses working in this industry, it was not surprising that Drexel identified this population of advanced practice nurses and sought to market Drexel's new DrNP degree to them. Chiefly, the Clinical Scientist role was devised to attract two different types of prospective doctor of nursing practice students: (1) students either active in the clinical trials/pharmaceutical research industry who needed a clinical research-oriented doctorate to better position them in the field, or for students interested in seeking typical industry positions; or (2) students who, for whatever reason, could not or did not want to attend a full-time PhD program (or lengthy part-time PhD program), but who wanted a greater focus on clinical nursing research than is typically available in the few research-oriented DNP programs across the country. This chapter will describe the evolution of the Clinical Scientist doctoral advanced practice role at Drexel University. Two students who enrolled in the track for both role aims above will also describe their journey through selection of the role to meet their own professional goals.

NEED FOR THIS INNOVATIVE ROLE: EVOLUTION OF THE CLINICAL TRIALS NURSE

Nurses have been involved in clinical trials for a long time, but until 1995 the formal role of the clinical trials nurse as a clinical research coordinator was vague (Raybuck, 1997). There was also no uniform job description or degree standard recognized for the role. The rapid emergence of the pharmaceutical research industry in the 1980s and need for more complex drug trials and more safety studies on new medical devices has paved the way for more nursing professionals in the clinical trials research industry. The numerous clinical drug trials that have mushroomed with the search for more effective drugs and drug combinations to treat those infected with the HIV/AIDS pandemic and the ongoing burgeoning cancer drug research industry have led to an enormous need for the skills and expertise of clinical research nurses, now identified largely as "research nurse associates" (Dore et al., 1995; Lenoble, 2000). To emphasize the role and need for more nurses in this growing specialty field, in 2004 the pharmaceutical research industry was generating some estimated $235.4 billion in United States domestic sales and had grown to an estimated $700 billion globally by 2009 (Rosen, 2009; Stephens-Lloyd, 2004; York University, 2008). Similarly, the global medical device industry generated an estimated $250 billion in sales in 2009 (Rosen, 2009). This enormous amount of revenue in the health care industry, one of the few growing job sectors during the global economic recession of 2008–2010 (Gaulin, 2008) has meant there were continuing job opportunities for the Registered Nurse who had the skills and expertise to work on one of the thousands of clinical research units (both inpatient and sometimes outpatient) across the United States and around the globe. Examples of such clinical research units include the Cornell Clinical Trials Unit in New York City, founded in 1986, which has conducted landmark studies for HIV/AIDS infection resulting in effective therapies, as well as research for the treatment and prevention of opportunistic infections. This center also has been a leader in recruiting diverse populations with HIV including women, people of color, and people exposed to HIV through needle sharing. Another example is the Covance Clinical Research Unit in Austin, Texas, which is equipped with 90 beds, including 12 beds for safety monitoring, and specializes in long-term confinement trials in healthy normal volunteers as well as special populations and in renal impairment studies, including patients on hemodialysis. Literally thousands of these research facilities would be completely nonfunctional if they did not employ research nurses engaged in all aspects of the clinical research enterprise.

A UNIQUE DOCTORAL ADVANCED PRACTICE NURSING ROLE
AT DREXEL UNIVERSITY

In 2000, nursing faculty in Drexel University's College of Nursing and Health Professions began to explore an alternative doctoral degree for advanced practice nurses as an option to the PhD. The Drexel nursing faculty were skeptical that the PhD should be the only degree option for advanced practice nurses, especially those who wanted to continue active practice while pursuing the doctorate (and why not?). The faculty were particularly interested in designing a rigorous nursing doctorate that focused both on practice and practical clinical research. Further, they wanted to construct it so that it would simultaneously allow for less than full-time matriculation for those who could not quit work (or who did not want to forego employment and lose valuable clinical skills) and attend PhD study full time, which is often required. Because Drexel's curricular development work on its doctor of nursing practice degree model preceded the 2004 vote by the

AACN to require the DNP degree for entry-level practice for all advanced practice nurses (nurse practitioners, midwives, nurse anesthetists, and clinical nurse specialists) by 2015 instead of the master's degree, Drexel elected to remain committed to its original DrNP degree first initiated in 2005 (Dreher, Donnelly, & Naremore, 2005). As one of the first doctor of nursing practice programs in the country, Drexel faculty believed firmly that all its doctoral degree graduates needed basic clinical research skills. Thus, a requirement to complete a clinical dissertation was included as part of the normal degree requirements.

THE CLINICAL SCHOLAR IN NURSING AND HEALTH RESEARCH: THE CLINICAL SCIENTIST

While the DrNP at Drexel was developed in 2005 chiefly for prospective doctoral students who wanted to obtain a nursing doctorate for career advancement as a practitioner or educator, the Clinical Scientist Track was also conceived as appropriate for individuals who desired to become independent investigators, conduct meaningful nursing research, and gain beginning skills as a Clinical Nurse Scientist. The genesis of this unique role originated in focus groups of APRNs working in large urban medical centers with strong research missions in Philadelphia. In our focus groups in 2003 and 2004, APRNs complained that while many of them were involved in clinical trials on a regular or infrequent basis, most were routinely left off the publication team, even after disclosing their substantive clinical research efforts to the PIs of the respective projects on which they were working or even coordinating. As educators, we were saddened and disappointed that even master's-prepared APRNs were being marginalized and excluded from the publication team, even while being the "workhorses" of the clinical research team. Our view was that the only way APRNs could claim a legitimate right to authorship and be considered an equal partner in the generation of new knowledge, was if they were equipped with (a) a doctorate and (b) credible, practical clinical research skills. In our focus groups, the concept of a "clinical dissertation" was not frowned upon by the participating APRNs. Instead, the prevailing view was that practical clinical research skills would give them increased leverage and enhance their career opportunities. Faced with a substantial number of APRNs who were routinely involved in funded federal and private research studies, our faculty determined this prospective population did not fit into any of our original tracks—practitioner, clinical executive, or educator, and thus, this the clinical scientist track was conceived.

One example of a student in this track could be an Oncology Clinical Nurse Specialist who wants to gain the research skills to serve as a Primary Investigator (PI) on NIH, private sector, or other types of oncology-focused clinical trials at her teaching hospital and magnet institution. Without a doctorate, this APRN could not do this. Furthermore, having a professional nursing doctorate without the dissertation or final research project would still not give this APRN the necessary research skills to credibly conduct or lead a clinical research team. However, the CNS pursuing the Drexel DrNP could potentially do a Clinical Practicum with any relevant population, such as working in a cancer genetics clinic, and then doing a research Role Practicum focusing on clinical trials development and management with an experienced clinical trials scientist mentor. Upon graduation, this student would be highly encouraged to pursue a career in the oncology clinical research/pharmaceutical industry or even pursue a postdoctoral research fellowship if she decided to pursue a primarily academic nurse scientist career trajectory. The critical element of the graduate from the Clinical Scientist track in the Drexel doctor of nursing practice program is a strong clinical dissertation, focusing on a practical, very clinically oriented problem in the nursing discipline. Because physicians with the MD degree routinely submit research grants without any formal research training in medical school (aside from electives in research or apprenticeship opportunities), we think it is illogical to assume a DNP or DrNP graduate, who has taken formal research methods coursework and has conducted a rigorous, practical clinical study, would be considered unqualified to pursue federal grant funding. Indeed, the National Institutes of Health has just announced that doctor of nursing practice graduates are now eligible for the Mentored Patient-Oriented Research Career Development Award (Parent K23) grant reissued December 17, 2009. The precise language used for those eligible to apply is:

> *Degree and Research:* Candidates for this award must have a health-professional doctoral degree. Such degrees include but are not limited to the MD, DO, DDS, DMD, OD, DC, PharmD, ND (Doctor of Naturopathy), as well as a doctoral degree in nursing research or practice.
>
> —*NIH, 2009, p. 1*

To be clear, the doctor of nursing practice degree *is not* designed to prepare the nurse scientist. However, we are aware that some graduates, simply based on their talent, ability, training, and mentoring in practice doctoral study, may actually be positioned to conduct rigorous scientific inquiry from a strong practice orientation.

Nevertheless, the inclusion of empirical research in the doctor of nursing practice degree remains controversial. Indeed, the AACN's 2006 *Essentials of Doctoral Education for Advanced Nursing Practice* states "For practice doctorates, requiring a dissertation or other original research is contrary to the intent of the DNP. The DNP primarily involves mastery of an advanced specialty within nursing practice. Therefore, other methods must be used to distinguish the achievement of that mastery" (p. 20). Nonetheless, a new doctoral degree is not crystallized overnight and this issue, whether original or empirical research ought to be permitted in DNP programs, continues to be hotly debated by the profession. Even one DNP Program, the University of Connecticut, has revised its curricula and added courses in research methods (they were absent originally) and has instituted a clinical practice dissertation focusing on quality improvement problems in nursing (Cusson, 2010). The University of Illinois-Chicago is also exploring changing their DNP Synthesis Project to a "Clinical Thesis" (Dr. Connie Zak, personal communication, July 13, 2010). We are actually aware of DNP students all around the country conducting empirical, practical clinical research in their respective degree programs, even if it is not formally endorsed or recognized. In reality, doctoral degrees around the world almost always include a research project, and it is only in the United States that there are a plethora of doctoral degrees that do not. Some of the health professions doctoral degrees in the United States that do not require an original research project include the MD (Doctor of Medicine), DPT (Doctor of Physical Therapy), PharmD (Doctor of Pharmacy), DDS (Doctor of Dental Science), the majority of DNP programs, and many others in the fields of occupational therapy, audiology, and more. These degrees are best described as *professional doctorates* and differ from the PhD degree, which is entirely a research intensive academic doctoral degree. There is another type of professional doctorate in the United States that *does* include research and while these degrees are in the minority, they are prevalent. These degrees are typically described as *hybrid professional doctorates*, because they combine the professional doctorate and the research doctorate (Dreher, Fasolka, & Clark, 2008; Smith Glasgow & Dreher, 2010). Some of these degrees in the health professions include the DrPH (Doctor of Public

Health), PsyD (Doctor of Psychology), DSW (Doctor of Social Work), DScPT (Doctor of Science of Physical Therapy), and the DrNP degree (Doctor of Nursing Practice).

We believe Clinical Scientist doctor of nursing practice students need to be comfortable with acquiring and developing basic clinical research skills, as this is what the clinical research/pharmaceutical industry is about—the generation of new findings, new devices, new knowledge, and ultimately the improvement of health. It seems odd to us that some DNP students would be restricted from this mission and only trained or educated to evaluate, translate, and disseminate clinical research findings. That is what the MSN graduate was educated to do. Certainly, this is great fodder for classroom discussion in your own doctor of nursing practice program. Because this still remains a new degree (remember the first PhD in Nursing was established in 1934), such intellectual discussions about what curricular content belongs in a doctor of nursing practice degree ought not to be quickly resolved or even mandated by any national nursing organization. Instead, best practices ought to evolve as both the market and academic forces shape this new doctoral nursing degree based on real program outcome data.

With many advanced practice nurses working in the industry (as evidenced by the Oncology Nursing Society's Pharmaceutical/Industry Special Interest Group), we envision an enhanced role for the doctorally prepared APRN in the clinical research/pharmaceutical research industry (Pence, 2008). However, the DNP/DrNP graduate will need to present with advanced clinical research skills that are comparable to the research skills that other doctorally prepared members of the clinical research team possess. A doctorally prepared RN in this industry with no experience at conducting or facilitating empirical research would likely have a narrower and limited career trajectory. Thus, there are those who disagree that the DNP degree should have no focus on conduct of empirical research, but instead believe the *degree of emphasis on research* should be what best differentiates the DNP degree from the PhD—not the complete elimination of the conduct of the research enterprise (Smith Glasgow & Dreher, 2010; Webber, 2008). As most DNP programs do not permit empirical clinical research in the "Final Project," we strongly encourage master's-prepared APRNs in this industry who are seeking the right DNP program to match their career interests and to be very discriminating. There are DNP programs (not just the Drexel DrNP program, which requires a clinical

TABLE 8.1
Sample Doctor of Nursing Practice Programs With Formal Research Projects

University	DNP or DrNP	Final Project Format
Case Western Reserve University	DNP	DNP Thesis (option)
Drexel University	DrNP	Clinical Dissertation
Fairfield University	DNP	Practice Dissertation
Oakland University	DNP	DNP Research Project
Sacred Heart University	DNP	Practice Dissertation
Shenandoah University	DNP	Clinical Research Implementation Project
University of Connecticut	DNP	Clinical Practice Dissertation
University of Illinois-Chicago	DNP	Clinical Thesis (in development)
University of Washington	DNP	Clinical Investigative Research Project

Note: This list in not comprehensive, and there may be other DNP programs that permit students to complete a formal research project.

dissertation) where students indeed can complete an empirical clinical research project (see Table 8.1).

Currently, there are many MSN degree programs across the United States that educate RNs at the master's degree level to assume various positions within the clinical trials industry: research coordinator; clinical scientist; clinical trials manager, coordinator, and developer. We think the positioning of a Clinical Scientist Track in a clinical research-oriented doctor of nursing practice degree is both an innovative idea and a way to enhance the career development of any master's-prepared nurse aspiring to or currently working in the clinical research/pharmaceutical industry. However, to be a full and equal partner at the table with other doctorally prepared clinical trials professionals, credibility and comfort with the clinical research process is critical.

PERSPECTIVES FROM TWO CLINICAL SCIENTIST TRACK STUDENTS

Case I: The Role of a Clinical Research Nurse Coordinator

The role of a clinical research nurse coordinator is frequently an "on the job" learning experience that evolves as the RN or Advanced Practice Nurse (APN) moves from the traditional nursing experience into the role of research coordinator (Hill & MacArthur, 2006; Mueller, 2001; Pitler et al., 2009). This transition frequently occurs in relationship to the respective employer, whether it is a private physician practice, academic medical center, or hospital setting. It is mostly in these diverse settings that physician researchers who are active in the clinical trials industry need the expertise of nurses to take on more clinical trial responsibility. In a 2004 health care workforce survey conducted by the U.S. Department of Health and Human Services, only 0.3% (76 of 30,233) of registered nurses stated their primary role was conducting clinical research. However, the percentage of nurses actually working in clinical research is estimated to be much higher, with many nurses working in the clinical trials industry with little or no formal training (Hill & MacArthur, 2006; Mueller, 2001).

My own personal experience is much the same. I started out helping researchers in the medical center where I was employed as an inpatient Pediatric Nurse Practitioner on a locked child and adolescent inpatient psychiatric unit and was the only APN in the hospital. My experience began when the physician investigators I worked with would bring the children (subjects) to my office on the inpatient unit so that I could assist them in study-related procedures such as drawing blood or performing ECGs and physical exams. At the time, the investigators did not have a nurse coordinator or study nurse on their research teams to assist with the procedures. As time went on, it was evident that having a nurse coordinator was much more efficient than hiring non-nurse coordinators, and I was eventually recruited to a full-time research position by one of the researchers I had been assisting on the unit. My title was changed to Clinical Research Nurse Practitioner, and the training and education that followed was what I like to call "baptism by fire" or "learn as you go." Now into my eleventh year as a research coordinator, I still see new research nurse coordinators struggling to learn a much more complicated role than they may have been led to believe when they were recruited for the position. Also, in my experience, *new* clinical research coordinators working with *new* principal investigators can be a recipe for disaster, and one that is not unfamiliar to the clinical research industry. Because the position is frequently much more autonomous and is conducted in isolation without support of other nurses (Hill & MacArthur, 2006;

Mueller & Mamo, 2002), many times unbeknownst to everyone involved, protocol and human subject violations occur and data are not collected and lost forever. This is slowly changing as formal clinical research training programs are becoming much more available to nurse coordinators (Mueller & Mamo; Pitler et al., 2009); however, many individuals still enter the field with little to almost no training or experience in clinical trials.

As an APN, I have always believed in continuing education and view my role on the research team as important and crucial for the team's ultimate success. The clinical research coordinator role is critical to the success of a research program, and continuing education in the clinical research field plays a major role in this success. As I have evolved from clinician to clinical research coordinator to subinvestigator, and in my DrNP program, to principal investigator (PI), I have had to seek out educational programs in all aspects of running a clinical trial. Some areas of additional training included human subject training, good clinical practice and federal guidelines, development and management of clinical trial budgets, and management and leadership of a clinical trial team. At present, I have two post-master's certificates: one in Clinical Trials Research and one in Epidemiology and Biostatistics from Drexel University. At present, I am completing the DrNP program of study in the Clinical Scientist track. Each educational endeavor has exposed me to the extensive amount of information available in the vast clinical trials industry and allowed me to choose what was necessary to learn in order to excel in my career. In my DrNP program, however, I find myself better prepared not only to excel in my present role, but also to grow and evolve to the role of principal investigator and run a study of my own one day. Indeed, my physician collaborators see me evolving into this role as I pursue doctoral study, and they heartily endorse it. Certainly, if I am bringing in research dollars to the practice, this is a "win-win" for all.

It is also important to emphasize that in my DrNP program (or in DNP programs that emphasize clinical or empirical research), education and training in research methods and mentoring in the conduct of good science are all part of my evolution from a research coordinator to principal investigator. For the most part, floor nurses take on roles in clinical research as study nurses or clinical nurse research coordinators (Mueller, 2001). Some nurses leave the clinical side and become monitors for clinical research organizations and pharmaceutical companies. Possessing increased knowledge in clinical research, however, does not lead one to change roles or move up the career ladder easily in the clinical trials industry. Most study nurses who evolve from clinician to coordinator never evolve past this role to the role of subinvestigator or PI, even though they may have the necessary knowledge base. The requirements set by academia and the clinical trials industry generally encourage only physicians, PhD-prepared scientists, and dentists to become PIs. However, the guidelines for becoming a principal investigator *do not require* the principal investigator to be a physician or a dentist. According to the Guidance for Industry E6 Good Clinical Practice (Food and Drug Administration [FDA], 1996), the requirements are that to be a principal investigator, one must be qualified by education, training, and experience to run a clinical trial and knowledgeable in the product (drug or device) under investigation. At Drexel University (2009), the Office of Regulatory Research Compliance required qualifications for a PI (as noted in the November 2009 *Guidelines for Biomedical and Behavioral Research Involving Human Subjects*) are that the investigator's professional development should be equal to the degree of protocol complexity and risk to human subjects. Proposals that require skills beyond those held by the PI can be modified by the IRB by requiring additional qualified personnel (e.g., in a drug trial a physician as a subinvestigator may be required). Only faculty and staff members may serve as the PI. Students, medical research residents, fellows, and postdoctoral fellows are always coinvestigators at Drexel. With this broad of a definition, however, many APNs with the skills learned in a doctoral program can move into the role of PI with ease. Convincing others, however, may take longer, and individual graduates of a Doctoral Nursing Practice Program will need to market their unique skills, experience, and education.

Increased leadership skills are also a necessary part of evolving from coordinator to PI. The ability to lead a team is crucial to a team's success in clinical trials, and it is mandated by the FDA and GCP (Good Clinical Practice) that the PI takes responsibility or delegates appropriately to other qualified members of the team but remains responsible for the outcome of the trial. The DrNP program instills in its students the need to move into leadership roles, and certainly a substantial amount of time in the curriculum is directed at preparing us for this daunting task. As I have seen significant growth in my ability to think critically, make decisions, and lead and teach others, my confidence in my ability to run a research team has increased as well. I have been forced to write and present and to learn to be critical of my work, as well as the work of others through peer review. If I had not been challenged to do all this, I may not have developed the confidence I have now to be a leader in my field, to move from a coordinator to a leader and educator in the field of clinical research. This combination of increased knowledge, leadership skills, and overall confidence allows for a smooth transition from the role of a nurse coordinator in clinical trials to designing and leading clinical trials in the role of Principal Investigator or Clinical Scientist.

Case II: An Enhanced Focus on Clinical Nursing Research

Based upon years of experience as a community addictions specialist and years of experience as a former school health nurse, I entered the Drexel DrNP program as I realized the Clinical Scientist track structure would give me the level of education to make an impact on the problem of underage drinking and school violence. Previously a PhD student, I transferred to the DrNP program; I was attracted to its particular emphasis on advanced practice and clinical research, and it seemed at least philosophically a better match for my lifelong strong connections to practice. As students in the Clinical Scientist track were encouraged to use the two cognate electives to take advanced statistics courses beyond the normal curriculum or to complete a three-course sequence in Epidemiology and Biostatistics in the School of Public Health.[2] I was able to transfer in some of my advanced statistics courses from my previous doctoral program. Subsequently, I have been able to audit two more statistics courses to enhance my skill set in analytic methods—particularly important for my secondary data analysis study design. Some students in this track are oriented to clinical trials research and others of us simply want an enhanced doctorate with more clinical research. To be honest, a couple of my peers probably would have preferred a PhD program, but most PhD programs require full-time study, which is not an option for working adults. Further, with the average PhD nursing student taking 8.3 years to complete the degree part time (Valiga, 2004), I mean: "Who wants that?" I did not have that many years to expend to complete my doctorate, and so it was critical that I find a program that still believed that anyone who has a nursing doctorate has a responsibility to advance nursing knowledge. Students like myself, who select the Clinical Scientist track, are very eager to acquire the skills necessary to create new knowledge in our respective field and advance the nursing discipline. It simply never occurred to me that I would enter doctoral study, but not be part of the science of discovery.

Our program requires us to formulate a clinical research question by the end of our third quarter of study, and the doctoral nursing faculty then meet to approve all questions. Our Department Chair, Dr. H. Michael Dreher, actually gave a presentation at the 2009 Hilton Head Island DNP Conference that described this approval process that both students and faculty go through (Dreher, 2009). In contrast, for a PhD program, the faculty and student make the determination of what study the individual student will undertake. However, in a doctor of nursing practice program, it is essential that student clinical dissertations are grounded in practice and germane to our degree. And in our case, the proposed data collection method for our clinical dissertations cannot exceed 3 months. Following 2 full years of rigorous, demanding study, I arrived at the point where it was time to complete my clinical dissertation proposal, defend it, and submit my proposed study to the IRB. I thought it might be important to describe my clinical study. Because our DrNP program encourages pilot studies that explore innovative clinical questions, replication studies, and secondary analyses, I chose the latter.

Proposed Clinical Study & Clinical Problem

Underage drinking (under age 21 years) and school violence are identified as preventable priority health-risk behaviors contributing to the leading causes of morbidity and mortality among the nation's children (U.S. Department of Health & Human Services, 2001, 2006, 2007). Studies of motor vehicle crashes, the leading cause of death for American youths, revealed 22% of drivers aged 15–20 years involved in fatal crashes had been drinking (Transportation Research Board, 2008). Annual direct and indirect costs of underage drinking and youth violence are estimated at $60.3 billion and $15 billion, respectively (CDC, 2008; Institute of Medicine [IOM], 2003). Adverse outcomes of school violence range from bullying to death; for example, in the 2005–2006 school year, 17 school-associated violent deaths occurred (National Center for Education Statistics [NCES], n.d.). In addition, 628,200 children and adolescents (aged 5–18 years) were victims of sexual assault, robbery, aggravated assault, and nonfatal crimes (e.g., thefts), and accounted for 1.5 million cases of school violence (NCES, n.d.). Further complicating the problem is the age of initiation of alcohol use. Research has shown that youth who initiate alcohol use before the age of 15 are more likely to develop alcohol use problems later in life as compared to individuals who initiate alcohol use later than age 21 years (Substance Abuse Mental Health Services Administration [SAMHSA], 2004). Alcohol-related problems range from alcohol dependence, liver disease, and alcoholic cardiomyopathy (SAMHSA, 2009). Table 8.2 provides an overview of my study.

SUMMARY OF DrNP CLINICAL SCIENTIST PROPOSED CLINICAL STUDY

Networking and the Socialization of the Clinical Nursing Scientist

Finally, one critical component of developing a clinical scientist is the ability to establish a network of regional, national, and international colleagues. With focused networking, any doctoral clinical nursing scholar can begin to meet scholars and researchers who may be important in one's career and these relationships may even lead to research collaborations. One distinguishing feature of the Drexel's Doctor of Nursing Practice

TABLE 8.2
Summary of DrNP Clinical Scientist Proposed Clinical Study

Clinical research question	What is the relationship between underage drinking on school property, age of initiation of alcohol use, and school violence among high school students at the national level in the United States?
Research design of proposed study	The proposed study is an exploratory, cross-sectional, nonexperimental, correlational study design that performs secondary data analysis of the NHTSA's *2007 Youth Risk Behavior Survey* data.
Theoretical perspectives	The study is rooted in the postpositivism worldview that retains elements of empiricism, yet admits that the verification of truth is not possible. Second, the clinical study accepts the philosophical tenets from the theory–observation distinction as proffered by Van Fraassen (2000), wherein theoretical entities may or may not exist, or may be observable or unobservable, or may only be observable under certain conditions. Third, the proposed study accepts assumptions from the Public Health Theory of Drug Abuse and psychometric theory. This study adopts the nursing conceptualization of "man" as a multidimensional being, holistic, value-laden; and as an open-system that interacts with elements in the environment (Cody, 2006; Creswell, 2009; King, 1992; Munhall, 2007).
Ethical considerations	The proposed study is guided by Kant's principle of categorical imperative, "act only according to the maxim whereby you at the same time will that it should become a universal law" (Encyclopedia Britannica, n.d.) and adheres to the American Nurses Associations (ANA, 2001) code of ethics.
Potential implications for nursing practice	Of course implications for nursing practice hinge on the results of the proposed clinical study; however, it is projected the findings will add to the extant literature and serve as a educational resource for school nurses in particular and across practice settings for use in intervening in the problem of underage drinking and school violence.

(DrNP) program is the curriculum requirement to study abroad. Each spring quarter in the second year of study the DrNP student lives abroad for 2 weeks in London or Dublin to attend classes, conferences, and educational field trips that highlight global nursing (e.g., visit to local hospital). Drexel's DrNP program promotes a philosophy emphasizes today's doctorally prepared clinical scholar needs a more 'real' perspective on global health and global nursing issues" (Dreher, Lachman, Smith Glasgow, & Ward, 2008). This DrNP clinical scientist student found these words to be very true and without a doubt my "study abroad" in Dublin experience has contributed to my growth as a Clinical Scientist student and as a doctoral-prepared APN.

I fully enjoyed my two weeks of studying abroad. Our Trinity College class day experience was an outstanding feature of the Dublin experience (see Figure 8.1 for a view of Trinity College). Attending classes and conferences in the hallowed halls of Trinity College of Dublin provided me an invaluable opportunity for scholarly growth. Each speaker shared a wealth of information from his or her area of expertise. As a Clinical Nurse Specialist in adult psychiatric mental health nursing, of special interest to me was the presentation by graduate student Mark Monahan titled *Ethnography of Psychiatric Nursing Care*. Monahan demonstrated an impressive degree of commitment to his doctoral studies for he will have spent 18 months being "immersed in the field" to observe his population. Chatting with Monahan following his presentation, he discussed the specifics of sample selection and study location for his study. He viewed the study's location and the demographics of the participants as a "micro" synopsis of the emerging

FIGURE 8.1
Trinity College, Dublin, Ireland founded 1592.
Source: Personal photograph provided by Sandra N Jones © 2009

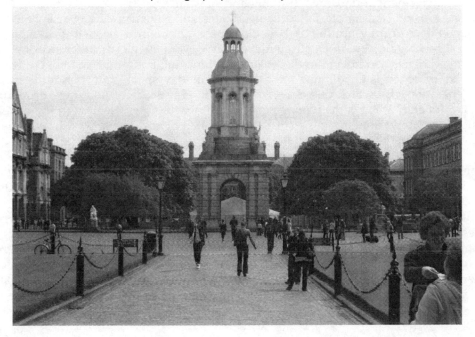

multicultural Ireland. An interesting dialogue ensued about the differences between the United States and Ireland in the treatment of preadolescent children with mental health diagnoses. For example, I have worked with 8-year-old children, diagnosed with schizophrenia who were medicated with the full psychotropic mediation regimen used in the treatment of the adult schizophrenic. In contrast, Monahan stated it would be a rarity to find children with diagnoses of schizophrenia in Ireland, nor would one find children treated with the same degree of psychotropic medication regimen used for adults. What a wonderful exchange of information we had—such contrasting views from a global perspective of mental illness and treatment between the United States and Ireland. Graduate student Frances O'Brian conducted an equally impressive presentation. She described how she will implement a random controlled trial study for her doctoral dissertation titled *An Individualized Educational Intervention for Patients with ACS[3] Symptoms*. Her detailed discussion of the study design was thorough and again indicated a commitment to her doctoral studies with 12–16 months devoted to data preparation and collection. I must note that while they were PhD students and we were DrNP students, we both shared our commitment to advanced nursing knowledge, and we learned from each other. We did not experience "You are not a PhD student so why are you conducting research?" If I am correct, in the British and Irish higher-educational system, all master's candidates must complete a thesis. So these students (and faculty) were very interested that our non-PhD degree and program had a particular focus on "practice-oriented research."

Because my research focus is the health-risk behavior of underage drinking, I was curious to learn whether or not underage drinking is a problem in Ireland. Subsequently, during the afternoon sessions at Trinity College I raised the question to Trinity faculty, and an interesting dialogue ensued with faculty and an audience member who works with adolescents with the problem of alcohol and drug abuse. Similarities and differences in the management of underage drinking and substance use between the two countries were examined; for example, in the United States underage drinking is designated and managed as a priority health-risk behavior but is not defined as such in Ireland. The study abroad experience in Dublin widened my eyes to the global differences between the United States and Ireland in the treatment of mental illness and underage drinking. My plan of action is to continue the dialogue. The day spent with Irish nurses led to the generation of research questions: What is the prevalence of underage drinking in Dublin, Ireland? What is the role of alcohol and tobacco advertisement in the development of underage drinking in Dublin? In the United States? In the world? What is the role of nurses in the prevention of underage drinking worldwide?

In summary, I know this innovative track might be controversial to some. One might ask, "Are you not trying to be a PhD?" My response is simple. I have an inquiring mind. I have a thirst to learn new things. I feel it is also my responsibility to contribute to my discipline.[4] Physicians or MDs routinely complete medical school and submit NIH grants with no formal preparation in research methods or the research enterprise unless they take an elective during medical school. But *no one* questions their right to submit proposals as Principal Investigators for federal funding. I actually have more formal academic preparation in research than most MDs. So why would some, including other nursing academics, discourage me? If our profession requires a PhD to *properly advance nursing knowledge*, then our drive to create more evidence-based practice is going to stall.

SUMMARY

It is important to realize that Drexel began development of its practice degree model starting in 2000 and had submitted its proposed curriculum to the Pennsylvania Department of Education even before the 2004 American Association of Colleges of Nursing vote. Our market research indicated that there were many nurses involved in clinical trials who needed a doctorate to credibly integrate them into the clinical research team. Further, we met many practicing nurses who just were not able to attend full-time PhD study and who winced at the endless number of years of part-time PhD study. As a result, this innovative track was created for them. We look forward to following these graduates as their careers progress and hopefully flourish. We are committed to tracking all the outcome data of our current and future DrNP graduates, and we look forward to reporting on accomplishments and career trajectories for this distinctive doctor of nursing practice track.

NOTES

1. Drexel's impetus to create an Educator Track really preceded the AACN's 2004 vote on the DNP degree. The Drexel nursing faculty thought a practice doctorate that included a nursing education emphasis was an innovative way to respond to the severe nursing faculty shortage then and now. In 2004, we projected that possibly 40% of all our graduates might eventually enter the teaching profession and Zungolo's (2009) data indicating some 33% of DNPs nationally are entering the professoriate indicate our projections were not far off.

2. Certificate in Epidemiology and Biostatistics: "This program provides research-oriented training in the theory and tools of core public health disciplines. Students build the statistical background needed to conduct research and learn how to develop hypotheses, analyze data, interpret and communicate results" (Drexel School of Public Health website: http://publichealth.drexel.edu/Academics/Degrees/Epi_and_Bio_Certificate/193/, 2010). The three course sequence includes—PBHL 701 (Introduction to Descriptive Epidemiology), PBHL 702 (Introduction to Analytic Epidemiology & Biostatistics), and PBHL 703 (Design & Analysis of Epidemiological Studies). The program is available online.
3. Acute coronary syndrome.
4. As DrNP students we are encouraged to collaborate with our faculty mentors and publish with them. Besides co-authoring this chapter, I have just had a manuscript title "An Evolutionary Concept Analysis of School Violence: From Bullying to Death" (co- authored with my two supervising professors) accepted for publication.

REFERENCES

American Association of Colleges of Nursing (AACN). (2006). *The essentials of doctoral education for advanced nursing practice.* Retrieved from http://www.aacn.nche.edu/DNP/pdf/Essentials.pdf

American Nurses Association (AAN). (2001). *Code of ethics for nurses with interpretative statements.* Silver Spring, MD. Retrieved from www.nursingworld.org/ethics/code/protected-nwcoe813htm#13

American Psychiatric Association. (2006). *Diagnostic and statistical manual of mental disorders: Test revision* (4th ed.). Arlington, VA: American Psychiatric Association.

Centers Disease Control and Prevention. (2008). *Understanding youth violence. fact sheet.* Retrieved from http://www.cdc.gov/ncipc/pub-res/YVFactSheet.pdf

Cody, W. (2006). Nursing theory-guided practice: What it is and what it is not. In W. K. Cody (Ed.), *Philosophical and theoretical perspectives for advanced nursing practice* (4th ed.) (pp. 19–26). Sudbury, MA: Jones and Bartlett.

Creswell, J. (2009). *Research design: Qualitative, quantitative, and mixed methods approaches* (3rd ed.). Los Angeles, CA: Sage.

Cusson, R. (2010). *The practice doctorate: Musings and methods of establishing the credibility of a new degree with multidisciplinary implications.* Paper delivered at the 2010 Drexel DrNP Summer Residency, Philadelphia, Pennsylvania, Drexel University College of Nursing & Health Professions, June 23, 2010.

Dore, C., Stark, K., Wood, H., Beckerleg, R., Craig, P., & Miller, J. (1995). *The clinical trial nurse: An emerging discipline.* Annual Conference of the Australasian Society of HIV Medicine, 1995, Nov. 16 19; 7: 52, Abstract No. 41.

Dreher, H. M. (2009). *A novel way to approve DNP projects and clinical dissertation topics.* Paper presented at the Second National Conference on the Doctor of Nursing Practice: The Dialogue Continues . . . Hilton Head Island, SC, March 24–27, 2009.

Dreher, H. M., Donnelly, G., & Naremore, R. (2005). Reflections on the DNP and an alternate practice doctorate model: The Drexel DrNP. *Online Journal of Issues in Nursing, 11*(1). Retrieved from http://www.nursingworld.org/MainMenuCategories/ANAMarketplace/ANAPeriodicals/OJIN/TableofContents/Volume112006/No1Jan06/ArticlePreviousTopic/tpc28_716031.aspx

Dreher, H. M., Fasolka, B., & Clark, M. (2008). Sky's the limit: Navigating the decision to pursue an advanced degree. *Journal of Men in Nursing, 3*(1), 51–55.

Dreher, H. M., Lachman, V. D., Smith Glasgow, M. E., & Ward, L. S. (2008). *Educating the global clinical scholar: The first doctoral nursing program to institute a mandatory study abroad program.* AACN Doctoral Education Conference, Captiva Island, FL, January 2008

Drexel University, Committee for the Protection of Human Subjects Institutional Review Board. (2009). *2009 guidelines for biomedical and behavioral research involving human subjects.* Retrieved from http://www.research.drexel.edu/forms/compliance/irb/IRB_Guidelines_2009.pdf

Encyclopedia Britannica. (2010). *Categorical imperative.* Retrieved from http://www.britannica.com/EBchecked/topic/99359/categorical-imperative

Food and Drug Administration. (1996). *Guidance for industry E6 Good Clinical Practice: Consolidated guidance.* Rockville, MD: Center for Drug Evaluation and Research. Retrieved from http://www.fda.gov/downloads/Drugs/GuidanceComplianceRegulatoryInformation/Guidances/ucm073122.pdf

Gaulin, P. (2008). Recession proof jobs and best industries for employment. *Associated Content, Inc.* Retrieved from http://www.associatedcontent.com/article/861875/recession_proof_jobs_and_best_industries.html

Hill, G., & MacArthur, J. (2006). Professional issues associated with the role of the research nurse. *Nursing Standard, 20*(39), 41–47.

Institute of Medicine (IOM). (2003). *Reducing underage drinking: A collective responsibility: Report brief.* Retrieved from http://www.iom.edu/~/media/Files/Report%20Files/2003/Reducing-Underage-Drinking-A-Collective-Responsibility/ReducingUnderageDrinking.pdf

King, I. (1992). King's theory of goal attainment. *Nursing Science Quarterly, 5*(1), 19–26.

Lenoble, E. (2000). Nurses in clinical trials research. *BNET: CBS Interactive.* Retrieved from http://findarticles.com/p/articles/mi_qa3916/is_200002/ai_n8898825/

Mueller, M. (2001). From delegation to specialization: Nurses and clinical trial co-ordination. *Nursing Inquiry, 8*(3), 182–190.

Mueller, M., & Mamo, L. (2002). The nurse clinical trial coordinator: Benefits and drawbacks of the role. *Research & Theory for Nursing Practice, 16*(1), 33–42.

Munhall, P. (2007). A phenomenological method. In P. L. Munhall (Ed.), *Nursing research: A qualitative perspective* (4th ed.) (pp. 145–210). Sudbury, MA: Jones & Bartlett Publishers.

National Center for Education Statistics. [NCES] (n.d.). *Indicators of school crime and safety: Key findings.* U.S. Department of Education Institute of Education Services. Retrieved from http://nces.ed.gov/programs/crimeindicators/crimeindicators2007/#top

National Highway Traffic Safety Administration. (2007). *Young drivers: Traffic safety facts.* Retrieved from http://www-nrd.nhtsa.dot.gov/pdf/nrd-30/NCSA/TSF2005/810630.pdf

National Institutes of Health. (2009). *Mentored patient-oriented research career development award (parent K23).* Retrieved from http://grants2.nih.gov/grants/guide/pa-files/PA-10-060.html

National League for Nursing Accrediting Commission. (2005). *NLNAC statement on clinical practice doctorates.* Retrieved from http://www.nlnac.org/statementClinPrac.htm

Pence, C. (2008). Sandy Smith speaks to the pharmaceutical/industry nursing SIG at 2008 ONS congress. *Oncology Nursing Society's Pharmaceutical/Industry Special Interest Group Newsletter, 8*(2), 1.

Pitler, L., Pompei, R. A., Malarick, C., Sutherlin, R. G., Leamy, J. H., & Larkin, M. E. (2009). Demystifying clinical research nursing. *The Monitor, 23*(5), 31–34.

Raybuck, J. (1997). The clinical nurse specialist as research coordinator in clinical drug trials. *Clinical Nurse Specialist, 11*(1), 15–19.

Rosen, M. (2009). Global medical device industry: Solid growth, with midwest companies leading the way. *WTN News: Wisconsin Technology News.* Retrieved from http://wistechnology.com/articles/6390/

Substance Abuse and Mental Health Services Administration. (2004). *Alcohol dependence or abuse and age at first use. National Survey on Drug Use and Health: The NSDUH Report.* Retrieved from http://www.oas.samhsa.gov/2k4/ageDependence/ageDependence.htm

Substance Abuse and Mental Health Services Administration. (2009). *Results from the 2008 National Survey on Drug Use and Health: National Findings* (Office of Applied Studies, NSDUH Series H-36, HHS Publication No. SMA 09-4434). Rockville, MD: US. Department of Health and Human Services, Substance Abuse and Mental Health Services Administration.

Smith Glasgow, M. E., & Dreher, H. M. (2010). The future of oncology nursing science: Who will generate the knowledge? *Oncology Nursing Forum, 37*(4), 393–396.

Stephens-Lloyd, A. (2004). The extended role of the clinical research nurse: Building an evidence base for practice. *Journal of Research in Nursing, 9*(1), 18–27.

Transportation Research Board. (2008). *Travel safety facts 2008: A compilation of motor vehicle crash data from the fatality analysis reporting system and the general estimates system.* Retrieved from http://144.171.11.107/Main/Blurbs/Traffic_Safety_Facts_2008_A_Compilation_of_Motor_V_163509.aspx

U.S. Department of Health and Human Services (DHHS). (2001). *Youth violence: A report of the Surgeon General.* Retrieved from http://www.surgeongeneral.gov/library/youthviolence/links.htm

U.S. Department Health and Human Services (DHHS). (2006). *Healthy people 2010 midcourse review.* Retrieved from http://www.healthypeople.gov/data/midcourse/html/focusareas/FA26Introduction.htm

U.S. Department of Health and Human Services. (2007). *The Surgeon General's call to action to prevent and reduce underage drinking.* Department of Health and Human Services, Office of the Surgeon General. Retrieved from http://www.surgeongeneral.gov/topics/underagedrinking/calltoaction.pdf

Valiga, T. (2004). *The nursing faculty shortage: A national perspective.* Congressional briefing presented by the A.N.S.R. Alliance, Hart Senate Office Building, Washington, DC.

Van Fraassen, B. (2000). Constructive empiricism. In T. Schick , Jr. (Ed.), *Readings in the philosophy of science: From positivism to postmodernism* (pp. 267–272). Mountain View, CA: Mayfield.

Webber, P. (2008). The Doctor of Nursing Practice degree and research: Are we making an epistemological mistake? *Journal of Nursing Education, 47*(10), 466–472.

York University (2008). Big pharma spends more on advertising than research and development, study finds. *ScienceDaily.* Retrieved from http://www.sciencedaily.com/releases/2008/01/080105140107.htm

Zungolo, E. (2009). *The DNP and the faculty role: Issues and challenges.* Paper presented at the Second National Conference on the Doctor of Nursing Practice: The Dialogue Continues . . ., Hilton Head Island, South Carolina, March 24–27, 2010.

CHAPTER EIGHT: Reflective Response

Diane J. Mick

The notion of a clinical scientist prepared via the path of a nursing practice doctorate is both innovative and controversial. According to the AACN *Essentials of Doctoral Education for Advanced Nursing Practice* (2006), both research-focused and practice-focused nursing doctorates share a scholarly approach to the discipline of nursing with a concurrent commitment to the advancement of the profession. Historically, doctoral programs in nursing have been viewed from a dichotomous perspective. Practice-focused doctoral programs have placed emphasis on educating clinicians to identify quantifiable problems, and to propose and implement solutions that result in measurable performance improvement in clinical practice. Via the attainment of the practice doctorate, and its accompanying credibility for the practitioner, the expert master's-prepared nurse has the opportunity to exert additional influence on systems and patient outcomes.

Research-focused doctoral programs, on the other hand, place emphasis on theory, metatheory, quantitative, and qualitative research methods, and advanced statistics for the analysis and application of findings from health care and social science literature (AACN, 2006). Collectively, the understanding and experience gained via these courses serve as a foundation for the generation of new knowledge by supporting the nurse researcher in designing and implementing a research dissertation that is both underpinned and explained by the application of theory.

What are some other differences? Research-focused doctorates typically have, as a milestone, one to two sets of qualifying examinations that serve as a threshold to candidacy for the degree. These qualifying examinations, held at the end of Year I and Year II of study, or after a prescribed set of courses have been completed successfully, serve to demonstrate that the student: (1) has mastered the advanced content of doctoral coursework; (2) is prepared to move into the next phase of developing a research proposal; (3) will be able to defend the proposal before a panel of faculty and peers; and (4) begins to collect data on the phenomenon of interest, whether it is clinical or patient and family focused. Practice doctorate programs, by virtue of their abbreviated length, do not ordinarily have a candidacy threshold. However, these programs do require a clinical or practice-oriented capstone project that demonstrates mastery of coursework and clinical expertise via accumulation of advanced practice clinical practicum hours beyond the requirement for the master's degree.

Where do the two types of doctorates intersect? Drexel University has developed a pioneering option for a research-oriented doctorate in nursing practice, a DrNP, analogous to other hybrid professional practice doctorates (e.g., DrPH, PsyD), that offer a student the advantage of obtaining advanced graduate education in both practice and research while studying for one degree. The impetus for this research-oriented practice doctorate came from the recognition of the desire of baccalaureate- and master's-prepared nurses who work as clinical research nurses and project coordinators to advance and apply their work-related experience at an increasing level of credibility. It is a known fact that study nurses and project coordinators bear the brunt of much of the "scut work" of a clinical trial, yet may not always reap the benefit of recognition as a coauthor on a study publication, or even receive acknowledgment for their often-substantive contributions to a research study or clinical trial. However, an understanding of what constitutes authorship may help to heal the wounds of those feeling slighted. While Bailey (2000) gently noted that a person who collects data does not qualify as an author, he provided criteria to help understand the author's role as one who conceptualizes and designs a project, analyzes and interprets data, drafts or critically revises the manuscript, and/or provides the final approval of the version to be published. Many baccalaureate- and masters'-prepared research nurses seize the opportunity to develop a portion of a clinical trial or research project into a professional poster for local or regional dissemination, and indeed, at times, study staff who are nurses may be invited by the principal investigator (PI) to present study findings at scientific sessions of a clinical practice organization such as the Society of Critical Care Medicine (SCCM) or the American Association of Critical Care Nurses (AACN). Such are prime opportunities for inclusion and recognition of the contribution made by research nurses and project coordinators.

As a PhD-prepared researcher and nurse practitioner with a long track record as principal investigator for industry-sponsored device trials, I believe that the clinical scientist prepared via the research track of a practice doctorate such as the DrNP or DNP can make a valuable contribution as a principal investigator for similar trials. A nurse prepared with a practice doctorate possesses the clinical expertise and acumen to identify clinical practice problems at the point of care, has the clinical networking skills necessary to interact and negotiate with representatives of device and pharmaceutical companies, and owns the experience and knowledge that is needed to see the "big picture" of activities required to get a clinical trial project up and running (Mick & Ackerman, 2005). These actions range from having a conversation with the institutional Office of Sponsored Research, to developing a study proposal and informed consent that is acceptable to the Institutional Review Board, and promoting nursing and medical staff awareness and acceptance of the clinical trial that will be taking place in the patient care area.

Because one of the fundamental differences between a research-focused doctorate and a practice-focused doctorate lies with the *generation* of new knowledge that is carried out by the PhD-prepared clinical researcher, it follows that the Clinical Scientist, prepared via the DrNP role, is the appropriate person to *test* new knowledge via the model of randomized controlled trials for both pharmaceuticals and devices. In this manner, new technology and new approaches can be compared to existing models of care, and be overseen by an expert clinical nurse who possesses value-added astuteness acquired via the coursework and experience associated with the practice-focused doctorate.

REFERENCES

American Association of Colleges of Nursing (AACN). (2006). *The essentials of doctoral education for advanced nursing practice.* Washington, DC: AACN.

Bailey, B. J. (2000). What is an author? *Laryngoscope, 110,* 1787–1788.

Mick, D. J., & Ackerman, M. H. (2005). Nursing and biomedical engineering transdisciplinary clinical trials collaboration. *Expert Review of Medical Devices, 2,* 131–133.

CRITICAL THINKING QUESTIONS

1. How might the clinical trials industry manage today globally without nurses?
2. How might the clinical trials industry benefit from having nurses doctorally prepared with a strong grounding in practice?
3. Why are some clinical trials nurses today, particularly those with master's degrees, left out of the publications that are the result of the clinical trial?
4. Describe your own experience, if any, with a hospital- or industry-based clinical trial.
5. Do you agree or disagree that any nurse with a doctorate should advance nursing knowledge? Discuss.
6. Who do you think is best prepared to create the evidence for nursing evidence-based practice: the PhD graduate, the DNP graduate, both equally, or both but differently?
7. Who do you think is best prepared to create *practice-based evidence* for the profession: the PhD graduate, the DNP graduate, both equally, or both but differently?
8. In what ways might global experiences enhance a doctor of nursing practice student's perspective or not?
9. If you could attend a short-term study abroad experience or even participate in an international doctoral practicum for your degree, what would it be and where?
10. Do you agree or disagree with this doctor of nursing practice degree Clinical Scientist Track role? Explain.

CHAPTER NINE

The Clinical Scholar Role in Doctoral Advanced Nursing Practice

Elizabeth W. Gonzalez and M. Christina R. Esperat

INTRODUCTION

The maturity of the nursing discipline and the challenges created by the market-driven environment that we live in today make clinical scholarship more important than ever before. The professional roles of nurses today require that nursing practice be consistent with the emerging knowledge. The roles and responsibilities of nurses will continue to expand as they become the key health care providers of the next decades. The new health care law emanating out of the Obama administration will make nursing increasingly outcome driven. To improve outcomes, clinical decision must be grounded in clinical inquiry where nurses who practice in a scholarly manner work directly and collegially with other health care providers in other settings, both in the discovery and the application of new knowledge. The integration of knowledge across disciplines and the application of knowledge to solve practice problems and improve health outcomes are alternative ways that new phenomena and knowledge are generated in nursing practice other than through research (AACN, 1999; Diers, 1995; Palmer, 1986; Sigma Theta Tau International [STTI], 1999). This chapter will address the kind of clinical scholarship that will be needed, created, and disseminated by advanced practice nurses with practice-focused doctorates.

HOW IS CLINICAL SCHOLARSHIP DEFINED?

The scholarly practice of nurses can be traced to Nightingale's work (1860, 1992) during the Crimean War in which data and statistical methods were used for clinical decision making. For several decades, nursing leaders have discussed the scholarship of practice (Benner, Tanner, & Chesla, 1996; Dickoff & James, 1968; Diers, 1995). Although discovery is central to expanding knowledge, linking discovery with application is an essential underpinning for practice disciplines (Riley, Beal, Levi, & McCausland, 2002). Therefore, the traditional belief that scholarship is primarily the conduct of original research is a serious limitation for a practice discipline such as nursing.

Boyer (1990) inspired most disciplines to engage in robust dialogues about the meaning of scholarship in modern times. Various nurse scholars have shared opinions on what a scholar and clinical scholarship means. In writing about clinical scholarship,

Diers (1995) argued that while clinical research in nursing is an accepted form of scholarly activity, clinical research and clinical scholarship are not the same. According to Diers, clinical scholarship offers an alternative way of extending knowledge about nursing practice. She conceptualized clinical scholarship in a practice profession as an intellectual activity that creates new understanding for practice. Clinical scholarship examines the practice itself and offers rich descriptions of the practice. Through clinical scholarship, the practitioner synthesizes practice knowledge and challenges the theories and procedures that we have learned and practiced.

Wright and Leahey (2000) argued that clinical scholarship requires an immersion in clinical practice while simultaneously finding ways to articulate, describe, and analyze what is occurring within clinical practice. Using a framework to describe the fundamental building blocks of clinical scholarship, they differentiated perceptual, conceptual, and executive skills related to the nursing of families. According to Wright and Leahey, perceptual skills focus on what the nurse observes, and conceptual skills involve how the nurse makes sense of what is observed, relying on his/her conceptual grounding and personal experience. In addition, there are executive skills which include what the nurse does. Specifically, how the nurse responds (communication skills) is based on how she or he conceptually makes sense of what is happening within the individual, family, and larger systems, as well as between herself and these systems. Clinical scholarship is refined through many hours of observation and participation in therapeutic conversations between nurse clinicians and families using written documentation that requires analysis of the therapeutic conversation between the clinician and families. Clinical scholarship requires intellectual maturity that comes from expertise and repeated experiences, which is reflected in careful analyses of situations and critical assessment of responses. The explanations and reflections offered by the clinical scholar are contextualized in her personal history and are enhanced by her well-supported interpretations.

Melanie Dreher (1999) argued that clinical scholarship is a value orientation about inquiry and implies a willingness to scrutinize nursing practice. Clinical scholarship is an intellectual process grounded in curiosity about why our clients respond the way they do and why we, as nurses, do the things we do. It includes challenging traditional nursing interventions, testing our ideas, predicting outcomes, and explaining both patterns and expectations. Clinical scholarship is rooted in observation on ways in which clients respond to their problems and to their treatments. Unfortunately, the observations nurses typically have documented often have not been for the purpose of improving patient outcomes, but rather for limiting liability. It is not sufficient to observe phenomena. Observations must be interpreted by comparing them with similar phenomena (whether or not those comparisons are drawn from personal clinical experience). Comparisons can also be accomplished by using what is known based on the literature. Synthesis builds on the analysis to create an understanding of why these patterns and/or exceptions exist. Synthesis in clinical scholarship is the process of explaining or attaching meaning to the observations and the use of comparisons in examining events or situations. Clinical scholars generate an interpretation of their observations through the process of discussion with colleagues within the nursing community and with other disciplines. Another example is the review of literature and the conduct of integrative reviews of nursing research that incorporate the informed and expert clinical knowledge of the clinician (Ganong, 1987). At another level, understanding meta-analyses of the science literature provides stronger evidence of practice phenomena under consideration.

In addition to observation, analysis, and synthesis, clinical scholarship includes application and dissemination—all of which result in a new understanding of nursing phenomena. With the current explosion of knowledge, there is an expectation that relevant knowledge must be translated to benefit societies. Various nurse scholars argued that clinical scholarship requires the ability to engage in critical theoretical discourse and discern gaps in knowledge related to clinical practice (Dracup, Cronenwett, Meleis, & Benner, 2005). Knowledge of different theoretical frameworks with various assumptions and theoretical propositions is critical for clinical scholars when choosing different types of evidence and in translating evidence into clinical practice. The DNP-prepared nurse can discover new ways of refining or transforming practice by using or adapting constructs and concepts in existing theoretical frameworks to solve everyday problems.

The scholarship of application encompasses translation of knowledge to solve problems for individuals, families, or society. This type of scholarship requires integration of knowledge of best practices in achieving best outcomes. Building on Boyer's (1990) perspective on scholarship, Palmer (1986) described the scholarship of application as a complex activity and synthesis of observations of clients and patients ... "a complex activity that has as its purpose, the discovery, organization, analysis, synthesis, and transmission of knowledge resulting from client-centered nursing practice" (p. 318).

STTI's Clinical Scholarship Task Force (1999) defined clinical scholarship as an approach that enables evidence-based nursing and development of best practices to meet the needs of clients efficiently and effectively. Clinical scholarship requires that desired outcomes are identified and systematic observation and scientifically based methods are utilized to identify and solve clinical problems. Additionally, scientific principles, current research, consensus-based guidelines, quality improvement data, and other forms of evidence are used to support clinical practice and clinical decisions. Evidence-based practice stresses the use of research findings as well as other sources of reliable data from quality improvements, consensus of recognized experts, and affirmed clinical experience (Stetler et al., 1998). The recent movement in nursing toward "evidence-based practice" has been articulated by leaders like Melnyk and Fineout-Overholt (2005), and has been widely adopted by the DNP program. Further, the faculty at the University of Washington have developed and launched a practice-focused doctorate that includes practice inquiry in the curriculum, addressing the appraisal and translation of evidence into practice and evaluation with the potential for collaborative clinical research endeavors (Magyary, Whitney, & Brown, 2006). Both evidence-based practice and practice inquiry are likely to impact DNP clinical scholarship in the future.

The clinical scholar with a practice-focused doctorate will provide leadership for evidence-based practice with skills in translational research. Clinical scholarship is informed by reading, by thinking, by discussing with colleagues (interdisciplinary efforts), and by mentoring so as to generate possible explanations on a clinical problem. Clinical scholars seek validation with fellow clinicians on their documented observations regarding patients' goal-related progress. Interdisciplinary efforts are necessary skills for the translation of research findings. The value of shared reflections on practice and experience is critical. These reflections can be developed formally through written clinical narratives (Benner, 1984). Reflection, self-scrutiny, and subsequent dialogue form the basis for personal growth and mutual learning among peers.

Despite the variations in the definition of what scholarship means, the following are common themes that describe a scholar. Clinical scholars are characterized by a high level of curiosity, critical thinking, continuous learning, reflection, and the ability to seek and use a spectrum of resources and evidence to improve the effectiveness of clinical interventions. They consistently bring a spirit of inquiry and creativity to their practice to solve clinical problems and improve outcomes (STTI, 1999).

HOW SHOULD CLINICAL SCHOLARSHIP DIFFER BETWEEN THE TRADITIONAL MSN-PREPARED APN AND THE DNP APN?

In an era of unprecedented accountability for the delivery of quality, cost-managed health care, nurses are challenged to demonstrate effective and efficient care. Well-informed consumers are demanding greater access to quality health care. Rising patient acuity, escalating complexity in health care needs, and the increasing infusion of technology in health care systems are creating daunting challenges for nurses. Additionally, nurses are practicing in environments with limited financial resources. As these challenges increase, nurses can no longer rely on traditional nursing practices or base their clinical decisions on intuition and years of clinical experience to plan and implement care required in today's patients. Responding to this challenge requires collective knowledge, clinical expertise, and commitment to base patient care decisions on evidence and involvement of patients. Clinical scholarship is particularly important for advanced practice nurses with practice-focused doctorates to provide leadership in establishing clinical excellence and inform health care policy.

The master's degree (MSN) historically has been the degree for specialized advanced nursing practice. With the development of DNP programs, a practice-focused doctorate, the DNP degree will become the preferred preparation for specialty nursing practice. According to the National Organization for Nurse Practitioner Faculties (2006), the competencies for the DNP are similar to the MSN competencies (with mastery of an advanced specialty within nursing practice), but the DNP competencies are formulated with more emphasis on leadership, quality improvement, health care delivery systems, and health care policy. The implementation of a model for evidence-based practice has been documented to promote clinical scholarship among clinical nurse specialists in various institutions such as Baystate Medical Center in Massachusetts, the University of Texas Medical Branch, Kaiser Permanente and California Pacific Medical Center, and the University of Iowa Hospitals and Clinics and College of Nursing (STTI, 1999). Clinical scholarship among nurse specialists provides opportunities to generate reflective thinking to improved clinical practice and heightened awareness for a new standard for evidence-based thinking (STTI). The Sigma Theta Tau International sponsored clinical scholarship programs for MSN-prepared APNs is well documented, including the Clinical Scholars Mentor Program, Clinical Fellowships, and celebrations of clinical scholarship which were some of the mechanisms used for advancing clinical scholarship for masters'-prepared APNs. Clinical scholarship for the practice-focused doctorate should build on what has been started by clinical scholars with the MSN degree to provide leadership for evidence-based practice. This requires the application of knowledge to solve clinical problems and generate evidence through their practice to guide improvements in practice, outcomes of care, and participation in collaborative research (DePalma & McGuire, 2005; Magyary et al., 2006). Evidence-based practice should result in better outcomes leading to a better quality of life for all citizens.

HOW IS EXPERTISE IN THE USE OF EVIDENCE-BASED PRACTICE ACHIEVED?

In practice, the utilization of research evidence does not occur in vacuum. Multiple contextual factors influence the diffusion of practices that carry the weight of evidence borne of scientific inquiry. Funk, Tornquist, and Champagne (1995) identified four categories of barriers perceived by nurses to the utilization of research in clinical practice: those related to nurses' research values and skills, those related to limitations in the setting, those related to how the research is communicated, and those related to the quality of the research itself. The DNP role's impact on facilitating evidence-based practice needs to be conceived as successfully overcoming those barriers. Because DNP competencies are formulated at a higher level with more emphasis on leadership, quality improvement, health care delivery systems, and health care policy, the DNP-prepared nurse will be expected to provide leadership in creating working environments for evidence-based practice, with the expectation necessitating a certain level of skills and competency in translating science into practice.

In terms of nurses' research values and skills, the DNP nurse can become a role model for change and transformation not only for the workplace environment, but also for the individual nurses working in that environment. This can occur at two levels by: (1) increasing the nurse's confidence in evaluating the quality of the research evidence, and (2) changing perceptions regarding the benefits of changing practice with the use of research evidence. The nurse leader who is prepared at the doctoral level can actively participate in formal or informal discussions on evaluating interventions reported in the research literature using the opportunity to increase nurses' knowledge and ability to evaluate research findings more wisely and logically. By taking on the role of an innovator, as an early adopter, the DNP nurse can create the climate for changing perceptions to one of increased respect and value for the scientific process and its outcomes.

As a leader in clinical practice, the DNP nurse can overcome limitations within the setting for practice. By allowing implementation of innovations through active support and provision of the needed structure and processes, the DNP administrator brings authority and accountability to bear in facilitating the workplace environment for these innovations. This includes focusing on overcoming the limitations in how research is communicated. By providing the resources needed for the nurses and health care team to develop skills in reading, understanding, and evaluating research reports accurately and efficiently, the DNP administrator can promote, sustain, and maintain the implementation of evidence-based practice. In terms of barriers related to the quality of the research evidence, the DNP nurse can lead the effort to contribute further to the knowledge base by replicating investigations that evaluate the effectiveness of interventions. This requires a step beyond simply implementing and measuring the outcomes of interventions, to formally testing hypotheses regarding the impact of such interventions on nursing and health care. In effect, it requires the DNP-prepared nurse to be skilled in the conduct, use, and dissemination of translational research.

In various leadership roles, the DNP-prepared nurse is uniquely positioned to innovate and experiment with various models for increasing utilization of research in practice settings. With administrative authority that comes with these leadership roles, the DNP-prepared nurse should have multiple options available for integrating research into the workplace environment. Whether it is increased and more effective use of existing resources or the deployment of external support and expertise, the DNP nurse can raise the organization to higher levels of application of translational science into practice. Particularly in promoting the translation of science into practice, the DNP nurse can engage in action research, which leads to the solution of everyday practical, as well as clinical, problems.

IS ACTION RESEARCH ORIENTED FOR DNP CLINICAL SCHOLARSHIP?

Methods to increase the quality and rate of research translation are increasingly becoming the focus of clinical practice. Leadership in clinical practice requires recognition that evidence-based practice is central to the achievement of effective and efficient health care delivery and to obtaining positive client outcomes (Mohide & Coker, 2005). Traditional approaches to building the evidence predominate in the current research enterprise. Be that as it may, there is increasing pressure upon the scientific community to look at alternative paradigms to increase the uptake of research evidence into community- and population-wide practice. Action research, one such alternative paradigm, is science designed to obtain practical results to solve a specific challenge. Engagement in action research is one in which the DNP nurse is optimally positioned, with the strong leadership skills in community-based initiatives that is one of the hallmarks of the education and preparation for DNP practice. In addition to the basic steps in traditional research of design, data collection, analysis, and communication, this alternative paradigm requires action, which is developmental in nature and has a wide range of applications in health care. This showcases the strengths and talents of the DNP nurse; it highlights the natural skills of the practitioner for practical solutions to real and actual problems in the clinical setting as they occur. In addition to skills and competencies in the application of multidimensional and multifaceted designs of participatory action research, the DNP nurse is prepared to lead communities to form collaborative partnerships with the academic scientists in community-based initiatives that aim to solve problems facing vulnerable populations (Stringer, 2007).

WHAT IS THE ROLE OF PRACTICE DOCTORATE CLINICAL NURSING SCHOLARS IN DISSEMINATION?

The role of the DNP nurse as clinical scholar has within it an inherent obligation and responsibility to disseminate knowledge and expertise gained from practice to various audiences. There are many reasons for engaging in the dissemination process. These include the sharing of ideas and new knowledge for the improvement of health care delivery to influencing outcomes of health care. In addition, for practical purposes, dissemination activities are essential job requirements, including requirements for promotion and tenure in any work setting. Thus, DNP preparation includes experiences aimed at developing and increasing skills in manuscript writing as well as in oral presentations in the dissemination of ideas. In leadership roles, the DNP nurse can create the climate for scholarship for those with whom she or he works. Increasingly, the endeavor to produce manuscripts for publication is carried on by writing teams who are engaged in common activities in health care delivery. Likewise, the tasks of preparing and delivering oral as well as poster presentations become less daunting and onerous if undertaken by teams of colleagues engaged in similar activities of dissemination. The DNP nurse provides the needed leadership to get the initiative started, to provide the resources for people to engage in these activities, and to encourage the work of continued and active scholarship. This also provides opportunities for mentoring and mentorship among nurses and other health care professionals who work together to achieve health care goals for groups of patients.

SUMMARY: THE FUTURE OF THE DNP CLINICAL SCHOLAR

Whether the creation of this new degree enhances the progress of the clinical scholarship for the profession of nursing and furthers the quality of patient care depends entirely on the nursing profession's willingness to address the critical issues related to educational quality, outcomes, and standards. Focusing on the issue of the preparation of the DNP as a clinical scholar is of particular importance. At the current time, when standards of DNP education are continuing to evolve, it is critically important that the skills and competencies that have been articulated to prepare the DNP for this role be coupled with specific parameters for identifying the outcomes of this preparation relative to this role. Learning experiences in the educational and training curricula must emphasize increasing skills in the application of translational research, while at the same time the development of higher levels of competencies in the conduct of evaluation research and dissemination of critical findings must be facilitated and monitored before the DNP is granted the degree.

Nursing leaders and state and national organizations have spent considerable time and finances ensuring the public, legislators, and other members of the health care community that the education that nurses currently possess results in high quality care. Although it is intuitively appealing that educational requirements and standards will address the Institute of Medicine's concerns about patient safety and health care quality (IOM, 2000, 2001, 2003), there are inconsistencies in the educational preparation of DNP nurses that may not fulfill the promise on the quality of patient care and progress in the nursing profession. Studies relating educational preparation and quality at the entry level do support that more and different education results in higher quality (Stanley, 2005). However, these data are not generalizable to advanced practice, and the suggestion that better patient care will result from this preparation, although intuitively appealing, must be documented based on evidence. These challenges must encourage continuous dialogue about the best educational preparation for doctorally prepared APNs who will assume the role of clinical scholars. This is critical as changing technology, changing health care delivery systems, changing science, and changing and evolving roles for nurses all require that the nurse of tomorrow be prepared to participate in the health care system as it evolves. Additionally, employers and professional organizations should provide mechanisms for exercising leadership that support activities for clinical scholarship for DNPs. It is imperative that professional nursing groups and organizations endorse a call for more prolific clinical scholarship in this new cadre of DNPs as central to their mission and philosophy and as a rationale for a practice-focused doctorate. Furthermore, the workplace also needs to state its commitment through tangible means of support to enhance clinical scholarship.

REFERENCES

American Association of Colleges of Nursing (AACN). (1999). *The essential resources for nursing's academic mission.* Washington, DC: Author. Retrieved from http://www.aacn.nche.edu/Education/pdf/ClinicalEssentials99.pdf

Benner, P. (1984). *From novice to expert: Excellence and power in clinical nursing practice.* Menlo Park, CA: Addison Wesley.

Benner, P., Tanner, C., & Chesla, C. (1996). *Expertise in nursing practice: Caring, clinical judgment and ethics.* New York, NY: Springer.

Boyer, E. (1990). *Scholarship reconsidered: Priorities of the professoriate.* Princeton, NJ: Carnegie Endowment for the Advancement of Teaching.

DePalma, J., & McGuire, D. (2005). Research. In A. B. Hamric, A. Spross, & C. Hanson (Eds.), *Advanced practice nursing: An integrative approach* (3rd ed.) (pp. 257–300). Philadelphia, PA: Elsevier Saunders.

Dickoff, J., & James, P. (1968). A theory of theories: A position paper. *Nursing Research, 17*(5), 197–203.

Diers, D. (1995). Clinical scholarship. *Journal of Professional Nursing, 11*(1), 24–30.

Dracup, K., Cronenwett, L., Meleis, A., & Benner, P. (2005). Reflections on the doctorate of nursing practice. *Nursing Outlook, 53*, 177–182.

Dreher, M. (1999). Clinical scholarship: Nursing practice as an intellectual endeavor. In Sigma Theta Tau International Clinical Scholar Task Force. *Clinical Scholarship Resource Paper*, (pp. 26–33), Retrieved from http://www.nursingsociety.org/aboutus/PositionPapers/Documents/clinical_scholarship_paper.pdf

Funk, S. G., Tornquist, E. M. A., & Champagne, M. T. (1995). Barriers and facilitators of research utilization: An integrative review. *Nursing Clinics of North America, 30*(3), 395–407.

Ganong, L. H. (1987). Integrative reviews of nursing research. *Research in Nursing & Health, 10*, 1–12.

Institute of Medicine (IOM). (2000). *To err is human: Building a safer health system.* Washington, DC: National Academies Press.

Institute of Medicine (IOM). (2001). *Crossing the quality chasm.* Washington, DC: National Academies Press.

Institute of Medicine (IOM). (2003). *Health professions education: A bridge to quality.* Washington, DC: National Academy Press.

Magyary, D., Whitney, J. D., & Brown, M. A. (2006). Advancing practice inquiry: Research foundations of the practice doctorate in nursing. *Nursing Outlook, 54*(3), 139–151.

Melnyk, B., & Fineout-Overholt, E. (2005). *Evidence-based practice in nursing and healthcare. A guide to best practice.* Philadelphia, PA: Lippincott, Williams & Wilkins.

Mohide, E., & Coker, E. (2005). Toward clinical scholarship: Promoting evidence-based practice in the clinical setting. *Journal of Professional Nursing, 21*(6), 372–379.

National Organization of Nurse Practitioner Faculties. (2006). *Practice doctorate entry level nurse practitioner competencies.* Retrieved from http://www.nonpf.com/NONPF2005/PracticeDoctorateResourceCenter/CompetencyDraftFInalApril2006.pdf

Nightingale, F. (1860/1992). *Notes on nursing.* New York, NY: Lippincott, Williams & Wilkins.

Palmer, I. (1986). The emergence of clinical scholarship as a professional imperative. *Journal of Professional Nursing, 2*(5), 318–325.

Riley, J. M., Beal, J., Levi, P., & McCausland, M. (2002). Revisioning nursing scholarship. *Journal of Nursing Scholarship, 34*(4), 383–389.

Sigma Theta Tau International. (1999). *Clinical scholarship resource paper.* Clinical scholarship task force, Sigma Theta Tau International, Indianapolis, IN: Author.

Stringer, E. (2007). *Action research* (3rd ed.). Thousand Oaks, CA: Sage.

Stanley, J. (2005). Evaluating the doctorate of nursing practice: Moving toward a new vision of nurse practitioner education. *Journal of Nurse Practitioners, 1*(4), 209–212.

Stetler, C., Brunell, M., Giuliano, K., Morsi, D., Prince, L., & Newell-Stokes, V. (1998). Evidence-based practice and the role of nursing leadership. *Journal of Nursing Administration, 28*, 45–51.

Wright, L., & Leahey, M. (2000). *Nurses and families: A guide to family assessment and intervention* (3rd ed.). Philadelphia, PA: F. A. Davis.

CHAPTER NINE: Reflective Response

Marie Annette Brown

Doctoral preparation for advanced practice nurses (APNs) is expected to trigger a dramatic rise in professional commitment to clinical scholarship. Drs. Gonzalez and Esperat offer a very timely analysis about this core responsibility and provide important guideposts for this new cohort of clinical scholars. They remind us that Nightingale epitomized clinical scholarship. In today's language, we might say that her reflective practice contributed to her success in "improving outcomes" for Crimean soldiers. The foundation for launching exciting new avenues of clinical scholarship was strengthened over the past several decades. Clinical scholarship is an idea that has now come of age.

Drs. Gonzalez and Esperat affirm the key contribution of Boyer (1990) to broaden the discourse about scholarship, particularly in light of the scholarship of application. Had Boyer been a nurse, the scholarship of practice would surely have been an essential component of his seminal work to change the research focused paradigm of scholarship! As our dialogue about scholarship expands, would this be the time to refine our language and move from clinical scholarship to practice scholarship in the same way the preferred title became the practice doctorate instead of the clinical doctorate? As nursing more clearly articulates its scope of influence, "practice at the individual, family, and community level" is becoming the preferred language.

Drs. Gonzalez and Esperat analyze clinical scholarship in a way that embraces a broad view of what constitutes evidence-based practice (EBP), including both clinical expertise and patient perspectives. The most current study from Benner, Sutphen, Leonard, and Day (2010) calls for a radical transformation in nursing education to better utilize this clinical expertise. They assert that "practice is a way of knowing in its own right ... innovation and new questions flow bidirectionally, from theory and science to and from practice" (p. 30). Furthermore, the essential contribution of patient perspectives must continue to be emphasized in APN education and viewed as a central dimension of EBP. Careful attention to patient/family values, concerns and choices must be the hallmark of nursing practice (Benner & Leonard, 2011). EBP must always be contextualized in the patient's unique situation.

The practice doctorate provides the impetus for advancing nursing's goal of clinical scholarship. Many nursing leaders celebrate the courage shown by this pioneer generation of advanced practice nursing doctoral students. They are committed to becoming clinical scholars to enhance the quality of care in a fractured and complex health care environment. The deep desire of the pioneer nurse practitioners of the 1970s to make "a difference for patients" (Brown & Draye, 2003) is manifest in the Doctor of Nursing Practice (DNP) pioneers who are creating new approaches to clinical scholarship.

Expertise in practice inquiry will be required to fuel this rise in clinical scholarship. Practice inquiry as conceptualized by Magyary, Whitney and Brown (2006) is emerging as an exemplar to address the realities and complexities of everyday APN practice

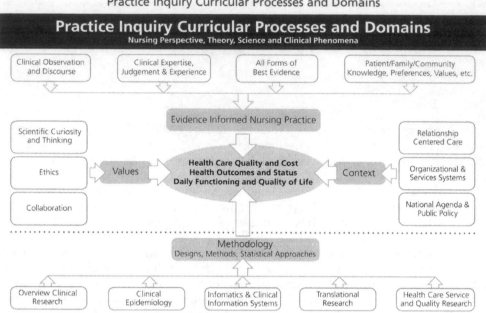

FIGURE 9.1
Practice Inquiry Curricular Processes and Domains

Reproduced with permission from Magyary, Whitney & Brown, "Advanced Practice Inquiry: Research Foundations for the Practice Doctorate in Nursing," *Nursing Outlook*, 2006; 54:139–151.

(see Figure 9.1). It bridges the responsibility of DNP APNs to observe, describe, understand, and appraise clinical phenomena with theoretical and empirical knowledge (Magyary et al., 2006). Practice inquiry has been defined as an:

> . . . ongoing systematic investigation of questions about nursing therapeutics and clinical phenomena with the intent to appraise and translate all forms of "best evidence" to practice, and to evaluate the translational impact on the quality of health care and health outcomes.
> —*Magyary et al., 2006, p. 143*

Establishing practice inquiry competencies as core to doctoral advanced practice will change how APNs view their practice. We found that *Thinking Differently About Practice* was a major theme from our research:

> I think the DNP helped me think systematically. . . [about] real practice inquiry versus asking a colleague 'Oh what do you do, Okay that's what I'll do.' [Instead I ask] what is the evidence that drives that policy, is it up to date, and how can we be sure that we're doing what's best for our patients based on the evidence and our patient population?[1]
> —*Research study participant (from Brown & Kaplan, 2010)*

and is exemplified by the statement of the DNP graduate above.

Drs. Gonzalez and Esperat suggest that the clinical scholarship of this new cadre of APNs can provide a model to inspire colleagues. Use of research evidence, particularly translational science about the most effective way to approach specific practice changes, will strengthen DNP APNs, effectiveness. The authors assert that by taking on the role of innovator and early adopter, DNP nurses can help create a climate of increased respect and value for the scientific process and its outcomes. These APNs will also have insight into their colleagues' practices that is drawn from their own practice and practice environment.

Drs. Gonzalez and Esperat urge clinical scholars with a practice focused doctorate to develop skill in the conduct, use, and dissemination of translational research and provide leadership for EBP. These scholars will be key to the creation of a paradigm shift to EBP in advanced practice nursing. The more completely this paradigm shift occurs, the more supportive practice environments are likely to be of clinical scholarship. A similar paradigm shift for APN educators will prompt movement from the traditional research education to prepare research generators to the curricular goal of proficiency in EBP (Fineout-Overholt, Stillwell, Williamson, Cox, & Robbins, 2011) and practice inquiry. It is critical that DNP APNs, who are educated during the emergence of this EBP paradigm, bring their values about practice inquiry to a health care environment that is in desperate need of leadership for EBP. Cultivation of a deep understanding of this phenomenon (APN use of EBP) is where change begins. Additionally, a commitment to reflective practice, essential in doctoral level practice, can prompt insight about the challenges and successes in EBP that we each experience in our own practice. Intuitively, we assume that most health care professionals would support the premise that practice should have a scientific foundation. Why, then, is the implementation of evidence-based practice so difficult?

Drs. Gonzalez and Esperat illuminate potential barriers that have slowed the application of research to practice. Little data exist, however, about the extent to which APNs understand and utilize the essentials of EBP and the barriers and facilitators involved. Nelson (2009) found that distribution of guidelines to health care providers specifying venous thromboembolism prevention did not stimulate adherence to guidelines. Barriers detailed in this project included lack of supportive systems, lack of individual responsibility for implementation, lack of acceptance, perceived lack of need in some clinical areas, no oversight or incentives, and conflicting guideline recommendations. To what extent are these barriers shared across disciplines? It is interesting to note that even EBP utilization studies that included NPs and physicians do not seem to report their data according to provider type (Flanagan, Ramanujam, & Doebbeling, 2009). Filling this gap could be a fruitful avenue for clinical scholarship among doctorally prepared APNs with the practice inquiry skills to initiate and lead "ongoing investigations of nursing therapeutics and clinical phenomena" (Magyary et al., 2006, p. 143).

An interesting exemplar of this type of work addressed the contextual influence of professional culture on EBP on certified nurse midwives' (CNMs). The study explored CNM knowledge of and reliance on evidence-based practice. The insights of Bogdan-Lovis and Sousa (2006) about power, tradition, and practice are instructive across APN specialties. For example, there was considerable variability among the nurse midwives with regard to their accurate understanding of EBP, ranging from solid expertise to less than a superficial understanding. Despite some indication to the contrary, some nurse midwives were "certain that their own practice protocols were based on best evidence . . . not uncommonly they mistakenly conflated the good intentions to deliver the best care to women with the 'best medicine' concept" (Bogdan-Lovis & Sousa, 2006, p. 2688). Some inaccurately portrayed EBP as "simply a new concept applied to an old standard" (Bogdan-Lovis & Sousa, p. 2687). The authors noted that in light of their findings "such misguided certainty could effectively reduce incentive to incorporate EBM into practice protocols" (p. 2788).

A closer look at EBP utilization issues in all APN specialties is warranted. To what extent are the issues about understanding and utilization of EBP that were highlighted in the CNM study similar to NPs? What are the unique and shared issues about utilization of EBP across APN specialties? What are the similarities and differences between master's and doctorally prepared APNs' utilization and depth of understanding of practice guidelines? What are common perspectives and values about clinical guidelines that may be subtly or overtly communicated in APN continuing education? To what extent do doctorally prepared APNs use current data from translational research to plan strategies that address the need for EBP in their practice settings?

How can their expertise in practice inquiry serve as the essential launching pad to investigate commonly asked questions across all health care professionals? For example, a critical question posed across disciplines is: To what extent do competencies in EBP and practice inquiry influence patient outcomes and the quality of care?

Quality of care delivered by APNs has been described and is becoming more systematically studied. Ironically, until the past decade a considerable amount of research about NPs (much of which compared NPs and physicians) was not conducted by APNs or by nurse researchers. The specific nature of interventions by APNs remains less understood. Wells' (2002) discussion titled *When a Dose of Advanced Practice is the Treatment* reminds us that "the nursing role, an early focus of research, is seldom an emphasis today, as investigation is more linked to patient outcomes." (p. 2092). Knowledge generation in this area has been undervalued and clinical scholarship in this area has had limited visibility, however new partnerships between DNP-PhD nurses can help answer salient questions about APN practice. The current emphasis on EBP, quality of care and patient safety among all health care professionals may help cultivate collaboration (Woods & Magyary, 2010).

The recent landmark integrative review of research on advanced practice nursing by a nurse researcher showcases new advancements in this area (Ingersoll, 2010). In response to the demand for changes in health care system financing, accountability, organization, and delivery, there is an urgent need for APNs to justify their contributions to health care and demonstrate the value they provide to their care environment. To respond to the call from employers, consumers, insurers, and others, Ingersoll synthesizes the growing body of vital evidence about multiple specialties within advanced nursing practice. These data are presented based on the emerging categories of role descriptions or characteristics, care delivery processes, process (or performance), improvement activities, program evaluation, disease management activities, outcomes management programs, or outcomes research (Ingersoll, 2010, p. 681). These data serve as a core element in the toolbox of doctorally prepared APNs, particularly as they launch their own clinical scholarship endeavors and promote the widespread utilization of APNs.

Drs. Gonzalez and Esperat suggest that clinical scholarship for doctorally prepared APNs be built on that of masters-prepared APNs. An alternative approach could be asking questions about new directions in clinical scholarship, such as those posed earlier, that arise from doctoral preparation for APNs. Questions about the "value added" in doctoral preparation could be answered by examining their clinical scholarship. Pioneer DNP APNs "have only just begun" to create and implement their new approach to practice. The development of a program of research in this area is urgently needed to understand and support their journey. The elaboration of research competencies as fundamental (master's) or expanded (doctoral) presented in the most recent work of DePalma (2010) can inform unfolding questions about the emerging contributions of DNP APNs.

In conclusion, Drs. Gonzalez and Esperat discuss how generative reflective thinking, inherent in clinical scholarship, is intended to raise the level of evidence-based care. If doctoral preparation for advanced practice has EBP as the core and the next generation of APNs brings enthusiasm about practice inquiry to their work, a new powerful force to guide advanced practice may emerge. An analogy comes from living on the shores of Puget Sound. The widely desperate fluctuations of the tides can determine how we approach daily life. Calculating when the tides allow for a beach walk becomes necessary. While on the beach, ocean tides may seem magical, the force that drives them is the powerful gravitational pull produced by the moon and the sun. If everyday APN practice was guided by the gravitational pull of practice inquiry, the strength of the goal of doctorally prepared APNs to enhance the quality of life for patients, families, and communities across the country could be realized.

NOTE

1. This quote is from a poster session and not yet published. The poster had quotes from multiple study participants. Dr. Brown can be emailed for further details.

REFERENCES

Benner, P., & Leonard, V. W. (2011). Patient concerns, choices, and clinical judgment in evidence-based practice. In B. W. Melnyk, & E. Fineout-Overholt (Eds.), *Evidence-based practice in nursing and healthcare* (pp. 167–185). Philadelphia, PA: Wolters Kluwer/Lippincott Williams & Wilkins.

Benner, P., Sutphen, M., Leonard, V., & Day, L. (2010). *Educating nurses: A call for radical transformation*. San Francisco, CA: Jossey-Bass.

Bogdan-Lovis, E. A., & Sousa, A. (2006). The contextual influence of professional culture: Certified nurse midwives knowledge of and reliance on evidence based practice. *Social Science & Medicine, 62*(11), 2681–2693.

Boyer, E. (1990). *Scholarship reconsidered. Priorities of the professorate*. Princeton, NJ: Carnegie Endowment for the Advancement of Teaching.

Brown, M. A., & Draye, M. A. (2003). The experiences of pioneer nurse practitioners in establishing advanced practice roles. *Journal of Nursing Scholarship, 35*(4), 389–395.

Brown, M. A., & Kaplan, L. A. (2010). The practice degree that changes practice. Poster presented at the National Organization of Nurse Practitioner Faculties Annual Meeting, Washington, DC.

DePalma, J. A. (2009). Research. In A. B. Hamric, J. A. Spross, & C. M. Hanson (Eds.), *Advanced Practice Nursing: An Integrative Approach*, (4th ed.) (pp. 681–732). Philadelphia, PA: Saunders Elsevier.

Fineout-Overholt, E., Stillwell, S. B., Williamson, K. M., Cox, J. F., & Robbins, B. W. (2011). Teaching evidence-based practice in academic settings. In B. W. Melnyk, & E. Fineout-Overholt (Eds.), *Evidence-based practice in nursing and healthcare* (pp. 291–329). Philadelphia, PA: Wolters Kluwer/Lippincott Williams & Wilkins.

Flanagan, M. E., Ramanujam, R., & Doebbeling, B. N. (2009). The effect of provider- and workflow-focused strategies for guideline implementation on provider acceptance. *Implementation Science, 4*(71), 1–10. Doi: 10.1186/1748-5908-4-71.

Ingersoll, G. (2010). Outcomes evaluation and performance improvement: An integrative review of research on advanced practice nursing. In A. B. Hamric, J. A. Spross, & C. M. Hanson (Eds.), *Advanced practice nursing: An integrative approach* (pp. 681–732). Philadelphia, PA: Saunders Elsevier.

Magyary, D., Whitney, J., & Brown, M. A. (2006). Advancing practice inquiry: Research foundations doctor of nursing practice. *Nursing Outlook, 54*(3), 139–142.

Nelson, W. J. (2009). Venous thromboembolism: What is preventing achievement of performance measures and consensus guidelines? *Journal of Cardiovascular Nursing, 24*(Suppl. 6), S14–S19.

Wells, T. J. (2002). When a dose of advanced practice nursing is the treatment. *Journal of the American Geriatric Society, 50*(12), 2092–2093.

Woods, N. F., & Magyary, D. (2010). Translational research: Why nursing's interdisciplinary collaboration is essential. *Research and Theory for Nursing Practice: An International Journal, 24*(1), 9–24.

CRITICAL THINKING QUESTIONS

1. Explain the differences in the clinical scholarship of a practice-focused doctorate from a research-focused doctorate.
2. Describe the kind of clinical scholarship you believe is most appropriate for the practice-focused doctorate.
3. Explain why knowledge in theoretical frameworks is critical for clinical scholars with a practice-focused doctorate.
4. Why is clinical scholarship for advanced practice nurses with practice-focused doctorates important?
5. How should clinical scholarship differ in advanced practice MSN from the DNP APN?
6. How does a DNP APN achieve expertise in use of evidence-based practice?
7. Explain the importance of action research for a clinical nursing scholar.
8. Explain how dissemination activities could be achieved by the DNP clinical scholar.
9. Discuss issues/barriers in the development of a DNP clinical scholar.
10. Explain the role of administrators in supporting DNP clinical scholars.

CHAPTER TEN

Role Strain in the Doctorally Prepared Advanced Practice Nurse

The Experiences of Doctor of Nursing Practice Graduates in Their Current Professional Positions

Mary Ellen Smith Glasgow and Rick Zoucha

INTRODUCTION

It is suggested that a role is the manifestation of behavior appropriate to an individual's position (Sveinsdottir, Biering, & Ramel, 2006). The Doctor of Nursing Practice (DNP) degree is a relatively new degree; therefore, the role for the Doctoral Advanced Practice Nurse is not yet clearly defined in many settings. As a result, these pioneers, new doctoral advanced practice nurses, may experience role stress in their new role. Psychologists, sociologists, and empirical researchers have conceptualized role stress from different perspectives (Kahn, Wolf, Quinn, Snock, & Rosenthal, 1964; Lazarus, 1967; Hardy & Conway, 1978). Hardy and Conway (1988) classified the dimensions of role stress specifically for health care professionals. These dimensions are role conflict, role ambiguity, role overload, role incompetence, and role incongruity. Among the many dimensions of role stress, most researchers have focused on the impact of role ambiguity or role conflict on personal or organizational outcomes; however, the role of the nurse has not been the focus of the research (Chen, Chen, Tsai, & Lo, 2007).

Role stress can arise from different patterns of mismatch in expectations, resources, capabilities, and values about the role (Chen et al., 2007). In an organization, an individual's role stress refers to "stress formed by the combined expectations of an individual's behavior from all circles" (Sveinsdottir et al., 2006). *Role strain* is a state of emotional arousal when an individual experiences role-related stress events, whereas role stress is external to the person in the role and results from societal demands. Role strain is conceptualized as one's perceived difficulty or angst in fulfilling role obligations. For example, a new DNP-prepared nurse executive who is unable to fulfill his obligations as defined by the Chief Executive Officer (CEO) would experience role strain. The role expectations may be beyond what he is able to achieve or the CEO may push him to the limits of his abilities. It must be noted that role stress has not been differentiated from role strain in previous nursing studies, causing confusion as to whether results reflected perceptions external to the individual or internal responses over stressful events (Chen et al., 2007).

Role strain is in contrast to *role conflict*, where tension is felt between two or more, competing roles. Role conflict results when an individual encounters tensions as the result of incompatible roles. For instance, a mother who is employed full-time as a DNP-prepared faculty member may experience role conflict because of the norms that are associated with the two roles she has. She may be expected to spend a great deal of time taking care of her children while simultaneously trying to advance her career as a teacher, scholar, clinician, and university citizen (Macionis, 2006).

Role ambiguity is defined as the lack of clarity related to one's position or role. A metasynthesis study by Jones in 2005 reviewed 14 relevant studies on role development and advance practice nurses in the United States and United Kingdom. Jones (2005) suggested that when advanced nursing roles were first introduced, clear role definitions and objectives needed to be developed and communicated to relevant key personnel to reduce role ambiguity. Interprofessional relationships and role ambiguity were the most important factors that enhanced or hindered performance. When one considers the various socio-political issues that presently face new doctoral advanced practice nurses, given the newness of the role, they will confront an array of reactions and situations. For the purposes of this chapter, the term *role strain* will be used as an umbrella term to discuss the perceived difficulty or angst in fulfilling role obligations experienced by DNP-prepared nurses for a variety of reasons.

In terms of role strain, organizational engagement efforts certainly play a key role in long-term solutions in the workplace. Engagement efforts require promoting job–person fit by matching individual and organizational profiles with six domains of work life: sustainable workload, feelings of choice and control, appropriate recognition and reward, supportive work community, fairness and justice, and meaningful and valued work (Shirey, 2006). Furthermore, the role for the doctoral advanced practice nurse, irrespective of whether the individual is a nurse practitioner, midwife, anesthetist or clinical nurse specialist, clinical executive, nurse educator, or clinical scientist, will demand a significant amount of the individual's time and attention. When one considers the multiple competing roles of the doctoral advanced practice nurses today (e.g., mother, father, caregiver, spouse or partner, professional, scholar, citizen), there are many demands for the doctoral advanced practice nurses' time in this fast-paced chaotic culture. The authors would be remiss if they failed to address the multiple roles of the doctoral advanced practice nurse outside of his/her professional role, which can place great demands on the individual's time as well as serve as a great source of stress as the doctoral advanced practice nurse attempts to achieve life balance and fulfill many competing demands.

DNP ROLE DESCRIPTIONS

In the workplace, doctoral advanced practice nurses (practitioner, clinical executive, nurse educator, or clinical scientist) experience role strain for different reasons based on their respective roles. The following sections provide a descriptive overview of the prospective role strain for each role.

The DNP-Educated Practitioner

Doctoral advanced practice nurses (DAPRN) who are nurse practitioners provide expert primary health care or specialty health care to diverse populations in various health care agencies and venues. DAPRNs who are nurse midwives, nurse anesthetists, and clinical nurse specialists also fullfill their professional roles. With health care reform looming, the future is bright for DAPRNs, especially if they innovate, design, or create efficient models of health care delivery. They may serve as leaders of nurse-managed clinics, private practices, convenient care clinics, or urgent care centers. They may serve as expert practitioners with additional confidence and knowledge to positively impact patient outcomes.

DAPRN's practice includes not only direct care, but also a focus on the needs of a panel of patients, a target population, a set of populations, or a broad community. These graduates are distinguished by their abilities to conceptualize new care delivery models that are based in contemporary nursing science and that are feasible within current organizational, political, cultural, and economic perspectives. Graduates are skilled in working within organizational and policy arenas and in the actual provision of patient care by themselves and/or by others. For example, DAPRNs understand principles of practice management, including conceptual and practical strategies for balancing productivity with quality of care. They are able to assess the impact of practice policies and procedures on meeting the health needs of the patient populations with whom they practice. DAPRNs are proficient in quality improvement strategies and in creating and sustaining changes at the organizational and policy levels. They have the ability to evaluate the cost effectiveness of care and use principles of economics and finance to redesign effective and realistic care delivery strategies. In addition, DAPRNs have the ability to organize care in a way that addresses emerging practice problems and the ethical dilemmas that emerge as new diagnostic and therapeutic technologies evolve (AACN, 2006).

It is clear that the DAPRNs can contribute significantly to the health and welfare of our nation; what is not clear is whether the role of the practitioner will change as a result of the DAPRN's additional knowledge and skills. If the workplace environment does not change, doctoral advanced practice nurses may feel frustrated in their role. They may also experience professional jealousy or other less than supportive behaviors from colleagues as a result of this new role, as well as role overload based on the sheer amount of work to be accomplished.

The DNP-Educated Clinical Executive

The DNP Clinical Executive (Chief Nursing Officers, Vice Presidents, and other executive-level nurse leaders) is called to address emergent and challenging issues for nursing practice, as well as to create opportunities that will shape and implement innovative changes in the health care system. Today, the DNP Clinical Executive is in short supply. Future doctoral level nurse administrators and executive leaders are also charged to improve health and health care outcomes through evidence-based practice in diverse clinical and health care settings. The DNP Clinical Executive emphasizes evidence-based approaches for quality and safety improvement in practice settings, applies research processes to decision making, and translates credible research findings to increase the effectiveness of both direct and indirect nursing practice. Some of the specific competencies outlined in the "essentials document" for the DNP Clinical Executive include the abilities to use sophisticated, conceptual, and analytical skills in evaluating the links between clinical, organizational, fiscal, and policy issues; establish processes for interorganizational collaboration for the achievement of organizational goals; design patient-centered care delivery systems or policy-level delivery models; collaborate effectively with legal counsel and financial officers around issues related to legal and regulatory guidelines; and demonstrate advanced levels of clinical judgment, cultural sensitivity, and systems thinking (AACN, 2006). The responsibilities for the DNP Clinical Executive may be daunting. As the leader, the DNP Clinical Executive will most likely not have a DNP-prepared CEO or role models to guide him/her as he or she navigates this senior executive role. He/she may experience the loneliness associated with a senior administration position. Fellow senior administrators and physicians may feel threatened with the credentials, power, influence, and position of the DNP Clinical Executive who traditionally did not hold a doctorate to serve in that leadership role.

The DNP-Educated Educator

Today, many nursing faculty are divorced from clinical practice. Current expectations of the tripartite nursing faculty role in relation to teaching, scholarship, and service are not realistic in advancing nursing science, clinical practice, or education. Nursing faculty juggle large teaching and service loads while attempting to engage in scholarship. For those nursing faculty who are research active, the juggling act is even more pronounced. In addition, few nursing faculty have formal practice appointments as part of their faculty role allowing them to stay clinically current to inform their teaching. For example, many Nurse Practitioner, Nurse Midwifery, and Nurse Anesthesia faculty have outside practice obligations to maintain their clinical hours/expertise for specialty certification, in addition to their full-time faculty appointments. With the introduction of the DNP Educator, the profession has an opportunity to reexamine the various roles of nurse faculty and create a model that encourages the faculty to master one or two areas rather than the current "jack of all trades" approach. The authors suggest three roles for the nurse in academic positions: Nurse Scientist, Educator Clinician, and Clinician Educator. Nursing education must redefine the expectations of the nursing faculty with a primary focus of research, teaching, or clinical. The DNP Educator is in a unique position to serve in the Educator Clinician role (e.g., 75% education and 25% practice) or Clinician Educator role (e.g., 75% practice and 25% education) as they are able to integrate the knowledge they present in the classroom with a clinical practice context, yet also have the educational theory to draw upon in the classroom. However, this will not be easy as the academy is an institution ensconced in tradition and may not embrace the DNP Educator role as an equal. Therefore, the DNP Educator may be viewed as a second-class citizen in the academy causing additional role strain as well as experience role overload from the tripartite role in academe and additional practice requirements.

The DNP-Educated Clinical Scientist

A DNP Clinical Scientist in the clinical trials industry will be a force for new innovation, specifically for nursing sensitive health care outcomes. This new role is a DNP degree innovation that is designed to support both the clinical nurse scientist in the clinical trials/pharmaceutical research industry and as a more intensive clinical research track option for DNP students who desire a greater focus on research than what is typical in a DNP curriculum. With health care remaining a growing field, there is no reason to believe that the consumer will not demand higher-quality health care services which translates to more research, more funding for new drugs and devices, and more innovation. The DNP Clinical Scientist can spearhead these clinical trials and serve as patient advocate, primary investigator, and leader in the clinical trials/pharmaceutical research industry. Although this is a potentially very valuable doctoral role for the DNP Clinical Scientist in the clinical trials industry, he or she may experience some internal angst and external obstacles as a pioneer in this area. The DNP Clinical Scientist will most likely not have DNP-prepared role models as guides as they navigate this new leadership role. Subsequently, the DNP Clinical Scientist may experience professional jealousy from non-DNP nurse peers. In addition, physicians and other PhD-prepared scientist colleagues may feel threatened with the DNP Clinical Scientist's new knowledge and influence.

A STUDY IS CONDUCTED: "THE EXPERIENCES OF DNPs IN THEIR CURRENT PROFESSIONAL POSITIONS"

Due to the novel and innovative nature of the various DNP roles, the authors sought to understand the experiences of DNP-prepared nurses who currently hold faculty, advanced practice, or executive positions in nursing by conducting a study on the lived experience of the DNP in his/her new professional role. This study titled, "The Experiences of DNPs in Their Current Professional Positions" was unique in that no current studies sought to understand the role of the DNP were found in the literature.

Purpose and Significance of the Study

The American Association of Colleges of Nursing (AACN) member institutions voted in October of 2004 to champion the DNP degree as the desired preparation for future nurses prepared for advanced nursing specialty practice, including the four most recognized advanced practice nursing (APN) roles of nurse practitioners, clinical nurse specialists, nurse midwives, and nurse anesthetists (AACN, 2009). Additionally, the AACN offered the DNP for advanced practice preparation of the Clinical Executive (AACN, 2006). The AACN recommended that academic institutions that prepare nurses for advanced practice prepare them at the doctoral level, instead of the current master's level, by the year 2015 (AACN, 2009). According to AACN's latest data (Fang, Tracy, & Bednash, 2010), there are 118 DNP programs currently enrolling students at schools of nursing nationwide, and an additional 100 DNP programs are in the planning stages (AACN, 2010). There are now DNP programs in 37 states plus the District of Columbia (AACN, 2010). From 2007 to 2008, the number of students enrolled in DNP programs nearly doubled from 1,874 to 3,415 and the number of DNP graduates increased from 122 to 361 (AACN, 2009).

The change in level of desired advanced practice nurse preparation has also led to a change in educational requirements and focus on evidence-based practice as noted in the *Essentials of Doctoral Education for Advanced Nursing Practice* published by the AACN in 2006. The major emphasis of the DNP is advanced practice, as opposed to the PhD, which emphasizes research (AACN, 2006). Loomis, Willard, and Cohen (2007) found that the majority of DNP students reported considering the PhD educational route, but chose the DNP over the PhD because of their disinterest in research and desire to become clinical experts. They reported that in these DNP students, 55% identified nursing education was their professional goal, and 61% reported that they considered eligibility to be a nursing faculty member as an advantage of the DNP degree (Loomis et al.). Schools and Colleges of Nursing are rapidly developing more DNP educational programs, and increased numbers of students are enrolling in these new APN programs. It is imperative that research is conducted to understand this possible transition in nursing education and practice, and the potential effect on nursing as a profession. Because the role of the DNP is so new and many are now beginning to enter into the employment arena, there is a gap in the literature as to what actual positions these new DNPs are pursuing and how they are experiencing their new roles. A research study that investigates the current role choices and experiences of DNP graduates can increase nursing knowledge about the role and experiences of the newly established position. The findings can be disseminated through publication with the intention of closing the gap in the literature and contribute to future discussions about the role and educational preparations for DNP students. The authors of this chapter conducted a qualitative study to initiate this area of inquiry.

Research Design and Procedures

The following research question guided the focus and method for the study: What is the lived experience of the DNP-prepared nurse who currently holds faculty, advanced practice or administration position in nursing? Nurses holding the DNP (or DrNP) degree were sought for this study to explore and understand their experiences in their current professional contexts using a descriptive, interpretive phenomenological approach in the tradition of the Dutch (Utrecht) School of Phenomenology. The Dutch approach to phenomenology is both descriptive and interpretive, and was used to guide this research. The research process focused on what informants verbally expressed regarding the meaning in the context of their particular DNP role. Prior to beginning the interviews, the researchers bracketed their presuppositions about the role of the DNP by discussing their presuppositions with each other. The process of bracketing was done to ensure that the researchers did not influence the informants and their responses during the study (Cohen, 1995). The research process allowed the researchers to engage in dialogue and discussion with the informants to clarify, verify, and interpret the data.

Instruments

An investigator-designed open, unstructured interview guide was used to understand the experiences of DNPs who currently hold faculty, advanced practice, or executive positions in nursing. In addition, demographic data were gathered to understand the context of the informants and assist with data analysis.

Informant Recruitment and Informed Consent

Once IRB approval was obtained from the University Institutional Review Board, informants were purposefully sought out through the snowball method in the nursing community in Pennsylvania and New Jersey. Ethical considerations related to data collection were included in the procedures that honored the privacy, feelings, and dignity of the informants and were intended to minimize any risks from the research process. The informants were informed of their rights and their willingness to participate in the study by reading and signing the informed consent. They were also informed that they had the right to withdraw from the study at any time. A voluntary, purposeful sample of nine nurses who held a doctor of nursing practice degree and who were currently employed either in nursing education, in clinical practice, or administration in nursing were recruited for this study. Nursing education DNPs were included if they were currently employed full time in a tenure or nontenure track position at a School of Nursing in a college or university setting offering a minimum of a BSN. DAPRNs were included if they were employed full-time as a nurse practitioner, clinical nurse specialist, nurse midwife, or nurse anesthetist. Nursing administration DNPs were included who had full-time employment as a nurse executive in a health care institution.

Collection of Data and Method of Data Analysis

The informants were interviewed in a place of their choosing providing privacy and comfort. The in-depth interviews lasted up to one and one-half hours and a second interview was requested by one informant for confirmatory purposes. Saturation of the data occurred after seven interviews, and two additional informants were sought for confirmation of the data.

The interviews were audio taped and the data transcribed verbatim for analysis. Concurrent data collection and analysis occurred, allowing the data to guide the analysis and further data collection. Analysis followed the procedures outlined by scholars from the Dutch (Utrecht) school (Barritt, Beekman, Bleeker, & Mulderjif, 1984). The data analysis process called for a two-part analysis of identifying common forms and shared themes or themes. In using this method, the researchers constructed a thematic analysis of the narrative through identifying the experiential (van Kaam, 1991). Nvivo 8 qualitative data manager was used to assist with the data analysis.

Findings

The findings of this study are being presented according to the process of analysis. There were 9 informants interviewed for this study. There were 8 women and 1 man. The ages ranged from 38 to 64, with the median age being 49. The majority of informants ($n = 7$) were from Pennsylvania and the remainder ($n = 2$) from New Jersey. All the informants identified their culture or race as white with five more specifically identifying themselves as either Italian American or one Polish American. All the informants received doctor of nursing practice degrees and all started as post-master's students. The length of the doctoral program varied from 1.5 years to 4 years, with the average length of time being 2.8 years. The focus of the doctor of nursing practice program for the informants included 5 with a focus in nursing education, 3 in advanced practice, and 1 as a clinical scientist in clinical research. The major focus of the *current job* of the informants was 1 nurse midwife, 3 nurse practitioners, 1 nurse executive, 3 nurse educators, and 1 in a dual role of nurse practitioner and nurse educator.

The focus of the analysis was on both description and interpretation of the phenomena of interest. The first step was to identify *common forms* after an analysis of the narrative (Barritt et al., 1984). The following were identified for this study:

1. Advise and goals
2. Confidence

3. Empowerment
4. Acceptance in the workplace
5. Context
6. Difference in roles
7. Misunderstandings about the role by peers
8. Multiple roles
9. Role
10. Tension
11. Barriers
12. Finding place
13. Opportunities

Further and more in-depth analysis of the common forms revealed shared themes or themes from the informant's experiences in their current role as a DNP. The following are themes:

1. Changing context and environment of the workplace involving the real and perceived role of the DNP; supported by the following common forms:
   (a) Misunderstanding, tension, multiple roles, difference in roles, context, acceptance, role
2. Feelings of confidence and empowerment in the role as a DNP; supported by the following common forms:
   (a) Advice and goals, confidence, empowerment
3. Finding my way by finding and responding to opportunity; supported by the following common forms:
   (a) Barriers, finding place, opportunity

Theme 1: Context of the DNP Role

The first shared theme interpreted from the data was the changing context and environment of the workplace involving the real and perceived role of the DNP. The context for this theme can be defined as the changing work environment and context of the informants. This includes hospital, school or college of nursing, and private and collaborative practice. Informants very clearly defined, and described the content of their professional lives as DNPs. Many of the DNPs interviewed for this study described not being completely certain about the scope of their role and engaged in working in multiple roles either in their primary place of employment or taking on a second job. One informant said: "I always have to explain what my role is;" another said, "I am always introduced as a PhD nurse and then have to explain that I do not have a PhD." Many worked primarily in either advanced practice nursing education, and took second jobs in the other. The nurse executive worked at one place, but the role has expanded due to obtaining the DNP. Many of the informants in the study took on additional roles in their current work place because they were not sure of their role and wanted to carve out a special place.

Many of the informants in the study shared that there was misunderstanding and tension from their peers in the work place. One informant said, "I think in my current position they are not used to the DNP." Another said, "there are NPs . . . they all kind of think it's a waste of time to have a doctorate in nursing and be a practitioner." The DNPs working primarily in advanced practice would hear from peers about why they did not need the DNP because their practice role has not changed. Many found that in some cases their peers would joke with them about having a doctorate, and that it really was not needed in their role. Nurses working in nursing education shared that they were not sure about their role (how their role was the same or different from their PhD colleagues) and their peers were equally unsure. There was no clearly identified role for them in nursing education. One informant said, "They don't know what to do with me now." Many were able to discuss a role that included teaching both theory and clinical, with the ability to bring evidence to support practice, and other informants also saw themselves as researchers. Overall, they were unsure of how the future would look regarding their role in nursing education. The nurse executive was the clearest about his/her role. The institution was very accepting of the individual in the role as a DNP. There appeared to be pride among peers and acceptance in the role overall.

In almost all cases, there was a general level of acceptance for the DNPs in their roles despite some instances of misunderstanding and tension. Peers in the context of the work setting were generally accepting of these individuals in their new roles, especially for the nurse executive.

Theme 2: Feelings of Confidence and Empowerment in the Role as a DNP

The second major shared theme from this study was "Feelings of confidence and empowerment in the role as a DNP." The majority of informants in the study shared that because of the DNP degree and educational process they felt a level of confidence about their preparation and current role. The majority of informants in the roles of advance practice, nurse administrator, and nurse educator expressed confidence and empowerment in their current role. Along with the sense of confidence, informants felt empowered in their role because of the degree. One informant said: "And for myself I feel very good about the whole thing." Another said, "Certainly it does have an impact on me and how I look at things but also in my degree of confidence in proposing what I think." The degree has helped many of the informants feel well prepared and confident about how they both perceive their role and how they work in their role. One informant said, "I'm a couple of years out from it and I can say that I feel it was worth it and that I'm starting to get the payoff in terms of confidence and career opportunities." Another informant reported that, "I certainly feel more confident about standing up in front of a group saying to a group of executives, senior leadership . . . this is the problem, this is the solution and this is the recommendation . . . this is why I feel more confident about my role." Some informants felt that the degree and preparation have helped them feel more confident in a specific role function such as research. This is supported when one informant said, "I know how to conduct research and I feel more confident in having looked at research, my conclusions, and because I have had the rigorous academic exercises over and over." In addition, the degree has assisted the informants in feeling empowered to make decisions with confidence about their work in their role. One informant said, "I thought it gave me a sense of empowerment to go out on my own and do things." Many informants felt that confidence in their role will ultimately assist the profession in being empowered. This statement was supported by data expressed by one informant as, "It gives you a different perspective on nursing. And I think it increases your pride in nursing, it increases your respect for nursing and respect for yourself and it's just totally empowering." Another informant said, "And I think the training itself helps you have a different voice in your practice."

Overall, the informants in this study felt that the DNP program prepared them with a sense of confidence and empowerment for their current role. Many felt that they perform their role with a sense of confidence—how they interact with peers, patients, students, and others in their role. Many informants felt they were well prepared by their program to do their respective jobs. For many, it means that the degree has helped them feel confident and empowered. Many informants felt that because they feel confident in their role "today" they will continue to grow and feel more confident and empowered in the future.

Theme 3: Finding My Way by Finding and Responding to Opportunity

The third major theme described by the informants in this study was "finding my way by finding and responding to opportunity." This particular theme was evident in almost all the informants' experiences as they described their current role as a DNP. This shared theme is closely linked to themes one and two for many reasons. One clear connection was the fact that many informants were involved in multiple roles in their current role or primary and secondary jobs as a DNP. It is as if the informants in the study were seeking to find the right fit for their new-found confidence and sense of empowerment by trying out a variety of roles. One informant said, "And then I really had a hard time finding where my place was going to be. I guess you can probably tell by the several career paths that I chose, education, and clinical practice." Another informant shared that: "I kind of was, you know, trying to reinvent myself." One informant added, "And I think some of it, too, was we were the very first class. And you're, you know, finding your way, and, you know, trying to figure out."

Informants in this study expressed hope that they will find their way as evidenced by one informant who said, "No, and that is the scary part. And I feel that I am shooting darts, but I don't really know where the bull's eye is. That does cause some angst. But what's the plan and how am I going to get from here to there? I'm going to try to find some people to help me to get from here to there." Another informant expressed a similar sentiment: "I think the hardest part for me is that I went from a position of 15 years of being on top of my game, knowing what I was doing, know who to contact, very autonomous, to being at the bottom and having to feel my way around. I felt like a baby learning to crawl."

The majority of the informants in this study felt that part of finding their way is to look for and take advantage of opportunity. One informant felt that, "And—and I was the only nurse. I was the only doctorally prepared nurse on the board. And the rest were physicians. The pharmaceutical company picked me and one physician to help them with this feedback on their product development. So that was actually really interesting. And I knew that every Joe Blow wouldn't get that opportunity." Another informant expressed hope about the future of his/her role as well as nursing in the following statement: "We're a dynamic profession in a dynamic environment. So who knows where we're all going to end up in the next 5 to 10 years?" Informants in the study were clear that they wanted the role to be transparent from the very beginning, starting with the accrediting body and schools of nursing. This view was expressed multiple times similar to the following statement by one informant: "I think that if the DNP is going to move forward, there really needs to be three tracks: practice, administration, and education. And that you would be able to come out saying it's a DNP 'with a focus in . . .' And all of the tracks need to have more of a focus on research dissemination."

In summary, theme three seem to be the theme that connected and linked the three themes together. Overall, informants in this study expressed concern about not being clear about their role in advanced practice and nursing education. Nursing administration seemed to have the clearest view of their role and the most support from their context or work environment. Informants felt hopeful about the future even though there is still a need to define the role of the DNP. However, they would also like the profession, schools of nursing, and employers to be clear about the expectations of the DNP in advanced practice, nursing education, and nursing administration. Informants felt that their programs prepared them in a manner that has helped them to feel confident and empowered in their role. *They also expressed concerns that in some cases, the work environment is not always accepting of the DNP especially in advanced practice.* For those in nursing education, the environment appeared to be supportive *if there was a need for faculty.* There was still a sense of not knowing the expectations in relation to teaching, tenure, and promotion in the academic setting. Again, the informants wished for clarity in the role. Overall, they were attempting to make their own way as there is a lack of clarity concerning the role of the DNP both in the context of the profession and workplace.

DISCUSSION AND CONCLUSIONS OF STUDY

As previously mentioned, there have been no published studies on the lived experience of the DNP graduate. The DNP graduates are truly pioneers in practice, education, and administration as they bring their advanced knowledge and skill to the table. The informants' confidence and sense of empowerment is refreshing and very much needed in today's nursing environment to effect change, as well as being consistent with the AACN's vision for the degree (AACN, 2006). They were enthusiastic about their advanced knowledge and wanted to apply that knowledge in their respective roles. However, many of them experienced role strain as they reported a lack of clarity and angst related to their new position or role. This phenomenon is consistent with the findings by Jones (2005) that clear role definitions need to be developed for new roles and communicated to all stakeholders over time to reduce role ambiguity and/or strain.

When the researchers reflect on the findings in this study, the experiences of some DNP graduates are not necessarily surprising in lieu of nursing's history. In this study, DNP graduates employed in advanced nursing practice roles have expressed concern that in some cases, the work environment is not always accepting of the DNP especially in advanced practice settings. From our history, we know that nursing practice, and to some degree education, has been slow to recognize or come to terms with the distinct differences of the associate degree-level (AD) graduate versus the baccalaureate-level (BSN) graduate (Moltz, 2010). Today, there are more health care institutions than not that do not distinguish the AD graduate from the BSN graduate in terms of initial salary or work responsibilities in the practice arena (Benner, Sutphen, Leonard, & Day, 2009). At present, the doctoral advanced practice nurse's role and expectations are no different than that of the master's-level advanced practice nurse's role and expectations. One hopes that the lack of differentiation in practice roles in the clinical arena may be due to the "newness" of the degree; however, it may also be due to the similarities in the scope of practice of the two degrees or, sadly, an anti-intellectual mentality or propensity for professional jealousy that exist for some in the profession.

If the practice arena does not distinguish the role, competencies, and expectations of the DNP versus the MSN advanced practice nurse in the future, *nursing may very well find itself in the same position as we are with the lack of differentiation between the AD and BSN graduates in clinical practice.* Based on the findings of this study, the informants feel that doctoral advanced practice nurses can contribute significantly to the advancement of the profession and are confident about its role in the future. It is not clear, however, whether the role of the doctoral-level advanced practice nurse will actually change as a result of the doctoral advanced practice nurse's additional knowledge and skills. The informants have sought opportunities to utilize their advanced knowledge and skills, as they have not felt "fulfilled" in their present role. It is not clear whether doctoral advanced practice nurses will continue to seek other positions or secondary positions to meet this need, or if they will push for change in the practice setting to accommodate their advanced knowledge as they attempt to find their way as doctoral advanced practice nurses. If the workplace environment does not change, doctoral advanced practice nurses may feel frustrated in their role, as they are not permitted to expand their scope concomitant with their new knowledge and skills. Based on the informants' experiences, the struggle to be accepted for one's contributions is not new in nursing's history and will require more renegades, rebels, and trailblazers to advance the profession (Dunphy, Smith, & Youngskin, 2009).

The informants in the educator role felt accepted by colleagues, yet they were unsure about their future in nursing education. The positive news is that the informants saw themselves able to bring evidence to support current practice back into the classroom. This is not surprising as the DNP graduate in the educator role is well suited to integrate the classroom content and the practice context as called for in the recent Carnegie Foundation Study, *Educating Nurses: A Call for Radical Transformation* (Benner et al., 2009). DNP educators are in a unique position to serve as faculty members, as they are able to integrate the knowledge they present in the classroom with a clinical practice context. There is still some uneasiness as to where they "fit" in the academy. One hopes that the academy will value their connection to practice which is sorely needed (Benner et al., 2009).

In this study, the nurse executive felt the most valued and accepted. One can hypothesize that senior administration "sees" the value of the doctoral-level nurse executive and is not as threatened by his/her new credential and advanced knowledge. High-performing organizations closely scrutinize leadership capacity and embrace talent (Wells & Hejna, 2009). These organizations look to doctoral-level nurse executives to shape their institution through their leadership and to address emergent and challenging issues for nursing practice as well as create opportunities that shape and implement innovative changes in the health care system (AACN, 2006; Upenieks, 2003). One must note that the doctoral level nurse executive is in a unique position in health care institutions; he or she is usually the only nurse among a group of senior, non-nurse leaders. The doctoral-level nurse executive may not face the same issues of professional jealousy that a doctoral-level advanced practice nurse may face in the practice arena.

SUMMARY

In summarizing this chapter, the study informants spoke to the need for differentiating the three distinct roles of the DNP graduate: advanced practice, educator, and executive in the educational and practice environment and the need for role clarity. Although there are core courses necessary for all DNP graduates, there is specialized knowledge required for each of the distinct roles. Will the DNP have less of a generalist curriculum in the future and have more emphasis on the specific advanced role? With the increase in

DNP programs across the nation, will we reach a critical mass of DNP graduates who will have a sufficiently strong voice in the education and practice settings to effect change? Time will tell if this critical mass of graduates can achieve what the BSN-level graduates were unable to do at a national level for themselves; yet, MSN-prepared advanced practice nurses were able to accomplish much and truly transform the landscape of nursing practice by creating a new role highly valued by society. Ultimately, will the DNP have similar success and achieve or surpass the AACN's vision of the DNP degree (AACN, 2006, 2009). The authors assert that DNP graduates will need to differentiate their practice from MSN graduates in order to substantiate their value to the profession, health care community, and public, or else the forces of role strain will likely persist and perhaps worsen. Health care reform and other market forces may also drive the need for the DNP going forward as we see a growing need for innovation and evidence to improve care.

REFERENCES

American Association of Colleges of Nursing (AACN). (2006). *The essentials of doctoral education for advanced nursing practice.* Retrieved from http://www.aacn.nche.edu/DNP/pdf/Essentials.pdf

American Association of Colleges of Nursing (AACN). (2009). *Fact sheet: The doctor of nursing practice (DNP).* Retrieved from http://www.aacn.nche.edu/Media/FactSheets/dnp.htm

American Association of Colleges of Nursing (AACN). (2010). *Doctor of nursing practice (DNP) programs.* Retrieved from http://www.aacn.nche.edu/DNP/DNPProgramList.htm

Barritt, L., Beekman, T., Bleeker, H., & Mulderij, K. (1984). Analyzing phenomenological descriptions. *Phenomenology and Pedagogy,* 2(1), 1–17.

Benner, P., Sutphen, M., Leonard, V., & Day, L. (2009). *Educating nurses: A call for radical transformation.* Stanford, CA: The Carnegie Foundation for the Advancement of Teaching.

Chen, Y., Chen, S. H., Tsai, C. Y., & Lo, L. Y. (2007). Role stress and job satisfaction for nurse specialists. *Journal of Advanced Nursing,* 59(5), 497–509.

Cohen, M. Z. (1995). The experience of surgery: Phenomenological clinical nursing research. In A. Omery, C. Kasper, & G. Page (Eds.), *In search of nursing science* (pp. 159–174). Thousand Oaks, CA: Sage.

Hardy, M. E., & Conway, M. E. (1978). *Role theory perspectives for health professionals* (1st ed.). New York, NY: Appleton-Century-Crofts.

Hardy, M. E., & Conway, M. E. (1988). *Role theory perspectives for health professionals* (2nd ed.). Norwalk, CT: Appleton & Lange.

Dunphy, L. M., Smith, N. K., & Youngkin, E. Q. (2009). Advanced practice nursing: Doing what has to be done—Radicals, renegades, and rebels. In L. A. Joel, *Advance practice nursing: Essentials for role development* (2nd ed.) (pp. 2–22). Philadelphia, PA: FA Davis.

Fang, D., Tracy, V., & Bednash, G. D. (2010). *2009–2010 Enrollment and Graduations in Baccalaureate and Graduate Programs in Nursing.* Washington, DC: American Association of Colleges of Nursing.

Jones, M. L. (2005). Role development and effective practice in specialist and advance practice roles in acute care hospital settings: Systematic review and meta-synthesis. *Journal of Advanced Nursing,* 49(2), 191–209.

Kahn, R. A., Wolfe, P., Quinn, R., Snock, J., & Rosenthal, R. (1964). *Organizational stress: Studies in role conflict and ambiguity.* New York, NY: Wiley & Sons.

Lazarus, R. S. (1967). *Psychological stress and the coping process.* New York, NY: McGraw-Hill.

Loomis, J. A., Willard, B., & Cohen, J. (2007). Difficult professional choices: Deciding between the PhD and the DNP in nursing. *Online Journal of Issues in Nursing,* 12(1), 16. Retrieved from http://search.ebscohost.com/login.aspx?direct=true&db=cin20&AN=2009526632&site=ehost-live

Macionis, J. J. (2006). *Society the basics* (8th ed.). Saddle River, NJ: Person Prentice Hall.

Moltz, D. (2010). Nursing tug of war. *Inside Higher Education*. Retrieved from http://www.inside-highered.com/news/2010/01/07/nursing

Shirey, M. (2006). Stress and burnout in nursing faculty. *Nurse Educator, 31*(3), 95–97.

Sveinsdottir, H., Biering, P., & Ramel, A. (2006). Occupational stress, job satisfaction, and working environment for Icelandic nurses: A cross-sectional questionnaire survey. *International Journal of Nursing Studies, 43*, 875–889.

Upenieks, V. V. (2003). What constitutes effective leadership? Perceptions of magnet and nonmagnet nurse leaders. *JONA: The Journal of Nursing Administration, 33*(9), 456–467.

Van Kaam, A. (1991). *Formation of the human heart*. New York, NY: Crossroads.

Wells, W., & Hejna, W. (2009, January). Developing leadership talent in healthcare organizations. *Healthcare Financial Management*, 66–69.

CHAPTER TEN: Reflective Response

Courtney Reinisch

The role for Doctoral Advanced Practice Nurses (DAPRNs) is evolving. The authors address the concern of role strain for DAPRNs. DAPRNs in the nurse practitioner, clinical executive, nurse educator, or clinical scientist role may experience role strain for different reasons. The authors make the point that the DNP degree has not solely focused on providing direct patient care but has rather expanded to include administrators, executives, and clinical scientists. Thus, the needs of health care, society, and DAPRNs at large are not being best utilized and may result in role strain for these graduates.

To avoid the negative effects of DAPRN role strain, I believe DNP educational programs should focus on the terminal goal of the DNP as expert clinician. This is supported by the Institute of Medicine (IOM) (2001), and the American Academy of the Colleges of Nursing's (AACN) *Essentials of Doctoral Education for Advanced Nursing Practice* (2006) and fact sheet on the doctor of nursing practice (2009). The IOM report *Crossing the Quality Chasm: A New Health System for the 21st Century* (2001) stresses that the health care system as currently structured does not make the best use of its resources. The aging population and increased client demand for new services, technologies, and pharmaceuticals contribute to both the increase in health care expenditure and waste of resources. A recommendation in the report calls on all health care organizations and professional groups to promote health care that is safe, effective, client centered, timely, efficient, and equitable (IOM, 2001, p. 6). In a follow-up report, *Health Professions Education: A Bridge to Quality*, the IOM Committee on the Health Professions Education (2003) states, "All health professionals should be educated to deliver patient centered care as members of an interdisciplinary team, emphasizing evidence-based practice, quality improvement approaches, and informatics" (p. 3). The development of a practice doctorate is supported in the National Research Council's report titled *Advancing the Nation's Health Needs: NIH Research Training Programs* (2005). That report notes the need for the nursing profession to develop a nonresearch practice doctorate to prepare expert practitioners who can also serve as clinical faculty. I believe that the DARPN educated as the expert clinician is well suited to be a part of an interdisciplinary team delivering health care that is patient centered, cost conscious, and evidence based.

AACN recognizes the DNP as an academic degree that prepares nurses for a variety of advanced specialty nursing roles, including the four recognized Advanced Practice Registered Nursing (APRN) roles: Certified Nurse-Midwives, Certified Registered Nurse Anesthetists, Clinical Nurse Specialists, and Certified Nurse Practitioners. The AACN (2004a) has conceptualized practice as "any form of nursing intervention that influences health care outcomes for individuals or populations, including the direct care of individual patients, management of care, administration of nursing and health care organizations, and the development and implementation of health policy" (p. 2). In issuing this statement, the AACN allowed programs of study to expand beyond the needs identified by the IOM and National Research Council reports which support the need for expert practitioners. In response to the AACN's definition, disparate educational programs have emerged. I believe that this contributes to the problems of DNP role ambiguity, role strain, and stress as identified by the authors of this chapter.

The authors of the chapter propose that the DNP-Educated Educator serve in a dual role combining clinical practice and classroom education. The authors propose the Educator Clinician role with 75% education and 25% practice commitment or the Clinician Educator role with 75% practice and 25% education commitment. I question how these percentages were determined. To enroll as a primary care provider with most insurers, a clinician needs to be in practice at least 2 days per week which implies a 40% time commitment to practice. I support the Educator Clinician role as truly engaging in the tripartite mission of nursing education which includes teaching, scholarship, and practice. The collaboration between academia and practice can be positively influenced when lines between faculty and clinical staff blend, with each serving the dual role of practitioner and academician, resulting in the development of new educational models that evaluate new and emerging nursing roles.

In this chapter, the authors present their original research of the "Experiences of DNPs in Their Current Professional Roles." In my opinion, the findings of the study are limited. The methodology requires more detailed description. I question the use of snowball sampling as 7 of the respondents are from Pennsylvania and 2 from New Jersey. Perhaps the experience of the DAPRNs differs by geographic location. Additionally, all respondents were Caucasian and 8 of the 9 were women. It would be interesting to have information about the focus of their educational programs and aspirations prior to enrollment. The participants included educators, administrators, and clinicians. While the authors state that they reached data saturation with seven participants, this does not address the nuances of the different roles that may have benefited from a larger sample. There is no discussion on the trustworthiness, credibility, dependability, confirmability, and transferability of the data (Lincoln & Gruba, 1985).

As a practicing DAPRN and educator, I agree with the authors. There is tremendous role strain due to ambiguity, rapid expansion of DNP programs, and lack of a clear professional direction for DAPRNs. In July 2008, AACN's Board of Directors endorsed the *Consensus Model for APRN Regulation*. This consensus supports APRN certification through a nationally recognized nursing certifying body, and will be used by state boards to grant APRNs the authority to practice. I am also in favor of certification for DAPRNs in the area of Comprehensive Care. The Columbia University Center for Clinical Practice (2010) defines the DNP who provides comprehensive health care to be "an expert clinician, knowledgeable in individuals' health care needs across the lifespan, practices in all clinical settings, analyzes and interprets evidence as the basis for health care choices, and engages the patient in a collaborative relationship in the provision of continuous, coordinated services that include health promotion, disease prevention, and definitive disease management" (p. 1). Certification in Comprehensive Care for these DNP graduates will provide support and criteria for clear role delineation and minimize the effects of role strain.

REFERENCES

American Association of Colleges of Nursing. (2004a). *AACN position statement on the practice doctorate in nursing.* Retrieved from http://www.aacn.nche.edu/dnp/pdf/DNP.pdf.

American Association of Colleges of Nursing (AACN). (2006). *The essentials of doctoral education for advanced nursing practice.* Retrieved from http://www.aacn.nche.edu/DNP/pdf/Essentials.pdf

American Association of Colleges of Nursing (AACN). (2009). *Fact sheet: The doctor of nursing practice (DNP).* Retrieved from http://www.aacn.nche.edu/Media/FactSheets/dnp.htm

Columbia University Center for Clinical Practice. (2010). *Advanced practice registered nurses and comprehensive healthcare.* Retrieved from http://cpmcnet.columbia.edu/dept/nursing/clinPracCtr/comprHealthCare.html

Institute of Medicine (IOM). (2001). *Crossing the quality chasm: A new health system for the 21st century.* Washington, DC: National Academies Press.

Institute of Medicine (IOM). (2003). *Health professions education: A bridge to quality.* Washington, DC: National Academies Press.

Lincoln, Y., & Guba, E. (1985). *Naturalistic inquiry.* New York, NY: Sage.

National Research Council of the National Academies. (2005). *Advancing the nation's health needs: NIH research training programs.* Washington, DC: National Academies Press.

CRITICAL THINKING QUESTIONS

1. Please address factors that may contribute to role ambiguity and role stress.
2. Discuss how job fit is a key factor in organizational engagement.
3. Discuss the multiple competing roles of the DNP graduate.
4. Discuss the role strain experienced by the doctoral advanced practice nurse (DAPRN).
5. Discuss the role strain experienced by the DNP executive.
6. Discuss the role strain experienced by the DNP educator.
7. Discuss the role strain experienced by the DNP clinical scientist.
8. How can the results of this study, "The Experiences of DNPs in Their Current Professional Positions," assist new DNP graduates in acclimating to their new roles? What can the profession learn from the informants' experiences?
9. How can DNP graduates differentiate themselves from MSN graduates in their roles?
10. How will health care reform and other market forces impact the role of the DNP-prepared nurse in his/her respective roles?

CHAPTER ELEVEN

Career Development Strategies to Support Nurses Engaged in Doctoral Advanced Nursing Practice

Understanding Trends and Mining Opportunities

Mary Ellen Smith Glasgow and Gloria F. Donnelly

INTRODUCTION

It is the year 2020! Bob Anderson and Jacqui Nolan have just earned Doctor of Nursing Practice degrees concentrating in Family Practice. Bob passed the certification examination for family nurse practitioner (NP) and applied for licensure as an advanced practice nurse in Montana where nursing regulation enables NPs to practice independently of physicians. Jacqui decided to remain in Pennsylvania where she joined a physician-owned Family Practice Group in the suburbs. Scope of practice for NPs in Pennsylvania was expanded in 2008; however, physician collaboration is required for diagnosis, treatment and prescription. Jacqui looks forward to someday being a partner owner in her current practice or moving to rural Pennsylvania to practice independently if regulation changes. The 2010 Health Care Reform legislation has created so many career opportunities for advanced practice nurses, especially doctoral advanced practice nurses. Choosing one's path involves both analysis and skill.

DNP: ADVANCED PRACTICE EVOLVING

In 2009, the *Advance for Nurse Practitioners* biennial national survey of NPs reported the following "typical" profile: a 47-year-old, master's-prepared, family NP with an average of 9 years of experience, working full-time in a family practice or hospital setting and reporting to a physician (Rollet, 2009). This same survey reported that overall average salaries for all NPs, both masters and doctorally prepared, rose from an average of $81,397 in 2007 to $89,597 in 2009. Further, NPs with DNPs had a median salary of $95,000 in 2009 compared with $84,786 in 2007, and all types of NPs who own their own practices had a median salary of $100,000 in 2009 compared to $89,634 in 2007 (Rollet, pp. 26 & 30).

Fast forward to 2020—with the proliferation of Doctor of Nursing Practice programs, since their inception mostly in 2005, the typical profile of the Advanced Practice nurse is likely to evolve to a younger, doctorally prepared NP working full-time in a nurse-managed health center, a convenient care center, or a hospital setting. In some of the more conservative states, the DNP will still need a collaborating agreement with a physician. However, more physicians will have come to the realization that DNPs not only provide high-quality care, but also add economic stability and advantage to a practice. In states where there is great demand for primary care services, DNPs will own their own primary care practices, their own convenient care centers, and will increasingly manage the health issues of a growing geriatric population. After nearly 50 years since the inception of the NP role, the perfect storm is gathering to drive the career trajectory of DNPs as independent practitioners, valued collaborators and innovators in health care delivery.

THE PERFECT STORM

While academics endlessly debate the structure and function of DNP programs and others idly deliberate whether or not DNPs should be called "doctor," market forces and changing legislation regulating NP practices across the United States are aligning to create the perfect storm of career opportunities for advanced practice nurses, particularly those with DNPs. This perfect storm is displayed in Figure 11.1.

First, the U.S. population is aging rapidly. Seventy-eight million boomers, born between 1946 and 1964, will increasingly demand age-related health care services (Lloyd, 2009). The most rapidly growing segment of the U.S. population is the group over 85, adding even more burden to the demand for elder care, particularly for chronic illnesses.

Second, the number of new physicians selecting primary care as a career has dropped dramatically since 1997, a 51.8% decrease as reported by the American Academy of Family Physicians. Further, newly graduated physicians, ridden with debt, are choosing higher paying specialties instead of the long hours and low reimbursement associated with family practice. Advanced practice nurses are increasingly filling the gap created by the dearth of family physicians (Johnson, 2010).

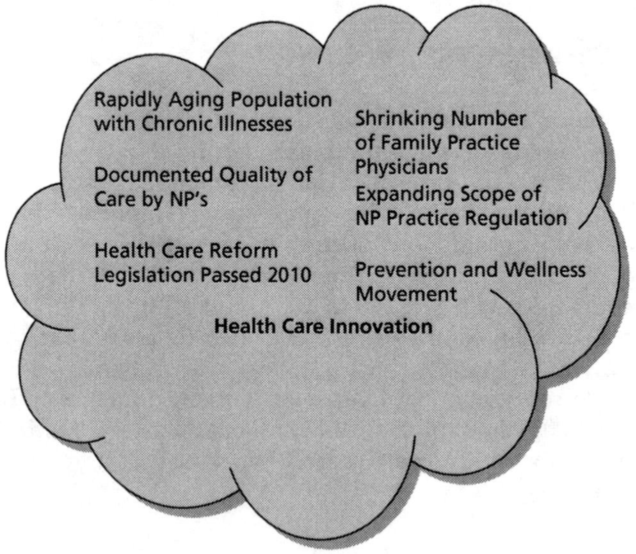

Rapidly Aging Population with Chronic Illnesses

Shrinking Number of Family Practice Physicians

Documented Quality of Care by NP's

Expanding Scope of NP Practice Regulation

Health Care Reform Legislation Passed 2010

Prevention and Wellness Movement

Health Care Innovation

FIGURE 11.1
The perfect storm: Factors driving career opportunities for DNPs.

Third, the quality of care delivered by NPs in the United States is firmly established. Studies over the last two decades have repeatedly demonstrated no difference in quality of care or patient outcomes between primary care physicians and NPs (Mundinger et al., 2000; Pearson, 2010).

Fourth, The Pearson Report (2010) documents a continuous expansion of the scope of practice for advanced practice nurses in the United States, particularly NPs and, in some states, Clinical Nurse Specialists. For example, by mid-2010, there were 44 states in which it was legal for NPs holding DNPs to be addressed as "Dr." There were 22 states in which the NP could diagnose and treat conditions without physician involvement, and 16 states in which NPs could prescribe with no physician involvement.

Fifth, health care reform legislation passed on March 21, 2010 the Patient Protection and Affordable Care Act (HR 3590, P.L. 111–148), which requires that in the future all U.S. citizens carry health insurance. This translates into more than 30 million previously uninsured individuals seeking primary and other forms of care.

Sixth, there is a growing, formalized movement focusing on the prevention of illness, wellness maintenance, and enhancement. The recently passed health care reform legislation will create a National Prevention, Health Promotion, and Public Health Council that will coordinate prevention policy and practices at the federal level. Christensen, Grossman, and Hwang (2008) have developed a model of chronic illness care in which they categorize chronic illnesses along three continua: chronic diseases with either immediate or deferred consequences, chronic diseases whose management is dependent on medical technology to varying degrees, and chronic diseases whose management is dependent on behavioral change. They also factor into their model rule-based chronic illnesses where there is a deep evidence base for management, such as diabetes, obesity, and depression. NPs and DNPs with a deepened knowledge and skill base can effectively manage behavioral-dependent illnesses, which may contribute to the evidence on best practices. Many nurse managed health centers in the nation are already using Christensen's et al. (2008) recommended approach and have been recognized for their efforts to infuse behavioral health, wellness programs, and complementary and integrative therapies into traditional medical primary care. This assists patients in making those behavioral changes that will improve health and wellness (Donnelly, 2009).

Seventh, innovation in health care will continue to proliferate as health care reform takes hold. Advanced practice nurses are involved in the proliferation of not only urban and rural nurse managed health centers for the medically underserved, but also in convenient care clinics, health coaching services and new approaches to delivering primary care to the homebound or institutionalized elderly. Future DNP graduates will need to understand the concept of "disruptive innovation" in order to effectively mine career opportunities.

THE DNP: DISRUPTIVE INNOVATION RECONSIDERED

In the 1990s, Christensen (1997) described a business phenomenon called "disruptive innovation," a product or service that enters a market at the low end, is more cost effective than the current, dominant product or service and eventually, through consumer satisfaction and demand, dominates the market. The prediction was that NPs, sometimes referred to as mid-level practitioners, would eventually become the disruptive innovation that dominates the health care market in the delivery of primary and chronic care services. The 2010 passage of the national health care reform bill and the proliferation of DNP programs are likely to accelerate Christensen's prediction. Nurse-managed health centers will grow in number, given their outstanding record in providing quality, cost-effective, community-based care. Tine Hansen-Turton, MGA, JD, CEO of the National Nursing Centers Consortium foresees opportunity for advanced practice nurses to fill the growing need by primary care providers, particularly physicians. Hansen-Turton asserts,

> The current shortage of primary care physicians is likely to increase during the next twenty years, resulting in a shortage of as many as 44,000 physicians in the fields of general internal medicine and family medicine by the year 2025.
> —*Hansen-Turton, Philadelphia Health Management Corporation, March 25, 2010*

Convenient care centers, also considered a disruptive innovation in health care, will continue to multiply across the United States as more and more individuals seek rapid, low-cost intervention care for nonemergent conditions. Evidence of the trend of more widespread use of convenient care clinics is demonstrated in numerous health care articles published since 2006, when the first wave of retail clinics was established. The Deloitte report projects exponential growth for this industry through the year 2014, with close to 3,200 convenient care clinics operating across the United States, as compared with 1,200 at present (Keckley, 2009).

It is likely that DNPs with an entrepreneurial bent will design, capitalize, and own a variety of health services and companies. Primary and convenient care are but two of the many areas in which the DNP can develop a career trajectory in addition to the more traditional roles of nurse educator and nurse administrator. Career planning strategies should be an integral part of the DNP's preparation to identify trends, mine opportunities, and make decisions about the best role and environment fit for one's career.

PERSONAL READINESS STRATEGIES IN PLANNING A CAREER TRAJECTORY

> *To achieve all that is possible, we must attempt the impossible . . . to be as much as we can be, we must dream of being more.*
> —*Gale Baker Stanton*

Case I: A DNP Graduate Goes into Academia

Maura McNamara, DNP, CRNP is a seasoned Family Nurse Practitioner who recently graduated from a Doctor of Nursing Practice Program (DNP) from a local college. Dr. McNamara has spent most of her career working in an emergency room in a busy academic health center, both as a staff nurse and NP. More recently, she has held a joint appointment at the university teaching Health Assessment and overseeing the management of the Student Wellness Center. Upon graduation from her DNP Program, she accepted a position as a Director of a DNP Program at the university where she is employed. Dr. McNamara has strong administrative, organizational, and clinical skills. However, she lacks knowledge of curriculum development, evaluation, and the academic culture. During her first year of serving in an academic administrator role, Dr. McNamara has struggled in her new role. Perceived by faculty as overly confident and directive, Dr. McNamara is perceived as a delegator with limited knowledge in NP education. In working with Dr. McNamara to be successful in her new role and plan a realistic, productive career, it is suggested that she would benefit from a variety of internal and external assessments, mentoring from a senior academic administrator, networking experiences with fellow DNP department chairs/directors, and leadership coaching and education.

As a Doctor of Nursing Practice (DNP) graduate, one needs to prepare for his/her first position as a DNP in addition to thinking about one's professional long-term career trajectory. The first step is one of critical self-reflection both in terms of oneself and one's practice. Critical examination of the role that one aspires to fulfill is essential in order to determine if one has the requisite knowledge and skills to fulfill the role. In terms of oneself, it is necessary to obtain the feedback of trusted colleagues related to one's strengths, weaknesses, professional persona, and learning needs. It is equally important to be open to the feedback no matter how difficult it may be to hear, and to seek advice from other trusted colleagues to confirm or refute findings. External assessments, such as the Myers–Briggs Trait Inventory (MBTI), 360-degree feedback assessment, and the FIRO-B Interpretive Report for Organizations can also prove helpful in gaining insight into one's leadership traits, assets, and needs (Lombardo & Eichinger, 2009; Myers & Myers, 1995; Pfau & Kay, 2002; Schnell & Hammer, 1997). These tools are designed to collect information related to personality preferences, colleagues' perceptions of the DNP's leadership skills, and interpersonal needs. The discussion of the MBTI, 360-degree feedback, and FIRO-B Interpretive Report for Organizations is mentioned briefly in this chapter to introduce the reader to relevant instruments that can assist a DNP graduate in his/her career trajectory.

The MBTI provides the DNP with a report of his/her personality preferences. The Myers–Briggs Type Indicator (MBTI) assessment is a psychometric questionnaire designed to measure psychological preferences in how people perceive the world and make decisions (Myers & Myers, 1995). The 360-degree feedback, also known as multirater feedback, multisource feedback, or multisource assessment, is feedback that comes from all around an individual. Here, "360" refers to the 360 degrees in a circle, with an individual figuratively in the center of the circle. Subordinates, peers, and supervisors provide feedback. It also includes a self-assessment and, in some cases, feedback from external sources such as other interested stakeholders. The results from 360-degree feedback are often used by the person receiving the feedback to plan career training and development. Results are also used by some organizations in making administrative decisions, such as pay or promotion (Pfau & Kay, 2002). The 360-degree feedback can provide the DNP graduate with insight as to how others view him/her in terms of personal leadership operating style, competence, communication effectiveness, ethics, and other qualities. The FIRO-B Interpretive Report for Organizations provide insight into one's own interpersonal needs that can assist the DNP graduate in evaluating career opportunities, whether the individual is seeking a new career or seeking to improve his/her satisfaction with a current position. The DNP graduate can evaluate an opportunity by considering how well it matches with his/her interpersonal needs. For example, if the DNP graduate has a high need for inclusion, he/she may wish to seek an organization that values teamwork and a position that provides a lot of opportunities to interact with others. In understanding his/her interpersonal needs, the DNP graduate can seek a position that is a "good fit" for his/her organization (Lombardo & Eichinger, 2009).

Although Dr. McNamara has been employed by the university and academic health center, she was not enmeshed in the academic culture. Her role as Director of the Student Wellness Center did not intersect with the faculty directly and did not entail any involvement in any curricular or faculty department meetings. Quite frankly, Dr. McNamara was not aware of what she did and did not know related to curricular knowledge as well as academic practices and culture. Although her background is certainly not ideal for an academic leadership role, Dr. McNamara does have some of the leadership qualities essential for a Director of Doctor of Nursing Practice Program. She has a strong clinical background and has solid administrative skills. In addition, Dr. McNamara has a keen sense of operations and logistics. Dr. McNamara needs to work with a mentor or executive coach to leverage her strengths and develop a plan to gain knowledge related to teaching, curriculum, evaluation, and academic culture. She also needs to share her expertise with faculty, immerse herself in DNP education via formal and informal learning, and role model other effective academic leaders.

It is wise for the new DNP graduate to secure a mentor to learn the political landscape of advanced practice nursing, expand his/her network, gain professional insights, and foster his/her personal and professional growth. Grossman and Valiga (2005) define a mentor as an individual who provides support and guidance during times of stress while assisting in the development and enhancement of professional skills. The mentoring relationship is generally consultative and constructive in nature (Sauter & Applegate, 2005). The DNP will particularly need consultation in navigating the workplace. The Doctor of Nursing Practice Degree (DNP) is a relatively new degree; therefore, the role for the Doctoral Advanced Practice Nurse is not yet clearly defined in many settings. As a result, these pioneers, new doctoral advanced practice nurses, may experience role stress in their new position. The "newness" of the doctoral advanced practice role may place additional stress on the DNP graduate, thus necessitating the need for additional mentoring and support. It may be challenging for the novice DNP to acquire a DNP-prepared mentor with significant knowledge and experience with respect to the same role. Alternatively, the DNP graduate can find a doctorally prepared mentor who is connected to his/her respective new role, whether it is in the education, practice, or executive arenas, and who also possesses the following key attributes. These fundamental attributes include:

- Knowledgeable about the role
- Willing to invest in mentee
- Willingness to give feedback
- Strong networking capabilities
- Ability to motivate
- Integrity
- Respectful and respected
- Professional demeanor

A mentor should invest a great deal of time and effort into the advancement of the mentor–mentee relationship. The mentor–mentee relationship should also be conscious, purposeful, and authentic (Grossman & Valiga, 2005).

Case II: A DNP Graduate Remains in Practice

Robin Johnson DNP, CRNP is a skilled acute care NP in a large cardiology practice in an academic health center. Upon completion of her DNP degree, Dr. Johnson assumes an administrative position overseeing the other NPs in the practice, many of whom who are masters'-prepared. Dr. ("Robin") Johnson also struggles in her new role, but for different reasons. The attending physicians make it very clear that she is not to refer to herself as "Dr. Johnson" as to not to confuse patients in thinking that she is a physician. Dr. Johnson did not intend to represent herself as a physician, but rather as a doctorally prepared NP. Her colleagues call her "Dr. Robin" in a joking manner, but Robin senses that there is some malice behind the smiles. When assuming a leadership role, she notes that she is getting much more "push back" from her former colleagues when she establishes the call schedule, attempts to establish a journal club, or involve the NPs in a clinical research project. Dr. Johnson tends to be reserved and uncomfortable with conflict. Given her personality preferences and current work issues, Dr. Johnson is questioning her own ability to serve as the Lead Nurse Practitioner in the practice. It would benefit Dr. Johnson to conduct an in-depth assessment of her leadership qualities as well as her "fit" with the organization. Although it is probably too early to obtain a 360-degree feedback assessment from her supervisor, colleagues, and subordinates, it would be appropriate to obtain a MBTI and FIRO-B Interpretive Report at this juncture. These assessments could assist Dr. Johnson with insight into her psychological preferences in how she perceives the world and makes decisions, as well as provide a perspective into her own interpersonal needs and "fit" with the organization. An executive coach can assist Dr. Johnson in interpreting these reports, provide feedback to improve Dr. Johnson's confidence, and raise her leadership consciousness. As a DNP and administrator, Dr. Johnson may also feel isolated and need to network with other DNP practitioners via list serves and professional organizations to seek professional support. Fellow doctoral-level nurses and professional organizations can provide an opportunity to promote the position of doctoral-level nurses in clinical practice settings, thereby fostering the development of the doctoral-level nurses in addition to integrating practice, research, and education. Professional networks for doctoral-level nurses will promote opportunities for doctoral-level nurses to conduct research and disseminate research findings to the public, clinicians, educators, and policy makers (Berlin & Sechrist, 2002; Hinshaw, 2001). Further, professional networks can be extremely valuable to a new DNP graduate who is attempting to launch his/her career post-professional doctorate. A mentoring relationship with a well-respected clinically connected, doctoral-level practitioner is strongly suggested to direct the new DNP graduate in his/her career trajectory. If the DNP graduate does not have access to an appropriate mentor, involvement in professional networks and organizations is highly recommended to seek doctoral-level practitioners with similar abilities and interests.

A proactive leadership assessment and support plan is critical to the DNP graduate's success. Transitioning from master's-level practitioner to doctoral-level practitioner is quite challenging for this doctoral-level practitioner, as she now has new knowledge and increased intellectual curiosity in a practice setting that has not changed. In her DNP Program, Dr. Johnson was taught to think creatively, strategically, and to challenge and question practice. She desires to be the conduit to change practice and improve patient outcomes (Dreher & Montgomery, 2009). In working with Dr. Johnson to be successful in her new role and plan a realistic, productive career, it is suggested that Dr. Johnson would benefit from a variety of internal and external assessments, mentoring from a senior doctoral-level practitioner serving in a comparable role, networking experiences with fellow DNP practitioners/administrators in the clinical setting, leadership coaching, and continuing professional education. Dr. Johnson is establishing herself as a DNP lead practitioner. It is important for Dr. Johnson and Doctor of Nursing (DNP) graduates to truly see themselves as future leaders and to understand the difference between their unique personality preferences and the role requirements of a leader. For example, Dr. Johnson's personality preference may be avoidance of conflict, but in her role as a leader she is required to hold people accountable for clinical outcomes. The goal is to support Dr. Johnson in her doctoral advanced nursing practice role and to also communicate that there are visual, vocal (pitch, tone, pace), and verbal cues of leadership and that these affect one's credibility as a leader. In leadership, the role responsibilities must overshadow personality preferences when there is a difference between personal preference and role expectations. Dr. Johnson has the capacity to effect change; however, she needs to first *see herself as leader* in order to have others see her as a leader.

Throughout the career development journey, the DNP graduate needs to bear in mind that he/she should not fall into the trap of becoming self-important or arrogant. He or she is a servant leader and not a self-serving leader. As a servant leader, the DNP graduate devotes him/herself to serving the needs of organization, focuses on meeting the needs of those he/she leads, develops and facilitates the growth of his/her staff, and listens and builds a sense of community (Blanchard & Hodges, 2003).

The key to success, and this is not world shattering, is to embark on a career based on one's passion. In order to find one's passion, the DNP graduate needs to reflect on what he/she enjoys as well as his/her capabilities. This endeavor will take time, research, some trial and error, and soul-searching. After identifying the ideal career based on one's passion, the DNP graduate needs to establish his/her personal brand or professional reputation (Lair, Sullivan, & Cheney, 2005). Although it seems rather simplistic, building and maintaining a solid professional reputation requires authenticity and vigilance. Does the DNP graduate have a strong work ethic, treat all individuals respectfully, act ethically, have a professional image, and possess the requisite knowledge and skills? Marketing oneself as a DNP graduate is the first step in establishing a personal brand. During this effort, the DNP graduate needs to articulate the new, enhanced knowledge and skill set of the doctoral advanced practice nurse and the value of doctoral education (Dreher & Montgomery, 2009). The major new skill sets would include:

1. Integrate nursing science with knowledge from other disciplines as the basis for the highest level of nursing practice;
2. Use science-based theories and concepts to determine the nature and significance of health and health care delivery phenomena;
3. Describe the actions and advanced strategies to enhance, alleviate, and ameliorate health and health care delivery phenomena as appropriate; and evaluate outcomes;
4. Develop and evaluate new practice approaches/models based on nursing theories and theories from other disciplines; and
5. Design, select, use, and evaluate programs that evaluate and monitor outcomes of care, care systems, and quality improvement, including consumer use of health care information systems (AACN, 2006).

Doctoral education that blends integrative nursing roles, leadership, and research skills will position advanced practice nurses to answer the needs and challenges facing the health care system (Draye, Acker, & Zimmer, 2006). As the DNP graduate seeks his/her first position post-DNP, he or she needs to consider the organizational philosophy, job/position description, salary and benefits (both compensated and uncompensated), advancement potential, and unit/organizational culture.

PUTTING IT ALL TOGETHER: FINAL SUGGESTIONS

The DNP graduate should not only prepare one's career for today's health care environment, but also for the health care system of the future. Examining the health care and political landscape for trends and opportunities and preparing oneself in the best way to operate and work in it effectively is vital for success. It is essential that the DNP graduate create an "action plan" to develop him/herself. There are many measurable characteristics related to one's success at work, ranging from intelligence, optimism, work ethic and positive boss relationships. These competencies can be grouped into six areas: (1) strategic skills; (2) operating skills; (3) courage; (4) energy and drive; (5) organizational and positioning skills; and (6) personal and interpersonal skills. Through a reflective and comprehensive assessment processes, the DNP graduate can recognize personal limitations and development opportunities. The DNP also needs to determine if the skill that he/she needs to acquire or strengthen is critical for his/her position for today or tomorrow (Lombardo & Eichinger, 2009). At the same time, the DNP graduate needs to be cognizant of career stallers and stoppers. These deficiencies are grouped into two areas: (1) *trouble with people* (does not relate well to others, self-centered, does not inspire or build talent) and (2) *trouble with results* (too narrow or does not deliver results). In creating a development plan, the DNP graduate should determine what is critically important for his/her position. He or she should obtain detailed behavioral feedback on his/her developmental needs and create an "action plan" as to what to stop doing, keep doing, and start doing. The DNP graduate should also search for individuals who are strong in the particular skill that he/she needs to acquire. It is important to remember that rarely does one mentor embody every skill that the mentee wishes to acquire. It is important, therefore, for the DNP graduate to seek out multiple individuals and sources (e.g., books, courses, and people) from which to learn and develop. As one acquires more knowledge, he or she should "stretch" him/herself by assuming responsibilities that will build this particular skill. It is important to set goals, track progress, and obtain feedback on one's skill building plan. For example, if the DNP graduate appears insensitive (distant, and aloof), he or she may make a concerted effort to disclose some personal information about him/herself to connect with employees as a "person" and offer to coach or mentor new staff or faculty. He or she should ask for feedback from others as to how he/she is perceived. A powerful resource for the DNP graduate's professional career development is: *FYI: For Your Improvement, A Guide for Development and Coaching* (Lombardo & Eichinger, 2009), which will serve to provide real-life examples, remedies, and assignments to assist with one's developmental needs.

SUMMARY

In terms of career progression, the DNP graduate needs to be open to career possibilities and seek career advancement opportunities with his/her strengths and weaknesses in mind. Seeking the support of trusted colleagues and mentors about the next steps in one's career trajectory is critical. The DNP graduate needs to have credibility in his/her new role and, therefore, needs to possess the requisite knowledge and skills for each new position. Balancing ambition and caution is necessary so that the DNP graduate does not advance too quickly, as there is a risk the DNP graduate may not have the necessary job requirements or the right credibility. Conversely, one should also be wary of advancing too slowly, and thus missing career opportunities.

> There are risks and costs to a program of action. But they are far less than the long-range risks and costs of comfortable inaction.
>
> —*John F. Kennedy*

REFERENCES

American Association of Colleges of Nursing (AACN). (2006). *The essentials of doctoral education for advanced nursing practice*. Retrieved from www.aacn.nche.edu/DNP/pdf/Essentials.pdf

Berlin, L. E., & Sechrist, K. R. (2002). The shortage of doctorally prepared nursing faculty: A dire situation. *Nursing Outlook, 50*(2), 50–56.

Blanchard, K., & Hodges, P. (2003). *The servant leader: Transforming your heart, head, hands, & habits*. Nashville, TN: Thomas Nelson Inc.

Christensen, C. M. (1997). *The innovator's dilemma: When new technologies cause great firms to fail*. Cambridge, MA: Harvard Business School Press.

Christensen, C. M., Grossman, J. H., & Hwang, J. (2008). *The innovator's prescription: A disruptive solution for health care*. New York, NY: McGraw-Hill.

Donnelly, G. (2009). Needs-based care for a community: Innovation or common sense. *Holistic Nursing Practice, 23*(3), 127.

Draye, M. A., Acker, M., & Zimmer, P. A. (2006). The practice doctorate in nursing: Approaches to transform nurse practitioner education and practice. *Nursing Outlook, 54*, 123–129.

Dreher, H. M., & Montgomery, K. A. (2009). Let's call it "doctoral" advanced practice nursing. *Journal of Continuing Education in Nursing, 40*(12), 530–531.

Grossman, S. C., & Valiga, T. M. (2005). *The new leadership challenge: Creating the future of nursing*. Philadelphia, PA: F. A. Davis.

Hinshaw, A. S. (2001). A continuing challenge: The shortage of educationally prepared nursing faculty. *Online Journal of Issues in Nursing, 6*(1), Manuscript 3. Retrieved from wwww.nursing-world.org/ojin/topic14/tpc14_3.htm

Johnson, C. K. (2010, April 16). Facing doctor shortage, 28 states may expand nurses' role. *USA Today*. Retrieved from www.usatoday.com/news/health/2010-04-16-nurse-doctors_N.htm

Keckley, P. (2009). *Survey of health care consumers: Deloitte Center for Health Solutions*. Retrieved from http://www.deloitte.com/view/en_US/us/Insights/centers/center-for-health-solutions/5735e23a4b101210VgnVCM100000ba42f00aRCRD.htm

Lair, D. J., Sullivan, K., & Cheney, G. (2005). Marketization and the recasting of the professional self. *Management Communication Quarterly, 18*(3), 307–343.

Lloyd, J. (2009, August 8). Doctor shortage looms as primary care loses its pull. *USA Today*. Retrieved from www.usatoday.com/news/health/2009-08-17-doctor-gp-shortage.htm

Lombardo, M. M., & Eichinger, R. W. (2009). *FYI for your improvement: A guide for development and coaching* (5th ed.). Minneapolis, MN: Lominger International: A. Korn/Ferry Company.

Myers, I. B., & Myers, P. B. (1995). *Gifts differing: Understanding personality type*. Mountain View, CA: Davies-Black Publishing.

Pfau, B., & Kay, I. (2002). Does 360-degree feedback negatively affect company performance? Studies show that 360-degree feedback may do more harm than good. What's the problem? *HRMagazine, 47*(6), 54–60.

Philadelphia Health Management Corporation. (2010, March 25). Health care reform package includes unprecedented investment in nurse-led health clinics. PR Newswire. Retrieved from http://www.prnewswire.com/news-releases/health-care-reform-package-includes-unprecedented-investment-in-nurse-led-health-clinics-89122187.html

Rollet, J. (2009). National salary and workplace survey: Good news in troubled economy. *Advance for Nurse Practitioners*. Retrieved from www.advanceweb.com/np

Sauter, M. K., & Applegate, M. H. (2005). Educational program evaluation. In D. Billings, & J. Halstead (Eds.), *Teaching in nursing: A guide for faculty* (pp. 543–599). St. Louis, MO: Elsevier.

Schnell, E., & Hammer, A. (1997). Integrating the FIRO-B with the MBTI: Relationships, case examples, and interpretation strategies. *Developing Leaders*. Palo Alto, CA: Davies-Black Publishing.

CHAPTER ELEVEN: Reflective Response

Sister Rosemary Donley

In this chapter, experienced nurse educators Smith Glasgow and Donnelly explore how newly prepared doctors of nursing practice (DNPs) will fit into nursing's hierarchy. The discussion is timely because this question is on the minds of physicians, the American Medical Association, the leaders of academic nursing, nurse executives, credentialing agencies, the State Boards of Nurse Examiners, and rank and file nurses, not to mention patients, and the newly minted DNPs themselves. The questions to be answered over time are: what will doctorally prepared advanced practice nurses do; where will they be employed; how will they be identified, recognized and rewarded in their first jobs and in their future careers; and, most importantly, what difference will they make in the health status of people and the cost of care?

Nursing has a mixed history of success in changing titles, roles, and educational requirements of professional nurses. What we know from studying a classic failure to assure that the title professional nurse was reserved for nurses with baccalaureate preparation may provide clues to predicting the future of men and women who hold the Doctorate in Nursing Practice degree (Donley & Flaherty, 2002). Smith Glasgow and Donnelly identify in their chapter many factors in the contemporary environment that will influence the employability and the acceptance of DNPs. One factor that is not thoroughly discussed by the authors is the growing competition among other health professionals to play more aggressive and expanded roles in the delivery of primary care. This group includes not only old rivals, physician assistants, but also new kids on the primary care block: pharmacists, social workers, and physical therapists. Many of these practitioners hold doctoral degrees, have command over a body of knowledge and a skill set, are recognized in the health care delivery system, and use the title "doctor" in their practices. Physicians seem not to be that interested in pursuing careers in primary care; osteopaths and dentists seem to track the career pathways of their medical colleagues (Lakhan & Laird, 2009). Some members of the allied health professions also own and manage their own businesses, providing direct health care services to the public. If the number of physicians remains relatively constant and they continue to prefer the specialized practice of medicine, will there be a sufficient number of DNPs to meet the needs of aging Americans and the new recipients of federal health care reform, some 30 million Americans who will have access to some form of heath care insurance? Will other members of the health professions compete with doctorally prepared advanced practice nurses to control primary care delivery? Is nursing and the DNP community ready for this competition?

Some 45 years after the American Nurses Association released its famous "Position Paper," the educational confusion in nursing still exists. One force that worked against the realization of the goals of the Position Paper was the number of nurses who had been educated in diploma programs of nursing. They, their teachers, and their employers were not willing to say that they were not professional nurses. With the rapid development of the associate degree (AD) educational movement, the number of supporters of AD and diploma nursing drowned out the voices of those who promoted baccalaureate education as the only pathway for entry into nursing practice (Donley & Flaherty, 2002). The professional landscape of 2010 is remarkably similar (Donley & Flaherty, 2008). There are approximately 250,527 advanced practice nurses. The majority of these nurses are masters-prepared NPs, nurse anesthetists, nurse midwives, and clinical nurse specialists (DHHS, 2010). If the American Association of Colleges of Nursing's (2004) timetable is to be achieved, only nurses with a new DNP degree will be able to call themselves advanced practice nurses after 2015. What will be the response of these men and women who were pioneers in the advanced practice role?

Then there is the question of employment and salary of nurses engaged in doctoral advanced nursing practice. In 1965, a significant obstacle to the achievement of the ANA Committee on Nursing Education's goals was the stance of American hospitals, the major employer, then and now, of nurses (DHHS, 2010). In most institutional settings, a staff nurse is/was a staff nurse. Historically, nurses have not been rewarded financially for earning baccalaureate degrees and continuing to engage in direct patient care, although they may be more eligible for promotion and job mobility. Smith Glasgow and Donnelly devote a significant portion of their article to the importance of DNPs engaging in planning their career development, emphasizing the importance of finding and consulting with mentors. To support this recommendation, they present case studies and discuss how the new DNP may not be prepared for the role of faculty member or ready to assume the directorship of a clinical practice or an educational program. While young physicians often begin their residencies with few marketable skills, on the job training from nurses, other physicians, and residents soon prepares them for increasing responsibility and leadership. Young physicians who join practices are helped to be successful by their future partners and the office staff. However, assuring the success of new DNPs may take more than career planning and mentoring, as supports available for physicians have not traditionally been available to nursing's new graduates. There is no evidence that DNP graduates will be welcomed and helped to succeed in either the academic or clinical practice environments by medical colleagues or other nurses. The not-so-silent message of Smith Glasgow and Donnelly is sobering. Failure of the DNP experiment will be a failure for nursing and will limit clinical choice for the American public.

REFERENCES

American Association of Colleges of Nursing (AACN). (2004). *AACN position statement on the practice doctorate in nursing October 2004*. Retrieved from http://www.aacn.nche.edu/DNP/pdf/DNP.pdf

Department of Health and Human Services (DHHS). (2010). *Registered nurse population: Initial findings from the 2008 National Sample Survey of Registered Nurses*. Washington, DC: DHHS.

Donley, R., & Flaherty, M. J. (2002). Revisiting the ANA first position on education for nurses. *Online Journal of Issues in Nursing, 7*(2). Retrieved from http://www.nursingworld.org/MainMenuCategories/ANAMarketplace/ANAPeriodicals/OJIN/TableofContents/Volume72002/No2May2002/RevisingPostiononEducation.aspx

Donley, R., & Flaherty, M. J. (2008). Revisiting the ANA First Position on Education for Nurses: A comparative analysis of the first and second position statements on the education of nurses. *Online Journal of Issues in Nursing, 13*(2). Retrieved from http://www.nursingworld.org/MainMenuCategories/ANAMarketplace/ANAPeriodicals/OJIN/TableofContents/vol132008/No2May08/ArticlePreviousTopic/EntryIntoPracticeUpdate.aspx

Lakhan, S., & Laird, C. (2009). Addressing the primary care physician shortage in an evolving medical workforce. *Internal Archives of Internal Medicine, 2*(14). Doi: 10.1186/1755-7682-2-14. Retrieved from http://www.ncbi.nlm.nih.gov/pmc/articles/PMC2686687/pdf/1755-7682-2-14.pdf

CRITICAL THINKING QUESTIONS

1. Describe the market forces driving career opportunities for DNPs.
2. Discuss how the Doctor of Nursing Practice degree is a disruptive innovation.
3. Please elaborate on health care reform as a disruptive innovation.
4. Please elaborate on new practice arenas for the DNP: (1) urban and rural nurse-managed health centers for the medically underserved; (2) convenient care clinics; (3) health coaching services; (4) and new approaches to delivering primary care to the homebound or institutionalized elderly.
5. What new skills will be required for the DNP to successfully navigate his/her career in the future?
6. What external assessments can the DNP utilize to gain insight into one's leadership traits, assets, and needs?
7. How can a DNP use a mentor or executive coach to leverage his/her strengths and develop a professional development plan?
8. Discuss the benefits of a proactive leadership assessment and support plan for a new DNP graduate.
9. Discuss the role requirements of the DNP graduate in a leadership role.
10. How can the DNP graduate effectively establish his/her personal brand or professional reputation?

CHAPTER TWELVE

Leadership and the DNP-Educated Nurse Executive

Revisiting the AACN's Eight Essential Competencies

Albert Rundio and Linda Scott

INTRODUCTION

Educational preparation for nurse executives has been a debatable issue for decades. As the standards of practice for nurse administrators continue to evolve amidst a rapidly changing, increasingly complex, technologically advanced health system, it is imperative that we end the controversy. The purpose of this chapter is to identify the leadership principles necessary for advanced administrative nursing practice and to advocate for the best curricular model that would prepare individuals to practice effectively in today's health care milieu.

REVISITING OUR PAST

Henry (1989) eloquently described the educational crisis in nursing administration. During the 1960s and 1970s, as health care institutions transformed into complex organizations and business entities, nurse executives were inadequately prepared to enact their roles. As a result, confidence in their effectiveness waned, graduate enrollments decreased, and the number of graduate nursing administration programs declined. The availability of qualified nurse executives continued to decline during subsequent decades. As we entered the 1990s, individuals seeking graduate education began to choose clinical specialty and practitioner programs, rather than programs with a nursing administration emphasis (Haynor & Wells, 1998). Further compounding the problem, nurse executives were replaced by non-nurses in clinical and boardroom settings, often to the detriment of nursing service and clinical practice leadership. Those interested in nursing administrative practice roles sought alternative education preparation in master's programs such as health administration (MHA), business administration (MBA), public administration (MPA), or dual-degree programs (MSN/MHA, MSN/MBA, MSN/MPA) to obtain the competencies required to function in or compete for administrative positions, as well as achieve credibility among their administrative colleagues.

As we fully enter this new millennium, we began to see a resurgence of graduate nursing administration programs. Curricula were revamped to include and standardize content believed to be essential to administrative practice. The Council on Graduate Education for Administration in Nursing (CGEAN) recommended four curricular areas to provide breadth and depth of knowledge for administrative practice: (1) nursing science and social science cognates; (2) nursing administration/management; (3) business administration/public administration/health care administration; and (4) methodology (Dienemann & Aroian, 1995). Likewise, in 1997, building on the American Association of Colleges of Nursing's (AACN) *Essentials of Master's Education for Advanced Practice Nursing* (1996), the American Organization of Nurse Executives (AONE) endorsed 14 core content areas for specialty education in nursing administration:

- Strategic management;
- Organizational development/business planning;
- Leadership;
- Policy development;
- Continuous quality improvement;
- Financial management/cost analysis/microeconomics and macroeconomics;
- Information systems;
- Human resource/outcomes management;
- Managed care and integrated delivery systems;
- Systems analysis;
- Environmental issues;
- Marketing and sales strategies;
- Negotiation strategies; and
- Public health/community-based systems.

While these organizations perceived this identified content as integral to effective administrative practice, it was recognized that a number of factors may hinder the ability to incorporate them in master's programs, including time constraints, resources, practica sites, and faculty expertise.

MASTERS VS. DOCTORAL PREPARATION

The complexity of nursing administrative science begs the question of the level of educational preparation for nurse administrators. Given the need for nurse administrators to practice, lead, and navigate within a fragmented and failing health care system, does master's education prepare them with the required competencies to be effective in their roles? Furthermore, as the standards of practice and competencies for nurse administrators continue to evolve, and their spheres of influence expand (American Nurses Association [ANA], 2009), it is imperative that they have the educational preparation necessary to represent our profession, advocate for nursing practice, and implement advanced administrative interventions that maximize the delivery of quality care, positive health outcomes, and patient/employee safety. In light of this, should we continue to support nursing administration preparation at the masters level? Contrary to members of AONE and CGEAN who believe that it is critical to have nursing administration programs at both the masters and doctorate levels (Herrin, Jones, Krepper, Sherman, & Reineck, 2006), we would argue that it is time to support the Doctor of Nursing Practice (DNP) as the terminal practice degree for nursing administration.

Complicating this issue is the diverse continuum of administrative roles in health care. Is it realistic to think that all nurse administrators (executives and managers) obtain doctoral preparation? According to the ANA (2009), a nurse administrator is "a registered nurse who orchestrates and influences the work of others in a defined environment, most often health care focused, to enhance the shared vision of an organization or institution" (p. 3), and whose broad-level thinking and efforts result in quality, safety, and requisite infrastructures that fulfill the expectations of the nursing profession, consumers, and society at large. Given the depth and breadth of the multifaceted nursing administrative role, it is not surprising that the ANA standard of practice should be that any nurse practicing in a management role needs to have a graduate degree. Furthermore, the ANA strongly recommends a doctoral degree for those with institutional authority or engaged in executive practice (2009). Therefore, we do everyone a disservice when we place individuals in administrative roles who do not have appropriate qualifications.

Sadly, some think that anyone with leadership ability or desire can be a nurse administrator. Likewise, others think that anyone can teach nursing administrative content in nursing curricula. Counter to these beliefs, nursing administration is a unique specialty that synthesizes nursing science, business principles, organizational theory and behavior, and resource management to lead, manage, and design systems of care. To our fortunate delight, nursing administrative practice was included as an advanced specialty practice when AACN endorsed the DNP as the terminal degree for advanced specialty practice in nursing in 2006 (AACN, 2006).

At this pivotal point in health care, it is time to embrace the recognition of administrative practice as an equitable counterpart to the clinical specialties, instead of relegating it to remain at the masters level. Furthermore, the move to DNP programs for nursing administration is congruent with the call to action to have nurses educated at the highest possible level for their practice specialty (Benner, Sutphen, Leonard, & Day, 2010). By doing so, we would be able to offer curricula that prepare individuals to meet the changing demands of society and health care in a reasonable timeframe for doctoral education, to be able to implement evidence-based administrative strategies at all levels of health care (micro, meso, and macro), and to award a degree that has parity with other disciplines.

THE LANDSCAPE FOR THE DNP CURRICULUM AND THE NURSE EXECUTIVE

There has been monumental change in our nation that will affect the future of DNP programs. The economic down turn that began in 2007 and is projected to last through 2010 and beyond has certainly begun the process of changing health care delivery in our nation. Because many Americans do not have health care insurance, the current President of the United States and Congress have just wrestled with a national health care reform plan that will provide many Americans with much needed coverage. The economy has certainly affected how health care services are delivered. Health care organizations have had to focus on the delivery of more cost-efficient care and have had to restructure their delivery systems. Several hospitals have closed across the nation, and it is predicted that many more will follow suit. It was reported from 1990 to 2000, that approximately 500 hospitals closed nationally (Medical Infrastructure, 2010). The Robert Wood Johnson Foundation completed a study of hospitals in 52 mid-sized and large cities and found that nearly 28% of hospital beds were eliminated from 1980 to 1997 (New Jersey Hospital Association, 2008). Viewing New Jersey as a microcosm of the nation from 1992 through 2007, there were 18 hospital closures in the state. Closure applications that were pending from 2007 to 2008 included another three hospitals, and in 2008, five hospitals had filed for bankruptcy (New Jersey Hospital Association, 2008).

As patients enter a hospital primarily for nursing care, nurses with the DNP degree are in a pivotal position to reshape the nation's health. It is clear that health care in the United States must shift from a disease-intervention model to a health-promotion model and no group better than nurses is in position to affect such change. But such reengineering of health care service delivery will take time and significant, yet controversial, reallocation of resources.

According to Chism (2009), the DNP clinical practice-focused doctorate needs to be grounded in clinical practice and demonstrate how research has an impact on practice. Rather than conducting primary research, the practice doctorate translates research into practice with the ultimate goal of achieving improved patient outcomes. There is controversy over this issue, however, as some colleges and universities have primary research as a component in their DNP programs. The most significant question that needs to be raised is the following: If primary research is both a component of the PhD and the DNP, then what is the separating factor of these two degrees (i.e., what makes them different from each other)? Perhaps the major difference in DNP programs with a primary research focus is that the research centers on clinical practice. This debate will no doubt continue into the foreseeable future. Nurse Executives with a DNP are in a pivotal role to effect such change and improvement in care through the reshaping of health care delivery systems. Fitzpatrick and Wallace (2009) state that DNP programs are based on the AACN's 2006 *The Essentials of Doctoral Education for Advanced Practice* (AACN, 2006). The AACN report details eight essentials that DNP programs should have as foundational.

These essentials are:

Essential I: Scientific underpinnings for practice

Essential II: Organizational and systems leadership for quality improvement and systems thinking

Essential III: Clinical scholarship and analytical methods for evidence-based practice

Essential IV: Information systems/technology and patient technology for the improvement and transformation of health care

Essential V: Health care policy for advocacy in health care

Essential VI: Inter professional collaboration for improving patient and population health outcomes

Essential VII: Clinical prevention and population health for improving the nation's health

Essential VIII: Advanced nursing practice

Note: The components of Essential VIII are delineated by national specialty organizations (AACN, 2008; Fitzpatrick & Wallace, 2009).

The question that must be raised is the following: Are the eight essentials outlined by the AACN for the DNP still current in lieu of what is occurring in our nation? When considering the DNP essentials document, one must realize that these were published in 2006 and are thus 5 years old at the time of this writing. This document was based on projections, rather than on factual outcomes. It is important to present both sides of the equation so that individuals can make rational conclusions based on the information at hand. It is also important to mention that initially the DNP essentials were for traditional advanced practice nursing roles only (AACN, 2004a). The nurse executive role evolved into DNP programs after publication of the official October 2004 AACN position statement on the practice doctorate (AACN, 2004b). It is also known that the Collegiate Commission on Nursing Education (CCNE) will not accredit nurse educator tracks in DNP programs as they state "The CCNE Board determined at its April 10–12, 2008 meeting that DNP programs with a nursing education track (major) will *not* be eligible to pursue accreditation . . ." (AACN, 2009, p. 1). One then must question why are nurse executive tracks accredited and nurse educator tracks excluded? Thus, should consideration of all types of nursing practice (e.g., clinician, educator, executive, and researcher) be included in DNP educational programs? Is nursing again "mudding the water," so to speak, by including some forms of practice and not others? Again, these issues will be debated for some time to come. Some educators agree with the CCNE position, and others do not.

There is no question that some of the essentials for the DNP Nurse Executive Track are current, as they are broad enough in scope and take a global perspective of what is and what might be. For example, in Essential I, scientific underpinnings must be the foundation and basis of any doctoral-level program. Work at the DNP level must be as scholarly as any at the PhD level. The primary difference between the degrees is that of primary research (PhD) and the translation of research into practice (DNP). Related to this, Essential III is also necessary as the work of the DNP must include clinical scholarship as well as analytic methods in order to evaluate and improve the nation's health. Essential II and IV also are closely related. Nurse Executives must be in a position to evaluate and change, where necessary, organization-wide systems in an effort to improve the quality of care that is delivered. As defined in Essential IV, information systems/patient care technology can have a profound effect on changing a system that delivers improved quality of care. For example, a patient was recently admitted to a community hospital for intravenous therapy for antibiotic administration for a resistant *Staphylococcus* infection. The patient was placed on an IV pump. The pump had to be programmed and contained all of the antibiotics utilized by the hospital's pharmacy. The menu in the pump included not only the medication, but also the amount and type of solution the medication was mixed in, as well as what time period the antibiotic was to be infused. The IV pump was positioned at a remote location in the patient's room, and once turned on and programmed, was also monitored simultaneously by the pharmacist located in the hospital's pharmacy while the patient's IV drip was running. This provided a double-check system for patient safety.

Another example would be a computer system that incorporates bar coding for medication administration. With a wand device the patient's identification bracelet is scanned prior to the nurse's selecting and administering a medication. The medication that the nurse is going to administer is also scanned. If the medication is not the correct medication, the computer alarms alert the nurse that she/he has selected the incorrect medication for that patient. This is another excellent example of how informatics can change a system for the improvement of patient care and safety. Nurses who work with such technology feel much safer with their practice, as there is a check and balance to the human component where errors can occur so frequently. The nurse executive needs to ensure that such technology is incorporated into practice, so that patient safety and improved patient outcomes are the net result.

Essential V, which centers on health care policy, is still necessary and vital to the reformation of any health care delivery system. Nursing has the largest number of care providers compared to other health care professions. For example, in the year 2000, there were 2,201,800 registered nurses compared to 782,200 physicians (Health Research Services Administration, n.d.). As a result, nursing could be a strong political voice at the national level. The major problem is that nurses do not unite as one voice. As a united force, nurses could drastically change health care in our nation. Schools and colleges of nursing have incorporated health policy courses into the curriculum in order to educate nurses to the political process and grass roots advocacy. This essential is still relevant and vital, and needs to incorporate a global perspective on health policy.

We have a global society, and we have learned that the world is very small. With the advancement of air travel one can be in any country generally within a day or two, and some countries within a few hours. Certainly what affects other countries has an effect on this nation. A recent example is the H1N1 flu epidemic. As we are a nation of diversity, it is incumbent upon DNP programs to foster an understanding of other countries' health care delivery and funding systems, so that nurses in this country can learn and apply such learning in our own health care delivery system.

Another example is the recent health reform efforts and the legislation *Title 1 Quality Affordable Health Care Bill* and the *Title 1 Amendments* that were signed into law by the President of the United States in 2010. This legislation will cover an estimated additional 32 million people in the United States out of the approximately 50 million individuals who have no health insurance. The ANA was politically involved in supporting and moving this legislation forward. The World Health Organization most recently tracked health rankings on quality and cost in 2000. This process had been completed every 10 years, but the WHO has decided that this tracking process is too cumbersome to continue. However, in the year 2000, the United States ranked 37th in health care outcomes. France ranked first, and Italy ranked second (World Health Organization, 2000). We can learn much from other nations regarding what their health policies are in relation to improving our own system of health care. Two major contributing factors very likely why other countries ranked higher than the United States were secondary to their focus on prevention and having a national health system where all individuals have access to health care.

Essential VI addresses interprofessional collaboration for improving patient and population health outcomes. This essential is still relevant, as the essential really is addressing communication, collaboration, and the importance of teamwork in the provision of patient care and quality outcomes. The Institute of Medicine (IOM) (1999, 2003, 2007) has reported nearly 100,000 iatrogenic events that occur in health care facilities on an annual basis. Since 2003, the goal of the IOM is to decrease these iatrogenic events with a resultant increase of quality care provided to patients. The IOM has concluded that communication is one of the major problems contributing to such negative patient outcomes (IOM, 1999, 2003, 2007). The majority of DNP programs do not incorporate communication courses in the curriculum and/or have communication threaded as a key component of all courses throughout the DNP program.

Of those that do, Chatham University in Pittsburgh, PA, for example, has a course that is titled *Communication for Nurse Executives*. Thomas Jefferson University in Philadelphia, PA, has a course that is titled *Leadership and Interprofessional Collaboration*. One must communicate in order to collaborate. Waynesburg University in Pittsburgh, PA, has a course titled *Interprofessional Collaboration and Team Facilitation*. And, the University of San Francisco has a course titled *"Communication."*[1] As the nation is still addressing iatrogenic events that result from poor communication, such as hand-off communication at the change of shift report, this essential is still vital to the nurse executive role and the improvement of patient safety and care.

Essential VI also addresses the importance of collaboration and team work. Drucker (2006) states that "the modern organization cannot be one of boss and subordinate. It must be organized as a team" (p. 150). Team building is defined as a process of deliberately creating and unifying a group of individuals into a functioning work unit, so that specific goals and objectives are accomplished (Huber, 2010). Groups only become a true team by doing the collective work. Teams progress through a developmental process, and this takes time and an investment of energy in order for this to materialize. Team building involves collaboration and creativity. The purpose of team building and collaboration results in greater problem solving, increased morale of team members, and improved coordination of work. Such teamwork is fundamental to the achievement of improved patient outcomes, and in this day of rising health care costs, improved cost control. Teamwork and collaboration have a positive effect on patient care by improving patient safety, reducing errors, and improving the quality of nursing care to the patient. Nurse executives must foster an environment of collaboration, teamwork, and excellent communication strategies. The nurse executive is in a pivotal position to ensure that good teamwork is implemented, so that the goals of the organization are accomplished. With the knowledge and skill set gained in a DNP Nurse Executive Program Track, these individuals should be positioned to accomplish this. These strategies not only improve the care to the patient, but they also improve the job satisfaction of the nurses who are led by DNP-educated nurse executives.

Essential VII focuses on clinical prevention and population health in order to improve the health care to the nation. This essential is still a vital component and should be a primary focus in all DNP curriculums. Our current system of health care has been focused on intervention rather than prevention. Some Americans view our health care system as the best in the world. There is no question that when it comes to the intervention side of health care, we do excel in technology and state-of-the-art health care facilities for those who can access the services. The question to consider is whether we really are doing what is best for patients by utilization of an intervention model rather than a prevention model?

Compared to other nations, our health care outcomes are deplorable. Our health care system costs billions of dollars and consumes a large percentage of our nation's gross national product (World Health Organization, 2000). Therefore, it is incumbent that our efforts as nurses focus on prevention and population health outcomes. Nurses are best positioned to educate and promote prevention and health. This is what mainly separates us from other professions including medicine.

Changes to Medicare reimbursement, national patient safety goals, and the institution of core measures are also driving this initiative. For example, acute care hospitals now must assess patients to see if they will take the influenza vaccine and, if the patient is of a certain age, the pneumococcal vaccine. Patients must sign a *declination form* if they do not elect to take the influenza vaccine. A recent patient who had been hospitalized in an acute care hospital also had his physician discuss and administer tetanus, diphtheria, and pertussis booster as it had been nearly 10 years since this patient had this type of vaccination. The patient had, however, not been hospitalized for a tetanus prone wound. These examples just demonstrate the move of hospitals and providers to institute primary prevention strategies in the acute care hospital setting. Nurse executives have to be at the center of such measures and ensure that their respective organizations are focused on such population-based health prevention measures. The DNP-prepared nurse executive can best implement such systems of care, as they have had education on population-based health, epidemiology, leadership, communication, collaboration, systems thinking, statistics, research, evidence-based practice, and health policy. Such executives have also completed either a capstone project or a clinical dissertation that focuses on clinical outcomes.

Essential VIII addresses advanced nursing practice. It is obvious that this essential is the basis for the AACN's (2004) recommendation to move advanced practice to the DNP level as entry into advanced practice by the year 2015. It has been known by those in the field that the AACN, through their CCNE accreditation process of DNP programs, will accredit program tracks for advanced practice nursing and nurse executives in DNP curriculum. Although the recommendation to have the DNP as the entry level into advanced practice by the year 2015 is the AACN's recommendation, it will be necessary for every state to change their individual legislation in order to meet this goal. Most of us are all too familiar with the ANA's recommendation to change the entry level of professional nursing practice to a BSN by 1965. However, only one state in our nation has accomplished this goal. This does not imply that we should not focus our efforts on accomplishing the AACN's recommendation. This again ties to Essential V, where we as advanced practice nurses, educators, and administrators must be politically active in our respective states to ensure that this goal becomes a reality.

However, one must question what is the reality of moving advanced practice nursing education to the DNP as the entry level to practice? As previously mentioned in this chapter, one of the major events that recently occurred was the implementation of health reform in the United States. With more individuals receiving insurance, access to care should dramatically improve. This should result in more individuals seeking health care, will to place further strain on an already overburdened health care system. Many states may be reluctant to move the DNP as the entry level into advanced practice nursing, as they will require more health care providers at the advanced practice level. The "baby boomers" are at or nearing retirement age, so the reality will be less service providers in the very near future. Most nurses also are well aware of the high average age of the nurse and that this "average age" can vary from state to state. Buerhaus, Auerback, and Staiger (2009) describe that most of the employment in the past few years have resulted from nurses who are in their 50s. Nurses under the age of 35 contributed to an increase of only 6% employment rates to hospitals.

The other reality is the question of whether an individual with a DNP earns a higher salary. For example, what would the cost be if an entire health system's nursing practitioner staff were all prepared at the DNP level, if salaries significantly rose for those individuals who obtained the DNP credential? Secondary to a constrained economy, most health systems are trying to lower costs, not increase costs. However, should not professionals with the highest educational credentials be compensated for such? For any of us who have been in education, I think that most of us realize we did not go into education for increased salaries. These are certainly considerations that must be taken into account. Such considerations may also provide a rationale as to why some states will be reluctant to implement the DNP as the entry level for advanced practice nursing.

SO WHAT IS MISSING IN THE DNP NURSE EXECUTIVE TRACK CURRICULUM?

In order for DNP curriculum to take a more contemporary approach to the education of nurse executives, it is our recommendation that two other elements be incorporated, not only in the curriculum of DNP programs, but into the AACN's *Essentials* (2006) as well.

These two core elements would be strategic management and succession planning. Each one of these core elements will be addressed separately.

Proposed Essential IX: Strategic Management

As health care has changed dramatically over the past decade or so, it is necessary for health care systems, especially acute care facilities, to embrace the concept of strategic management. Many such facilities have changed their focus from long-range planning, which was once required for a certificate of need process, to that of the development of strategic plans. Now, the strategic plan is the first bridge to strategic management. By strategic management, we are referring to a much broader concept. Strategic management involves the incorporation of a department that specifically focuses on strategy to grow the business. According to Huber (2010), strategic management evolves from the organization that wants to establish its competitive position in the market place. For example, one large tertiary acute care facility in Philadelphia, PA has implemented a position of a strategic administrator. They hired a former nurse executive to fill this role. In her role, she bonds with organizations throughout the region to grow the business of her organization. One community hospital needed radiology services, and the tertiary facility now provides the radiology services to this community hospital. The trade-off is that the community hospital refers their tertiary care to the tertiary center providing their radiology services.

Strategic management is both an art and a science. According to Huber (2010), strategic management begins with the organization's mission and vision. Development of the organization's vision and mission should include all levels of staff in the process, as well as key stakeholders in the community. It involves the development of relationships with other organizations and individuals, as well as the need to critically analyze strategic maneuvers. For example, if there were perceived need to have off-site radiology procedures for a certain community, the community and surrounding areas would be assessed to see what other similar facilities exist, what potential market share could be captured by the organization, and at what cost it would take to add such a facility. If the analysis projected a loss of revenue and/or that the population size was not really there to serve, an off-site radiology facility would not be implemented. Another example would be an organization that wants to achieve Magnet status or the Malcolm Baldrige Award for quality. One example of this is the AtlantiCare Health System in southeastern NJ. This health system had the vision to be a premiere quality organization and achieve these two top award designations. They have achieved Magnet status for the second time, and in 2009, was one of two health systems in the nation to receive the Malcolm Baldrige Award for quality.

Strategic management also ties to Essential IV: Information systems/technology and patient technology for the improvement and transformation of health care, and Essential VI: Inter professional collaboration for improving patient and population health outcomes. Information technology is utilized that maps out geographic regions identifying what services are available in that region and the population demographics. Such informatics assists in the decision-making process. Interprofessional collaboration is essential in forming alliances for implementing strategy.

Strategic management will become more critical, especially as health systems evolve from an intervention to a prevention model. Most health systems are in the infancy stages in this process. It is critical that DNP programs incorporate strategic management into nurse executive program tracks.

Proposed Essential X: Succession Planning

Once upon a time, it seemed that nurse executives felt that the organization could not survive without them. Little attention was paid to those who would fill the shoes of the nurse executive should the person leave, retire, or be terminated. This not only left nursing to flounder, but oftentimes during leadership change, negative outcome was the net effect. The goal of all nurse executives should be to ensure patient care continuity and continued survival of the organization beyond their tenure at the organization. Good executives recognize that succession planning is critical to the process of organizational growth and survival. Collins (2001) states that organizations need to begin succession planning by looking at the individuals within the organization itself. There is now a move toward succession planning in health care organizations. A recent visit to a hospital in Connecticut provides an excellent example. At this hospital, the CEO was retiring after 30 years of service. He mandated that not only he, but that each executive including the nursing executive, develop a succession plan for their position. The CEO appointed his successor, a physician from within the organization, and for the last year of his tenure as CEO, the CEO mentored and gave the incoming CEO one of his departments to manage each month. By the time the CEO had retired, the new CEO was essentially doing his job. The nurse executive (Chief Nursing Officer) had a plan to retire within 3 years. She had already identified who would replace her. This person already was the director of several of the nursing units. The CNO's plan was to have this director take the reins of the nursing department when she retired; however, the exiting CNO planned to remain on staff in a different position for a year or two so that she could be available to help the new CNO if needed.

Beyers (2006) interviewed six nurse executives from five different practice settings. The purpose of this study was to evaluate how succession planning is being conceptualized in today's world of practice. These nurse executives recognized that succession planning takes different forms in different facilities. In other words, there is no one right way in which to do succession planning. The overriding finding and theme of this study was that succession planning is critical to nurse executive practice, and that succession planning is critical to quality patient care outcomes. Succession planning is critical and all nurse executives, as well as leaders in all types of organizations, need to embrace and implement this concept. It is critical that DNP nurse executive track programs address succession planning in the curriculum.

SUMMARY

Our chapter has focused on DNP curriculum as it relates to nurse executive program tracks and our exploration of the current AACN *Essentials* (2006) as they relate specifically to leadership. We have traced the evolution of contemporary nursing administration program tracks and have attempted to identify what is still current and what needs to be added to the curriculum. We also recognize that these recommendations will change over time as health care in our nation continues to evolve. However, what will remain the same is the need to have nurses educated at the highest level for administrative practice. If we want to close the quality chasm (IOM, 2003), we must raise the bar!

NOTE

1. These DNP curricula can be viewed at the following websites: Chatham University: http://www. chatham.edu/ccps/dnp/; Thomas Jefferson University: http://www.jefferson.edu/jchp/ nursing/dnp.cfm; Waynesburg University: http://www.waynesburg.edu/?q=Doctor_of_ Nursing_Practice; University of San Francisco: http://www.usfca.edu/nursing/dnp/

REFERENCES

American Association of Colleges of Nursing (AACN). (1996). *The essentials of master's education for advanced practice nursing.* Washington, DC: Author.

American Association of Colleges of Nursing (AACN). (1997). *Joint position statement on nursing administration education.* Retrieved March 28, 2010, from http://www.aacn.nche.edu/ Publications/positions/nae.htm

American Association of Colleges of Nursing (AACN). (2004a). *AACN draft position statement on the practice doctorate in nursing January 2004.* Washington, DC: Author.

American Association of Colleges of Nursing (AACN). (2004b). *AACN position statement on the practice doctorate in nursing.* Retrieved from http://www.aacn.nche.edu/Publications/positions/ index.htm

American Association of Colleges of Nursing (AACN). (2006). *The essentials of doctoral nursing education for advanced practice nursing.* Retrieved from http://www.aacn.nche.edu

American Association of Colleges of Nursing (AACN). (2009). *Frequently asked questions DNP programs & CCNE accreditation.* Retrieved from http://www.aacn.nche.edu/accreditation/ dnpFAQ.htm

American Association of Colleges of Nursing & American Organization of Nurse Executives. (1997). *Joint position statement on nursing administration education.* Retrieved from http:// www.aacn.nche.edu/Publications/positions/nae.htm

American Nurses Association (ANA). (2009). *Nursing administration: Scope & standards of practice.* Silver Spring, MD: Author.

Benner, P., Sutphen, M., Leonard, V., & Day, L. (2010). *Educating nurses: A call for radical transformation.* San Francisco, CA: Jossey Bass-Carnegie Foundation for the Advancement of Teaching.

Boyer, M. (2006) Nurse executives' perspectives on succession planning. *The Journal of Nursing Administration, 36,* 304–312.

Buerhaus, P. I., Auerback, D. I., & Staiger, D. O. (2009). The recent surge in nurse employment: Causes and implications. *Health Affairs, 28,* 657–668.

Chism, L. A. (2009). *The doctor of nursing practice: A guidebook for role development professional issues.* Boston, MA: Jones & Bartlett.

Collins, J. (2001). *Good to great: Why some companies make the leap . . . and others don't.* New York, NY: Harper Collins.

Dienemann, J., & Aroian, J. (1995). *Essentials of baccalaureate education for nursing leadership and management and master's nursing education for nursing administration advanced practice.* University of North Carolina, Chapel Hill, NC: Council on Graduate Education for Administration in Nursing (CGEAN). Retrieved from http://www.cgean.org/documents/essentials_of_bac_ nursing11.pdf

Drucker, P. F. (2006). *Classic Drucker.* Cambridge, MA: Harvard Business Review Publications.

Fitzpatrick, J. J., & Wallace, M. (2009). *The doctor of nursing practice and clinical nurse leader: Essentials of program development and implementation for clinical practice.* New York, NY: Springer Publishing Company.

Haynor, P. M., & Wells, R. W. (1998). Will nursing administration programs survive the 21st century? *JONA, 28*(1), 15–24.

Henry, B. (1989). Education for administration: The crisis in nursing administration education. *JONA, 19*(8), 6–7, 28.

Herrin, D., Jones, K., Krepper, R., Sherman, R., & Reineck, C. (2006). Future of nursing administration graduate curricula, Part 2. *JONA, 36,* 498–505.

Health Research Service Administration. (n.d). *National Center for Health Workforce Analysis: U.S. Health Workforce Personnel Factbook.* Retrieved from http://bhpr.hrsa.gov/healthworkforce/reports/factbook.htm

Huber, D. L. (2010). *Leadership and nursing care management.* Maryland Heights, MO: Saunders Elsevier.

Institute of Medicine (IOM). (1999). *To err is human: Building a safer health system.* Washington, DC: National Academies Press.

Institute of Medicine (IOM). (2003). *Crossing the quality chasm. A new health system for the 21st century.* Washington, DC: National Academies Press.

Institute of Medicine (IOM). (2007). *Preventing medication errors.* Washington, DC: National Academies Press.

Medical Infrastructure—Hospital Closures and Access to Health Care. (2010). Retrieved from http://social.jrank.org/pages/1202/Medical-Infrastructure-Hospital-Closures-Access-Health-Care.html#ixzz0nN0JD2Wy

New Jersey Hospital Association. (2008). *NJ hospital crisis.* Retrieved from http://www.njha.com/njhospitalcrisis.pdf

World Health Organization. (2000). *The world health report 2000.* Retrieved from www.who.int/whr

CHAPTER TWELVE: Reflective Response

Joyce J. Fitzpatrick

The authors have provided a detailed discussion of current issues confronting nursing in the development of the necessary curricula for preparation of nurse executives. They outline the eight curriculum essentials for Doctor of Nursing Practice (DNP) programs specified by the American Association of Colleges of Nursing (AACN, 2006) and describe the relevance of each of these essentials to the preparation of nurse executives. They then propose two additional essentials for the DNP Nurse Executive Track: Strategic management and Succession planning. They have raised important issues that require consideration by all concerned about the preparation of nurse leaders for the future of health care delivery. Also, they have added to our understanding of the core content required for the nurse executive of today and tomorrow.

I agree with the primary argument of Rundio and Scott that the DNP is the most appropriate preparation for the nurse executive. Importantly, in contrast to the authors, I strongly recommend a total revision of the 2006 AACN *Essentials* rather than only the addition of essentials specific to the nurse executive track. Core content should be delineated for all advanced areas of nursing, including advanced clinical practice, administration, education, and informatics. Once the core content dimensions are outlined then there should be specific "essentials" for each of the specialties. The areas that should be included are those in which one can receive advanced certification. AACN's current position is to not include nursing education as a specialty for the DNP, which, in my opinion, is a mistake. Many nurse educators are opting for the DNP degree. Early in the development of the national discussions regarding professional doctorates in nursing, I argued for the professional/clinical doctorate as the most appropriate degree for clinical nurse educators for preparation of nurses for beginning and advanced clinical practice (Fitzpatrick, 1989, 2003). Further, there is advanced content in nursing education that should be essential for nurse educators prepared at the DNP level.

In relation to the preparation of nurse executives, all of the eight existing AACN essentials statements are general enough that the relevance can easily be inferred, yet some are more central to the preparation of the nurse executive than others. For example, Essentials II: Organizational and systems leadership for quality improvement and systems thinking; IV: Information systems/technology for the improvement and transformation of health care; V: Health care policy for advocacy in health care; and VI: Interprofessional collaboration for improving patient and population health outcomes, are all directly relevant to the preparation of nurse executives. Some of the other essentials are more directly related to the traditional definition of advanced practice nursing (i.e., the preparation of clinicians for one of four roles: nurse practitioner, clinical nurse specialist, certified nurse midwife, or certified registered nurse anesthetist).

The problem, and sometimes the resultant confusion, seems to stem from the original deliberations of the DNP as entry-level preparation for advanced practice nursing. This idea was originally presented within the structure of the narrower definition of advanced practice, namely advanced clinical practice for the four specialty practice roles noted above. As programs were implemented, nursing informatics, administration, and public health nursing were added as meeting the requirements for "advanced practice." Yet, the AACN (2006) *Essentials* were not revised to reflect the inclusion of these added areas of advanced practice.

The addition of these other areas further complicates discussions of the requirement of the DNP degree for advanced practice by 2015 (AACN, 2004). This position statement is relevant to only the advanced clinical areas of nursing, namely those of nurse practitioner, clinical nurse specialist, nurse midwife, and nurse anesthetist. These are the only advanced practice areas that have received title recognition in state legislation governing advanced practice nursing. Furthermore, there is some variation across states as to which of these advanced specialties are included. For example, in some states, the title recognition does not include clinical nurse specialists. As Rundio and Scott have noted, changing the regulations throughout each of the states is no easy task. None of the current advanced practice state legislation includes nurse informaticians, nurse executives, nurse educators, or public health nurses. These are roles that are different from those of advanced clinical practice.

The dilemma seems to be that the original proposal for the DNP was meant to be specific to advanced clinical practice, a replacement for the masters level clinical nursing practice programs. And with that proposed change, the transition to the 2015 requirement for DNP entry level seemed to be a straightforward goal, one that would require the agreement of the specialty organizations in nursing that concern themselves with the four advanced practice clinical roles. Even so, there has not been agreement from these specialty organizations. For example, even though the American Association of Nurse Anesthetists (AANA) has supported the requirement for doctoral education as preparation for nurse anesthetist practice by 2025, they have not specified that this is to be the DNP degree (AANA, 2007).

The content that Rundio and Scott identify under the two new essentials that they propose can arguably be subsumed under the AACN's Essential II: Organizational and systems leadership for quality improvement and systems thinking. System leadership and system thinking lead to strategic management, and succession planning is one aspect of strategic management that responsible leaders do. Granted that succession planning is rarely done within organizations (Cantor, 2005). Yet, excellent leaders have their eyes on the future of the organization and plan for its future, including the time when they are no longer in the leadership role. The example of succession planning provided by Rundio and Scott is an excellent illustration of how this long-range planning can be implemented.

As a result of a longstanding commitment to the professional doctoral for executive nurse leaders, together with colleagues, I implemented a cohort model in the DNP program at Case Western Reserve University for preparation of nurse leaders in several acute care hospitals. The impetus for this program was described by Donahue (2009), a senior nurse executive who was searching for the best program for preparation for nurse leaders within the hospital where she was the chief nursing officer. From a collaborative relationship with one hospital, this program grew into a partnership with seven hospitals and health systems, and was supported by a grant from the Health Resources and Services Administration (HRSA) Division of Nursing. More than 50 nurse executives have completed the program and several others are currently completing coursework. Their positions range from chief nursing officer in major medical centers to quality directors and directors of specialized services. Many of the projects that were initiated as part of their DNP program have resulted in publications, thus contributing to the science of nursing management and administration (e.g., Alvarez & Fitzpatrick, 2007; Armellino, Quinn Griffin, & Fitzpatrick, 2010; Cajulis & Fitzpatrick, 2007; Donahue, Piazza, Quinn Griffin, Dykes, & Fitzpatrick, 2008; Garber, Madigan, Click, & Fitzpatrick, 2009; Piazza, Donahue, Quinn Griffin, Dykes, & Fitzpatrick, 2006; Porter, Kolkaba, McNulty, & Fitzpatrick, 2010; Scherer & Fitzpatrick, 2008).

One of the health care systems, North Shore Long Island Jewish Health in NY, has supported more than 50 nurses in leadership positions to obtain their DNP degrees through this cohort model. Another institution, Mount Sinai Medical Center in NY, has supported two cohorts of nurse leaders in the pursuit of the DNP. These nurse executives are passionate about the work they do, and equally passionate about the centrality of the DNP to their current leadership and future goals for moving health care forward in their environments.

So now that we in nursing have collectively significantly modified (some might say homogenized) the original proposal, what is the best way forward? The Tri-Council for Nursing (which consists of representatives of the four major nursing professional organizations: the American Nurses Association, the American Organization of Nurse Executives, the American Association of Colleges of Nursing, and the National League for Nursing) should convene a workgroup to address the current situation and make recommendations for the future professional preparation of nurses for all roles that require advanced education. This alternative is preferable to the current approach where decisions are made based on the initiatives of individual associations or schools of nursing or education accrediting bodies. Rundio and Scott have presented many strong arguments for the fact that the nurse executive of the future should be prepared with a professional doctorate. Similar arguments could be provided for the preparation of nurse educators. This would be an ideal time for consensus and scholarly debate to advance the discipline and prepare the leaders of tomorrow for a wide range of leadership roles.

REFERENCES

American Association of Colleges of Nursing (AACN). (2004). *AACN position statement on the practice doctorate in nursing.* Retrieved from http://www.aacn.nche.edu/Publications/positions/index.htm

American Association of Colleges of Nursing (AACN). (2006). *The essentials of doctoral nursing education for advanced practice nursing.* Retrieved from http://www.aacn.nche.edu

American Association of Nurse Anesthetists (AANA). (2007). *AANA position statement on doctoral preparation of nurse anesthetists: Adopted June 2, 2007.* Retrieved from http://www.aana.com

Alvarez, C., & Fitzpatrick, J. J. (2007). Nurses job satisfaction and patient falls. *Asian Nursing Research, 1*(2), 82–94.

Armellino, D. A., Quinn Griffin, M. T., & Fitzpatrick, J. J. (2010, in press). Structural empowerment and patient safety culture among Registered Nurses working in adult critical care units. *Journal of Nursing Management.*

Cajulis, C. B., & Fitzpatrick, J. J. (2007). Levels of autonomy of nurse practitioners in an acute care setting. *Journal of the American Academy of Nurse Practitioners, 19*(10), 500–507.

Cantor, P. (2005). Succession planning: Often requested, rarely delivered. *Ivey Business Journal,* January, February 1–10. Retrieved from http://www.iveybusinessjournal.com/view_article.asp?intArticle_ID=531

Donahue, M. (2009). The doctor of nursing practice degree: Reaching the next level of excellence. In J. J. Fitzpatrick, & M. Wallace (Eds.), *The doctor of nursing practice and clinical nurse leader: Essentials of program development and implementation for clinical practice* (pp. 61–66). New York, NY: Springer.

Donahue, M., Piazza, I., Quinn Griffin, M., Dykes, P., & Fitzpatrick, J. J. (2008). The relationship between nurses' perceptions of empowerment and patient satisfaction. *Applied Nursing Research, 21*(1), 2–7.

Fitzpatrick, J. J. (1989). The professional doctorate as an entry level into professional practice. In National League for Nursing's, *Perspectives in nursing, 1987–1989* (pp. 53–56). New York, NY: National League for Nursing.

Fitzpatrick, J. J. (2003). The case for the clinical doctorate in nursing. *Reflections on Nursing Leadership*, First Quarter, pp. 8–9, 37, 52.

Garber, J., Madigan, E. A., Click, E., & Fitzpatrick, J. J. (2009). Attitudes toward collaboration and servant leadership among nurses, physicians, and residents. *Journal of Inter-Professional Care, 23*(4), 331–340.

Piazza, I., Donahue, M., Quinn Griffin, M., Dykes, P., & Fitzpatrick, J. J. (2006). Differences in perceptions of empowerment among nationally certified nurses and nurses who are not nationally certified. *Journal of Nursing Administration, 36*(5), 277–283.

Porter, C. A., Kolkaba, K., McNulty, R. M., & Fitzpatrick, J. J. (2010). The effect of a labor management partnership on nurse satisfaction and turnover. *Journal of Nursing Administration, 40*(5), 205–210.

Scherer, D., & Fitzpatrick, J. J. (2008). Perceptions of patient safety culture among physicians and RNs in the peri-operative area. *AORN Journal, 87*(1), 163–175.

CRITICAL THINKING QUESTIONS

1. What are two reasons why some people would disagree with the transition of nursing administration educational preparation to the Doctor of Nursing Practice?
2. Using one of the reasons from the above question, what would your argument be for the transition of nursing administration practice to the DNP?
3. Of the eight essentials cited by the AACN, which one of these essentials do you feel is the most important for nurse executive practice? Explain your selection.
4. There is no question that the nurse executive role has become more and more data driven. In what ways can an informatics system assist the nurse executive in this "data-driven" world?
5. As policy is vital to what a nurse executive does, how could you utilize policy and politics to make the DNP as the entry level to nurse executive practice a reality in your respective state by the year 2015?
6. What are some potential problems with communicating vision and strategy internally in your organization?
7. Moving the DNP forward as the entry level in nurse executive practice incurs some risks. How does one take risks today in a cost-focused, competitive environment?
8. Leaders "challenge the process"—how do nursing leaders today seek out opportunities and risks? What if the risk fails?
9. Do you view the DNP as entry level into nurse executive practice as both an opportunity and a risk? Explain why or why not?
10. Because nurse executives are visionary, what do you see the future holding for the educational preparation of nurse executives?

CHAPTER THIRTEEN

Executive Coaching to Support Doctoral Role Transitions and Promote Leadership Consciousness

Beth Weinstock and Mary Ellen Smith Glasgow

INTRODUCTION

This chapter addresses the many challenges inherent in professional work transitions. It speaks to the need for heightened leadership consciousness during times of change, and describes how executive coaching can support new leaders in making effective transitions that develop their best gifts, talents, and strengths.

As a doctorally prepared nurse, the Doctor of Nurse Practice (DNP) graduate is in a position of leadership. As the nursing profession itself becomes more and more central to our health care system, the DNP will increase its importance and scope of influence. This role expansion involves transitions and challenges for the individual DNP graduate and also for the discipline itself. Understanding the challenges and preparing to meet them will help the DNP graduate realize her or his full potential.

Transitions in the work place can be personally and professionally satisfying and yet be difficult to manage. Switching roles and increasing responsibilities entails not only adjustments to new task assignments, but also to a new relationship with ourselves, and with those around us. As in a kaleidoscope, when we turn just one small part of the design, the entire structure transforms. When we move into new roles, it feels as if the world has gone on tilt until we find ourselves fully settled in the new design. Transitions need time and attention for all parts to integrate and realign with one another. This chapter will shed light on the often hidden aspects of work transitions for the DNP graduate, with the intent to help those individuals evolve as leaders in practice, education, administration, and/or clinical research.

The DNP graduate's new leadership role will require expanded ways of thinking and being, best summed up in the concept of *leadership consciousness*. Leadership consciousness is a constant and pervasive awareness that one's actions have impact that matters. This consciousness holds awareness that all behavior influences its environment, and that the influence needs to be carefully tracked. As a frame of mind and attitude it colors all thought and behavior. Its wisdom reminds those in leadership that success is never solely about oneself, but about a contribution reflected in the people and systems that are being led. Leadership, at the simplest level, is about the execution of defined leadership tasks. At a more complex level, it is about how we develop and embody leadership consciousness. This chapter will explore the route toward leadership consciousness by mapping its many domains.

Executive coaching is a leadership development intervention that can guide the new DNP through role transitions and into greater leadership consciousness. It focuses on helping clients perform to the best of their potential, both in successfully achieving their role responsibilities, and in finding their own best way of accomplishing this goal. The process of executive coaching involves a relationship of mutual respect and engagement between the coach and coaching client (or coachee) which leads to feedback and support for the client's growth and development. This chapter will define executive coaching, describe what it entails, and clarify how it works. A case example will be presented as an illustration of a successful executive coaching project at a College of Nursing.

TRANSITIONS IN PROFESSIONAL DEVELOPMENT

We are living in turbulent times. On the global front, threats to safety have generated widespread anxiety. On the home front, the current economic crisis has created fear and disruption. In the midst of our domestic upheaval lies uncertainty about the state of national health care, creating worry in the general population and stress within the nursing profession. The DNP is opening new possibilities for the nursing profession and health care; however, this new degree will lead the profession into uncharted territory where there are no clear maps for moving forward. The DNP graduate and our health care system are transitioning at the same time, heightening the challenges for managing change. It is of paramount importance that attention is placed on DNP professional development during such times of transition.

The academic, corporate, and practice world is accustomed to change and transition. As doctoral-level nurses transition into leadership roles, DNPs must develop skills to negotiate the politics and hierarchies of the workplace setting. Given the shortage of DNP leaders, there will be few comparably educated role models in the discipline. As new DNPs are promoted to advanced practice, faculty, and executive positions, a broader spectrum of new competencies will be required. As the role is defined, many challenges will emerge.

With each shift, there are different skill sets for DNPs to develop. Some of these skills are grounded in content related to a nursing specialty, but many fall under the umbrella of management and leadership. It is the goal of DNPs as leaders to: (1) earn the trust of the organization; (2) be deeply engaged with professional colleagues; (3) earn legitimacy and mobilize people around a focused agenda; (4) devote considerable efforts to develop employees and build the organization's collective leadership capabilities; and lastly, (5) strive for high performance that is committed to the larger institution (Eisenstat, Beer, Foote, Fredberg, & Norrgren, 2008). Clearly, major shifts in the role from clinician to leader create the demand for change on many fronts for the DNP.

Role shifts create change in all our relationships, both personal and professional. They create change, as well, in how we see ourselves. There is no external promotion without an internal shift; no new leadership position is embodied without personal growth and development. This transformation can be both invigorating and also disorienting. In addition to the excitement, delights, and satisfactions of new leadership positions, transitioning into them involves a labyrinth of twists, turns, and invisible obstructions. The hidden challenges are rarely addressed, which ultimately can be detrimental. Too often, it is simply assumed that if one is competent in one job with a high degree of responsibility, the same person will excel when given increased and different responsibilities. This is not necessarily true. Even extremely competent leaders need adjustment time to become firmly grounded in their new roles. Success often hinges on understanding and addressing the many factors that impede or support smooth transitions (Elsner & Farrands, 2006).

THE HIDDEN CHALLENGES IN PROFESSIONAL TRANSITIONS

The Boundary Challenge

When one gets promoted from a cohort group or achieves a higher level of status among one's peers, the shift into authority can create confusion and conflict in relationships. Peers may become resentful because they think they should have been chosen for the promotion. They may feel unseen and undervalued by the authority who determined the promotion. Their work will now be evaluated by a former peer, and this may raise the fear that personal information that is already known will be used against them. They may know the weaknesses of the promoted peer and think the promotion was unjustified. Resentment can lead to distancing in the form of complaining to other colleagues or withholding information from the new leader that previously would have been openly shared.

Making the transition into a *boss* who remains open and available, but at the same time, can shut the door, give hard feedback when necessary, or make unpopular mandates can be a daunting task. Once in a position of authority over others, there are decisions to make that are challenging:

- "How much insider information should I share with my peers?"
- "How do I close my door without offending people who previously had easy access to my time?"
- "How do I make sure my former peers feel respected and valued?"
- "How do I give critical feedback in a way that can be heard and processed?"
- "How do I demand greater work productivity?"

For each individual, the boundary challenge will play out differently. No matter how it is negotiated, it will require conscious behavior designed for positive impact that can maintain good relationships, while at the same time initiate changes in those very relationships. In addition to the boundary challenge of supervising former peers, the DNP will likely encounter being supervised by non-nurses. Non-nurses are likely to bring different approaches to the health care domain and have varying philosophies and histories with different contexts. This change will also present a range of boundary renegotiations.

The Loneliness Challenge

Once new boundaries are set, one may feel isolated or even lonely. New leadership positions entail shifting alliances from peers to the next level of group leadership. In the course of being coached, new leaders often report that they feel alone, unsure of whose information to trust, unclear about who to go to for input and answers, and uncertain how much personal disclosure is appropriate in their new cohort group. It takes time to find the answers to these questions and to feel securely situated.

The Competency Challenge

Competency in one professional area does not necessarily translate into all aspects of new roles or assignments. Each shift in role involves new content-related areas of skill development and also new leadership demands. For example, one coaching client was a top-notch teacher and a highly responsible taskmaster in all parts of her faculty responsibilities. When promoted to an academic administrative role, she was surprised to learn that part of her actual job was to spend time nurturing and maintaining relationships with her colleagues. She had formerly dismissed such activities as a waste of time, but now needed to practice the art and competency of relationship building. With awareness and determination, she learned to maintain connections with her colleagues in new ways—asking about people's children, stopping by people's desks during the day, hosting people in her office when it was not time for a meeting. As a newly promoted executive, she gained leadership skills beyond her academic excellence and increased collaboration with her own and ancillary departments.

The Confidence Challenge

If we have been at our job long enough, we usually feel settled and confident. We know the rules of the game. We know how to speak up within our work group. We have gotten feedback about how well we perform. Just when we feel proud of accomplishments and comfortable with an existing level of responsibility, a shift in role, even when positive, can create a crisis in confidence. For example, one coaching client who was formerly accustomed to being outspoken with her professional peers, suddenly experienced great fear about speaking up in her new leadership group. She worried that her strong voice would be seen as too aggressive. She feared exposing herself as not knowing all that others expected her to know. Struggling with these doubts, she inhibited her expressions and contributions until her confidence was once again established.

The Identity Challenge

As we move into different roles, we undergo a transformation. How we see ourselves, how we feel, how we dress, how we move—all these aspects of who we have been start to shift. For some, the shift in identity is quite subtle and may take place with no noticeable attention. For others, the shift is unsettling and as tumultuous as for *Alice in Wonderland*, as she slips through the looking glass.

> "Who are you?" said the caterpillar . . . .
>
> "I-I hardly know, Sir, just at the present," Alice replied rather
> shyly. "At least I know who I *was* when I got up this morning, but I
> think I must have been changed several times since then."
>
> —*Lewis, 1981, p. 34*

Changing our perception of ourselves and our external reality usually takes place slowly over time. Sometimes we do not even notice that a shift has happened until time has passed. When we notice the shift, we may even be surprised that it has happened at all. This phenomenon is probably best expressed by writers and poets. The poet Juan Ramon Jimenez (1995) wrote:

> I have a feeling that my boat
> Has struck, down there in the depths,
> Against a great thing.
> And nothing happens!
> Nothing … Silence … Waves …
> —Nothing happens?
> Or has everything Happened,
> And are we standing now, quietly, in the new life?
>
> —*Jimenez, 1995, p. 105*

Once we live through uncertainties and come out on the other side, we find ourselves different in ways that are sometimes hard to name or even recognize. We have shed a layer, or grown one. We connect the dots and discover a new design. We have a new pair of inner glasses that creates an altered vision of our realities. As we move through the many and diverse challenges inevitable with professional transitions and integrate our new awareness with the tasks of leadership, we can move into the realm of leadership consciousness.

MYTHS ABOUT TRANSITIONS INTO LEADERSHIP ROLES

Elsner and Farrands (2006) researched the experience of many leaders who moved from one position of great corporate responsibility into another. In their book *Lost in Transition*, they identify what they call *myths* about leadership transitions which are applied to the DNP experience below. These *myths* can generate considerable distress if left unrecognized. With heightened awareness of them, however, transitions can be much smoother.

Myth # 1. The job matches the job description. Most often the realities of high level positions involve work tasks and organizational complexities that were never in the job description (Elsner & Farrands, 2006). As DNPs find their place in more and more organizational settings, this is bound to be true. Time and support will be needed to gain clarity on the actual territory and boundaries of their job description and new role.

Myth # 2. Leaders in new positions need to make a mark early on in order to be seen as worthy of their appointment. In a magazine interview written by Clements, Farrands is quoted as saying, "The key to success for the incoming leader is to not hit the ground running, but to spend time thinking, reflecting, watching, listening and questioning" (Clements, 2006, p. 34). DNPs are vulnerable here in seeking to prove the utility and wisdom of both the new role and the new degree. Quick action and early visibility must be carefully considered options and not merely strategies for managing anxiety.

Myth # 3. Leaders should demonstrate independence and not need help. The nursing field is predominantly female dominated, which may make it more collaborative than male-dominated professions. To the extent that this is true, the collaborative attitude may render this myth less powerful in nursing than in other parts of corporate America. Nonetheless, across fields, new leaders are often fearful of asking for help lest they be seen as indecisive or weak. This issue may arise for DNP graduates who report to non-nurse supervisors who may be a physician, senior hospital executive, or academic administrator. In light of this new working relationship, DNPs may try to prove themselves prematurely.

Myth # 4. Bosses can be friends and trusted work colleagues. It is tempting to think that the person who does the hiring or promoting can be a trusted support, mentor, and/or ally. The reality is that new DNP leaders need to determine how safe it is to share work-related concerns with their boss, in this case a supervisor. They must learn how to "manage up," identify their supervisor's style, and communicate in a way that gets heard. In some instances, the supervisor will have a different educational background and discipline, thus requiring DNPs to translate their message into language that their supervisors can easily comprehend.

Myth # 5. The Leader does not change: everything else does. As we have seen above, this is not true. Leadership roles, inevitably, involve personal as well as professional change.

Myth # 6. Leaders should not show emotions at work. In many work settings, this myth is beginning to change. However, women leaders in particular need to assess their work context and determine how, when, and where it is safe to show emotion. When it is not safe, they need to learn ways to contain and manage their feelings at work.

Myth # 7. New leaders should be well situated and comfortable within 100 days. The fact is that for many new leaders, it takes up to a year to truly understand the new systems where they are working, the boundaries of their power, and the culture and politics of their organization (Elsner & Farrands, 2006). For the DNP, the challenges of becoming situated are parallel for the individual, as well as for the profession itself, and this will take time.

These seven myths can be landmines waiting to explode if the new leader remains unaware of and/or does not attend to them. Citing them, hopefully, works to debunk them before they take new leaders off course.

As leaders transition from one leadership position to another, they are bound to encounter the challenges mentioned above. As the DNP position expands its field of influence in the nursing profession, these challenges will be amplified. Increased leadership consciousness and attention to the rich potential of each individual's leadership capacity will be even more critical.

LEADERSHIP CONSCIOUSNESS

The leadership role requires vision, analysis, decision making, conflict management, action, influence, and the ability to inspire others, track impact, and give rewards. These are skills which can be taught and learned in leadership training programs where methods and techniques are practiced. Embodying these skills and carrying them forth with leadership consciousness is the challenge of a great leader. Davis Kyle (1998) said "Leading, then, is not primarily about doing something, but rather about being something" (1998, p. viii). Les Omatoni quotes Walt Whitman expressing a similar sentiment: "We convince with our presence" (Omatani, 2007, p. 34). When we infuse the discrete tasks of leadership with who we are, our personal passion, our unique presence, our particular way of moving through daily actions, and our commitment to outcomes that benefit the most number of people, all bring us into our fullest power as leaders.

A leadership story is told about a man named Zusia. Originally from the Hebrew tradition, it now has many variations as a teaching tale and is adapted below:

Zusia was a highly regarded member of his community who decides to climb his spiritual mountain and face his Gods. He goes with great fear and trembling in spite of his community's assurances that he, of all people, who has given so much, should not be concerned.

But Zusia knows better. When he returns, he appears ashen and shaken to his core. His people inquire as to what the Gods could have said to disturb him so. Zusia tells them, "The Gods did not ask me why like Moses I did not part the Red Sea. Nor did they ask me why like Gandhi I did not go on a hunger strike for people. Nor did they ask why like Rosa Parks I did not refuse to go to the back of the bus. They asked me, 'Zusia, why have you not been more like Zusia'?"

—*Hassidic Stories, 2010*

The lesson from Zusia's Gods is that we must finely and deliberately hone in on who we are and then deliver our services based on our truth. We do this by increasing our self-awareness in many domains. As we increase this awareness and weave together self-knowing and authenticity, we move toward leadership consciousness.

Leadership consciousness is not only about what we do as leaders. It is certainly about performing actions that benefit most of the people, about working for long-term gains over short-term successes, and about considering a legacy left for future generations (Barret Values Centre, 2009). Those are the external results that come from conscious and responsible leadership. Leadership consciousness speaks, in addition, to the interior life of the leader—a state of being that is mindful of and quests to merge individual meaning with community benefit. David Whyte (1994), poet and organization consultant, said "We cultivate an inner life knowing that what is most important to us must be spoken and made real in the outer world "(p. 142). The route toward developing leadership consciousness will vary for each DNP according to individual style differences, histories, cultural backgrounds, age, gender, and work contexts, but this will always involve increased awareness in the multiple domains described below.

DOMAINS OF SELF-AWARENESS

We, ourselves, are the instruments of change. We therefore need to know who we are and who we are not. This means insight into our gifts and talents, how to use them, what blocks their potency, and what support and guidance we need for further development. It means knowing how we differ from others, that we cannot be all things to all people, and that we have limits to our gifts and strengths. Once we are clear and accept who we are and who we are not, we can move forward to actualize our leadership potential.

Awareness of Personal Styles and Strengths

Many cultures throughout time have created systems for mapping different character types. Land-based cultures, those that are literally dependant on geography, seasonal changes, and weather, have traditionally differentiated people by how they represent qualities of the seasons and the directions of the earth. These divergent qualities, when put together, reflect balance and harmony with the environment. The ancient Celtics from Ireland and Scotland referred to the Wheel of Being (Baggott, 2000), and many Native American peoples refer to the Medicine Wheel to reflect archetypal ways of being (Arrien, 1993). These two different cultures, developed thousands of miles away from one another, have astonishing parallels in identifying character types. When we translate these types into our modern way of thinking, they describe four archetypes as follows: the *Leader* or *Warrior*, represents the North; the *Visionary* represents the East; the *Healer* represents the South; and the *Teacher* represents the West (Arrien, 1993).

In our Western culture, there are many personality templates that help identify and differentiate character type and therefore raise self-awareness. One of the most widely known and used in work settings is the Myers–Briggs Type Inventory (MBTI). It is a personality profile borrowed from Jungian theory that discerns if we are introverts or extroverts, if we are large systems thinkers or focused on details, if we make decisions based on objectivity or subjectivity, and if we move through the world creating closure or staying ever open to possibilities.

Another powerful vehicle for increasing self-awareness is the "360" feedback process (Lepsinger & Lucia, 1997). This involves a leader choosing several people within their current and past work experiences to answer the same questions about his or her for example, strengths, competencies, or areas of weaknesses. Thus, the "360" provides the leader with feedback on how he or she is viewed from several perspectives, revealing clear themes that speak to strengths and also areas of needed development.

Personality and character assessments help us to appreciate and value the ways in which we are unique, and appreciate and value the uniqueness of others. They lend insight into how we operate, as well as how we are experienced by others. This information is essential for any leader who values heightening self-awareness, deepening authenticity, and fortifying leadership consciousness.

Awareness of How We Behave Under Stress

Leaders need to know how they tend to operate when stressed and to determine if their behaviors are useful, or not, for accomplishing a given goal. What we do well, we tend to do more of when we are feeling stressed. If we tend to be decisive, we may become controlling. If we are good at creating collaboration and consensus, under stress we may take too much time and miss deadlines for decision making. A DNP who is generally decisive, action oriented, and a clear communicator may become aggressive and appear to bully others under pressure. If the work task is to design and develop a team approach to solving a unit's clinical problems, this behavior under pressure does not represent good leadership. If, however, the work task requires quick action in the ER, then the momentary aggression may be quite appropriate and acceptable.

Some of us lose the use of our greatest strength under pressure. For example, one coaching client realized that while she was incredibly gifted as a creative and visionary force, under pressure she often became fearful, lost her very gift, and made snap decisions that were not always the best for her team. In the process of executive coaching, she increased her awareness of this tendency under stress and learned to slow down, take the time she needed, and ask for input before making her final decisions.

Awareness of our Emotional Intelligence

In 1983, Dr. Howard Gardner, a professor of education at Harvard University, developed a theory of multiple intelligences which posited that the traditional notion of intelligence (based on the standardized I.Q. test) was a limited way of determining human potential (Goleman, 1996). He proposed eight different intelligences (linguistic, logical–mathematical, spatial, kinesthetic, musical, interpersonal, intrapersonal, and naturalistic) to represent a wide range of ways in which we demonstrate our mental attributes. Knowing our most and least developed intelligences provides important guidance, particularly in times of uncertainty and transition. When we become aware of an underdeveloped intelligence, we can work to strengthen it. For example, a DNP graduate who took a position in a nurse-managed health clinic was formerly a highly revered, inspiring lecturer of undergraduates. Her teaching skills were excellent. However, when she transitioned into administrative responsibilities where she needed to collaborate with peers, she was initially perceived as arrogant and unapproachable. Her interpersonal "intelligence" was underdeveloped until it improved as a result of the executive coaching process.

Awareness of Our Fit with the Work Environment

Regardless of our professional competencies, we need to know in what environments we can contribute and feel valued and to know those environments that are likely to stifle our creativity and productivity. We are not interchangeable parts, easily fitting into any work context. The following work story demonstrates this point. A DNP graduate sought coaching during her first year on a critical care team when she found herself challenged with the team's expectations. Passionate about helping patients understand their medical conditions and treatments, she would finish her administrative tasks and spend time with patients and their families educating them, drawing charts, and explaining how their medications worked. Her team members did not value spending this amount of time with families and criticized her for not being committed to her other responsibilities. The DNP became worried about her team's perception of her and even began to doubt herself, but at the same time questioned whether or not she could tolerate being on a team that believed that greater boundaries between the DNP and patient made for better care. Coaching sessions helped her understand that the criticism from her team was related to a culture clash, not her professional competencies. With clear understanding about the honest differences between herself and her team members, her anxiety diminished and she learned to support her own choices while managing time in such a way that her team was satisfied.

Awareness of Our "Inner Critic"

We all talk to ourselves silently inside our heads. The constant commentary is referred to as *self-talk*, and learning how we talk to ourselves is an important part of self-awareness. Some people are fortunate to have high levels of self-esteem that carry them through challenges with little self-criticism; they have encouraging and positive self-talk. Many of us, however, live with the internal voice of an "Inner Critic" that can hold us hostage to self-doubt (Shure & Weinstock, 2009). The "Inner Critic" can thwart spontaneity, limit freedom of expression, and create fear about what we have said or done. When we transition into new roles, the "Inner Critic" has fertile ground to get activated. Faced with a new role it is easy to wonder:

- "Am I doing what I should be doing?"
- "Would someone be doing this a better way?"
- "Am I looking foolish in meetings when I speak up? Or when I don't speak up?"
- "Will I learn the new job well enough to be successful?"

While the "Inner Critic's" voice may be strong, it can be tamed. Managing it and diminishing its negative effect starts with having an awareness that it exists, noting what it says and with what tone it says it, and then developing the voice of an "Inner Coach" that can counteract it. Developing a strong "Inner Coach" creates self-talk that is encouraging and compassionate, and over time will triumph over the "Inner Critic." The coaching process can assist leaders in strengthening this new voice which is an important asset for all leaders.

Awareness as Mindfulness

Mindfulness is the practice of focusing attention and awareness on the present moment, noticing thoughts, feelings, and bodily sensations as they appear and disappear. The goal of mindfulness is to help us observe and accept what appears in our mind without resistance, noting that our brain produces many reactions to our circumstance that, like clouds moving across the sun, continue to move and change. Mindfulness helps us to be grounded, clear, and able to let go of attachments to our own sometimes rigid ideas in order to be alert and available for what is needed at the moment.

A story from the Buddhist tradition teaches about holding on and letting go. A variation of its many renditions is adapted here as follows:

> Two Buddhist monks belong to a sect that prohibits physical contact with women. As they cross a rushing river, they come upon a woman who is struggling to make it to the other side. One monk picks her up and carries her safely across the torrent, deposits her, and moves on. The other was troubled and asked, "How could you carry that woman? You know we can't touch women." The first monk replied, "I left the woman at the rivers edge a long way back, but you are still carrying her."
>
> —*Personal Evolution, 2010*

The second monk is caught in a moment that has already passed. The first monk, attending to what is present at the moment of choice, makes a decision and moves on to the next choice point, unattached to what is now history.

Mindfulness is a form of self-awareness that helps us notice when we are bogged down in matters that have already passed, or are lost in concerns about the future rather than attending to the present. It originates from the Buddhist tradition of meditation practice and has become a highly researched stress management technique (Davidson et al., 2003; Kabat-Zinn & Chapman-Waldrop, 1998). In 1979, Dr. John Kabat-Zinn established an innovative Stress Reduction program at the University of Massachusetts based on Buddhist meditation techniques and has since brought Mindfulness to the general public (Kabat-Zinn, 1994). His teachings, have spread beyond his clinic, and there are now many programs throughout the country that teach mindfulness-based stress reduction using meditation.

Mindfulness, whether or not one actively practices meditation, is an important component of good leadership. It brings attention to what is at hand. It helps free the mind from extraneous thoughts and emotions, and it grounds one in space and time. It is one form of consciousness, and as such, it is an important component of leadership consciousness.

Leadership consciousness challenges us to use the best of our personal and professional selves for making the world a better place, reaching our organization's goals, and supporting the people who report to us, all while facilitating our own inner growth. If we do all this, we not only lead well, but also provide a leadership legacy for those who follow.

EXECUTIVE COACHING

In Arthur Koestler's "Janus" (1978), he tells a story about the captain of a ship who is instructed not to read his written orders until he is out on open sea. He looks forward to the moment that will end his uncertainty and confirm for him whether or not he has been on the right course. When he finally opens the envelope, he finds that the salt air has faded his instructions beyond recognition; that he will never know if he is in the right place on the high seas or following the right course.

Executive coaching is one form of support for leaders who transition through uncharted waters without a clear map, and for those who can use assistance to find their place when the mandate is unclear. In its different forms, coaching has been used throughout human history. Cave dwellers were probably coached on how to draw pictures of their hunt on cave walls, as were young medicine women on how to find medicinal herbs. The modern world of music and sports is accustomed to using one-on-one coaching to support peak performance, but only recently has executive coaching become a resource for leaders across a wide range of fields.

Susan Gatton (2008) provides a comprehensive definition of executive coaching as follows:

> Executive Coaching is a confidential one-on-one, mutually designed relationship between a leader and an executive coach. As a leader, coaching helps you address and resolve issues that limit your success, prepares you for additional responsibilities, or helps you jump-start your acclimation [sic] to a new position or culture.

> During the coaching process, you explore skills and knowledge needed to get you where you want to go—important areas such as leadership, management, communication, political savvy, career decisions, executive presence, social acumen, executive image, work/life balance, and others. You can examine your strengths, blind spots, and perceptions of others while getting a clearer view of how different adapted behaviors result in greater effectiveness.

> You may need to adjust to a different culture and a new team or quickly get a handle on a larger sphere of influence. Coaching can help you advance your skills and minimize the overwhelming feelings of added responsibilities. In today's sensitive and fast-paced workplace, coaching allows you to explore ways of dealing with "politically sensitive" hurdles or get back on track after losing focus. It may simply provide you with an objective viewpoint that is not encumbered by the executive coach being a part of your company and feeling pressured to say the "right" thing (Gatton, 2008, paragraph 1–3).

There are many variations in how executive coaching is done. Some coaches work only face to face, while others work on the phone or use modern technology like Skype. Some will collect data by surveys and interviews, while others will work only with the client's own identification of needs. Coaches who have an expertise in organization development may combine coaching with interventions that involve the client's team, or facilitate meetings with the coaching client and other key figures in the organization. Regardless of the specifics of the executive coach's methodology, all approaches involve the following steps:

- Identifying the client (coachee's) challenge;
- Identifying specific coaching goals that will address the challenge;
- Understanding the challenge in light of self-assessment;
- Creating and brain-storming strategies to achieve goals;

- Acting upon the strategies;
- Tracking success of the strategies, both the tangible outcomes and the client's subjective experience;
- Acknowledging successes; and
- Evaluating the coaching process.

The following is a case study of executive coaching in an academic setting that reflects these steps. It also illustrates many of the challenges addressed in this chapter—the tensions that arise for individual professionals when their institutions undergo changes, when those professionals transition into positions of greater authority, and when the new leader faces the tasks involved in developing not only leadership skills, but leadership consciousness.

EXECUTIVE COACHING CASE EXAMPLE

Case Study Background

This case example involves a nursing department at a large university that was undergoing huge expansion and the promotion of faculty with teaching excellence into positions of administrative leadership (Smith Glasgow, Weinstock, Lachman, Suplee, & Dreher, 2009). The new leaders had great competencies in their areas of clinical and academic expertise, but were new to administrative roles. The Associate Dean made an extraordinary move in providing executive coaching for all of her new academic nurse administrators in order to support them individually and to create a strong team. Since 2006, nine Department Chairs have been, or were currently being, coached. The Associate Dean's wise grasp of the complexities involved in times of transition, her trust in her new department chairs, and her commitment to the development of a strong team, all contributed greatly to the success of this executive coaching project.

Like most large nursing organizations, the college had, from an administrative perspective, a very large, complex undergraduate and graduate nursing program. There were three BSN tracks, ten MSN tracks, and one Doctor of Nursing Practice Program that collectively enrolled a total of 1500 nursing students and employed 60 full-time nursing faculty members as well as 200 adjunct faculty members per term. At that time, several experienced administrators were leaving. After conducting a search, the college hired or promoted faculty who had extensive teaching experience, but minimal administrative experience. In addition to a large group Leadership Symposium to support leadership development for these new leaders, the Associate Dean decided to provide executive coaching for the entire novice group of Department Chairs and Associate Chairs.

Not surprisingly, the new leaders faced all the transition challenges discussed above. For those promoted from within their peer group, they had to readjust boundaries and manage the emotions that accompany authority over former colleagues. Reassigning teaching schedules and clinical placements meant delicately managing a shift in relationships. Privileged information needed to be kept from former friends and discussed only with those in the leadership group. It was no longer appropriate to freely discuss personal feelings about colleagues or about administrative decisions. For some new Department Chairs, this generated the loneliness that can accompany leadership positions.

One Department Chair was brought in from outside the institution to be in charge of a large department undergoing huge growth involving administrative and structural changes. While she was learning systems that were totally unfamiliar to her, she was making decisions that affected large numbers of faculty and staff. Managing these changes meant learning to contain her own anxious emotions, discerning with whom it was safe to share high emotions while consciously working to maintain her self-confidence. Another newly appointed Department Chair came with a whole department that had been independent of the Nursing Department, but who would now report to the Associate Dean. She was faced with no choice but to integrate her department into a faculty group that felt more like a distant relative than immediate family. Thus, while each new Department Chair's story had unique elements, as a new leadership group, they faced the full range of challenges that go with leadership transitions.

Case Study Coaching Methodology

As stated above in the description of executive coaching, there are many different approaches to coaching that vary in how they collect and analyze data, involve other key players in the institution (or not), and establish the specified number of sessions, and time frame, in which the coaching process takes place. In this academic setting, assessing the new leaders' needs and identifying their coaching goals was done with a combination of approaches. A few new leaders were given a "360" feedback survey. All were administered the MBTI. There was also a team meeting of all the new Department Chairs where they shared their leadership style differences that were identified using the MBTI.

All Department Chairs moved through the following sequence of meetings to establish their individual coaching goals.

- The coach met alone with the Associate Dean to hear her assessment of the Department Chair's strengths and challenges.
- The coach met alone with the Department Chair to hear what he or she perceived about the primary challenges to his or her development.
- The coach, Department Chair, and Associate Dean met to share their perceptions and identify coaching goals.

Structuring these first three meetings in this way created the time and space for the Department Chair to identify his/her challenges separately from the Associate Dean's analysis of his/her strengths and challenges. If there were any discrepancies, these became important discussion points in identifying development needs and agreeing upon goals. This process created a three-way buy-in to the coaching goals, and left no room for differing perspectives to fall between the cracks.

Four to six to ten coaching sessions followed, lasting about an hour to an hour and a half. They were designed as individual face-to-face sessions, except for an occasional shared meeting between two Department Chairs to discuss their different leadership styles when this exploration was relevant to their coaching goals. Department Chairs were also encouraged to contact the coach between sessions should they want feedback, or time to discuss a current issue. Throughout the duration of the coaching process, the Department Chairs were encouraged to use the Associate Dean as a mentor—to feel free to ask for feedback on decisions, to stop by her office to ask a question, and/or to brainstorm alternative ways of handling situations. In this way, the Associate Dean was a positive part of the ongoing coaching process and methodology.

The Case Study Coaching Challenges

There were common leadership development themes that emerged with the new leaders in this academic setting, and also some that were unique to the individual coaching client. The following challenges emerged during the coaching process, many of which were targeted as specific goals for individual coaching clients:

- Learning to say 'No' and set boundaries;
- Letting go of perfection in the service of getting things done;
- Attending to relationships over task accomplishment;
- Learning when it is safe to ask questions and to not need to appear as an expert;
- Developing listening skills;
- Creating visibility outside the Nursing School and within the larger university;
- Managing time;
- Identifying patterns of self-sabotage and reversing them;
- Managing self-care in the midst of feeling overwhelmed;
- Creating strategies for stress reduction;
- Modulating emotional reactivity; and
- Finding and developing a personal style of leadership presence.

These themes, and the challenges that they bring, can be expected to appear in most institutions in which there are leadership transitions.

Individual Case Examples from the Case Study

The following two case examples describe the specific challenges and their contexts for two of the newly appointed leaders who generously allowed their stories to be told:

Case I:

Dr. Flynn was promoted to Department Chair after years of teaching excellence at the university. Her development needs included assertiveness, managing conflict, finding a leadership presence, performing responsibilities with greater confidence, articulating opinions within the executive nursing council, and becoming more visible within the larger university system. Dr. Flynn worked closely with Dr. Morgan, the Associate Chair, who had a big personality, had extensive administrative experience, but who was new to the college. Together they inherited a complex department that channeled large numbers of students into different specializations, at a time when the structure for these programs was in flux. Dr. Flynn felt responsible for helping Dr. Morgan learn the ropes and spent many hours in this role behind the scenes. She also let Dr. Morgan be the more visible presence. One year later, Dr. Flynn was seen only in Dr. Morgan's shadow. Coaching sessions with Dr. Flynn focused on her personal barriers to establishing autonomy and on strategies to assert her authority successfully. In the coaching process Dr. Flynn became more comfortable with conflict resolution. She established a separate identity and created greater visibility within the university.

Case II:

Professor Castle was promoted to administrative leadership with a reputation as an excellent teacher and an efficient task-master on any given professional assignment. Extremely introverted, she liked to work with her door closed with minimal social exchange and treasured quiet time alone at her desk. She spent long days at work and looked forward to renewing herself at home after hours. While she was liked by others and always socially appropriate, she maintained a strong personal boundary. Professor Castle was surprised to learn that her new role involved not just task accomplishment, but also informal attention to relationships which involved verbal and visible accessibility which, by nature, she had formerly considered a waste of time. Learning to converse casually in order to gain others' trust and comfort, making daily connections, and stopping by other peoples' offices all were aspects of leadership that had not been on her radar screen. Being more accessible, while also attending to her needs for working and being alone, became a focus for the coaching process. Professor Castle and the coach talked about ways to create greater ease with stopping by other Department Chair's offices, and how she could answer emails so they were to the point, but also made some personal references that would build connection between herself, her faculty reports, and other Department Chairs. They identified hours of the day she could most comfortably have an "open door policy," and other times that she would partially close her door. Over time Professor Castle felt more comfortable with the extroverted parts of her new role and learned to balance her interactive and solo work time (Smith Glasgow et al., 2009).

CONCLUSION

As we work to develop DNP leadership consciousness, we are aware that the DNP role is still in its early development with a wide range of challenges. To date, the nursing profession has not frequently engaged the use of executive coaching to help grow its future leaders. However, with the advent of this new role, it is the right time, and wise, for the DNP graduate and other leaders in the nursing world, as well, to seek support for leadership excellence. Executive coaching can help individuals manifest their talents and resourcefulness and maximize their personal and professional leadership potential. It can inspire and support the nursing profession as it attends to its mission of creating strategies and solutions that improve and heal the human condition.

REFERENCES

Arrien, A. (1993). *The four fold way.* San Francisco, CA: Harper Collins.

Baggott, A. (2000). *The celtic wheel of life.* Dublin, Ireland: Gill & Macmillan.

Barret Values Centre: Supporting Leaders in Building Values-Driven Cultures "The Seven Levels of Leadership Consciousness" (2009). Retrieved from http://www.valuescentre.com/leaders/sllconsciousness.htm

Carroll, L. (1865/1871/1981). *Alice's adventures in wonderland and through the looking glass.* New York, NY: Dell Bantam Books.

Clements, A. (2006, September). A lonely life. *Retail Week*, 34–35. Retrieved from http://www.theturningpoint.co.uk/?page_id=8

Davidson, R. J., Kabat-Zinn, J., Schmacher, J., Rosenkranz, M., Muller, D., & Santorelli, S. F. et al. (2003). Alterations in brain and immune function produced by mindfulness mediation. *Psychosomatic Medicine, 65*, 564–570.

Eisenstat, R., Beer, M., Foote, N., Fredberg, T., & Norrgren, F. (2008). The uncompromising leader. *Harvard Business Review. 86*(7–8), 50–57.

Elsner, D., & Farrands, B. (2006). *Lost in transition: How business leaders can successfully take charge in new roles.* London, UK: Marshall Cavendish.

Gatton, S. (2008). *Home page: What is executive coaching.* S. C. Gatton and Associates, Inc. Retrieved from http://indigoq.com/10029.htm#process

Goleman, D. (1996). *Emotional Intelligence and why it can matter more than IQ.* New York, NY: Bantam Dell.

Hassidic Stories. (2010). Retrieved from Hassidic http://www.hasidicstories.com/Stories/Other_Early_Rebbes/zusia.html

Jimenez, J. R. (1995). *News of the universe: Poems of twofold consciousness.* Bly, R. (Ed., trans.). San Francisco, CA: Sierra Club Books.

Kabat-Zinn, J. (1994). *Wherever you go there you are: Mindfulness mediation in every day life.* New York, NY: Hyperion.

Kabat-Zinn, J., & Chapman-Waldrop, A. (1998). Compliance with an outpatient reduction program: Rates and predictors of completion. *Journal of Behavioral Medicine, 11*, 333–352.

Koestler, A. (1978). *Janus.* New York, NY: Vintage Books.

Kyle, D. (1998). *The four powers of leadership.* Deerfield Beach, FL: Health Communications.

Lepsinger, R., & Lucia, A. D. (1997). *The art and science of 360 degree feedback.* San Francisco, CA: Jossey-Bass.

Omatani, L. M. (2007). Caring, serving . . . Leading. In P. Houston, A. Blankstein, & R. E. Cole (Eds.), *Out of the box leadership* (pp. 31–48). Thousand Oaks, CA: Corwin Press.

Personal Evolution: Health, Fitness and Personal Development. (2010). (Para 1–4), Retrieved from http://www.endlesshumanpotential.com/buddhist-monk-story.html

Shure, J., & Weinstock, B. (2009). Shame, compassion, and the journey towards health. In M. Maine, W. Davis, & J. Shure (Eds.), *Effective clinical practice in the treatment of eating disorders* (pp. 163–177). New York, NY: Routledge.

Smith Glasgow, M. E., Weinstock, B., Lachman, V., Suplee, P. D., & Dreher, H. M. (2009). The benefits of leadership program and executive coaching for new nurse administrators: One college's experience. *Journal of Professional Nursing, 25*(4), 204–210.

Whyte, D. (1994). *The heart aroused.* New York, NY: Doubleday.

CHAPTER THIRTEEN: Reflective Response

Margo A. Karsten

Health care reform, countless stories about the eroding ethics in leadership, lack of trust among front line staff with administration, and a disengaged workforce are ingredients for a perfect storm. However, Weinstock and Smith Glasgow provide a silver lining to this dark health care landscape, by articulating the importance of executive coaching for nursing leaders. They not only explored the many domains of leadership consciousness, but reinforced that executive coaching is an intervention that assists leaders, in this case DNP graduates, to achieve their full potential. The recognition of the impact executive coaching can have on a leader comes at a critical time in health care. Articulating the transition that health care and nursing are currently experiencing, they have highlighted the critical need to have a neutral person that a leader can candidly talk to about the various challenges that face them on a day-to-day basis.

My experience of more than 16 years of administrative practice, including over a decade as chief nurse in various medical centers and experience as a chief operating officer and chief executive officer, gives me firsthand knowledge of what it feels like to transition into various executive roles. The majority of my transitions have come from within the same facility. Learning how to manage former relationships in a new role is an art. New competencies are needed as a person accepts various roles. According to Anderson, organizations are transitioning from traditional paternal forms of organizations to high involvement, empowered partnership, and collaborative learning organizations (Anderson, 2000). These changes warrant a new set of competencies and behaviors. Weinstock and Smith Glasgow captured these new competencies and behaviors in their two case studies.

These two case studies highlight the need for an objective and supportive coach. Growing into a new position can be an awkward transition. Balancing the appropriate autonomy and authority is a challenge that many new leaders struggle to accomplish. As demonstrated in the first case study, an executive coach can assist in this balancing act. The second case study demonstrates another common challenge for leaders; new leaders find themselves at times in a role with high expectations of outgoing sociability. This new expectation of building relationships and creating connections can feel like foreign territory. It has been my experience that new leaders do not understand the importance and value of creating connections with their newly acquired direct reports. Successful leader takes time to create and nurture relationships throughout the work environment. Weinstock and Smith Glasgow highlight the importance of finding the balance of being accessible to a team with an open door policy and creating office time for the leader to be alone in the their second case study. In addition to finding their balance of creating relationships and finding the balance of being available to the team, I found additional challenges in transitioning from the bedside to a management position.

The hidden challenges in professional transitions reflect a previous reality that I experienced in the acute care setting. Loneliness, wavering confidence, boundary setting, questioning my own competency, and staying true to my own identity clearly haunted me as I made my various transitions from bedside to the boardroom. Over the past twelve years, having an executive coach allowed me to overcome these hidden challenges. I believe it is an art to learn how to find your own voice and ensure that it is heard in the appropriate settings. The executive coach is the person who encourages and supports you in finding your voice and reminds you that your main responsibility is *to speak the truth*. Coaching allows professionals to become neutral and objective persons who can be a mirror to reflect their true sense of self.

As Weinstock and Smith Glasgow mentioned, there are many different approaches to coaching. I have found that to be true in my experience as well. Each coach and client will establish how they collect and analyze data, involve other key players in the institution (or not), and establish the specified number of sessions and time frame in which the coaching process takes place. I have found that the use of a "360" feedback survey enriches the coaching experience. Thach (2002) utilized a 360-degree feedback instrument to determine the impact of executive coaching on leadership effectiveness. Two hundred and eighty one leaders participated in 360-degree feedback before and after an average of 6 months of coaching. The overall impact of leadership effectiveness, as perceived by direct reports, peers, and managers was an average of 55% and 60%, respectively, during the two phases of the study. I have experienced similar results when coaching was combined with a 360-feedback tool. Combining a tool that gives a leader insight into her style with an executive coach who can assist in further refining the leadership behaviors and competencies that are critical for success is a perfect formula for leadership effectiveness. Laske (2004) investigated the mental and emotional growth of 6 executives who were coached over 14 months. Coaches and participants' developmental and behavioral profiles were assessed before and after coaching. Three executives made significant developmental progress and were perceived to have improved their leadership effectiveness through the use of coaching. This type of developmental progress takes time and a willingness to reflect on your own personal growth opportunities.

It is important in this period of significant change that nursing leaders take the time to reflect upon their own journey. Weinstock and Smith Glasgow provide reflective questions which stimulate the reader to pause and become introspective about their own lives. As nursing leaders take the time to become introspective, having an executive coach at their sides will only accelerate their personal and professional growth. According to Wales (2002), coaching provides a space for profound personal development and enables leaders to understand how to translate personal insights into improved leadership effectiveness and, ultimately, organizational development. As these authors noted, executive coaching can inspire and support the nursing profession as it attends to its mission of creating strategies and solutions that improve, and heal, the human condition. I believe that creating caring, healing, and compassionate cultures for our team and patients we serve takes an incredible amount of stamina and resilience. The research and evidence is clear: executive coaching can have a profound impact on the conscientiousness of nursing leaders. This leadership intervention will help ensure we lead with our values intact.

REFERENCES

Anderson, J. (2010). The leadership circle. Retrieved from www.leadershipcircle.com

Laske, O. (2004). Can evidence-based coaching increase ROI? *International Journal of Evidence Based Coaching and Mentoring, 2*(2), 41–53.

Thach, E. (2002). The impact of executive coaching and 360 feedback on leadership effectiveness. *Leader Organizational Development Journal, 23*, 3–4.

Wales, S. (2002) Why coaching? *Journal of Change Management, 2*(2), 275–282.

CRITICAL THINKING QUESTIONS

1. What professional transitions have you already experienced in your career development? What were the challenges you faced in making those transitions?
2. If you were promoted into a position of authority over those who are current peers, what challenges do you think you would face?
3. What are the likely transition challenges that the DNP will face in the near future?
4. What expectations or *myths* about new leaders may inhibit smooth transitions into positions of increased authority?
5. How do you define leadership?
6. What do you consider your strengths and weaknesses as a leader?
7. Describe an experience of your professional "personal best." What have you accomplished professionally that you are most proud of? What leadership qualities of yours contributed to your success in this endeavor?
8. What does *leadership consciousness* mean to you? What role models do you have for leaders who embody leadership consciousness?
9. What is executive coaching? In what ways might executive coaching provide leadership development for you in your leadership position?
10. In the executive coaching case example described in this chapter, what interests you the most? Would you have wanted a similar intervention for your professional development?

CHAPTER FOURTEEN

Leveraging Technology to Support Doctoral Advanced Nursing Practice

Frances H. Cornelius, Gary M. Childs, and Linda Wilson

INTRODUCTION

The past decade has been defined by the rapid pace of change and innovation. We live and work in a technology-infused world that promises to become even more integrated with technology in the future. Technology is integral in our efforts to meet the challenges faced by our health care system today and in the future. The doctoral APN (advanced practice nurse) must be proficient in the use of technology to assume a leadership role in efforts to improve practice, and to conduct research to improve health care, systems, and patient outcomes. The doctoral APN will be using technology in a variety of roles—practitioner (and clinical expert), educator, clinical scientist, or nursing administrator—and must be competent in these technologies to be able to leverage their use in every role or setting. A strong recommendation is that the doctoral APN possesses a higher level of technical competency than expected of the master's-prepared APN.

OVERVIEW OF CURRENT ADVANCE PRACTICE NURSE TECHNOLOGY EXPECTATIONS

The Institute of Medicine (IOM, 1999, 2001, 2003) has led the intense scrutiny of our health care system and has focused attention on health care delivery, patient safety, and the education of health professionals. Recent reports have highlighted the need for comprehensive restructuring of the education of all health professionals, with an emphasis on evidence-based practice, quality improvement, and informatics, as well as an interdisciplinary approach to patient-centered care. Given these reports and emerging trends in the health care arena, particularly related to technology, there is a heightened awareness of the importance of essential informatics/technology competencies among nurses at all degree levels. The American Association of Colleges of Nursing (AACN, 2006) supports these recommendations and has proposed that doctorally prepared nurses be poised to assume *key leadership positions* to drive these changes in order to be actively participating in executive decisions to address these important issues. It is for these reasons that the doctoral APN must be prepared to take full advantage of all available technologies to support his/her practice.

EXPECTATIONS FOR THE MASTER'S-LEVEL PRACTITIONER

The AACN (2010) is currently updating its publication that has identified competencies that are essential for master's-prepared nurses to practice effectively (it was last revised in 1996). While technology is assumed to be integrated throughout all the competencies, this AACN draft document explicitly addresses in *Essential V: Informatics and Healthcare Technologies*—five broad areas that these competencies encompass. The masters-level practitioner must be proficient in: 1) Patient care and other technologies to deliver/enhance care; 2) Communication technologies to integrate/coordinate care; 3) Data management to analyze/improve outcomes of care; 4) Health information management for evidence-based care/health education; and 5) Facilitation and use of electronic health records to improve patient care (AACN, 2010, p. 17). No matter the practice setting of the master's-prepared nurse, proficiency in the utilization of technology is crucial to any effort to address health care needs, whether directly or indirectly. The focus at this level is *proficiency*. For the doctoral APN, the expectations are much higher.

RAISING THE BAR: EXPECTATIONS FOR THE DOCTORAL APN

Because the use of technologies to deliver, improve, and document care is changing rapidly in the current, dynamic health care arena, it is absolutely essential that the doctoral APN possesses high-level skills—basic proficiency is insufficient. It is expected that the doctoral APN will function in a leadership role in the use of technologies to support health care delivery (Chase & Pruitt, 2006; Otterness, 2006; Porter-O'Grady & Malloch, 2008; Webber, 2008). It is important that the doctoral APN not only possess these skills, but also take measures to ensure that these skills are kept up-to-date.

The doctoral APN is expected to leverage the skills and knowledge of information systems and technology in both academic and health care settings with the goal of improving patient care and the health care systems charged with providing this care. To accomplish this, the doctoral APN must not only possess technological skills, but also high-level practical research skills in order to be able to contribute to the body of scientific knowledge, and further, to serve as a catalyst for change. We admit this is and will continue to be a debatable point with regard to the practice doctorate—the graduate's role in knowledge development. We assert, however, that the overly simplified adage that the DNP graduate will only translate and disseminate research findings is problematic if it is assumed that all doctoral graduates should contribute to the evidence base of their respective discipline. In addition, he/she must be able to manage and use effectively an increasing volume of evidence to guide practice and establish new standards of care within health care systems. Technologies explored in this chapter will provide doctorally prepared nurses and those beginning doctoral studies an understanding of how these can be utilized effectively to support the advanced practice role and meet these expectations.

INFORMATICS AND TECHNICAL COMPETENCIES FOR THE DOCTORAL APN

The AACN's (2006) *Essentials of Doctoral Education for Advanced Nursing Practice* (AACN, October 2006) has identified specific competencies expected of a doctoral APN. Again, the use of technology is threaded throughout the document; however, Essential IV clearly speaks to expected proficiencies with information systems and patient care technologies. The AACN maintains that nurses at this level are "distinguished by their abilities to use information systems/technology to sustain and improve patient care and health care systems, and provide leadership within health care systems and/or academic settings" (2006, p. 12). The doctoral APN should be able to take a leadership role in: (1) the design, selection, use, and evaluation of technologies for care; (2) analysis and identification of critical elements to assist in the selection and evaluation process of these technologies; and (3) design and implementation of mechanisms to extract data from practice information systems and databases for the purpose of evaluation and improvement in "programs of care, outcomes of care, and care systems" (2006, p. 12). A key competency involves the ability to combine information from a variety of data sources to create new information, and possibly new knowledge, to support care delivery, decision support, and care outcomes. Dreher has recently termed the knowledge emanating out of doctor of nursing practice programs (by both DNP and DrNP graduates) as *practice knowledge* (Dreher, 2010).

Informatics Competencies

It is expected that the doctoral APN would have informatics competencies at an expert level. It is expected that he/she will be a role model to others in the integration and utilization of clinical data systems to support the development of "practice wisdom," the development and application of unified nursing documentation language, the utilization of information systems to improve quality and care outcomes, as well as demonstration of advanced troubleshooting skills (Barton, 2005; Gassert, 2008; Staggers, 2002; Westra & Delaney, 2008).

The Technology Informatics Guiding Educational Reform (TIGER, 2009) initiative has identified three categories of informatics skills: (1) basic computer competency, (2) information literacy, and (3) information management (Gugerty & Delaney, 2009). At an expert level, it is expected that the doctoral APN would possess advanced skills using word processing, spreadsheets, and presentation software. In addition, it is expected that he/she would possess high-level skills in distance learning technologies.

Essential information literacy skills include the ability to:

1. Determine the nature and extent of the information needed;
2. Access needed information effectively and efficiently;
3. Evaluate information and its sources critically and incorporate selected information into his or her knowledge base and value system;
4. Individually or as a member of a group, use information effectively to accomplish a specific purpose; and
5. Evaluate outcomes of the use of information (TIGER Informatics Competency Collaborative, 2009).

Knowledge Management Competencies

Knowledge management competencies are integral to health care and nursing practice (Dreher, 2009a). While it is a growing expectation that nurses at all levels possess knowledge management skills, the doctoral APN must take a leadership role in efforts to document and understand the impact of nursing care on the health of patients. It is through the use of knowledge management systems that these important data can be collected, stored, retrieved, and used to generate knowledge regarding nursing outcomes and improve patient care and safety. Integral to these efforts is the electronic health record (EHR), as it can provide a mechanism to record data collected at the point of care. The doctoral APN must have a good understanding of knowledge management systems in order to influence the design and management of these systems (Canadian Nurses Association, 2006; Contino, 2004; Hsia, Lin, Wu, & Tsai, 2006; Staggers et al., 2002).

In addition, the doctoral APN must champion efforts to have a unified nursing language system that is integrated with universal clinical care terminology. A unified nursing language makes nursing data more visible within health systems and can support the development of nursing knowledge (Coenen & Bartz, 2006). Fully integrated systems can "facilitate communication and data sharing across multiple practitioners, delivery settings, geographic settings and languages" (p. 2) as well as provide an "essential building block for the development of information systems that support clinical decision-making and evidence-based practice" (p. 2). (International Council of Nurses [ICN], n.d.).

TECHNOLOGICAL TOOLS THAT CAN SUPPORT THE DOCTORAL APN

As technological innovation continues, the list of tools continues to grow and can be organized into four categories that support (1) reference management, (2) data collection, (3) data analysis, and (4) report generation. Specific information regarding these tools is presented in Table 14.1.

Reference management tools can be divided into two subcategories: (1) basic reference management tools, and (2) integrated reference management tools. Basic reference management tools include web-based applications such as CiteULike, Connotea, and JabRef. These tools allow the user to collect, organize, and share personal bibliographies and information with colleagues. These resources permit access from any computer and can facilitate collaboration with colleagues who share a similar research interest. Zotero is similar to the other three; however, it offers the additional capability to cite your research sources. A key characteristic shared by these tools is that the bibliography can be accessed from any computer.

Integrated reference management tools take the basic reference management features one step further by integrating a literature database search with reference

TABLE 14.1
Selected Research Tools

Category	Tool	Web Site
Reference management	CiteULike	http://www.citeulike.org
	Connotea	http://www.connotea.org
	JabRef	http://jabref.sourceforge.net
	Zotero	http://www.zotero.org
	Endnote®	http://www.endnote.com
	RefWorks©	http://www.refworks.com
Data analysis and report generation	PSAW (formally SPSS)	http://www.spss.com
	SAS	http://www.sas.com
	Atlas	http://www.atlasti.com
	NVivo	http://www.qsrinternational.com
	Crystal Reports	http://crystalreports.com

management and the writing process. Using the advance functionalities of tools such as RefWorks$^{©}$ and Endnote$^{®}$, the doctorally prepared nurse can write a paper while automatically generating citations and reference lists in the correct format. These tools provide the option to easily switch style formats, such as APA to MLA sometimes required when submitting papers for publication. These tools/skills are useful to the doctoral student, and can also be useful for the clinical scholar beyond graduation given the expectation of dissemination of practice scholarship.

Data collection tools can range from simple Excel spread sheets or Access databases, to more complex electronic medical records (EMRs), to even more sophisticated system-wide data collection systems such as a health information system (HIS). The key consideration for the doctoral APN is that it is imperative that one has a clear understanding of how these various data collection mechanisms operate, how databases are organized, and how these can be utilized to improve patient outcomes and knowledge generation. Collecting and managing data using electronic data collection tools can improve accuracy, completeness, and timeliness of data, consequently ensuring data integrity. All of this then can efficiently supporting enhanced clinical decisions by practitioners/clinicians when delivering patient care or by supporting the nondirect care functions of doctoral advanced nursing practice.

Data analysis and report generation demands yet another skill set involving the use of programs such as PSAW (formally SPSS) or SAS for quantitative data analysis and Atlas or NVivo for qualitative data analysis. In the past, the majority of research conducted by APNs was quantitative. It is important to note that qualitative research in primary care settings is gaining acceptance and is more widespread in the literature (Aflague & Ferszt, 2010; Doherty, 2010; King, Muzaffar, & George, 2009; Tanyi, McKenzie, & Chapek, 2008; Thrasher & Purc-Stephenson, 2007).

Another valuable program for data analysis is Crystal Reports, which permits extraction of information from multiple data sources to create reports. A good understanding of these and similar tools and of how to present information meaningfully is essential. Using tools such as these can help the doctoral APN to not only manage large data sets but to conduct high-level analysis that can generate new knowledge.

PROFESSIONAL ORGANIZATIONS AND INFORMATICS EXPECTATIONS OF THE DOCTORAL APN

American Association of Colleges of Nursing (AACN)

The AACN published *The Essentials of Doctoral Education for Advanced Nursing Practice* in 2006, and some 5 years later it is critically apparent that the original essentials must be revisited. According to the AACN (2006) there are eight essentials including the following: (1) scientific underpinnings for practice; (2) organizational and systems leadership for quality improvement and systems thinking; (3) clinical scholarship and analytical methods for evidence-based practice; (4) *information systems/technology and patient care technology for the improvement and transformation of health care*; (5) health care policy for advocacy in health care; (6) interprofessional collaboration for improving patient and population health outcomes; (7) clinical prevention and population health for improving the nation's health; and (8) advanced nursing practice. We pose the following question: should the informatics competencies be different for students in doctoral advanced practice tracks versus students in the aggregate/systems//organizational tracks??

American Association of Nurse Anesthetists (AANA)

The AANA developed a task force to examine the appropriateness of the doctor of nursing practice degree for the nurse anesthetist. After investigation, the AANA decided to support doctoral education for entry into practice for the nurse anesthetist by the year 2025. In the AANA (2007) position statement on *Doctoral Preparation of Nurse Anesthetists*, it states their rationale: "to best position CRNAs to meet this ongoing challenge and remain recognized leaders in anesthesia care, the AANA believes it is essential to support doctoral education that encompasses technological and pharmaceutical advances, informatics, evidence-based practice, systems approaches to quality improvement, health care business models, teamwork, public relations, and other subjects that will shape the future for anesthesia providers and their patients" (p. 1). It should be noted, however, that the AANA was not exclusively endorsing the "DNP" degree, but other doctoral options for CRNAs as well.

American Academy of Nurse Practitioners (AANP)

The AANP has not specifically identified informatics competencies as an essential component in their official *Position Statement on Nurse Practitioner Curriculum* (2007) or in their *Discussion Paper: Doctor of Nursing Practice* (2010). There is an implication that the APN would possess advanced skills in the roles of manager and researcher who would effectively manage and negotiate health care delivery systems.

American College of Nurse Midwives (ACNM)

The ACNM in their publication *Position Statement: Appropriate Use of Technology in Childbirth* (2003) touches briefly on the use of technology by nurse midwives, but does not specifically address informatics competencies. Their official position is limited to the "use of appropriate technological interventions where the benefits of such technology outweigh the risks" during the childbirth process (ACNM, p. 1). In two other more recent publications, *ACNM Standards for the Practice of Midwifery* and *The Core Competencies for Basic Midwifery Practice*, the organization refers, respectively, to the responsibility of the nurse midwife to promote "a documentation system that provides for confidentiality and transmissibility of health records" (ACNM, 2009, p. 3) and that he/she possess the ability to "evaluate, apply, interpret, and collaborate in research" (ACNM, 2008, p. 3).

National Association of Clinical Nurse Specialists (NACNS)

The NACNS does specifically address informatics competencies in their publications *NACNS Update on the Clinical Nurse Leader* (2005a), *White Paper on Certification of Clinical Nurse Specialists* (2005b), and *Position Statement on the Nursing Practice Doctorate* (2009). However, demonstration of knowledge in the use of "technology, products, and devices that support nursing practice and contribute to improving patient outcomes" is a required component of the certification examination (AACN, 2009, p. 3).

Clearly, not all professional organizations have explicitly identified technological and informatics competencies expected of their professionals. However, given the emerging trends, it is inevitable that these will be forthcoming. It is our view that these will likely be in line with the competencies outlined by the AACN (2006). Competencies will be high level and universal, and easily transferred to a variety of practice settings.

OTHER FACTORS INFLUENCING EXPECTATIONS OF THE DOCTORAL APN

While professional organizations play a key role in influencing expectations of the doctoral APN, there are other entities that are also playing an important role.

The TIGER Informatics Competency Collaborative was created to develop informatics competency expectations and recommendations for all practicing nurses and graduating nursing students (TIGER, 2009). The doctoral APN will need to be competent in the following three primary areas: basic computer competencies, information literacy, and information management.

The Robert Wood Johnson Foundation (RWJF) funded the Quality and Safety Education for Nurses (QSEN) project with the broad objective of "preparing future nurses with the knowledge, skills and attitudes necessary to continuously improve the quality and safety of the health care systems in which they work" (Cronenwett et al., 2007, p. 122). The QSEN has defined six competencies for the professional nurse. These include: professional development, patient-centered care, teamwork and collaboration, evidence-based practice, quality improvement, and safety and informatics. Within each competency there are specific domains of knowledge that must be mastered, skills that must be developed, and attitudes that must be cultivated if a nurse is to deliver high-quality, safe, patient-centered care as a member of a health care team" (Cronenwett et al., p. 127).

The evidence-based practice movement has significant impact for the doctoral APNs. In the clinical expert role, it is imperative for the doctoral APN to promote the use of evidence-based practice, not only in one's own practice, but also as a catalyst for change. The doctoral APN is expected to assume a leadership role within his/her organization and, in this capacity, to spearhead the development of an evidence-driven organization. This requires an in-depth understanding of the organizational components including infrastructure, processes, and behaviors, which must be integrated into efforts to incorporate evidence into all aspects of clinical practice. "Evidence-driven practice is no longer optional and is now a fundamental leadership requisite in all clinical settings" (Porter-O'Grady & Malloch, 2008, p. 176).

ROLE AND RELEVANCE OF THE DOCTORAL APN AND TECHNOLOGY

There are many opportunities and roles within health care for the doctoral APN. While according to AACN (2006), the role of the doctoral APN is specifically in the clinical setting, some DNP programs do focus on the administrator role. Although controversial, some programs also emphasize the doctor of nursing practice's expanded role of clinical scientist in the clinical research industry and of nurse educator. Generally, within contemporary doctor of nursing practice programs, the APN must select one of these four tracks as they seek preparation for a new role.

In the clinical setting, the doctoral APRN (advanced practice registered nurse) works as a nurse practitioner, clinical nurse specialist, nurse midwife, or nurse anesthetist. In this role, the doctoral APRN is the clinical expert providing direct care to the patient. In the educator role, the doctoral APN can work in an academic setting, clinical setting, or staff development setting. The educator APN works with undergraduate students, graduate students, doctor of nursing practice students, and licensed nurses. In the administrator role, the doctoral APN serves in a position of nursing leadership, such as Director of Nursing, Vice President of Nursing, or any other nursing leadership role. In the clinical scientist role, the doctoral APN functions as a clinical researcher. The clinical scientist APN will conduct clinical research and assist staff nurses with activities for any ongoing clinical trials/clinical research activities. Table 14.2 identifies the representative technology competencies for these specific doctoral advanced practice roles.

BEYOND THE DNP DEGREE: STRATEGIES FOR DEVELOPING AND MAINTAINING ESSENTIAL SKILLS

Library Search Skills

Development of library database research-related skills among doctoral APNs is essential to success. Health care providers need to learn how to access and evaluate information used to make clinical decisions (Buus-Frank, 2004). Due to the overwhelming amount of information available and the technological skill that is required to become a thorough researcher, multiple library/research-related workshops are strongly recommended. Whether a formal component within a program or offered on an individualized one-on-one basis, this method allows the librarian to go into more depth and cover more material to build these essential competencies (Megaw & McClendon, 2003). Table 14.3 includes a selected database resource list that is essential for any graduate nursing student.

Both practicing doctoral APNs and students who are entering a doctor of nursing practice program require training to familiarize themselves with the primary academic library they have access to and ensure their database research skills are up-to-date. Components of comprehensive library training include an orientation to the physical as well as the electronic library, an overview of resources and services available, and in-depth database searching. Specific skills that must be developed and maintained include:

1. Use of keyword searching, truncation/wildcard symbols, subject heading searching, Boolean logic, the use of limits (including clinical queries) in databases such as Cumulative Index to Nursing and Allied Health Literature (CINAHL), LexisNexis, and Education Resources Information Center (ERIC).
2. Creation and maintenance of personal accounts within various databases to facilitate the retention of search strategies.
3. Use of the various publication styles such as *Publication Manual of the American Psychological Association* or *American Medical Association Manual of Style* for in-text citation style and references in writing for publication.
4. Use of bibliographic management tools such as RefWorks[C] and EndNote[®], described earlier in this chapter, to assist in organizing and managing writings.
5. Ability to locate evidence-based practice information using "Clinical Queries" in various databases such as PubMed/MEDLINE, the Cochrane Library, the National Guidelines Clearinghouse (NGC), and the TRIP Database (Turning Research into Practice).

TABLE 14.2
Representative Informatics Competencies for Specific Doctoral APN Roles

Practitioner/Clinician	Educator	Clinical Executive	Clinical Scientist
Identify the importance of health information systems (Tiger, 2009)	Identify the importance of health information systems (Tiger, 2009)	Identify the importance of health information systems (Tiger, 2009)	Identify the importance of health information systems (Tiger, 2009)
Demonstrate knowledge of various health information systems (Tiger, 2009)	Demonstrate knowledge of various health information systems (Tiger, 2009)	Demonstrate knowledge of various health information systems (Tiger, 2009)	Demonstrate knowledge of various health information systems (Tiger, 2009)
Recognize the importance of the confidentiality of patient information (Tiger, 2009)	Recognize the importance of the confidentiality of patient information (Tiger, 2009)	Recognize the importance of the confidentiality of patient information (Tiger, 2009)	Recognize the importance of the confidentiality of patient information (Tiger, 2009)
Utilize technology to assist with evidence-based projects and research	Utilize available evaluation and assessment technologies for curricular design/improvements and facilitating learning	Utilize available information technologies to manage organizational operations, guide strategic business development	Utilize evidence to drive improvements in nursing practice and maintain professional standards of practice
Examine the use of technology in clinical, education, and administrative settings	Utilize an evidence-based approach to design systems that support continuous improvement in nursing education	Analyze available systems and financial data to determine value, utility, and significance in the current and future for achieving desired outcomes	Utilize available technologies to collect and analyze patient care data to identify new approaches to improve patient safety and outcomes
Utilize available technologies to collect, store, and examine data	Utilize an evidence-based approach to incorporate instructional technologies, such as simulation into education while collecting and refining assessment data to improve student outcomes	Utilize information systems to conduct organizational assessments to enhance agility, effectively manage resources, and adhere to regulatory standards and industrial/legal responsibilities	Apply information systems knowledge and clinical expertise to participate in the design of clinical information systems
Examine information and its source critically (Tiger, 2009)	Examine information and its source critically (Tiger, 2009)	Examine information and its source critically (Tiger, 2009)	Examine information and its source critically (Tiger, 2009)
Demonstrate how to effectively access information from various sources (Tiger, 2009)	Identify and analyze appropriate student outcome measures to support curricular improvements	Determine the type and amount of information needed (Tiger, 2009)	Demonstrate the ability to access information efficiently (Tiger, 2009)
Examine outcomes of the use of information (Tiger, 2009)	Demonstrate the ability to access resources through library information systems (Tiger, 2009)	Utilize information to accomplish a specific purpose (Tiger, 2009)	Utilize information to accomplish a specific purpose (Tiger, 2009)

TABLE 14.3
Selected Database Resource List

Tool	Web Address
CINAHL (Ebsco Publishing)	http://www.ebscohost.com/cinahl
Cochrane Library (Wiley InterScience)	http://www3.interscience.wiley.com/cgi-bin/mrwhome/106568753/HOME
ERIC (Institute of Education Sciences—U.S. Department of Education)	http://www.eric.ed.gov
LexisNexis Academic (LexisNexis, a division of Reed-Elsevier Inc.)	http://academic.lexisnexis.com/online-services/academic-overview.aspx
National Guidelines Clearinghouse (Agency for Healthcare Research and Quality/U.S. Department of Health and Human Services)	http://www.guideline.gov
PubMed (U.S. National Library of Medicine/National Institutes of Health)	http://www.ncbi.nlm.nih.gov/pubmed
TRIP Database (Turning Research into Practice)	http://www.tripdatabase.com

In our own 2-day DrNP orientation we include a 1 hour tour of the physical library on day 1 to give students an overview of what they have access to. On day 2 they have a 3 hour technology workshop which introduces them to the topics listed above. They also have a 3 hour technology update workshop during their subsequent two summer residencies where they receive further training in the device they were given on entry into the program (e.g., smartphone, iPAD, Kindle, or ACER mini-laptop). Providing research-related training to develop and maintain skills is essential to success within an academic program and can assist with answering clinically related questions in the future.

Life-Long Learning: Keeping Skills Up-to-Date Long After Graduation

Life-long learning is a core value that must be embraced by the doctoral APN. New information that can improve health care, health care systems, and patient outcomes is made available daily. It is an overwhelming task to keep up with the flow of information. There are several strategies and technological tools that can assist doctoral APNs in keeping current. These include: (1) keeping research-related skills current; (2) reference alerts, also known as Selected Dissemination of Information (SDIs); (3) Web 2.0 tools such as RSS and Twitter; and (4) personal learning environments (Dreher, 2009a, 2009b). Some of the Web resources to explore these strategies are included in Table 14.4.

Keeping research-related skills up-to-date can be challenging. Bibliographic databases such as MEDLINE are not static works. New information is added on a routine basis. In addition, valuable features such as subject headings/controlled vocabulary and interfaces that allow researchers to more easily search for new information from endless sources that rapidly change. Furthermore, databases are not just often updated sometimes completely redesigned. Bibliographic management tools receive these updates when new versions are released. Moreover, even publication styles can change (e.g., the *second printing* of the new *Publication Manual of the American Psychological Association: Sixth Edition* [updated from the previous 5th edition] was released in October, 2009).

TABLE 14.4
Selected Web Resource List

Tool	Web Address
Active Worlds Educational Universe	http://www.activeworlds.com
Netvibes (Netvibes Incorporated)	http://www.netvibes.com
Scrapplet (radWEBTECH)	http://www.scrapplet.com/index.html
Second Life (Linden Research Incorporated)	http://secondlife.com
Twitter (Twitter Incorporated)	http://twitter.com
Wonderland (LeadingVirtually.com)	http://www.leadingvirtually.com

There are ways to address these needs in traditional or remote settings. Many libraries offer assistance via telephone, email, and instant messaging. Other forms of contact include collaborative learning software applications, such as Wimba or Adobe Connect, which allow information to be shared in a synchronous or asynchronous fashion via a recorded archive.

Reference alerts are very helpful in providing the busy practitioner an automated mechanism to receive notification of new publications related to a specific topic. After completing a search in a bibliographic database, users can sign up for individual accounts in order to save their searches, relevant citations, and receive current awareness alerts. Users can determine the frequency of alerts along with specifying how they would prefer to receive this type of information. Common formats include email notifications and RSS feeds.

Web 2.0 tools such as RSS feeds and Twitter provide yet another means to support life-long learning. RSS, "really simple syndication," is a mechanism by which individuals or organizations can publish and distribute content, audio, or video to the world. RSS feeds eliminate the need to constantly check to see if there is any new information available by "pushing" out information when it becomes available.

Twitter offers another way to receive updated information using a hybrid instant messenger transmitting 140 characters at a time to a select group. This technology can be useful to communicate with a research team, providing a mechanism to pose a question and get immediate responses. Twitter is a relative newcomer to the social networking arena but has had a major impact already, even on disseminating health information (Dreher, 2009b). Notable examples include an instance when a surgeon sent "tweets" from an operating room when a particularly innovative surgical procedure was underway at Henry Ford Hospital in Detroit, Michigan (Cohen, 2009) or reputable "Tweeters" such as the Center for Disease Control, Johns Hopkins University, Mayo Clinic, and World Health Organization. (Angeles, 2009; Mister Medicine Blog, 2010).

Personal learning spaces, such as NetVibes and Scrapplet, are gaining in popularity as a means to individualize one's web experience by creating a single, personalized page that has the capability to function as an aggregator collecting and organizing RSS feeds and other information from multiple sources. Information collected from news sources such as blogs, social networks, or podcasts will be organized and presented in a uniquely customized manner and automatically updated. One particularly valuable feature is the capability to setup a "watch" dashboard to keep track of subjects of interest. A personalized learning environment permits the user to access "mash up" information. The capability of combining and remixing information, media, content, and web applications and services opens up the opportunity to perceive information in new ways by enhancing life-long learning through a highly personalized experience.

Clearly there is tremendous value to be found in these tools. The strategies and tools described in this section offer the doctorally prepared nurses not only a way to stay up-to-date and support life-long learning activities essential in a dynamic health care arena, but a way to make it both highly personalized and relevant.

TECHNOLOGY FOR LEADERSHIP ROLES AND RESPONSIBILITIES OF THE DOCTORAL APN

The doctoral APN's academic preparation as a clinical expert and leader with an intimate understanding of health care practitioner information needs, places him/her in a position to play an important role in influencing the health care system. Important competencies to meet the challenges of this role include a broad understanding of basic information management, strong communication skills, and the ability to work collaboratively with interdisciplinary teams that include health care professionals, administration, and HIT.

Interfacing With Information Systems Teams

In a highly complex health care system, interprofessional collaboration is essential, and it is expected that the doctoral APN will be prepared to interface effectively with the information systems team in order to help shape organizations and to drive system changes essential in supporting APN needs and needs of evolving health care systems. This necessitates not only skills in communication and a keen understanding of organizational behavior, but it also requires a working knowledge of hospital information systems and systems, life cycles in order to participate in the ongoing dialogue to improve patient outcomes. The 4th and 6th DNP essentials identify this role for the APN as critical in efforts to transform the health care system (AACN, 2006; Smith & McCarthy, 2010). As Health Information Systems and Patient Care Technologies are becoming more and more central to health care delivery, the APN must be prepared to utilize these technologies, not only in practice, but also to actively participate in efforts to use these technologies to drive transformation. Owing to the dynamic nature of health care systems, interprofessional teams are fluid and adjust to accommodate system needs. The doctoral APN must be prepared to be an active member of the team, playing "a central role in establishing interprofessional teams, participating in the work of the team, and assuming leadership of the team when appropriate" (AACN, 2006, p. 14).

Interfacing With Libraries for Research-Based Support

Interfacing with key librarians for research-based support can be extremely beneficial. Libraries are variable, for example, in physical size, staff size, scope of subject coverage, access to resources, and classification schemes. Obtaining specific information from an institution's library related to materials/resources and available services allows beginning researchers to focus on locating data versus having to discover appropriate resources on their own. Connections to individual members of the library staff can be built and overtime can be critical to sustaining a research career. Our program has been fortunate to have a longstanding librarian assigned to work with our doctoral nursing students.

There may be subject specific reference librarians who can assist with navigating the library catalog, electronic databases (e.g., MEDLINE, CINAHL), and bibliographic management tools (e.g., EndNote®, RefWorks©). As indicated earlier, reference librarians have considerable expertise in this area and spend a large portion of their workday providing assistance to patrons who require skills related to database searching and associated technology. Due to their focus on these types of skills, reference librarians can provide assistance to beginning, intermediate, and advanced researchers.

EVOLVING AND EMERGING TRENDS TO ENHANCE DOCTORAL APNS

Simulation

There are many opportunities for the doctoral level APN to use simulation including education, clinical practice, and research. Typically, simulation activities utilize human patient simulators or standardized patients. On occasion, the two are combined to create a hybrid simulation experience.

The Human Patient Simulator is a simulation mannequin device. There are many different vendors and levels of fidelity available with the human patient simulators. An example of a low-fidelity human patient simulator would be a simulator that would be able to portray lung and heart sounds. A high-fidelity simulator would be a simulator that would be able to demonstrate realistic body functions and even diaphoresis. The varying levels of fidelity go along with varying levels of programmable software to be used to develop and run patient scenarios.

A standardized patient is an actor who is trained to demonstrate realistically a selected patient scenario. In this type of simulation, the scenario is developed very similarly to an actor's script. This scrip contains all the information needed by the standardized patient to act out the scenario including the following: (1) all questions that can be asked and the appropriate response; (2) emotions to be portrayed; (3) student or nurse items to be examined following the scenario; and (4) specific feedback to be provided to the simulation participant following the completion of the scenario.

Hybrid simulation is a simulation experience where there is a combined use of both the human patient simulator and a standardized patient. Examples of a hybrid scenario include the following: (1) a standardized patient portraying the mother of a child and the child represented by an infant human patient simulator; (2) a human patient simulator used as a patient and a standardized patient portraying a sibling or a significant other; and (3) an obstetrical patient with vaginal complications where the vaginal area is a simulator or task trainer.

Simulation to Enhance and Evaluate Competency

The doctoral APN (or student) can use simulation strategies to evaluate competencies in an academic educational program or in a clinical setting. Competencies can be assessed using human patient simulators, standardized patients, or task trainers. In each of these types of simulations, specific competency assessments or expected outcomes must be identified in advance. Then, depending on the type of simulation utilized, a competency evaluator must be identified such as the standardized patient, a faculty member, a clinical manager, or others. Simulation is a very effective tool that can be used to provide complex situations in a very safe environment (Kneebone, 2006).

Simulation for Research

The doctoral APN (and student) can also use simulation strategies in many types of research in the academic setting and the clinical setting. Simulation can be used to portray a limitless number of scenarios. These scenarios can be specific to a particular educational activity, an educational process, an interaction, or a self evaluation. A variety of research designs can also be included such as a pretest/posttest design or a posttest-only design. Simulation has many advantages such as control of extraneous variables, standardization of data collection procedures, and manipulation of variables of interest (Lanza, 1990).

TECHNOLOGIES THAT SUPPORT COMMUNICATION AND INFORMATION ACCESS IN MOBILE ENVIRONMENTS

Over the past decade, mobile devices (e.g., PDAs and Smartphones) have had an increasing presence in the health care arena. These devices have significantly improved "information access, enhance workflow, and promote evidence-based practice to make informed and effective decisions at the point of care" (Lua, Xiaoa, Searsb, & Jackoc, 2005, p. 409). Mobile devices provide "real-time" access to health care information and have transformed the way information is managed in the health care arena (Siau & Shen, 2006). It is expected these devices will be even more pervasive in health care as product and software improvements are released. The true value of these devices will not be fully realized until institutions provide seamless integration with hospital information systems permitting access to essential information at any place and any time via wireless networks.

One particular benefit of a widely dispersed, integrated system will likely be reduced medical errors resulting from improved access to vital information (Varshney, 2007). The doctoral APN must not only be proficient in the use of these technologies, but also be prepared to champion mobile initiatives as a means to "improving quality of care, enhancing patient services, increasing productivity, lowering costs, improving cash flow, as well as facilitating other critical delivery processes"(Lin & Vassar, 2004, p. 343).

VIRTUAL WORLDS FOR EDUCATION AND RESEARCH

Second Life, Active Worlds, Wonderland, and other virtual worlds offer extraordinary opportunities for education, simulation, and research. In education, a virtual world can provide an enriched learning experience, strengthen the sense of social presence, and utilize multilevel interaction and enriched multimedia resources employing a constructivist approach in the learning process (Wang & Hsu, 2009). Virtual worlds are important to higher education because these environments: (1) offer an immersive environment where users interact and construct knowledge; (2) shift from a traditional dissemination tool to one where users create and design content to add value and meaning; and (3) provide learners an array of opportunities for interaction within a multi-user environment (Skiba, 2007).

Virtual worlds have been utilized in health professions education with great success. Initial endeavors suggest that virtual worlds offer extraordinary opportunities for educators to enhance learning outcomes beyond that which is provided by more conventional online or face-to-face classroom experiences. Virtual worlds offer rich opportunities for postgraduate professional development activities, continuing education, professional certification or recertification, and much more. This very flexible environment can be utilized to stage experiences that help students and health care professionals build cultural competency and improve communication and patient interviewing skills. In addition, virtual worlds have been utilized to provide very realistic disaster simulation training (Simon, 2010; Wiecha, Heyden, Sternthal, & Merialdi, 2010; Young, 2010).

Virtual worlds provide opportunities for creativity that are not limited by the laws of physics, financial constraints, or geography. Realistic environments and simulation experiences can be designed to educate and conduct research by containing costs while simultaneously expanding your reach to vast numbers of students and potential research subjects.

While virtual worlds can be utilized for education, simulation, and research purposes, caution is advised. Due to the nature of massive multiplayer games, users may encounter some less-than-ideal occurrences including vandalism and other disruptions (Boulos, Hetherington, & Wheeler, 2007). One notable example mentioned in a previous work by Childs (2008) involved an online chat that was disrupted by digitally rendered, flying objects. These instances can be proactively managed effectively by using available security settings within the virtual environment. In addition, as a means to combat these malicious attacks, virtual worlds offer policing and enforce strict sanctions to offenders (Boulos et al., 2007).

WHAT'S ON THE HORIZON?

These are very exciting times. It is a time in which technological innovations are emerging rapidly and diffusion of these technologies is taking place at an unprecedented rate (Kittleson, 2009). Major shifts will involve: (1) a "smarter web" through parallel processing capabilities; (2) more personalization; (3) true portability of personalized web content via expanded access and cloud computing; (4) increasing data collection and analysis capabilities; and (5) interoperability.

A major innovation in the future will be a "smarter Internet." In the very near future, the parallel processing technology will make it possible for the Internet to "recognize" the relevance of information as it appears in real time. The convergence of "all of this data and these technologies will necessitate sophisticated algorithmic models to aid interpretation and decision making" (Newton, 2009, p. 1). The design of these models will require the input of health care professionals such as the doctoral APN.

A major benefit of expanded processing capabilities will likely be with more intelligent search tools that will be "smarter," functioning similar to a personal assistant who "knows" your likes and dislikes and "understands" the context of the information being sought. As a result, searches for information will deliver personalized and highly relevant information directly to your Personal Learning Environment (PLE) no matter where you are. Currently, the focus is upon social networking and connections to people. The shift in the future will be increased connections to information that will have limitless application for practice.

"Cloud computing" is here to stay, and this will further increase the portability of personalized web content. As more and more applications, content, and communities become web based, we will demand access to the web anytime and everywhere. It is expected that expanded bandwidths and the capabilities of smart phones and other wireless devices globally will continue to evolve and further expand opportunities to access and utilize data (Newton, 2009).

Another transformative change that is anticipated with the expanded functionality of the Internet (smarter web and ubiquitous wireless network access) is the ability to use widely dispersed sensors to collect all types of data. The data collection possibilities will thus be limitless. For example, sensors can collect "...vital signs, energy usage, soil moisture, traffic patterns, manufacturing efficiency ... it will all be tracked remotely and analyzed in real time and fed into the Smart Web" (Newton, 2009, p. 1). This opens the door for extraordinary research opportunities; however, consideration must be given to the privacy concerns that are bound to arise. The doctoral APN must be prepared to take a leadership role in supporting new research while championing the privacy rights of the individual.

It is reasonable to expect that all advances in technology described thus far will impact the heath care system. One major impact will be on system interoperability. Currently, hospital systems are not integrated and, consequently, system wide communication is impaired, making it difficult to provide seemless care. Improved data tracking and tightly integrated systems will transform health care by improving disease management and patient outcomes. Health care delivery will likely become more decentralized due to an extensive network-based system, high-tech equipment, and software permitting more sophisticated telemedicine encounters in one's home. This interoperability will spill over to other areas of the health care system and even our personal lives, bringing new levels of "life-wide" connectivity across the lifespan.

Second Life, Active Worlds, Wonderland, and other virtual worlds will become more sophisticated, and we will likely see overlap between virtual worlds and the real world via technologies that enable "augmented reality" interfaces. This blend will enhance our opportunities to provide rich simulated learning experiences for students, support continuing education among our practicing professionals, and conduct research. In addition, augmented reality technology will also provide the capability to provide enhanced clinical decision support in real time at the bedside where it is needed most and will have the greatest impact upon patient outcomes.

SUMMARY

This chapter provided an overview of technological tools that provide opportunities to work more efficiently and effectively to deliver, improve, and document care in our health system. It is absolutely essential that the doctoral APN possess high-level skills in the use of technologies to support health care delivery in order to function effectively in a leadership role (Chase & Pruitt, 2006; Otterness, 2006; Porter-O'Grady & Malloch, 2008; Webber, 2008). The APN must be able to utilize technology to better manage and use an increasing volume of evidence to guide practice and establish new standards of care within health care systems. The doctoral APN must *leverage these technologies* to generate more evidence-based and practice-based scientific knowledge and serve as a catalyst for change.

REFERENCES

Aflague, J. M., & Ferszt, G. G. (2010) Suicide assessment by psychiatric nurses: A Phenomeno-graphic study. *Issues in Mental Health Nursing, 31*, 248–256.

American Academy of Nurse Practitioners (AANP). (2007). *Position statement on nurse practitioner curriculum*. Retrieved from http://www.aanp.org/NR/rdonlyres/59523729-0179-466A-A7FB-BDEE68160E8E/0/NPCurriculum.pdf

American Academy of Nurse Practitioners (AANP). (2010). *Discussion paper: Doctor of nursing practice*. Retrieved from http://www.aanp.org/NR/rdonlyres/9DC9390F-145D-4768-995C-1C1FD12AC77C/0/AANPDNPDiscussionPaper.pdf

American Association of Colleges of Nursing (AACN). (2006). *The essentials of doctoral education for advanced nursing practice*. Retrieved from http://www.aacn.nche.edu/dnp/pdf/essentials.pdf

American Association of Colleges of Nursing (AACN). (2009). *Clinical nurse specialist core exam board certification*. Retrieved from http://www.nursecredentialing.org/Documents/Certification/TestContentOutlines/CNSCoreExamTCO.aspx

American Association of Colleges of Nursing (AACN). (2010, August 23). *Draft The Essentials of Master's Education in Nursing*. Retrieved from http://www.aacn.nche.edu/Education/pdf/DraftMastEssentials.pdf

American Association of Nurse Anesthetists (AANA). (2007). *AANA position on doctoral preparation of nurse anesthetists*. Retrieved from http://www.aana.com/uploadedfiles/members/membership/resources/dtf_posstatemt0707.pdf

American College of Nurse Midwives (ACNM). (2003). *Position statement: Appropriate use of technology in childbirth*. Retrieved from http://www.midwife.org/siteFiles/position/Approp_Use_of_Tech_05.pdf

American College of Nurse Midwives (ACNM). (2008). *The core competencies for basic midwifery practice*. Retrieved from http://www.midwife.org/siteFiles/descriptive/Core_Competencies_6_07_000.pdf

American College of Nurse Midwives (ACNM). (2009). *ACNM standards for the practice of midwifery*. Retrieved from http://www.midwife.org/siteFiles/descriptive/Standards_for_Practice_of_Midwifery_12_09_001.pdf

Angeles, R. (2009). *Health care professionals and organizations using Twitter*. Retrieved from http://socialmediaphilippines.com/health-care-professionals-and-organizations-using-twitter

Barton, A. J. (2005). Cultivating informatics competencies in a community of practice. *Nursing Administration Quarterly, 29*(4), 323–328.

Boulos, M. N. K., Hetherington, L., & Wheeler, S. (2007). Second Life: An overview of the potential of 3-D virtual worlds in medical and health education. *Health Information and Libraries Journal, 24*, 233–245.

Buus-Frank, M. E. (2004). What you don't know can hurt you. *Advances in Neonatal Care, 4*(1), 1–5.

Canadian Nurses Association. (2006). *Position statement: Nursing information and knowledge management*. Retrieved from http://www.cna-nurses.ca/cna/documents/pdf/publications/ps87-nursing-info-knowledge-e.pdf

Chase, S. K., & Pruitt, R. H. (2006). The practice doctorate: Innovation or disruption? *Journal of Nursing Education, 45*(5), 155.

Childs, G. M. (2008). Are you ready for Second Life: Primer for online virtual society software. *MLA News, 403*, 20.

Coenen, A., & Bartz, C. (2006). A unified nursing language system. *Nursing Outlook, 54*(6), 362–364.

Contino, D. S. (2004). Leadership competencies: Knowledge, skills, and aptitudes nurses need to lead organizations effectively. *Critical Care Nurse, 24*, 52–64.

Cronenwett, L., Sherwood, G., Barnsteiner, J. H., Disch, J., Johnson, J., Mitchell, P. et al. (2007). Quality and safety education for nurses. *Nursing Outlook, 55*(3), 122–131.

Doherty, M. E. (2010) Voices of midwives: A tapestry of challenges. *The American Journal of Maternal/Child Nursing, 35*(2), 96–101.

Dreher, H. M. (2009a). How do RNs today best stay informed? Do we need 'knowledge management'? *Holistic Nursing Practice, 23*(5), 263–266.

Dreher, H. M. (2009b). Twittering about anything, everything and even health. *Holistic Nursing Practice, 23*(4), 217–221.

Dreher, H. M. (2010). Next steps toward practice knowledge development: An emerging epistemology in nursing. In M. D. Dahnke, & H. M. Dreher, *Philosophy of science for nursing practice: Concepts and application.* New York, NY: Springer.

Gassert, C. A. (2008). Technology and informatics competencies. *Nursing Clinics of North America, 43*(4), 507–521.

Gugerty, B., & Delaney, C. (2009). TIGER Informatics Competencies Collaborative (TICC): Final report. *Technology Informatics Guiding Educational Reform (TIGER).*

Hsia, T.-L., Lin, L.-M., Wu, J.-H., & Tsai, H.-T. (2006). A framework for designing nursing knowledge management systems. *Interdisciplinary Journal of Information, Knowledge, and Management, 1,* 13–22.

Institute of Medicine (IOM). (1999). *To err is human: Building a safer health system.* Washington, DC: National Academies Press.

Institute of Medicine (IOM). (2001). *Crossing the quality chasm: A new health system for the 21st century.* Washington, DC: National Academies Press.

Institute of Medicine (IOM). (2003). *Health professions education: A bridge to quality.* Washington, DC: National Academies Press.

International Council of Nurses. (n.d.). *About ICN.* Retrieved from http://www.icn.ch/abouticn.htm

International Council of Nurses. (n.d.). *Nursing matters fact sheet: Nursing informatics.* Retrieved from http://www1.icn.ch/matters_informatics.pdf

King, T., Muzaffar, S., & George, M. (2009). The role of clinic culture in implementation of primary care interventions: The case of reach out and read. *Academic Pediatrics, 9*(1), 40–46.

Kittleson, M. J. (2009). The future of technology in health education: Challenging the traditional delivery dogma. *American Journal of Health Education, 40*(6), 310–316.

Kneebone, R. L. (2006). Crossing the line: Simulation and boundary areas. *Simulation in Healthcare, 1*(3), 160–163.

Lanza, M. L. (1990). A methodological approach to enhance external validity in simulation based research. *Issues in Mental Health Nursing, 11,* 407–422.

Lin, B., & Vassar, J. A. (2004). Mobile healthcare computing devices for enterprise-wide patient data delivery. *International Journal of Mobile Communications, 2*(4), 343–353.

Lua, Y.-C., Xiaoa, Y., Searsb, A., & Jackoc, J. A. (2005). A review and a framework of handheld computer adoption in healthcare. *International Journal of Medical Informatics, 74*(5), 409–422.

Megaw, A., & McClendon, J. (2003). One-shot to a full barrel. In J. K. Nims, & E. Owens (Eds.), *Managing library instruction programs in academic libraries* (pp. 113–115). Ann Arbor, MI: Pierian Press.

Mister Medicine Blog. (2010). *50 authoritative tweeters with daily health tips.* Retrieved from http://www.lvntorn.net/50-authoritative-tweeters-with-daily-health-tips.html.

National Association of Clinical Nurse Specialists. (2005a). *NACNS update on the clinical nurse leader.* Retrieved from http://www.nacns.org/LinkClick.aspx?fileticket=3%2bip4nbDLho%3d&tabid=116

National Association of Clinical Nurse Specialists. (2005b). *White paper on certification of clinical nurse specialists.* Retrieved from http://www.nacns.org/LinkClick.aspx?fileticket=%2ftvaTXjUbGY%3d&tabid=116

National Association of Clinical Nurse Specialists. (2009). *Position statement on the nursing practice doctorate.* Retrieved from http://www.nacns.org/LinkClick.aspx?fileticket=TOZlongI258%3d&tabid=116

Newton, T. (2009, November 25). Ten Trends for 2010. *Forbes.com.*

Otterness, S. (2006). Implications of doctorate in nursing practice—Still many unresolved issues for nurse practitioners. *Nephrology Nursing Journal, 33*(6), 685.

Porter-O'Grady, T., & Malloch, K. (2008). Beyond myth and magic: The future of evidence-based leadership. *Nursing Administration Quarterly, 32*(3), 176–187.

Siau, K., & Shen, Z. (2006). Mobile healthcare informatics. *Informatics for Health and Social Care, 31*(2), 89–99.

Simon, S. (2010, April 13). Avatar II: The hospital. *The Wall Street Journal*, p. R8. Retrieved from http://online.wsj.com/article/SB10001424052748703909804575124470868041204.html?mod=WSJ_topics_obama

Skiba, D. J. (2007). Nursing education 2.0: Second Life. *Nursing Education Perspectives, 28*(3), 156–157.

Smith, M., & McCarthy, M. P. (2010). Disciplinary knowledge in nursing education: Going beyond the blueprints. *Nursing Outlook, 58*(1), 44–51.

Staggers, N., Gassert, C. A., & Curran, C. (2002). Results of a Delphi study to determine informatics competencies for nurses at four levels of practice. *Nursing Research, 51*(6), 383–390.

Tanyi, R. A., McKenzie, M., & Chapek, C. (2009). How family practice physicians, nurse practitioners, and physician assistants incorporate spiritual care in practice. *Journal of the American Academy of Nurse Practitioners, 21*, 690–697.

Thrasher, C., & Purc-Stephenson, R. (2007). Integrating nurse practitioners into Canadian emergency departments: A qualitative study of barriers and recommendations. *CJEM: Journal of the Canadian Association of Emergency Physicians, 9*(4), 275–281.

TIGER Informatics Competency Collaborative. (2009). *TIGER informatics competencies*. Retrieved from http://tigercompetencies.pbworks.com/

Varshney, U. (2007). Pervasive healthcare and wireless health monitoring. *Mobile Networks and Applications, 12* (2–3), 113–127.

Wang, S.-K., & Hsu, H.-Y. (2009). Using the ADDIE model to design second life activities for online learners. *TechTrends, 53*(6), 76–82.

Webber, P. B. (2008). The doctor of nursing practice degree and research: Are we making an epistemological mistake? *Journal of Nursing Education, 47*(10), 466.

Westra, B. L., & Delaney, C. (2008, November 6). Informatics competencies for nursing and healthcare leaders. *AMIA Annu Symp Proc.*, 804–808.

Wiecha, J., Heyden, R., Sternthal, E., & Merialdi, M. (2010). Learning in a virtual world: Experience with using Second Life for medical education. *Journal of Medical Internet Research, 12*(1):e1, Doi: 10.2196/jmir.1337. Retrieved from http://www.jmir.org/2010/1/e1/

Young, J. R. (2010).After frustrations in Second Life, colleges look to new virtual worlds: The hype is gone, but not the interest, and professors think some emerging projects may have instructional staying power. *The Chronicle of Higher Education, 56*(23), p. A14.

Victoria M. Bradley

Informatics knowledge and skills are essential for all of the roles of the doctoral advanced practice nurse (APN) as technology increasingly permeates every component of the health care delivery system. The authors provide an extensive, informative review of the technology tools available to the doctoral APN and suggest ways they can be deployed to enhance practice and transform care. I absolutely agree that at the doctoral level advanced practitioners need a higher level of technical competency to practice and lead in this technology era. I also agree that DNP graduates should contribute to the evidence base of their discipline, through an ongoing measurement of both process and outcomes. I have, however, a few considerations and additions gained from my experiences as a DNP graduate with informatics as my specialty.

In the technological tools section, I would additionally suggest workflow and mind mapping software such as Smartdraw or Visio. In the technology drill down study Burnes, Glassert and Cipriano (2008) reported that 766 unique process issues (out of 946) were required to improve and enable nurses to spend more time at the bedside to address patient care needs. One of the most common reasons for lack of adoption of clinical information systems is that the system does not support the nurse's workflow. Routine consistent use of these tools may decrease the number of workarounds that evolve with implementations when changes in workflow patterns are not adequately addressed. Reference management and report writing tools are nice to know but suggest prioritization of workflow tools higher in the chain of what technologies support advanced practice. Having said that, with each new release of these tools, they have become increasingly user friendly, and so it will become much easier to be competent in their use.

I was delighted to see the Technology Informatics Guiding Educational Reform (TIGER) initiative reference. This is a rich resource of information for incorporating informatics into all levels of practice. Increasing knowledge about health information technology among practicing nurses is a recognized challenge and is also being addressed in a number of ways by the organizations within the Alliance for Nursing Informatics.

The authors describe one of the key competencies of the doctoral APN as interfacing with the information systems team. It is necessary that the doctoral APN understand what technologies are available and how these technologies can be deployed to improve the care delivery system. Stead and Lin (2009) describe four domains of information technology in health care: automation, connectivity, decision support, and data-mining capabilities. When seeking solutions for problem solving or ways to improve practice, the technology competent doctoral APN would be able to recommend how the technology could be deployed to resolve the issue, and then conduct an evaluation to see if the change is effective and if any unintended consequences occur. For example, the system can be used to calculate doses (automation) or decision support to warn a nurse if a prescribed dose is out of range based on age and/or weight. For connectivity, a device interface from mobile vital sign monitors to clinical documentation could eliminate delays in access to the information and eliminate transcription errors. The doctoral APN can determine what data are needed in a report or a dashboard to facilitate recognition and prioritization of issues by organizational units or by patient population. The doctoral APN does not need to be a programmer but needs to understand what the electronic health record can do for him or her, other members of the care delivery team, and consumers. By working collaboratively with the information system team, the doctoral APN can continue to discover the most effective technology strategy to meet patient care needs.

It was interesting to read about informatics competencies in some of the specialty groups. The National Association of Pediatric Nurse Practitioners (NAPNAP) position statement (2008) agrees with the development of the doctorate in nursing practice (DNP) as the appropriate credential and level of education for advanced practice nursing. They have a web page with a short list of technology resources for practice. In comparison, the American Association of Nurse Executives (AONE) has many more informatics resources. They support informatics as an essential competency for the nurse executive. The *AONE Position Statement Doctorate of Nursing Practice* (2007a) supports the DNP as a terminal degree option for practice-focused nursing; however, they also believe in the retention of the nursing master's-degree programs in nursing administration.

In 2005 AONE published their *Nurse Executive Competencies* which described five levels of competencies: Communication and relationship-building, knowledge of the health care environment, leadership, professionalism, and business skills. Included under business skills is information management and technology which contains 14 skills covering specifics such as email, word processing, spreadsheet, databases, and decision support to broader skills including evaluation of information systems and awareness of new technological and societal trends. It is interesting that they do not include reference management tools, nor do they include quantitative or qualitative data analysis tools, suggesting that there may be different competencies at the doctoral level for the different specialties of practice.

They also have published the *AONE Guiding Principles for Defining the Role of the Nurse Executive in Technology Acquisition and Implementation* (AONE, 2007b) and the *AONE Guiding Principles for the Nurse Executive to Enhance Clinical Outcomes by Leveraging Technology* (2009). These documents describe top priorities for the nurse executive to assure that there is a defined governance model that oversees technology: to define clear, measurable, clinical outcomes for each technology initiative/project, and to assume ownership of the process roadmap for future work redesign and the relationships that manage the process.

AONE (2010) also has a certification for the nurse executive "Certified in Executive Nursing Practice (CENP)." The examination content outline includes a section on information management and technology with the following content areas:

1. Identify effective uses of informatics resources for performance improvement
2. Identify effective uses of informatics resources for patient care processes and systems
3. Utilize informatics resources to analyze data from disparate sources
4. Participate in system change processes and utility analyses
5. Participate in evaluation of enabling technology in practice settings

6. Use data management systems to process administrative data
7. Identify technological trends, issues, and new developments as they apply to nursing
8. Demonstrate skills in assessing data integrity and quality
9. Lead implementation of information systems within the work setting
10. Advocate for adequate resources for implementing information systems

The American Nurses Credentialing Center (ANCC) offers Nurse Executive Board Certification (NE-BC) and Advanced Board Certification (NEA-BC) which includes informatics competencies for technology planning and management. NE-BC certification requires a Bachelors of Science in Nursing degree and covers five major topics: Delivery of Care; Legal, Regulatory and Ethical Issues; Healthcare Economics; Healthcare Environment; and Professional Practice (ANCC, 2008a). The NEA-BC content outlines five central domains of practice: 1) Quality Management/Care Management; 2) Professional Practice Environment; 3) Organizational Leadership; 4) Organizational Systems Management; and 5) Communication/Collaboration (ANCC, 2008b). It is noteworthy that the competencies from these two organizations are different. They both list evaluation as a competency. I would recommend that the nurse executive attain both sets of competencies.

One of the key roles of the doctoral APN is to support evidence-based practice. A competency, however, that is described but needs more attention for all doctoral APNs is the field of clinical decision support (CDS). As scientific knowledge continues to grow at an amazing rate, it has become impossible for a clinician to keep up—not to mention all the distractions occurring in the clinical environment. Use of clinical information systems provides an opportunity to integrate knowledge and decision support so that they are available to clinicians as needed. I would expect the doctoral APN to make recommendations from the review of the standard of care and best evidence on how CDS could be used to improve the care delivered. For example, are there components of the assessment that are routinely being missed? If so, should the data elements be rearranged on the form or reminders given when documents are submitted with missing data fields or fields made mandatory, to ensure collection of complete and accurate information? What alerts and reminders are helpful? Osheroff and colleagues (2005) described six primary ways that decision support can be provided to clinicians: Documentation forms/templates, relevant data presentations, order/prescription creation facilitators, time-based checking/protocol pathway support, reference information and guidance, and reactive alerts and reminders. Excellent resources can also be found on the Agency for Healthcare Research and Quality (AHRQ) web site on the HIT (Health Information Technology) CDS Initiative (2010). The majority of this work to date relates to physicians. Mitchell et al. (2009) have found little research examining what CDS systems are available to nurses or the characteristics the systems possess in comparison with physicians. Dowding et al. (2009) found that nurses used CDS systems to record information, monitor patients' progress, or confirm a decision that they had already made. Use was influenced by how well the nurse knew the patient, their experience, and how well it fit in their workflow. These studies were, however, conducted in the National Health Service in England. We need the assistance of doctoral APNs to both develop and further evaluate the use of CDS systems for nursing.

I would propose that there is a fifth doctoral APN role in the field of clinical informatics. Nurse informaticists are functioning in senior leadership roles such as chief nursing informatics (or information) officer (CNIO) or VP of Clinical Informatics (Swindle & Bradley, 2010). The CNIO is an expert in the field of *nursing informatics,* which has been recognized as a specialty by the American Nurses Association (2008) since 1992 and defined as

> a specialty that integrates nursing science, computer science, and information science to manage and communicate data, information, knowledge, and wisdom in nursing practice. Nursing informatics supports consumers, patients, nurses, and other providers in their decision-making in all roles and settings. This support is accomplished through the use of information structures, information processes, and information technology.
>
> —*American Nurses Association, 2008, p. 1*

There is, however, no advanced certification for the informatics role at present. Instead, the ANCC has a specialty certification for informatics only requiring a bachelor's degree in nursing or other relevant field. This certification covers seven major topic areas: System Life Cycle; Human Factors; Information Technology; Information Management and Knowledge Generation; and Professional Practice, Trends, and Issues; Models and Theories; and Management and Leadership (ANCC, 2007). There is therefore a need to establish competencies for the doctoral APN in informatics if this is to become a recognized advanced practice specialty. This role has many of the competencies in common with the other doctoral APN roles except that their specialty and field of research is informatics. I believe that the DNP course of study could prepare APNs in informatics.

I support the authors' emphasis on library search skills as critical to support lifelong learning. Further, I applaud their inclusion of social networking as the doctoral APN needs to be aware and keep abreast of what consumers and their patients are using to manage their health as well as identify ways these tools can augment their practice.

There is a lot of material to be covered in the informatics arena. The authors have provided an extensive informative review of the technology tools available to the DNP student and doctoral APN and have suggested ways in which they can transform care. This review is a good starting point for further discussion and development of the informatics competencies of the doctoral APN.

REFERENCES

Agency for Healthcare Research and Quality (AHRQ). (2010). *Clinical decision support initiative*. Retrieved from http://healthit.ahrq.gov/portal/server.pt/community/ahrq-funded_projects/654/clinical_decision_support_initiative/13665

American Nurses Association. (2008). *Nursing informatics: Scope and standards of practice*. Silver Spring, MD: NursesBooks.org

American Nurses Credentialing Center (ANCC). (2007). *Informatics Nurse Board Certification Test Content Outline*. Retrieved from http://www.nursecredentialing.org/Documents/Certification/TestContentOutlines/InformaticsNurseTCO.aspx

American Nurses Credentialing Center (ANCC). (2008a). *Nurse Executive Board Certification (formely Nursing Administration) Test Content Outline*. Retrieved from http://www.nursecredentialing.org/Documents/Certification/TestContentOutlines/NursingExecutiveTCO.aspx

American Nurses Credentialing Center (ANCC). (2008b). *Nurse Executive, Advanced Board Certification (formely Nursing Administration, Advanced) Test Content Outline*. Retrieved from http://www.nursecredentialing.org/Documents/Certification/TestContentOutlines/Nurse Executive AdvancedTCO.aspx

American Organization of Nurse Executives (AONE). (2005). *Nurse Executive Competencies 2005*. Retrieved from http://www.aone.org/aone/resource/home.html

American Organization of Nurse Executives (AONE). (2007a). *AONE Position Statement Doctorate of Nursing Practice.* Retrieved from http://www.aone.org/aone/docs/Position Statement060607.doc

American Organization of Nurse Executives (AONE). (2007b). *AONE guiding principles for defining the role of the nurse executive in technology acquisition and implementation.* Retrieved from http://www.aone.org/aone/resource/home.html

American Organization of Nurse Executives (AONE). (2009). *AONE guiding principles for the nurse executive to enhance clinical outcomes by leveraging technology.* Retrieved from http://www.aone.org/aone/resource/home.html

American Organization of Nurse Executives (AONE). (2010). *Certified in Executive Nursing Practice (CENP).* Retrieved from http://www.aone.org/aone/certification/CENP.html

Burnes, B. L., Gassert, C. A., & Cipriano, P. F. (2008). Technology solutions can make nursing care safer and more efficient. *Journal of Healthcare Information Management, 22*(4), 24–30.

Dowding, D., Mitchell, N., Randell, R., Foster, R., Lattimer, V., & Thompson, C. (2009). Nurses' use of computerized clinical decision support systems: A case site analysis. *Journal of Clinical Nursing, 18,* 1159–1167.

Mitchell, N., Randell, R., Foster, R., Dowding, D., Lattimer, V., Thompson, C. et al. (2009). A national survey of computerized decision support systems available to nurses in England. *Journal of Nursing Management, 17*(7), 772–780.

Osheroff, J. A., Pifer, E. A., Teich, J. M., Sittig, D. F., & Jenders, R. A. (2005). *Improving outcomes with clinical decision support: An implementer's guide.* Boca Raton, FL: Productivity Press.

National Association of Pediatric Nurse Practitioners (NAPNAP). (2008). *NAPNAP's position statement on the doctorate of nursing practice.* Retrieved from http://www.napnap.org/PNPResources/Practice/PositionStatements.aspx

Randell, R., & Dowding, D. (2010). Organisational influences on nurses' use of clinical decision support systems. *International Journal of Medical Informatics, 79,* 412–421.

Stead, W., & Lin, H. (2009). Computational committee on engaging the Computer Science Research Community in Health Care Informatics; National Research Council. *Computational technology for effective health care: Immediate steps and strategic directions.* Washington, DC: National Academies Press. Retrieved from http://books.nap.edu/catalog.php?record_id=12572

Swindle, C., & Bradley, V. (2010). The newest O in the C-suite: CNIO. *Nurse Leader, 8*(3), 28–30.

TIGER Initiative. (2010). *Technology Informatics Guiding Educational Reform (TIGER) initiative.* Retrieved from http://www.tigersummit.com/

CHAPTER FOURTEEN: Reflective Response 2

Rosario P. Estrada, and Cheryl Holly

In Chapter 14, Cornelius, Childs, and Wilson (authors) provide an overview of the expected informatics and technological competencies needed to support advanced nursing practice at the doctoral level. They differentiated the technological competencies for the doctoral advanced practice nurse and master's-prepared nurse practitioner and recommended that the doctoral APN must be proficient and have a higher level of technical competency compared to the APN with a master's degree. Subsequently, they identified the technical, informatics, and knowledge management competencies of the doctoral APN. Most importantly, the authors addressed technological tools, emerging innovations, and strategies to enhance the leadership role of the doctoral APN.

We are totally in agreement that there is a distinction of expected technological competencies between the doctoral APN and master's-prepared APN. However, we find the authors inconsistent in comparing the expected technological competencies for the doctoral APN and master's-prepared APN by using different sources of criteria in identifying these competencies. The authors first identified the expected technical competencies of the master's-prepared nurse from the draft of the AACN's Essential for Masters Education in Nursing (2010) Essential V: Informatics and Healthcare Technologies. They emphasize a higher level of proficiency expectation for the doctoral APN for the leadership role in the dynamic health care delivery system from citations of various authors. As a catalyst for change, they further proposed that the doctoral APN must have advanced technological and practical research skills for knowledge development. Although these are valid and valuable expectations from a doctoral APN, the comparison would have been more consistent and clear if the authors had used the AACN (2006) DNP Essential IV as a reference for identifying expected proficiencies with information systems and patient care technologies and made more distinct contrasts between the AACN (2010) *Draft Essential for Masters Education in Nursing*. We contend DNP just by reading the two AACN *Essentials* from similar sources (draft masters versus DNP), one can discern the difference and the level of competency expected for the doctoral APN and the master's-prepared APN. However, as nursing informaticists we believe there should be more differentiation, precision and detail as we expect DNP APNs to function with greater technological proficiency than with the MSN.

We concur with the authors that the doctoral APN needs informatics and knowledge management competencies. Therefore, we propose that the AACN (2006) Essential III: Clinical Scholarship and Analytical Methods for Evidence-Based Practice is a necessary inclusion. This expected competency requires knowledge development/application and, importantly, translation of knowledge into practice, which is congruent with the knowledge management systems competency identified by Cornelius, Childs, and Wilson. According to Magyary, Whitney, and Brown (2006), "the advancement of APNs' practice inquiry competencies is timely for it interfaces with the national scientific agenda's emphasis on translating science to clinical practice, health care delivery systems and policy" (p. 139). As knowledge management competency involves collecting/generating meaningful evidence that predicts and analyzes outcomes, it is necessary that the doctoral APN have the knowledge and skill necessary to perform a comprehensive systematic review of existing knowledge and the ability and competency to translate this knowledge to practice, policy, and system situations through the recommendation of best practice. Indeed, doctorally prepared advanced practice nurses have an opportunity to transform nursing care through informatics and knowledge management.

REFERENCES

American Association of Colleges of Nursing (AACN). (2006). *The essentials of doctoral education for advanced nursing practice.* Retrieved from http://www.aacn.nche.edu/dnp/pdf/essentials.pdf
American Association of Colleges of Nursing (AACN). (2010, August 23). *Draft the essentials of master's education in nursing.* Retrieved from http://www.aacn.nche.edu/Education/pdf/DraftMastEssentials.pdf
Magyary, D., Whitney, J., & Brown, A. (2006). Advancing practice inquiry: Research foundations of the practice doctorate in nursing. *Nursing Outlook, 54,* 139–151.

CRITICAL THINKING QUESTIONS

1. What weaknesses did you identify from the specialty nursing organizations' discussions of their goals for technology competency and utilization?
2. Perform a literature search on the Technology Informatics Guiding Education Reform initiative (TIGER). Discuss what kind of impact TIGER is making on nursing informatics and health care.
3. Discuss the similar and different technology needs of the four types of doctoral APNs in the clinical setting.
4. Evidence-based information can be located in PubMed/MEDLINE, and in the CINAHL database using certain search methods. Perform a search of one of your professors using each one of these databases and try and conceptualize what the focus of their scholarship is.
5. Describe some ways in which Twitter can be used in health care beyond what was discussed in this chapter.
6. Evaluate your own skill at "knowledge management." Discuss what your primary specialty area is and where you go for the most up-to-date content.
7. Go to the Cochrane database and browse. Retrieve a systematic review close to your specialty area and discuss its significance.
8. Go to "Second Life" at secondlife.com. Register (it's free) and request an Avatar (a name). What kind of health care uses might there be for Second Life?
9. Identify ways in which the use of the standardized patient could be used in doctor of nursing practice curricula.
10. Discuss whether DNP-prepared APRNs ought to have better technology proficiency skills than MSN-prepared APRNs.

CHAPTER FIFTEEN

Negotiation Skills for Doctoral Advanced Nursing Practice

Vicki D. Lachman and Cheryl M. Vermey

INTRODUCTION

Nurses engaged in doctoral advanced nursing practice (DNPs) are creating new frontiers in the field of nursing, and as practitioners, they are contributing significantly to the overall health care system. To fulfill this role, they will encounter many situations requiring negotiation skills. The realm of negotiation falls within both strategy and tactics. This chapter focuses primarily on the strategic role of the DNP and provides tactical examples that may be faced in actual practice.

This chapter begins with the context of organizational culture and systems theory as the place where negotiation takes place. Our discussion includes the traits of successful negotiators and the crucial elements for successful negotiation, sources of power, and the five-step process for negotiation. Since not all individuals approach negotiation from a collaborative stance, skills are required for negotiating at an "uneven table," when rank and privilege affects the strategies. The chapter ends with strategies for overcoming barriers to successful negotiation, such as the "Four Horsemen of the Apocalypse" and common mistakes in negotiation.

Negotiation is a crucial skill for successful relationships (Mayer, 2006; Shell, 2006). In order to have the necessary collaborative relations within and between disciplines, DNPs must have the skills and strategies known to diplomats. For example, individuals who take a win-win approach to conflict resolution view conflicts as problems to be solved and seek solutions that achieve both their own goals, as well as the goals of the other person. Individuals with this orientation see conflicts as opportunities for improving relationships by reducing the tension between two people (Katz & Pattarini, 2008). Therefore, the purpose of negotiation is to resolve differences over, for example, information, values, or goals. Fisher, Ury, and Patton (2003) provide the following working definition of negotiation as "two or more parties, with common and conflicting interests, come together to put forth and discuss explicit proposals for the purpose of reaching an agreement" (Video).

It is important in any negotiation to begin with common interests in order to create rapport. The purpose of negotiation is to reach an agreement that is based upon a thorough discussion of each party's ideas, where an agreement is reached to meet the needs of both parties. The solution is one that assures commitment to follow through to completion by each party. This differs from compromise, which is based upon both party's willingness to *settle* on an option. Compromise might be best described as "mini-lose, mini-lose."

THE ROLE OF THE DNP IN NEGOTIATION: THE STRATEGIC VIEW

Case I:

Dr. Schmidt, prior to completion of her DNP degree, was a nurse practitioner in the Stroke Center for an academic medical center. Because of her years of experience in the acute care of stroke patients, she decided to do her DNP clinical practicum in a rehabilitation unit. This rounding out of her experience with stroke patients and her evidence-based focus led her to conclude that stroke rehab needs to focus on all domains, social and functional, for patients to recover a sense of self and the roles in their lives and families. Unfortunately, she was met with resistance to this change by colleagues. What new ideas can we offer Dr. Schmidt in negotiation?

This section addresses (1) a systems context for using negotiation skills, (2) the organizational culture as a context for change, and (3) how gender and culture influence the DNP role. Helping Dr. Schmidt understand the organizational culture in which she finds herself and using the principles from the Center for Right Relationship (CRR) (2005), a systems approach described in the following paragraphs could help her better negotiate the change. Perhaps, because of her gender, she is more focused on maintaining a relationship than in clearly and directly arguing for change for the patient's sake (Donaldson & Frohnmayer, 2007).

SYSTEMS THEORY AS A CONTEXT FOR NEGOTIATION

The DNP role in negotiation requires a high level of systems thinking and an ability to apply expertise in systems theory and functioning. The role includes being a participant in the larger system and being a catalyst for systems change through negotiation. Therefore, there is a compelling leadership dimension to negotiation at this higher level. Historically, negotiation took place within top-down, patriarchal organizational systems. The current decade is unfolding a new dimension in systems work. The dimensions include: focus on the relationships within systems; organizational theory; and emotional, social, and systems intelligence (Goleman, 2004; Goleman & Boyatzis, 2008); seminal research on process and deep democracy (Mindell, 1995, 2001a, 2001b); and the empirical research conducted on relationships (Gottman, 1999, 2007). This new approach focuses on connections between and among members of a system and recognizes that people are in relationship, at all times, starting with ourselves.

The CRR (2005) has created a groundbreaking model, which is used internationally for coaching within organizations and groups to unfold the power and potential of relationship systems. This new methodology for facilitating human relationships is inspired by and combines the concepts from coaching, psychology, organizational development, mediation, quantum physics, process work, and general systems theory. All of these are directly applicable to the DNP's use in negotiation. In effect, the negotiation role includes managing and leading relationship systems.

The CRR (2005) systems approach is founded on the following principles that DNPs can use to create desired outcomes rather than focus on solving a problem. The *first principle* is creating a shift from "who is doing what to whom" to "what is trying to happen here." It creates a climate of being in right relationship with self, others, and the larger organization or system in which the DNP is functioning. In this view, all parties have a voice that needs to be heard and honored before a successful conclusion to any negotiation can occur. Every relationship system is characterized by various dynamic and evolving situations and human interactions. The DNP needs to be prepared to assess what is happening in the situation that creates the need for negotiation. Sometimes what is needed is to reveal that there is a system breakdown that is essential to address in order to move forward.

The *second principle* is that the relationship system is naturally creative and whole. In this view there is no "they;" rather there is "I, you, and we." Whenever one falls into a "they" view of a situation, the individual risks putting herself or himself in the place of victim, undermining their effectiveness and ability to resolve the situation. Assuming that all parties in the relationship form something larger than the whole, this change empowers members of the system to negotiate new ways of working together effectively.

A *third principle* is that the DNP will work with the whole system within a larger context, not just what appears on the surface. It is taking a metaview of the larger picture that is important here, much like an orchestra conductor. Think of a gestalt, where the whole is greater than the sum of its parts. For example, Dr. Schmidt needs to acknowledge that all opinions need to be voiced in order to uncover the real issues under the resistance to change. She can then articulate what is going on that may be impacting optimal patient outcomes negatively and use the collective knowledge and wisdom of the group to create better solutions for ensuring that a holistic framework is used. This means that the old way of working the system needs to yield to one that is more empowered toward collective interest versus individual self-interest.

In summary, the role of the DNP in a systems context is essentially to reveal the system to itself. In contrast to "fixing" what appears on the surface, the nurse can hold up a mirror to what seems to be happening so that others may be able to respond in ways that better meet the needs of the larger system. The metaphor for the principle is "the view of the eagle looking at the system versus the ant on the floor."

POLITICAL, CULTURAL, AND GENDER CONTEXTS WITHIN THE SYSTEM

Organizations may be viewed through various perspectives. Bolman and Deal (2008) describe the four frames of an organization from a systems perspective, which include the structural and human frames, as well as the unseen and often underappreciated political and symbolic or cultural frames through which the DNP must practice. Structure includes buildings, departments, technology, and equipment. Human resources include the people and hierarchy within the system. However, negotiation mostly takes place within the context of the political and symbolic frames.

Bolman and Deal (2008) use the metaphor of a jungle to view the political frame. This is where the intersection of power, conflict, and coalition takes place. A critical lens through which one views negotiation is to recognize that the system comprises of various political arenas including administration, governing bodies, medical groups, ancillary personnel, and nurses at all levels of education and experience. Therefore, individuals could argue that the DNP role is like that of a politician, but not in the traditional sense. For example, titles connote power in society and organizations. The title "doctor" has historically been seen as belonging to a physician or perhaps to a university professor. The title "doctor" when describing a nurse creates both confusion and conflict related to the power and political meaning of the term. The DNP needs to be prepared to respond to this issue.

Bolman and Deal (2008) also describe a symbolic frame, which includes the organizational culture and its symbols. A metaphor here is the system as theater, which includes many cues, symbols, and stories that create system norms that often resist challenge or change. The DNP role includes viewing the system from the metaview of both political and symbolic or cultural frame. Combining acute understanding of these frames, along with skill in being in the right relationship with self and others, distinguishes the role of the DNP from others. For example, DNPs who are using evidence-based practice may challenge organizational ways of practice (as will be seen in the next case example).

An examination of context would not be complete without including thoughts on the effect of gender and other measures of equity on the system, and the ability of the DNP to negotiate effectively. Today, 94% of the nurses are still women (American Association of Colleges of Nursing [AACN], 2009). The issues of gender also apply to issues of race, ethnicity, and other considerations of equity (Harris, Moran, & Moran, 2004).

In several studies on gender differences in negotiation strategies, it was found that men tend to view bargaining situations as short-term and episodic in nature, while women tend to view transactions with others as part of a long-term relationship (Babcock & Laschever, 2007). Consequently, saying that women adopted more flexible bargaining stances than their male counterparts can be explained by their attitude toward the length of the relationship. But this difference in negotiating behavior can also be explained as women's concern for the equity of interpersonal relationships. In another gender-related study, the results suggested that women report having obtained a good outcome when they felt they had a pleasant interaction with the other party, even though they did not resolve or even discuss the conflict between them (Donaldson & Frohnmayer, 2007). The results of these studies suggest that women need to learn that it is legitimate to say what they want, even if it conflicts with what they think the other person wants.

In summary, the leadership needed for successful negotiation requires the DNP to assess and balance the principles of the structural, human, political, and symbolic frames of organizations. This means going beyond the organizational structure, staff reporting lines and job descriptions, developing skills in political dynamics, and understanding cultural norms that have an often unseen but huge impact on negotiation outcomes. The four frames also need to be balanced with an understanding of the impact of gender and diversity on the issue at hand.

RANK AND PRIVILEGE

To delve deeper into the concept of rank and privilege requires distinguishing between rank, power, and privilege. Mindell (1995) describes rank as a way of indicating a level of status. Privilege and power can be derived from different bases or sources, such as educational, social, economic, or cultural. Therefore, a nurse with a doctoral degree has greater inherent privilege and implied power than that of a nurse with a baccalaureate degree. At present, society and organizational structures grant physicians greater rank and privilege than nurses, regardless of education or other forms of standing. It will be interesting to see if this will change when there are increased numbers of DNPs, especially those functioning specifically in clinical settings.

Case II:

Dr. Bowman completed his DrNP degree at Drexel University where he was enrolled in the Clinical Scientist Track. He was interested in conducting research on the "Role Strain in Family Caregivers of Persons Diagnosed with Alzheimer's Dementia," as his clinical focus was with patients with Alzheimer's disease. Up to this point, he had been the nurse collecting information for many physician-led studies. After conducting this study, he was now ready to be the primary or co-investigator of studies. He put forth research ideas and possible funding sources, but met with resistance. Apparently, members on his interdisciplinary team were having difficulty seeing him as the primary researcher and as a leader. What ideas and skills can we offer Dr. Bowman in negotiation?

Phyllis Beck Kritek (2002), in her groundbreaking book *Negotiating at an "Uneven Table,"* explored the process of resolving conflicts, similar to those facing DNPs, in situations where unacknowledged inequity influences disputes and their outcomes. It is an act of inner courage and conviction that allows the DNP to be authentic in any situation that requires the use of negotiation skills. Essential inner qualities include increasing inner awareness, being a truth teller, and standing in your own integrity.

Mindell (1995) further describes low rank as being devalued, disrespected, and excluded from influence, decision making, and conversely the benefits that come from having high rank. Because of this norm, nurses have historically been impacted in areas of self-esteem and self-worth. A source of conflict can be the unconscious use of rank. For example, a person in a higher position confronted with "pulling rank" or dismissing the concerns or needs of others often becomes angry or uses denial as a defense mechanism. The DNP has two critical roles here: the first is to know and effectively use skills and strategies for negotiation; the second is to use a systems approach to resolving issues involving negotiation strategies. In the example of Dr. Bowman, he was seen by his colleagues as having neither the rank nor the privilege to warrant being the primary investigator of the study. One successful outcome of his negotiation is acknowledging the contributions of his colleagues, choosing to take the first step as a coinvestigator of the study, and demonstrating how research builds evidence-based practice and the importance of implementation to improve patient outcomes.

THE ROLE OF THE DNP IN NEGOTIATION: THE TACTICAL VIEW

Case III:

Dr. Land is a recent DNP graduate, and she is negotiating for a promotion to a Chief Nursing Officer position in an academic medical center where she has been a Director of Cardiovascular Services for 10 years. She knows her competition all have either an MSN in nursing administration or an MBA and that they are from out of state. She decides to leverage her DNP degree and her understanding of the organization's culture and goals, which will allow her to hit the ground running. Since many on the search committee will not understand what knowledge and skills a DNP degree brings, she decides to provide them with two brief articles outlining the MSN and DNP curriculum differences. She also plans to use her organizational power by having one of her recommendations come from the chairperson of surgery. She knows all her years as a critical care nurse will help her think clearly under the stress of the interview. Her reputation as a person of integrity and her willingness to be assertive in conflict situations, with a focus on problem resolution, will stand well for her. What ideas and skills can we offer Dr. Land in her negotiation?

The following section focuses on the specific tactics and strategies used in negotiation, which fit within the strategic thinking or systems framework where the DNP functions. The literature describes the traits of successful negotiators and the strategies for a win-win outcome (Lewicki, Barry, & Saunders, 2006; Lewicki & Hiam, 2006). Dr. Land (Case III) is already applying some of the crucial traits and elements for successful negotiation, and the following section should prove helpful as she plans her next steps.

TRAITS OF SUCCESSFUL NEGOTIATORS

When we study the diplomatic styles of individuals, we are able to identify seven traits in individuals that we would rate as key to their success (Malhorta & Bazerman, 2007; Raiffa, Richardson, & Metcalfe, 2007). The *first trait* is having strong planning skills. Successful negotiators will often state that they spend 50% or more of their time planning what will be said in their interactions. Such planning includes not only the content, but where they will meet, who else should be present, whether information should be sent prior to the meeting, and even what time of the day the meeting should occur. Successful negotiators want to maximize their opportunities for success; therefore, they recognize that the process and place is equally as important as the concrete words stated.

The "ability to think clearly under stress" is the *second trait* of successful negotiators. Being prepared is one way to reduce the stress in any negotiation process. Two other ways are staying focused on problem-solving, not on individual personalities, and recognizing at any point you can back away from the negotiation and come back at a later time. Diplomats tend to project an air of confidence; therefore, when an attack occurs, their positive self-regard holds them in good stead.

A *third trait*, and often an undervalued trait, is the "ability to use common sense." The most common meaning of this phrase is good sense and sound judgment in practical matters. Taking the time to establish rapport, providing sufficient information upon which to base a decision, and remembering the basics about positive interpersonal relationships are all utilizing common sense.

The individual's "verbal ability" is the *fourth trait*. This is the ability to state one's ideas and opinions assertively, as well as to clarify the other party's ideas and opinions (Benum, 2006; Bishop, 2006; McClure, 2007). The abilities to manage other people's defensiveness, side-stepping of issues, or overt hostility in a nondefensive manner are also the key verbal skills. An example of success using these persuasion skills is that agreement is facilitated when the desirability of the agreement is stressed.

"Content knowledge" is the *fifth trait* found in successful negotiators. For example, if Dr. Land was going to negotiate a union contract that involved changing the role of nurse aides in the institution, she would certainly come to the table having already investigated licensure laws, how other institutions have handled such a change, and the present attitude of the staff.

The *sixth trait* is "personal integrity." In truth, if one is not perceived as trustworthy and credible, the person will not be seen as an individual with integrity. Being seen as trustworthy requires that the person be honest, open instead of defensive, consistent in standards and approach, and someone who treats individuals with the respect that they deserve.

The final and *seventh trait* of successful negotiators is "the ability to perceive and use power." Power is the ability and willingness to affect the outcome. There are multiple sources of power that are available for use in negotiation. For now, suffice it to say, that successful negotiators keep their eye on the outcome that they desire and use multiple sources of power to move the negotiation to the conclusion they seek (Aquilar & Galluccio, 2007).

In the case example, Dr. Land needed to be consciously aware of and apply the traits or skills of planning, think clearly under stress, use her common sense and verbal skills, and have strong knowledge of the content or information required in the situation. To this she needed to balance her own sense of personal integrity with her ability to perceive and use power in an effective way. This is not "power over," but the courage and willingness to step forth and do what is needed in the situation.

THREE CRUCIAL ELEMENTS FOR SUCCESSFUL NEGOTIATION

Power, time, and information are the three interrelated variables in any negotiation process (Cohen, 2003; Thompson, 2007). Power is the capacity to get things done, to exercise control over people, events, or situations. Usually when knowledgeable people complain about power, it is for one of the two reasons: (1) they do not like the way power is being used—it is often power over an individual; and (2) they do not approve of the goal of the person exerting control—power should never be a goal in and of itself, but should be a means of transport to a desired outcome.

In any negotiation, the second variable of time needs consideration. Expect the most significant concession behavior in any settlement action to occur close to the deadline. It is crucial that both parties know the deadline. However, deadlines are more flexible than most people realize. DNP clinicians need to utilize this misunderstanding of the time dimension to negotiate for outcomes that support excellence in patient care, quality education, or crucial changes in organizational effectiveness.

Information is the third crucial element in negotiation process. During the actual negotiating event, it is often a common strategy for one or both sides to conceal their true interests, needs, and priorities. The rationale is that information is power, particularly in situations where one cannot trust the other side fully.

It is important to gain information by asking questions every time you are given answers. A way to test the credibility of the other side is to ask questions, the answers to which are already known. The more information one has about the other person's priorities, deadlines, and real needs, the better one can bargain. A key piece of information that all negotiators want to know is—what are the real limits of the other party, or just how much will they sacrifice in order to make a deal? Very often this can be ascertained by observing the pattern of concession behavior on the part of the other side.

Turning back to the case of Dr. Land, one can see how she has used the above principles. She established her background and credentials early in a negotiation. She demonstrated the kind of expertise that is required for most negotiations by asking intelligent questions to know whether the responses are accurate. It is important for Dr. Land to remember that she brings to the table clinical and managerial expertise in a negotiation process. For example, the search committee may state that they want their candidate to have had previous experience as a Chief Nursing Officer, whereas their real need is that the candidate knows how to work effectively in a complex academic medical center. The more Dr. Land can acquaint herself with the committee's needs, the better her position to negotiate a possible resolution for their real need. An example of using the power of identification is when Dr. Land mentions that a well-respected academic medical center had just hired their internal candidate last year and she has been very successful. If the organization has had a precedent of promoting from within, Dr. Land can use the power of precedent. The best outcomes employ a systems approach where the parties rise above individual interests to view the greater good. While holding the strategic view, it is also important to use the tactical skills needed in a negotiation process (see Table 15.1).

BARRIERS TO SUCCESSFUL NEGOTIATION

Barriers to successful negotiation are multidimensional and involve behaviors that people use, often at an unconscious level, to thwart resolution. This section will also include descriptions of "The Four Horsemen of the Apocalypse" (Gottman, 1999) and individual common mistakes (ChangingMinds.org, n.d.) that the DNP will need to understand to be successful in negotiating. Individuals, like Dr. Ross, will need to overcome these barriers for successful negotiation.

Case IV:

Dr. Ross began her academic teaching career after she completed her DNP degree last year. Prior to this she had been a women's health NP in a busy practice connected to an academic medical center for ten years. It became quickly apparent that several of the other professors with a background in women's health were unhappy with her appointment as track coordinator. Her initial efforts at inclusion in curriculum planning were met with stonewalling and disrespect. It appeared her questions about the present curriculum were taken as criticism, rather than her effort to understand the rationale used for the inclusion of specific content in some of the courses. The nonverbal responses included eye-rolling, silence, or looks of shock when she suggested changes. What ideas and strategies could we offer Dr. Ross in negotiation?

THE "FOUR HORSEMEN OF THE APOCALYPSE"

Dr. John Gottman (1999, 2007) has conducted empirical research on healthy and unhealthy marriages and his work is now being extrapolated and further validated for use in organizations (Gottman, 2007). There are four toxic behaviors that doom

TABLE 15.1
Five Steps in Negotiation Process

The Negotiation Process Steps	Key Points to Include
1. Preparation	Know the facts
	Know what self and other wants
	Develop the strategy
	Identify the "must have"
2. Develop Objective Criteria	Includes laws, policies, precedence, moral standards and community norms as possible criteria
	Consider accreditation standards
	Seek benchmark models for comparison
3. Communicate Interests and Needs	Communication includes both clear dialog and a heartful connection to others
	Body language sends messages that others will see
4. Search for Mutually Acceptable Solutions	Look for areas of agreement and common ground
	Be willing to accept mutually accepted options not previously considered
5. Finalize the Agreement	Ensure clear agreement on the details
	Who will do what and in what time frame
	Distribute a summary with the agreed upon outcomes
	Identify areas for future discussion

Source: Compilation of sources: Fisher et al. (2003); Mayer (2006); and Raiffa et al. (2007)

relationships, regardless of the setting, that are called "The Four Horsemen of the Apocalypse." These behaviors include:

1. Blame/criticism, consisting of attacking or blaming other instead of his or her own behavior;
2. Defensiveness, in response to being criticized, which is really another way of blaming;
3. Contempt, which is the use of sarcasm, belittling, cynicism, hostile humor, and belligerence; and finally
4. Stonewalling, which includes cutting off communication, silent treatments, refusals to engage, withdrawal, or in some cases just not directly expressing what you are thinking.

Gottman (1999) found that 69% of all problems are perpetual, meaning that they can be managed through dialog, but resist ultimate resolution. Therefore, the role of the DNP is not to "fix" the issue, but to engage in negotiation strategies that will: (1) increase positive dialogue; (2) reduce any negative affects during conflict, particularly the difficult challenge of working with contempt; and (3) increase positive affects during conflict resolution. Exhibit 15.1 includes some antidotes that are effective in working with the Four Horsemen.

EXHIBIT 15.1   Antidotes to "The Four Horsemen of the Apocalypse" Behaviors[a]

Toxic Behaviors	Strategies to Deal with Them
General Behaviors	Name it and educate the parties on the negative impact/destructiveness. Review what happened and discuss alternative behaviors/strategies. Increase positive behaviors and attitudes where possible with a soft approach, accepting influence, and noticing efforts to "repair" what has happened. Encourage that there are alternative ways to negotiate through a situation or conflict.
Blame/Criticism	Ask: Are you willing to resolve this without blame? Address the behavior, not the person. Try a soft start up to lessen the impact. Look for the request behind the criticism. Encourage the use of "I want . . . ., I feel . . . ." statements.
Defensiveness	Active listening and clarifying what the other person is hearing. Assume that 2% of what you or the other person is saying is true. Look for areas of truth behind the complaint.
Contempt	Ask: Are you willing to resolve this without sarcasm or name calling? Allow the parties to ventilate to you. Check for emotional flooding and soothe. Encourage the use of "I want . . . ., I feel . . . ." statements.
Stonewalling	Check for emotional flooding and soothe. Address fears of what will happen if the person speaks what is being thought or felt. Encourage moving beyond the edge that is keeping the person back and support the effort.

[a]Adapted from "*The Seven Principles for Making Marriage Work*," by J. M. Gottman (1999).

The "Four Horsemen of the Apocalypse" can lead negotiators to make common mistakes. Of the 15 mistakes listed (ChangingMinds.org, n.d.), the most recurrent ones are accepting positions, hurrying, issue fixation, and missing strengths. Creative thinking needed for win-win solutions will not occur if others will not change their positions and not look for innovative solutions, but remain fixated on their chosen solutions. Many beginning negotiators fail to see the strengths they have, often because they are hurrying to a solution to please others (see Exhibit 15.2).

An important role for the DNP is to first assess what is going on within the system that requires negotiation. Taking a systems view, understanding issues of rank and privilege, using the skills needed to negotiate effectively, and having a clear understanding of what gets in the way of resolution, all of these approaches arm the practitioner with the background to be an effective negotiator. It is also important to be grounded in a strong sense of self and know what values one brings to the situation. Using the approaches delineated in Exhibit 15.1 enables the DNP to be effective in dealing with toxic behaviors.

Based on the work of the CRC (2005), overcoming barriers is predicated on the principle of finding common interest. The following questions are useful: (1) Are you willing to resolve this without blame? (2) Why is it important to resolve this? and (3) What do you agree on? A *caveat*: if the parties are unwilling to resolve the issue without blame, there is no point in proceeding further. One will need to develop another strategy for resolution.

EXHIBIT 15.2   Common Mistakes that Negotiators Make[a]

1. *Accepting positions*: Assuming the other person won't change their position
2. *Accepting statements*: Assuming what the other person says is wholly true
3. *Cornering them*: Giving them no alternative but to fight
4. *Hurrying*: Negotiating in haste (and repenting at leisure)
5. *Hurting the relationship*: Getting what you want but making an enemy
6. *Issue fixation*: Getting stuck on one issue and missing greater possibilities
7. *Missing strengths*: Not realizing the strengths that you actually have
8. *Misunderstanding authority*: Assuming that authority and power are synonymous
9. *Misunderstanding power*: Thinking one person has all the power
10. *One solution*: Thinking there is only one possible solution
11. *Over-wanting*: Wanting something too much
12. *Squeezing too much*: Trying to gain every last advantage
13. *Talking too much*: Not gaining the power of information from others
14. *Thinking in absolutes*: Assuming that there are only a few possibilities
15. *Win-lose*: Assuming a fixed-pie, win-lose scenario

[a]Adapted from Changing Minds.org http://changingminds.org/disciplines/negotiation/mistakes/mistakes.htm.

SUMMARY

Negotiation is a complex process where individuals are seeking an agreement to which all parties can make a commitment to follow through to completion. In this context, the role of the DNP includes holding a strategic or systems view of the negotiations process. How to negotiate and with whom one can negotiate is largely determined by the organizational culture in which negotiators find themselves. There are cultural and gender variables to be aware of in the process. The CRC speaks directly to possible strategies to right the system.

The role of the DNP is also to be skilled in and use effective tactical strategies for negotiation. The five steps in the negotiation process are fraught with possible complications, from "The Four Horsemen of the Apocalypse" to the common errors in negotiation. The DNP graduate, in his or her leadership role, may also be responsible for facilitating negotiation between two other individuals.

Note: The authors gratefully acknowledge the support and permission from the CRR in the use of their model and the select materials in the preparation of this chapter.

REFERENCES

American Association of Colleges of Nursing (AACN). (2009, February 26). *Despite surge of interest in nursing careers, new AACN data confirm that too few nurses are entering the healthcare workforce.* Retrieved from http://www.aacn.nche.edu/media/NewsReleases/2009/workforcedata.html

Aquilar, F., & Galluccio, M. (2007). *Psychological processes in international negotiations: Theoretical and practical perspectives.* London, UK: Springer.

Babcock, L., & Laschever, S. (2007). *Women don't ask: The high cost of avoiding negotiation—and positive strategies for change.* New York, NY: Bantam.

Benum, I. (2006). *Stop pushing me around: A workplace guide for the timid, shy, and less.* Franklin Lakes, NJ: Career Press.

Bishop, S. (2006). *Develop your assertiveness* (2nd ed.). London, UK: Kogan Page.

Bolman, L. G., & Deal, T. E. (2008). *Reframing organizations: Artistry, choice and leadership.* San Francisco, CA: Jossey Bass.

Center for Right Relationship (CRR). (2005). *Organization and relationship systems coaching manual.* Vallejo, CA: Author.

ChangingMinds.org. (n.d.). *Negotiation mistakes.* Retrieved from http://changingminds.org/disciplines/negotiation/mistakes/mistakes.htm

Cohen, H. (2003). *Negotiate this! by caring, But not T-H-A-T much.* New York, NY: Warner Books.

Donaldson, M. C., & Frohnmayer, D. (2007). *Negotiating for dummies* (2nd ed.). Hoboken, NJ: Wiley.

Fisher, R., Ury, W., & Patton, B. (2003). *Getting to yes: Negotiating agreement without giving in.* New York, NY: Simon & Schuster Audio (CD-ROM).

Goleman, D. (2004). What makes a leader? *Harvard Business Review, 76*(6), 93–102.

Goleman, D., & Boyatzis, R. (2008). Social intelligence and the biology of leadership. *Harvard Business Review, 86*(9), 74–81.

Gottman, J. M. (1999). *The seven principles for making marriage work.* New York, NY: Three Rivers Press.

Gottman, J. M. (2007). Making relationships work. *Harvard Business Review, 85*(12), 45–50.

Harris, P. R., Moran, R. T., & Moran, S. V. (2004). *Managing cultural differences: Global leadership strategies for the twenty-first century* (6th ed.). Los Angeles, CA: Butterworth and Heinemann.

Katz, N. H., & Pattarini, N. M. (2008). Interest-based negotiation: An essential business and communications tool for the public relations counselor. *Journal of Communication Management, 12*(1), 88–97.

Kritek, P. B. (2002). *Negotiating at an uneven table: Developing moral courage in resolving our conflicts.* San Francisco, CA: Jossey-Bass.

Lewicki, R. J., Barry, B., & Saunders, D. M. (2006). *Essentials of negotiation* (4th ed.). New York, NY: McGraw-Hill Higher Education.

Lewicki, R. J., & Hiam, A. (2006). *Mastering business negotiation: A working guide to making deals and resolving conflict.* San Francisco, CA: Jossey-Bass.

Malhorta, D., & Bazerman, M. (2007). *Negotiation genius: How to overcome obstacles and achieve brilliant results at the bargaining table and beyond.* New York, NY: Bantam.

Mayer, R. (2006). *How to win any negotiation: Without raising your voice, losing your cool, or coming to blows.* Franklin Lakes, NJ: Career Press.

McClure, J. S. (2007). *Civilized assertiveness for women: Communication with backbone not bite.* Denver, CO: Albion Street Press.

Mindell, A. (1995). *Sitting in the fire: Large group transformation using conflict and diversity.* Charlottesville, VA: Hampton Roads.

Mindell, A. (2001a). *The deep democracy of open forums.* Charlottesville, VA: Hampton Roads.

Mindell, A. (2001b). *The dream makers apprentice.* Charlottesville, VA: Hampton Roads.

Raiffa, H., Richardson, J., & Metcalfe, D. (2007). *Negotiation analysis: The science and art of collaborative decision making.* Boston, MA: Belknap Press.

Shell, G. R. (2006). *Bargaining for advantage: Negotiation strategies for reasonable people* (2nd ed.). New York, NY: Penguin.

Thompson, L. (2007). *The truth about negotiations.* Upper Saddle River, NJ: FT Press.

CHAPTER FIFTEEN: Reflective Response

Susan Baseman

The art of negotiation is central to nursing practice at all levels, from basic to advanced. Nurses must constantly engage in negotiations with patients, family members, other nurses, health care professionals, and physicians. Negotiation is a skill that is to some degree innate and then honed through learned experience; it is necessary not just for success as a nurse, but for basic survival as well. It is intrinsic to all we do.

Nurses in advanced practice roles must take this skill to another level. I agree with the authors that those of us with the Doctor of Nursing Practice (DNP or DrNP) degree encounter both higher expectations and greater challenges in professional negotiations. Upon achieving the doctorate, we find ourselves negotiating both in higher levels within our organizations and for higher stakes in terms of our professional success and credibility in the workplace. We have a responsibility to our patients, our employers, and the future success of the DrNP/DNP role to respond to the challenge and master the art of negotiation.

Given the current crisis state of health care in this country, I have found the advice of a well-known police expert in hostage/crisis negotiation, Dominick Misino (2002), to be highly relevant to my own experiences negotiating in the health care arena as a DrNP graduate. Many of his comments, strategies, and recommendations mirror those of Drs. Lachman and Vermey as described in this chapter.

In an article published in the *Harvard Business Review*, Mr Misino (2002) describes hostage negotiations as "applied common sense," in which he constantly asks himself, "What is the simplest thing I can do to solve the problem?" (p. 50). The skills he describes as essential to defusing a crisis situation are similar to those described in this chapter; specifically, understanding the other person's point of view, showing respect and sensitivity to the other party's needs, and giving something in the negotiation by creating a sense of obligation on the other party's part to give something in return (Misino).

Misino (2002) further describes a negotiation as a series of small agreements, in which it is important to use every possible opportunity to get the other party to agree with you on an issue or goal, no matter how small. The authors similarly advise beginning a negotiation by identifying areas of common interest to create rapport. Misino also articulates the need to be truthful, even if the truth is not what the other party wants to hear. Truthfulness leads to trust and credibility, laying the groundwork for progress in the negotiation (Misino). Nurses who must explain that a treatment will be painful, but will ultimately improve the condition and health of the patient, understand this perfectly. This is consistent with the authors' description of one of the key traits of a successful negotiator—that of personal integrity.

Misino (2002) describes other personality traits of a successful negotiator, which again dovetail with the descriptions offered by Drs. Lachman and Vermey. Key among these is that of being a good and active listener. He describes active listening as being attuned to the emotions of both the other party and yourself, identifying them, and helping the other party to work through them. He also describes the need to be attuned to the feelings being expressed behind the words, and to use "we" statements when negotiating—also strategies offered by the authors.

Misino (2002) offers several potential pitfalls to successful negotiation as well. One of these is to identify too strongly with the other party or individual, saying that you have "walked in his/her shoes" and "understand his/her point of view." This can infuriate the other party, particularly if they feel that you know very little about them personally or what they may have been through to get where they are today. This approach may damage both your credibility and the success of the negotiation. Another pitfall is to take the negativity expressed in the negotiation as a personal rejection. If you cannot step back and be objective, your rejection response will ultimately doom the negotiation. These pitfalls can be likened to several of the behaviors/barriers identified by the authors—specifically, defensiveness, blame, criticism, and contempt.

A key success strategy described by Misino (2002) that I find particularly relevant to my own experiences in negotiation as a DrNP graduate is that of a team approach. Misino describes how a team consisting of primary negotiator, commander, coach, scribe, and runner all work together in carefully defined roles to achieve a successful result. I liken this to the authors' description of the systems approach to negotiation, with its focus on "connections between and among members of a system" (p. 3). The tasks and responsibilities described by Misino for these team members correlate to the traits of successful negotiators described in this chapter. For example, the commander and primary negotiator exhibit strong planning skills and the ability to perceive and use power. The primary negotiator must demonstrate verbal ability and personal integrity, and he/she receives content knowledge from the runner and commander. All members of the team must have the ability to use common sense, to think clearly under stress, benefit from the moral support and encouragement of the coach.

Working as a team to share these roles and interact for a common goal is a strategy that DNPs can and should employ to achieve success in negotiations. Creating teams for negotiations can be highly effective. Teamwork and leadership are core competencies of a DNP who can utilize these skills to develop strong and effective negotiating teams to deal with the complex and difficult health care issues we all currently face.

In my current role, negotiation is required for almost every meeting and interaction. The skill that I employ most often is *active listening*—in my experience this is the most important negotiating skill in the toolbox, and often the most underutilized. If the party you are negotiating with is frustrated and on the offensive, listening and letting them vent their frustration can quickly diffuse the situation. An example from my personal experience follows.

My institution, like most others, is struggling to achieve 100% compliance with all the Core Measures—those evidenced-based indicators for key conditions which have been shown to improve outcomes and are associated with high quality of care. The burden for meeting the Core Measures for pneumonia falls largely on the ER staff and physicians, who have also been dealing with a number of other issues—a massive physical plant renovation, increasing patient volumes, most of whom are uninsured due to economic factors, and pressures to meet time-sensitive and specific standards of many other clinical programs and services.

At a meeting of ER staff and staff members in Performance Improvement (PI), one of the ER physicians gave a 10 minute introduction, and was at times agitated and angry about how the measures are arbitrary, they do not really relate to quality at all, and the ER doctors are impossibly burdened with all they are expected to do and to remember at any given time. I did not comment or interrupt and only listened attentively, nodding sympathetically. When he finished, I responded by agreeing with most of what he said, and that indeed, the burden does fall disproportionately on the ER. However, ongoing failure to achieve top scores in this measure results in the ER and the institution continually lagging behind our competitors in the public reporting on these measures. All agreed that this was not the image we want in the public eye, especially as it is not an accurate reflection of the excellent care we all know we provide. I suggested that we all work together to come up with some system supports that would enable the ER to better meet the measures without creating additional time or burden on an already over-burdened staff. The result was that we were able to come up with three or four specific strategies, including more on-site support from the PI department and use of the electronic medical record to support better compliance and documentation of the pneumonia measures. Our scores correspondingly improved, and the relationship between the ER and PI groups completely turned around—they became partners, rather than adversaries.

In summary, I concur with the authors that negotiation is a skill that is critical to the success of all nurses, and that those with a DNP degree require advanced skills and face particular challenges in negotiations. The authors clearly articulate those challenges and give specific advice and strategies to overcome them. I would further offer that in today's difficult, fast-moving and financially challenging health care environment, DNPs or DrNPs like myself can benefit from the lessons of crisis/hostage negotiation. These include using active listening, common sense, personal integrity, and expertly led teamwork to achieve success in professional negotiations.

REFERENCE

Misino, D. J. (2002). Negotiating without a net: A conversation with the NYPD's Dominick J. Misino. *Harvard Business Review, 80*(10), 49–54.

CRITICAL THINKING QUESTIONS

1. Why is it important to first focus on common versus conflicting ideas in negotiation process?
2. What are the three principles designed to resolve conflict in a system put forward by The CRRs?
3. Compare your present skills to the seven traits of successful negotiators. What are your strengths and areas for development?
4. Gottman describes the "Four Horsemen of the Apocalypse." What is necessary to resolve conflicts utilizing this model?
5. There are five steps in the negotiation process. Why is the first step, preparation, described as the most important step?
6. Common mistakes in the negotiation process involve cognitive and affective errors. Of this list, where are your vulnerabilities in negotiation in your workplace?
7. How would you describe the role of the DNP in facilitating the negotiation process between others?
8. What personal values are important to bring to situations requiring negotiation for successful resolution?
9. Think of a situation where a person was being defensive. What was the "2%" truth in that person's position? What strategies can one use to find common ground?
10. Review the case examples included in this chapter. Based on your experience, what are other effective strategies?

CHAPTER SIXTEEN

Seeking Lifelong Mentorship and Menteeship in the Doctoral Advanced Nursing Practice Role

Roberta Waite and Deena Nardi

INTRODUCTION

Recently, there has been a proliferation of *doctor of nursing practice* (DNP) programs within the United States. The DNP's unique academic preparation centers on a strong advanced clinical nursing practice focus not found in the nursing doctorate programs currently available. Many individuals within the profession, health organizations, and the public will need to be educated about the DNP, and why this new role was developed. Development and progression in the individual DNP's chosen field of practice is vital to his or her success; therefore, it is critical to examine how DNPs are mentored in their programs and the best approach for continued mentoring after they graduate. Consideration for mentoring needs to take into account the doctorally prepared scholar *and* the scholar's new role (e.g., clinician, educator, or executive). Engagement in a mentoring relationship is an important role that all nurses have to assume, formally or informally, sooner or later in their professional life. Meeting the demands of complex care environments requires a DNP-prepared nursing workforce that is committed not only to continued learning, but also to mentorship activities that improve their own professional skills. Moreover, for all new doctorally prepared nurses, including new DNPs, mentoring during the early stages of their careers may significantly influence career satisfaction and may guide the development of professional competence.

The word mentor is defined as both a noun ("a trusted counselor or guide") and a verb ("to serve as a mentor for") (*Merriam-Webster's Collegiate Dictionary*, 2001, p. 725). There are some differences of opinion about what constitutes a mentoring relationship both *within* and *across* disciplines. However, it is possible to identify several characteristic features of mentoring. First, it is a dyadic relationship between a more experienced person (a mentor) and a less experienced person (a protégé). Second, the relationship is reciprocal, yet asymmetrical. Although both mentor and mentee may benefit, the primary goal of mentorship is the growth and development of the mentee. Third, mentoring relationships are dynamic. The relational processes and outcomes associated with mentoring change over time. Finally, mentors are distinct from other potentially influential people, such as role models, advisors, teachers, supervisors, or coaches (Eby, Rhodes, & Allen, 2007). Karcher, Kuperminc, Portwood, Sipe, and Taylor (2006) report that mentoring is an interactive, facilitative process meant to promote learning and development that is based on educational and social learning theories. Mentoring has been studied largely within the context of large corporations where it is used for training and succession planning (Allen, Eby, & Lentz, 2006).

At various developmental points, professionals tend to identify and seek to learn from, and often emulate, their mentors. They become models for the development of effective problem-solving and decision-making techniques, the demonstration of technical skills, development of interpersonal abilities, and provision of personal guidance. How does this occur, as most DNP students will not be taught by faculty with this degree? Will the role modeling (by faculty) and the articulation (by faculty) of what comprises the graduates' new DNP role be accurate? The nursing profession in general, and DNP graduates and their employers in particular, have become more aware of mentoring. Organizations/employers of these professionals suddenly have before them new and unfamiliar challenges regarding expectations, utilization, and understanding of the DNP professional role. Undoubtedly, many of these individual graduates will also enter the workplace with differing levels of confidence and experience, thus creating great variability in their perceived need for mentoring. With the enormous growth of these programs, real concerns have been voiced about the quality of the mentoring that is going to take place (or not take place) for this cadre of professionals.

Therefore, this chapter will examine critical elements of mentoring and their relevance to both the DNP student and graduate, as well to those interested in mentoring DNPs; these critical elements include (a) the history of mentorship in nursing; (b) mentorship models, as well as the characteristics of mentors; (c) mentoring of underrepresented groups among DNPs; (d) preparation of mentors (institutional support for good mentoring as well as tips for mentees and mentors); and (e) future directions and recommendations for the profession about mentoring DNP professionals. The importance of addressing these concerns about mentorship is heightened, not only because of the increase in new DNPs, but also because of the substantial number of forthcoming retiring senior mentors.

HISTORY OF MENTORSHIP AND MENTEESHIP IN THE NURSING PROFESSION

If I am walking with two other men, each of them will serve as my teacher. I will pick out the good points of the one and imitate them, and the bad points of the other and correct them in myself.

—*Confucius*

The process of mentoring was named after Mentor, a family friend who was considered to be a surrogate parent, counselor, and guide for the apprentice-king Telemachus during his father Odysseus' absence during and after the Trojan War (Roberts, 1995). Since the Trojan War occurred about 1200 BC, this makes mentoring an established role for over 3,000 years. Historically, science-based professions have used networking and mentoring to identify, encourage, and support new students and colleagues as they become acculturated to a new organization, academic setting, and/or private practice (Rosser & Taylor, 2009).

Nursing as an occupation has been around since the dawn of time, when early mankind first picked up an aloe plant and used it to soothe a wound. But nursing as a profession has a much more recent genesis, first recognized as such through the works of Florence Nightingale (Nightingale, 1859). Advanced practice nursing (APNs) has evolved more recently as a response to regulatory requirements and rapid scientific advances and health care change, and it continues to evolve as a distinct and independent health profession. Because of this, the need for mentorship of doctorally prepared APNs is acute, yet the culture of mentorship in advanced nursing practice is still in its infancy.

We might consider Florence Nightingale as the first mentor of professional nurses. She mentored Linda Richards, considered the United States' first professional nurse, who trained in 1877 at Nightingale's training school St. Thomas Hospital in London (*Florence Nightingale*, 2007). Ms. Richards then returned to America and established several nursing schools in the United States. Now, mentoring is considered to be an important facilitator of nursing scholarship, as well as socialization to the advanced practice role (Chism, 2009; Scheetz, 2000). However, in recent years, advanced practice nurses have been faced with a paucity of mentors. This situation is due to a confluence of events, including the nursing shortage, the nursing faculty shortage, the proliferation of distance learning and online classes, and new roles for doctorally prepared nurses as primary health care providers. The American Association of Colleges of Nursing (AACN, 2006) emphasized the need for mentoring/precepting/supporting new doctorally prepared nurses, and has suggested that doctoral programs for nurses, including DNP programs, recruit faculty and preceptors from a wide variety of disciplines for these positions. In this way, all doctoral students have exposure to other role models and mentors when no nursing mentor is available. The Council of Graduate Schools also reported that during exit surveys, mentoring was identified as essential for doctorate completion (Council of Graduate Schools, 2006). Doctorally prepared APNs must take the lead in mentoring qualified candidates in order to establish a pipeline of competent and confident DNPs who are health care providers, scientists, educators, and researchers.

MODELS OF MENTORSHIP AND MENTOR–MENTEE PROFILE

Models of Mentorship

A number of mentoring models have been described in the nursing literature; however, none are universally accepted (Smith, McAllister, & Crawford, 2001). Traditionally, mentoring in nursing has either occurred informally or as a planned program where the individual is matched with an experienced nurse in a formal one-to-one program. While such programs can benefit nurses, many will miss out on the opportunity to support professional development of nurses, particularly new DNP graduates. Further, mentoring dyads do little to enhance a more collaborative atmosphere in professional nursing. Alternative mentoring approaches exist and can provide advantages to the traditional approach. Viewing how DNP graduates can best be supported is critical given the landscape of contemporary health care and the call for increased interdisciplinary collaboration (Clinton & Spearhac, 2006). Therefore, DNPs may need multiple mentors to develop their new roles, or they may need several mentors in succession, as they grow and develop new roles.

There are a few mentorship models particularly designed for doctorally prepared nurses. However, the Schumacher model provides a linear framework that emphasizes fostering scholarship and excellence in nursing and for recruiting and grooming new faculty. It articulates methods for nurse educators to capitalize on each other's strengths to work together to address the current shortage (Schumacher, Risco, & Conway, 2008). The model also encourages novice faculty to actively share expertise and to seek input from both individual mentors and entire faculty units as mentor. When a faculty unit has identified the specific strengths that each faculty member contributes, new faculty members are then given this list of individuals who can serve as specific resources to assist them in meeting their career objectives in teaching, excellence, and scholarship. The Schumacher model can help seasoned faculty mentors begin a working relationship with new faculty. Discussion related to documented shared vision, trust, respect, and commitment provides a unified foundation for the mentorship relationship (Schumacher et al., 2008). Finally, the Schumacher model offers a stated and integrated goal of fostering scholarship and excellence for the mentorship relationship. The new faculty member and protégé can work backward from the model's goals of fostering scholarship and excellence by starting with identification of the most important barriers for the new faculty member, and then prioritizing the strategies needed to address them. Mentors and novice faculty then collaborate regarding which specific actions are most significant for promoting the new faculty's success.

Rabionet, Santiago, and Zorrilla (2009) support a multifaceted mentoring model that strengthens research capacity. This model was specifically developed to contribute to greater productivity of researchers, especially minority researchers, in the fields of biomedical and social sciences. This multifaceted mentoring model includes establishing multiinstitutional collaborations (Ostlin, Braveman, & Dachs, 2005), offering systematic and continuous training based on competency development (Mullins, Blatt, Gbarayor, Keri-Yang, & Baquet, 2005), and creating cross-disciplinary research teams in which mentors and mentees work together (Green, Rivers, & Arekere, 2006). Rabionet et al. (2009) report that attention to these three facets produces synergy and provides the solid foundation needed to foster long-standing mentor–mentee relationships. Fundamental to this model is the understanding that mentoring is a process in which mentors and mentees jointly advance their commitment to scholarly pursuit; thus, mentoring is envisioned as a process for fostering systematic engagement, while inspiring and empowering both mentee and mentor (Fuller, 2000). Additionally, mentoring offers a platform for researchers from diverse disciplines to appreciate what they share and to explore what is beyond their disciplinary domains. Importantly, the multifaceted mentoring model has the potential to be replicated in varied contexts.

Given the emphasis on extensive clinical practice and strong scholarly and evidence-based practice, mentoring models from a practice perspective are central to DNP graduates. No models specific for DNP practice were found in the extant literature. However, Yoder (1990) proposed a clinical mentoring model with two dimensions: (a) instrumental or career functions (coaching, challenging assignments, protection, sponsorship, exposure, and visibility), and (b) psychosocial functions (counseling, acceptance, role modeling, and friendship). As such, the personal scenarios, anecdotes, case examples, and humorous stories shared by mentors can be foundational in the growth and development of new DNP graduates practicing in the clinical forum. Yoder's model mirrors the typology by Kram (1985) described in organizational literature, in which eight mentoring behaviors are described. Five are related to career development (sponsoring, exposure, teaching the job, teaching the informal system, and protection), and three are related to psychosocial support (role modeling, encouragement, and personal counseling).

Models that support leadership development for DNPs are critical. Leadership has been around for centuries beginning with Plato's belief that leaders are created based on their class position; current leaders are created based on their relationships with other individuals (Gregory-Mina, 2009). Leaders today must shape organizational culture, communicate value systems, model ethical behavior, engage and inspire followers, and manage diversity (Grant, 2010). Hoeger, Wilson, and Evans (2009) propose a Moses Cone Health System Critical Leadership Passages Link Model (MCHS) and a Leadership Competency Model (LCM). MCHS, the name of a health care system located in Greensboro, NC, has identified specific passages through which its nurse leaders must pass in order to advance to the next level along the administrative track (i.e., assistant director, department director, service director, vice president of nursing, and chief nursing officer [CNO]) (Succession Management Task Force, 2006, as cited in Hoeger et al., 2009). A core group of administrators who are invested in the growth and development of aspiring nurse leaders serve as mentors. Depending on the mentees' goals, they may keep the same mentor or have different mentors at varied levels to meet their needs. The guidance and mentorship being provided serves as both a motivation and a retention effort for aspiring leaders throughout the MCHS organization. The LCM encompasses three leadership dimensions: Leading and Managing Self, Leading and Managing Others, and Leading the Business of Health Care. As leaders move through the pipeline, key behaviors for each competency are necessary at each level (Hoeger et al.). Although the competencies are similar despite the level of leadership, behaviors that reflect the competency are dissimilar. For instance, behaviors that demonstrate competency in financial acumen are very different at the CNO level compared to the Director level. These differences are clearly identified and drive development for a potential leader, such as a DNP executive.

Finally, Cole and Wright-Harp (2005a, 2005b, 2006) propose a Multiple Mentor Model. This model supports novice professionals having multiple mentors of varied skills, ages, and traits who can meet their individual needs. Cole and Wright-Harp (2005a) purport that since no one mentor can address the varying needs of mentees as they transition into their new professional careers, one can never have too many mentors. The Multiple Mentoring Model was specifically developed for graduate students and highlights the fact that these students benefit from having the following types of mentors: academic, clinical, research, peer, and career/professional development (CPD) mentors.

The main role of the academic mentor is to establish both a professional and personal relationship that helps to facilitate the mentee's academic success. The academic mentor also makes a commitment to see that the student successfully completes the graduate program, thus decreasing the number of students with the status of "all but dissertation" and "all but master's thesis" (Wright-Harp & Cole, 2008). Ideally, the academic mentor serves as teacher and guide in an interactive partnership that is intended to enhance the mentee's self-awareness and fulfillment, with the ultimate goal of helping the mentee to have a positive and fulfilling graduate school experience (Wright-Harp & Cole, 2008). The academic mentor also provides an integrative experience to give support to students in the development of cognitive maps of the program, the discipline, and the profession; therefore, the mentee is better able to make the transition from academia into his or her chosen career path.

The clinical mentor is more relevant to the discipline of the mentee's selected profession that requires students to acquire practical training through a variety of clinical practicum experiences (e.g., university clinics, hospitals, rehabilitation clinics, and public and private schools). In the clinical domain, the ideal mentor would engage in continuing education efforts to remain current in the discipline and remain current on the most recent state-of-the-art approaches to clinical management. In addition, the clinical mentor: (a) provides continuous feedback to facilitate the mentee's development of clinical competencies, and (b) integrates the importance of using research and outcome data as part of the mentoring experience, which in turn would improve treatment efficacy (Wright-Harp & Cole, 2008).

> The ideal research mentor should have a record of successful research mentoring, be current in his or her discipline, conduct research that is relevant to the needs in the field, have a productive track record in research that is regarded as such by colleagues within the department and the discipline, and have a record of funded research and publications.
>
> —*Wright-Harp & Cole, 2008, p. 10*

Other factors that are important to this process include the research mentor's willingness to (a) allow research activities to be observed, (b) assume responsibility for research, (c) share mentoring responsibilities and rewards, (d) have a record of successful mentees, and (e) be genuinely interested in the success of the mentee. Finally, the research mentor must be willing to invest the necessary time to foster the development of a mentee's research capabilities and aid in the enhancement of the mentees professional self-confidence and esteem by providing opportunities for the mentee to disseminate his or her research through presentations and publications (Wright-Harp & Cole, 2008).

In the Multiple Mentor Model, peer mentors play a major part in the graduate school process. The ideal peer mentor has a desire to mentor, has high-quality interpersonal skills, is punctual and reliable, understands the significance of confidentiality regarding information discussed: with the mentee, and adheres to the university's code of conduct. Other important characteristics for peer mentors are (a) they usually have the same academic major as their mentees and are in the same professional training program or institution, and (b) they are normally in the advanced stages of their academic training or have a particular area of expertise to share with other students. Peer mentors also utilize strategies to help new students overcome challenges in their graduate school experience, serve as tutors, share their own learning experiences (e.g., professional successes as well as failures), and help motivate mentees on a routine basis and in challenging or trying situations. Students who serve as peer mentors during graduate school are provided opportunities to hone and develop their mentoring and leadership skills (Wright-Harp & Cole, 2008).

Of all the mentor types in the Multiple Mentor Model, the CPD mentor plays the most critical role in helping the mentee to successfully transition into his or her chosen career setting (Wright-Harp & Cole, 2008). Attributes to seek in a CPD mentor include patience, experience, availability, and expertise in the discipline. Additional characteristics CPD mentors should possess include: (a) patience in providing guidance to mentees based on their skill sets, (b) establishment of self as a model professional in the current employment setting, (c) ability and willingness to impart their knowledge relevant to the delivery of services to target populations, and (d) knowledge about the culture of the organization and ability to orient mentees to the politics of the employment setting. CPD mentors also help mentees develop the competencies necessary to advance along the career path and guide mentees in meeting their career goals.

Given the variation in mentorship models, DNP graduates need to incorporate relevant aspects of models that can support their growth. As the profession continues to refine the different tracks DNPs will pursue, models for mentorship can be developed that best fit meeting their career trajectories.

Mentor–Mentee Profile

Characteristics and preparation of mentors as well as the mentor–mentee profile are critical to successful mentee development. Young and Wright (2001) report that the following qualities are requisite to being good mentors: (a) being committed to their role;

(b) authentically accepting of the mentee, while being sensitive and understanding of their mentee's needs; (c) being skilled at providing support; (d) being knowledgeable in their specific area; and (e) being a model for continuous learning. Schwiebert, Deck, and Bradshaw (1999) also report that effective mentors should demonstrate the ability to: (a) make an investment of quality time in the relationship; (b) maintain supportive interaction; and (c) make a commitment to create time necessary to allow for in-depth discussions of the needs and goals of the mentee and the progress toward the goals. Thus, the ideal mentor possesses a multitude of attributes and skills. Moreover, mentors must be sensitive to cultural diversity (e.g., willing to understand the culture of individuals from diverse minority/marginalized groups and those from racial/ethnic backgrounds). Being able to understand factors that may be attributed to gender differences and societal mores (e.g., demands of being a wife and mother, of being single parent, and of being male in a predominantly female profession) that could influence the mentee's academic success is requisite. The styles which mentors use to carry out these responsibilities vary.

Research conducted by McNally and Martin (1998) identified three styles of mentorship: laissez-faire, collaborative, and imperial. The primary role of laissez-faire mentors is to nurture and provide support for novice professionals as they manage complex and often emotional challenges of learning their new role. While laissez-faire mentors may understand the difference between, and the need for, both challenge and support, they have a strong belief in the need for emotional support and reducing stress for the novice (McNally & Martin, 1998). Collaborative mentors combine support and challenge in ways which empower the novice professional to engage in learning as a critically reflective process. Mentors understand the pedagogy of mentoring and think about how to make the role more effective. They see their main task as one of being able to "tune in" to the individual novice's needs in a way that recognizes and respects the person as a future colleague, yet also seeks to extend the novice's experiences and thinking about this new professional role. The mentor is both proactive and reactive in shaping the novice's learning experiences (McNally & Martin, 1998). The imperial mentor is a person with strong beliefs about learning and a strong sense that the mentoring role provides an intellectual challenge to the novice as the person develops as a professional. The mentor's role is colored by the person's own level of expertise as a professional and by the person's status as someone in authority within his or her selected area. The needs of the novice are not seen as being as important as the goals and vision that mentors hold related to their mentees. The stress for the novice can come from the perceived gap between the novice's current level of development and the need to match the mentor's expertise. The role is strongly interventionist and proactive, as the mentor attempts to shape the novice's learning experiences (McNally & Martin).

Mentees with the following qualities are reported to be most successful. These include the mentee's ability to: (a) enter the mentorship relationship willingly; (b) exhibit responsibility by taking initiative and showing resourcefulness; (c) respect and trust the mentor; (d) listen to advice and respond in the most effective manner to meet his or her needs; and (e) develop a plan proactively for accomplishing goals (Young & Wright, 2001).

Given the particular attributes and skills needed by mentors, it is critical for someone (e.g., administrators, leadership) to invest in training and support individuals from varied professions to serve as mentors. This can take place in different contexts (e.g., academic organizations, health care institutions, political arenas, and primary care practices). Even more than a desire to mentor, financial commitment is requisite to build a foundation of effective, competent mentors who can take on responsibilities to develop nurses in the profession. Two vignettes illustrate a positive and negative mentoring experience.

Case I: David: A DNP Student

David was in his last year of doctoral study and was about to register for his culminating capstone course, which required him to design and conduct a clinically based study. He was having difficulty, deciding on a topic or population to study. His faculty advisor mentioned his difficulty to another faculty who was involved in a county-wide assessment of mental health needs in uninsured patients and their families. She approached David and asked him if he would like to join her at the planning meetings and decide if he would like to participate in the project. He agreed, and accompanied her to the next planning meeting, where she personally introduced him to several key people, and made sure he sat at the table with her. During the planning discussions at the table, she would seek his opinions, and explained some constructs and history to him when needed. She asked him if he would like to develop a questionnaire and interview a group of stakeholders, and he agreed. They met in her office several times during the first few months, during which she guided his process of coding, analyzing, and interpreting responses. David completed his capstone paper, and she then invited him to present his study at a regional research conference. During his presentation, David pointed to his mentor and thanked her for her help. She then asked him if he wanted to rewrite the paper for submission to a nursing journal, and he willingly agreed. He worked on the paper with her assistance for the rest of the summer, it was submitted to a nursing journal, was accepted, and published a year later. She incorporated the study into the literature review for a proposal she wrote a year later, which received full funding from the HRSA division of the U.S. Department of Health and Human Services.

Case II: Patricia: A New Faculty Member With a DNP Degree

Patricia returned to graduate school after 20 years of practice in acute care hospitals as a critical care nurse. Following graduation with a DNP degree, she accepted a position as an assistant professor at a small nursing school. This would be the first time she would assume the role of a nurse educator, although she had precepted many nursing students in hospital settings. She received a short orientation to her role, and was told that the department chair of the course to whom she was assigned would be her mentor. She had many questions and concerns about her role and about how to identify and access resources she would need to create and teach her courses. Her efforts to contact her mentor, however, were unsuccessful. They had not established any regular times to meet, her phone messages went unanswered, and her emails were either answered late or the chair's responses were so brief as to be useless. When she approached the chair at faculty meetings, the chair would complain about her workload and the students. Patricia reached out to other faculty, and found one who answered her questions and helped her as she negotiated her new role. But even this faculty did not seem to welcome her, or include her in any informal meetings or lunches. After the first semester, the chair told her that the three faculty who taught in the clinical course always met at her house to calculate final grades, so she would be expected to travel across the city to her chair's home, and bring her student's graded papers, which she did. The meeting took most of the day, although the actual time spent calculating students' grades was about an hour. At the end of the meeting, she picked up what she thought was all of her student papers, placed them in her briefcase, and traveled across town again to her house. Later that evening, she realized that a paper was missing when she went through her briefcase. She called the chair, who told her that the paper was not there. Patricia spent a sleepless night, and then the next morning she searched her home, car, and office but could not find that paper. As she prepared to contact the student, another faculty called her to tell her that the chair had the paper, but had decided to keep it for a few days to teach Patricia to keep better track of her student's papers. Patricia finished her semester at that nursing school, but quit at the end of the year. Years later, she once again accepted a position as an assistant professor at a different nursing school, this time with very different results. She is now enjoying an academic experience, and makes a point of welcoming and mentoring new faculty.

Professional development of DNP graduates will not occur solely by and/or with other DNP graduates. We must ask: "Given the state of cross disciplinary initiatives, is that really necessary and/or beneficial?" DNPs will operate in fluid, multidisciplinary environments; therefore, depending on their career specialization and trajectory, it will be useful to engage in diverse mentorship experiences with others outside of the nursing profession. While doing this, it is important to build a foundation of DNP mentors to refine practice among this cohort.

MEETING THE NEEDS OF UNDERREPRESENTED GROUPS OF DNPs

Professional nursing has a sad history of limiting or preventing access to leadership roles in academic programs and clinical practice for nonmainstream populations. This pattern of discrimination by a European-Caucasian dominant mainstream culture can be traced back at least to Ms. Nightingale, the same Nightingale who so successfully mentored Linda Richards, a Caucasian American nurse, in 1877. Mary Seacole, a Jamaican nurse, visited Ms. Nightingale in Scutari during the Crimean War and offered her services as part of the nursing staff; however, she was refused. Seemingly undaunted, Ms. Seacole established a British Hotel near the battlefield, where she tended to the sick and wounded from that war (Mary Seacole Centre, 2006). Although increased numbers of people from minority cultures are enrolling in doctoral programs, prior discriminatory practices have created a system of barriers to advanced practice and leadership in health care and academia. These barriers to upward mobility and practice for nurses from minority cultures challenge nursing today and are shown in:

- Lack of diverse mentors from nursing faculty (e.g., gender, ethnicity, and religion);
- Lack of mentors from underrepresented groups in doctoral programs (e.g., sexual orientation—lesbian, gay, bisexual, or transgender);

- No training or insufficient training in cultural sensitivity for faculty, providers, or administrators who serve as mentors;
- Doctoral programs that require on-campus residency making it impossible for many candidates with family obligations to attend; and
- Insufficient funding support for doctoral study, which impedes the career advancement of many nurses who are sole financial supports of their families (Marquand, 2008).

Mentoring has special significance for faculty of minority status. Without such help, these faculty members can have difficulty cracking "the old girls' network." A mentor can be very helpful in this regard, as successful mentoring can help minority and marginalized DNPs climb the professional ladder. For historical reasons, owing to their prominence in senior positions, middle-aged Caucasian women predominantly have fulfilled the role of mentor in the Western world. Even though they are capable mentors to members of minority groups, there may be instances where cultural differences can make the relationship difficult.

Of the over 2.6 million nurses in the United States, only 196,279 are educated at the graduate level and only 10–12% of these are APNs from minority cultures (Spratley, Johnson, Sochalski, Fritz, & Spencer, 2000). Membership by individuals from minority cultures in many professional nursing organizations is also disproportionate to their total number in the organization, which is now 34% and is estimated to be 54% of the population by 2050 (Demographics of the United States, 2009). For instance, 5.5% of the membership of the American Academy of Nurse Practitioners is African-American, 3.0% is Hispanic American, and 1.3% is American Indian/Native Hawaiian/Pacific Islander (American Academy of Nurse Practitioners [AANP], 2006).

The AACN (2008) has examined this disparity in minority representation in APNs. It calls for all nursing education programs to strive for ethnic and racial diversity in its faculty and students. To apply its goals to advanced practice, nurses from ethnic or racial minority cultures should make up 25% of the nation's estimated 17,256 doctorally prepared nurses (Spratley et al., 2000). Meeting this goal will take a combination of collective will, focused recruiting, support, networking, and mentoring of doctoral candidates, students, and DNPs who are new to a role or position. One of the strategies to accomplish this goal is to create formal mentoring programs to recruit and support nurses from underrepresented groups for DNP preparation in direct health care delivery, education, and research.

One of the most successful of these formal mentoring programs is the "Bridges to the Doctoral Degree," which is a program for mentoring students from underrepresented minorities sponsored by the National Institutes of Health (NIH) (Marquand, 2008). For example, the 5-year Bridges program consists of several partner schools collaborating with the University of Illinois-Chicago (UIC) to recruit, support, and mentor MSN students into UIC's PhD in Nursing program (Kim et al., 2009). Project coordinators guide and counsel students throughout the application process. Seminars and socials provide needed peer and faculty networking time. NIH research training grants support students' research experiences. Although this is a new and ongoing program at UIC, preliminary data show that faculty mentoring support, as well as financial support, are keys to retention. Other schools that have participated in this NIH-sponsored program include the University of Minnesota, Rutgers, North Dakota, and Oklahoma (Henley, Struthers, Dahl, Patchell, & Holtzclaw, 2006).

Another example of a formal mentoring program to increase minority prepa-ration for leadership positions in health care is the Leadership Enhancement and Development (LEAD) Project for Minority Nurses (Bessent & Fleming, 2003). Its goal is to strengthen the leadership skills of minority nurses through a series of workshops on leadership and race, and on strategies for confronting and overcoming barriers in the workplace. After attending these workshops, nurses can continue to attend these semi-nars led by nurse leaders from diverse backgrounds. Mentees have the option to select mentors from the nurse leaders at these workshops depending upon their needs and interests.

No matter which model of mentoring is used, or whether mentoring is provided through a formal program or informal process, DNP mentors must have as their goal to increase minority representation in leadership in health care as administrators, policy makers, faculty, and providers. Strategies must be developed to facilitate market-ing and target recruitment to specified populations or of nurses. For instance, ads can be placed in the journals and magazines directed to specific minority group readers, such as *Minority Nurse*. In addition, college recruiters can actively recruit and display at minority professional conferences, such as the National Black Nurses Association or the National Association of Hispanic Nurses. Mentors must advocate for closer access to doctoral programs, help with facilitation of the application process (which itself can be a barrier to access), target recruitment of minority students, and provide support for the many stu-dents who are also caring for senior parents as well as minors in their homes. This support includes financial aid, which is considered crucial for doctoral students (Marquand, 2008).

EFFECTIVE MENTORING

A supportive network of colleagues who "have your back" is recognized as a key com-ponent of job satisfaction and effective mentoring (Miller, Apold, Baas, Berner, & Levine-Brill, 2005; Jacelon, Zucker, Staccarini, & Henneman, 2003). Doctorally prepared nurses are usually over the age of 40 when they begin doctoral study, are experienced practitioners, and often supervise others. Their mentors should consider that these experienced practitioners would benefit from peer mentorship. This approach views the mentor and mentee more as a collegial relationship. That is, although the mentee is just starting in this new role, the mentee is also an experienced provider who has much to offer the organization. The mentor assists the mentee in navigating and using a new environment; both will learn from each other as peers and engage in a mutually beneficial, heuristic process of sharing ideas and resources. Peer mentoring can assist doc-torally prepared faculty in new careers to facilitate integration into a new work culture with its own routines, policies, and practices. This mentoring approach can be provided informally, or through a more formal, established peer mentoring program.

One example of peer mentoring is the process that newly hired faculty from one university developed to support each other's paths to tenure. Several faculty collaborated to participate in research projects, to network, and to support each other's scholarship. After one year, participants reported more mutual collaboration and individual productivity, and stronger professional relationships as outcomes from this process (Jacelon et al., 2003). Another example is the group of nursing faculty who developed a Western Writers Coercion Group to support and facilitate nursing faculty scholarship.

After two years, it evolved into a five-university and multidisciplinary peer support and mentoring program. Members used the group to focus, set, track, and attain goals and to encourage their fellow faculty members to do likewise (Cumbie, Weinert, Luparell, Conley, & Smith, 2005).

Yet another example of peer mentoring is the informal mentoring process at the University of St. Francis College of Nursing and Allied Health's DNP Program in Joliet, Illinois. Students in its post-master's DNP program begin their studies with mostly decades of experience as nursing leaders, many own their own businesses, others have published, are educators, or may have served in key positions in professional organizations or in acute care hospitals. They are new again to the graduate student role, and are acculturating to the new role of DNP, but they are board-certified practicing peers in their own right. They learn about the background, clinical, and research interests of faculty at orientation, and both faculty and doctoral students are encouraged to connect and share interests with each other in preparation for the student's scholarly papers at the culmination of their program of study. The purpose of this program is to encourage networking role model collegiality in APNs, and to build a system of mutual collaboration in scholarly projects.

Figure 16.1, developed by the coauthor of this chapter, depicts this dynamic process as a wheel, turning as the process of mentoring first moves from mutual introductions, commitment and contract formation, through anticipatory information sharing and exchanges, to the mentor actively supporting the student's scholarship, to the final collaborative relationship. Encircling this process is the required organizational support in terms of time, recognition, and resources, which enables this relationship to develop to its potential.

Anyone seeking to develop a mentoring program can learn from a wide variety of successful programs that could be adapted to doctoral education, or new careers, or research and nursing science positions. A formal program of mentorship not only requires willing participants and a plan, but also a supportive environment for mentor and mentee alike. The mentor invests considerable amount of time, effort, and persistence to advance and nurture the mentee. This investment ultimately benefits the organization in measurable outcomes of employee and student productivity, retention, and satisfaction. This investment should not only be recognized by the organization, but supported and rewarded if it is to continue. The following are key institutional mentoring resource elements that organizations such as universities, schools, hospitals, and other industries should provide to support the mentoring role of its employees. The Dean or Chief Nursing Officer can:

- Construct a written contract or signed agreement about the mentor's duties or role, which any mentor can use as a guide to keep the process on target.
- Provide training on the role of a mentor that includes cultural sensitivity training for all employees (e.g., administrators, staff, and faculty) to promote the value of this role to the organization. The emphasis on formal training conveys the organization's investment in the mentoring process.
- Support the mentoring process because mentoring relationships develop gradually, creating mutual trust and finding mutual interests. These relationships are guided by the goals of the mentee; create avenues for communicating interests for meeting new candidates and for mentees and mentors to view the work and backgrounds of potential mentors. *Avoid* arbitrarily assigning mentors to newly hired employees or to new doctoral students.

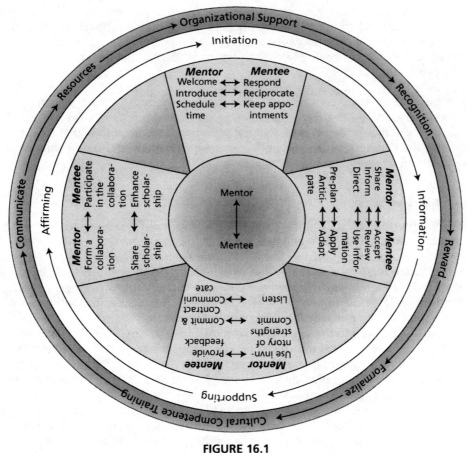

FIGURE 16.1
USF model of peer mentoring

- Provide release time from job-related duties and functions, so that the mentor can find the time to meet with the mentee, and will *not* ultimately view the role as overtime, overload, or extra work.
- Recognize the value of the mentoring role to the organization by communicating its goals, function, and benefits to the internal structure of the organization. This communication can be done in the form of written communication (e.g., newsletter article, posters), or formal events where mentors can be introduced to others in the organization, or in informal conversations.
- Formally recognize and reinforce effective mentoring. This recognition can come in many forms including a raise or stipend, a certificate or letter of support that can be added to a portfolio, or submission of the mentor's name to a professional organization for an award.
- Support the development of a process for mentors to identify and support each other. This process might come in the form of a support group, list serve, or monthly meeting. The goal of the supportive process is to nurture the nurturers, and to retain the leaders among us who choose to advance and support other APNs.

Organizational support for the mentoring programs, program objectives, degree of program oversight and ongoing relationship support, rewards for program participation, and the specific procedure used to match mentors and mentees is critical. When the organizational supports are in place, then the mentor and mentee can concentrate on creating productive relationships.

Effective mentoring is a process that includes the use of mutual respect, appreciation, a positive attitude, commitment, and honesty by both the mentor and mentee. The following are tips for effective mentoring for both the mentor and mentee. These tips can be used as a guide for any doctorally prepared nurse who is planning to serve as a mentor to a colleague or student or to any nurse who is entering a new role, accepting a new position, or opening a new practice.

Tips for the Mentor

- Since mentoring can occur through informal or formal processes, do not wait to be appointed or asked to be someone's mentor. If you see someone who is new to a role or career or setting or position or skill set, step up. Welcome, invite, introduce, and reinforce with your presence and new learning. Your mentoring actions will be rewarded through the growth of your colleagues in advanced practice.
- Mentoring is a heuristic process when done well, so consider that your mentoring actions will also be rewarded by your own self-growth.
- Make a commitment to the mentoring relationship. You can commit if you can decide what time, resources, and use of self you can offer to develop and support the mentoring relationship. If you do not have the time or resources, then do your prospective mentee and yourself a favor, decline the request/invitation and find another way to use yourself as a collegial resource.
- Conduct a self-inventory before you decide to be a mentor, and identify the strengths and attributes you bring to the role of mentor. You can then build upon these strengths for your mentees and for your own growth during the mentoring process.
- Take time — *time* to select a colleague or student who is new to your program or organization, *time* to listen, *time* to consider what the mentee wants, and *time* to decide what information your mentee needs in order to contribute and grow in your program or organization.
- Determine if your mentee also needs or would appreciate on-site consultation.
- Assist your mentee with setting the goals that can be met through the mentoring process, then regularly evaluate in what ways your mentoring has assisted in meeting those goals.
- Keep all appointments and commitments.

Tips for the Mentee

- Conduct a self-inventory before you meet with or contact your mentor. Identify the strengths you bring, goals, resources you will need, and information you should have in this new organization, academic setting, or professional practice.
- Communicate your needs clearly to your mentor early and often. Expect that these needs will constantly change, but do not expect that your mentor will recognize what they are or when they have changed, unless you have communicated that.
- If your mentor has helped you in negotiating the system, working within the organization, or learning within an academic setting, then acknowledge the help and thank the mentor. A simple acknowledgment in the way of a thank you is a powerful

reinforcer of effective mentoring, and lays the groundwork for continuing collaboration and support.

▓ Remember that you are a collaborative partner in the mentoring relationship.
▓ Keep all appointments and commitments.

Mentoring is conducted through a dynamic relationship forged between mentor and mentee. Just like any other organic phenomenon, it must be nourished and protected, or it withers and dies. As these tips for mentor and mentee illustrate, if both partners in this relationship are considerate of each other's time and talents, commit to some goal setting and preparation planning, and clarify their interactions, the relationship should flourish. The end product of this mentoring process can be improved professional skills, increased career satisfaction, and more confident doctorally prepared nurses committed to continued learning and collaborative practice.

FUTURE DIRECTIONS AND RECOMMENDATIONS

Mentoring the next generation of DNP graduates to generate leaders in the profession is requisite. Understanding how they are being mentored by senior faculty at their institutions is important for career guidance. Thus, collaborative relationships are requisite between DNPs and faculty with other academic degrees (e.g., EdD, DNS, PhD) if individual faculty are to be properly provided guidance about how to succeed either in practice, academia, research, and/or in leadership positions. If this does not occur, the advancement of DNPs can be stifled. To maximize the probability of success, DNPs need effective mentoring. Most successful individuals have one to four mentors (Arnold, 2005). In the academic world, there is clear evidence that good mentoring is associated with successful grant applications and academic publications (Hitchcock, Bland, Hekelman, & Blumenthal, 1995; Steiner, Curtis, Lamphear, Vu, & Main, 2004; Steiner, Lanphear, Curtis, & Vu, 2002). In the business literature, there are data that mentoring is associated with higher annual income and job satisfaction (Zachary, 2000).

Mentoring is particularly important to the development of this new professional cohort entering a complex socio-cultural, political, and health care structure. First, the evidence base is changing rapidly; therefore, DNP graduates need teachers and mentors to help them learn the cognitive, affective, and behavioral skills required to be competent DNP professionals. This means teaching both the formal knowledge and the informal art of DNP practice.

Second, the routes to career success for DNP graduates are fluid and still being defined. Newcomers to the advanced nursing practice profession need a host and guide who can give them advice about how to weigh the risks and benefits of different career options. Many DNPs may be linked through APN associations in their own field of interest. These networks may lend support to colleagues whereby they can recommend a prospective mentor who might help with their professional advancement.

Finally, at the same time that individuals are learning to be DNP professionals, it is likely they are going through other developmental tasks common to adulthood, such as developing long-term relationships, choosing a home, deciding whether to have children, supporting children through higher education, or caretaking of parents. It often helps to gain guidance by more senior personnel in the same field about these topics. Finding out about how others balance work and home may offer new options or reinforce one's views about how to manage one's life. This is especially important for DNP graduates who are more often women. This can have even higher stakes for DNP graduates from minority cultures who tend to have a narrower support system that can authentically relate to their professional and personal circumstances. There is a lot to learn (about both life and DNP professionals) during one's early years and having a mentor increases the chance that one will make this transition successfully. Truthfully, while mentoring relationships are important, it is not something that many individuals know how to do effectively. Moreover, the skills required to "pave the way" are different from the skills required to help others find their way. Individuals often succeed by charisma, intelligence, hard work, self-resolve, and determination. Mentoring requires listening to what others want and helping them achieve those goals, even if the mentor does not agree with them. Mentees need to know that their mentor is there for them and yet must learn ultimately to make independent decisions.

SUMMARY

The APN role has evolved as a response to regulatory requirements, rapid scientific advances, and health care change Illinois and is still evolving as a distinct and independent health professional. Because of this, the need for mentorship of doctorally prepared APNs is acute, yet the culture of mentorship in advanced nursing practice is still in its infancy. Doctorally prepared APNs must take the lead in mentoring qualified candidates in order to establish a pipeline of competent and confident DNPs who are health care providers, scientists, educators, and researchers. This chapter has described the need for mentoring DNP students and DNP graduates in new roles, and has recommended ongoing mentoring for advancement. Selected mentoring models can be used to guide the development and application of mentoring programs to support doctoral students and doctorally prepared nurses in new positions.

The major purposes of mentoring are to encourage networking, to role model collegiality, and to build a system of mutual collaboration in professional activities. A mentoring program not only requires willing student and faculty participants, but also a plan *and* a supportive environment for mentor and mentee alike. The successful mentor invests a considerable amount of time, effort, and persistence to advance and nurture the mentee. This investment ultimately benefits the organization in measurable outcomes of employee and student productivity, retention, and satisfaction. This investment should not only be recognized by the organization, but supported and rewarded if it is to continue. Institutional resources are keys in supporting the mentoring role of its doctorally prepared employees.

REFERENCES

Allen, T. D., Eby, L. T., & Lentz, E. (2006). The relationship between formal mentoring program characteristics and perceived program effectiveness. *Personnel Psychology, 59*, 125–153.

American Academy of Nurse Practitioners (AANP). (2006). *Member demographics*. Retrieved from http://aanp.org/AANPCMS2/MemberCenter/Individual+Members/Member+Demographics.htm

American Association of Colleges of Nursing (AACN). (2006). *AACN DNP tool kit: Template for the process of developing a DNP program*. Retrieved from www.aacn.nche.edu/DNP/toolkit.htm7

American Association of Colleges of Nursing (AACN). (2008). *Statement defines vision of nursing higher education for next decade*. Retrieved from http://www.aacn.nche.edu/Media/NewsReleases/visnstm.htm

Arnold, R. (2005). Mentoring the next generation: A critical task for palliative medicine. *Journal of Palliative Medicine, 8*(4), 696–698.

Bessent, H., & Fleming, J. (2003). Leadership enhancement and development project (LEAD) for minority nurses. *Nursing Outlook, 5*, 255–260.

Chism, L. (2009). *The doctor of nursing process: A guidebook for role development and professional issues.* Boston, MA: Jones and Bartlett.

Clinton, P., & Spearhac, A. (2006). National agenda for advanced practice nursing: The practice doctorate. *Journal of Professional Nursing, 22*(1), 7–14.

Cole, P., & Wright-Harp, W. (2005a, April). *Mentoring mechanisms for building pathways for success in graduate education.* Presentation at the annual convention of the National Black Association for Speech-Language and Hearing, Richmond, VA.

Cole, P., & Wright-Harp, W. (2005b, April). *Transcending barriers through mentoring: Building pathways for success in graduate education.* Presentation at the annual conference of the International Mentoring Association, Oakland, CA.

Cole, P., & Wright-Harp, W. (2006, April). *Ethics and research.* Invited mini-seminar presented at the annual convention of the National Black Association for Speech-Language and Hearing, Memphis, TN.

Council of Graduate Schools. (2006). *Exit surveys show mentoring essential to doctorate completion.* Retrieved from http://www.cgsnet.org/Default.aspx?tabid=240&newsid440=93&mid=440

Cumbie, S., Weinert, C., Luparell, S., Conley, V., & Smith, J. (2005). Developing a scholarship community. *Journal of Nursing Scholarship, 37*(3), 289–293.

Demographics of the United States. (2009). Retrieved from http://en.wikipedia.org/wiki/Demographics_of_the_United_States#Race_and_ethnicity

Eby, L. T., Rhodes, J., & Allen, T. D. (2007). Definition and evolution of mentoring. In T. D. Allen, & L. T. Eby (Eds.), *The Blackwell handbook of mentoring: A multiple perspectives approach* (pp. 7–20). Oxford, UK: Blackwell.

Florence Nightingale. (2007). *Florence Nightingale, 1810–1910.* Retrieved from http://www.solarnavigator.net/history/florence_nightingale.htm

Fuller, S. S. (2000). Enabling, empowering, inspiring: Research and mentorship through the years. *Bulletin of Medical Library Association, 88*, 1–10.

Grant, S. (2010). Diversity in healthcare: Driven by leadership. *Frontiers of Health Services Management, 26*(3), 41–45.

Green, B. L., Rivers, B. M., & Arekere, D. M. (2006). Mentoring: A framework for developing health disparities researchers. *Health Promotion and Practice, 7*, 336–345.

Gregory-Mina, H. J. (2009). Four leadership theories addressing contemporary leadership issues as the theories relate to the scholarship, practice, and leadership model. *Academic Leadership.* Retrieved from http://www.academicleadership.org/emprical_research/Four_Leadership_Theories_Addressing_Contemporary_Leadership_Issues_as_the_Theories_Relate_to_the_Scholarship_Practice_and_Leadership_Model.shtml

Henley, S., Struthers, R., Dahl, B., Patchell, B., & Holtzclaw, B. (2006). Research careers for American Indian/Alaska Natives: Pathway to elimination of health disparities. *American Journal of Public Health, 96*(4), 606–611.

Hitchcock, M. A., Bland, C. J., Hekelman, F. P., & Blumenthal, M. G. (1995). Professional networks: The influence of colleagues on the academic success for faculty. *Academy of Medicine, 70*, 1108–1116.

Hoeger, P., Wilson, J., & Evans, J. (2009). Cultivating nurse leaders from the bedside to the boardroom. *Nurse Leader, 7*(4), 41–45, 50.

Jacelon, C., Zucker, D., Staccarini, J., & Henneman, E. (2003). Peer mentoring for tenure-track faculty. *Journal of Professional Nursing, 19*(6), 335–338.

Karcher, M. J., Kuperminc, G. P., Portwood, S. G., Sipe, C. L., & Taylor, A. S. (2006). Mentoring programs: A framework to inform program development, research, and evaluation. *Journal of Community Psychology, 34*(6), 709–725.

Kim, M., Holm, K., Gerard, P., McElmurry, B., Foreman, M., Poslusny, S. et al., (2009). Bridges to the doctorate: Mentored transition to successful completion of doctoral study for underrepresented minorities in nursing science. *Nursing Outlook, 57*(3), 166–171.

Kram, K. (1985). *Mentoring at work: Developmental relationships in organizational life.* Glenview, IL: Scott Foresman.

Marquand, B. (2008). Going the distance. *Minority Nurse.* Retrieved from http://www.minority-nurse.com/minority-nurse-retention/going-distance

Mary Seacole Centre. (2006). *Mary Seacole, 1805–1881.* Retrieved from http://www.maryseacole.com/maryseacole/pages/

McNally, P., & Martin, S. (1998). Support and challenge in learning to teach: The role of mentor. *Asia-Pacific Journal of Teacher Education, 26*(1), 31.

Merriam-Webster's. (2001). *Merriam-Webster collegiate dictionary* (10th ed.). Springfield, MA: Merriam-Webster.

Miller, K., Apold, S., Baas, L., Berner, B., & Levine-Brill, E. (2005). Job satisfaction among nurse practitioners. *Journal for Nurse Practitioners, 1*(1), 30–33.

Mullins, C. D., Blatt, L., Gbarayor, C. M., Keri-Yang, H. W., & Baquet, C. (2005). Health disparities: A barrier to high-quality care. *American Journal of Health System-Pharmacy, 62,* 1873–1882.

Nightingale, F. (1859). *Notes on nursing (Commemorative Ed.).* Philadelphia, PA: J.B. Lippincott.

Ostlin, P., Braveman, P., Dachs, J. N., WHO Task Force on Research Priorities for Equity in Health, & WHO Equity Team. (2005). Priorities for research to take forward the health equity policy agenda. *Bulletin of the World Health Organization, 83,* 948–953.

Rabionet, S., Santiago, L., & Zorrilla, C. (2009). A multifaceted mentoring model for minority researchers to address HIV health disparities. *American Journal of Public Health, 99*(S1), S65–S70.

Roberts, A. (1995). *Homer's mentor: Duties fulfilled or misconstrued.* Retrieved from http://home.att.net/~OPSINC/homers_mentor.pdf

Rosser, S., & Taylor, Z. (2009). Why are we still worried about women in science? *Academe: Bulletin of the AAUP, 95*(3), 6–10.

Scheetz, L. (2000). *Nursing faculty secrets.* Philadelphia, PA: Hanley & Belfus.

Schumacher, G., Risco, K., & Conway, A. (2008). The Schumacher Model: Fostering scholarship and excellence in nursing and for recruiting and grooming new faculty. *Journal of Nursing Education, 47*(12), 571–576.

Schwiebert, V., Deck, M., & Bradshaw, M (1999). Women as mentors. *Journal of Humanistic Counseling Education and Development, 37*(4), 241–253.

Smith, L., McAllister, L., & Crawford, C. (2001). Mentoring benefits and issues for public health nurses. *Public Health Nursing, 18*(2), 101–107.

Spratley, E., Johnson, A., Sochalski, J., Fritz, M., & Spencer, W. (2000). *The registered nurse population: Findings from the National Sample Survey of Registered Nurses.* Retrieved from http://bhpr.hrsa.gov/healthworkforce/reports/rnsurvey/

Steiner, J. F., Lanphear, B. P., Curtis, P., & Vu, K. O. (2002). Indicators of early research productivity among primary care fellows. *Journal of General Internal Medicine, 17,* 845–851.

Steiner, J. F., Curtis, P., Lamphear, B. P., Vu, K. D., & Main, D. S. (2004). Assessing the role of influential mentors in the research development of primary care fellows. *Academic Medicine, 79,* 865–872.

Wright-Harp, W., & Cole, P. (2008). A mentoring model for enhancing success in graduate education. *Contemporary Issues in Communication Science and Disorders, 35,* 4–17.

Yoder, L. H. (1990). Mentoring: A concept analysis. *Nursing Administration Quarterly, 15*(1), 9–19.

Young, C., & Wright, J. (2001). Mentoring: The components for success. *Journal of Instructional Psychology, 28*(3), 202–207.

Zachary, L. (2000). *The Mentor's guide: Facilitating effective learning relationship.* San Francisco, CA: Jossey-Bass.

CHAPTER SIXTEEN: Reflective Response

Marlene Rosenkoetter

The authors have presented a noteworthy and in-depth discussion of the issues and conflicts surrounding the mentor–mentee relationship for DNP students and faculty. From my own experience, there seem to be several basic concepts that impact that relationship. The first is "willingness," namely willingness to be mentored and willingness to be a mentor. Many DNP students are well established and highly skilled practitioners, administrators, or faculty members. They have years of experience and now return to a novice level, of sorts, as students in an as yet not fully understood or accepted doctoral-level program. They are faced with returning to their workplace with a degree that may not be perceived to be equivalent to the PhD, may not provide them with credentials for tenure and promotion, and may not be deemed an essential degree for advanced practice by their peers. Questions continue to remain among some advanced practice nurses regarding the appropriateness of requiring them to hold the DNP and use the title "Dr" (Miller, 2008), and it may actually take years before the DNP is accepted by other disciplines as the equivalent of the PhD (Apold, 2008). Silva and Ludwick (2006) made a strong case for questioning the ethics of having the degree. The students may even have clinical skills that exceed those of some of their classroom teachers.

At the initial point of entry into the DNP program, students may experience role shock, role ambiguity, role confusion, and role changes. The faculty member as a mentor is possibly addressing some of these same issues, having been expected to take on the role of mentoring students in a program that is in its infancy and clearly continuing to evolve. Students must be willing to be mentored, to be challenged, and to take responsibility for a new level of practice in their own environment. Faculty members need to be intuitive, reflective, and sensitive not only to the needs of students, but also sensitive to and aware of their own strengths and weaknesses. The DNP student will most likely need and have several mentors across the span of the educational program. There may be one in a clinical subspecialty, evidence-based practice, research, teaching, or administration, to mention a few. The key to a successful relationship seems to evolve around the most basic principles of professionalism—collaboration, collegiality, cooperation, and commitment—all of which are based on mutual trust and ethical beliefs and practices.

Senior faculty can most easily assume the mentoring role, provided they are willing, receptive to the idea and, as the authors point out, have sufficient support within the School of Nursing to fulfill their responsibilities. Mentoring can take many forms, not just for coursework and projects, but also in assisting the DNP student to understand the mentor role (as future mentors), what being a faculty member or administrator in advanced practice is all about, as well as how to negotiate difficult agreements, resolve conflicts, and reach consensus in meetings. To achieve this, mentors may ask students and junior faculty to join them on publications, do research, attend meetings, present papers, and participate in most any scholarly endeavor. Providing a student with the opportunity to be the first author on a publication can foster self-esteem, while experiencing the process of getting a manuscript submitted, accepted, and published is learned. The ultimate goal in mentoring for many students is developing a long-range plan that will lead to Fellowship in the American Academy of Nursing. This needs to start early and may take years to fulfill, but can be a highly rewarding attainment in the end. This particular mentoring role may extend to both students and faculty in other schools of nursing, and even internationally.

The mentor–mentee relationship for international students becomes considerably more complex. Not only is the DNP student adjusting to a new doctoral program, but as well may be adjusting to a new culture and strange environment. This needs interactions with colleagues and interpersonal communication. It is predictable that international students will have even more challenges and changing needs than native students as they progress through the program.

Being a mentor is not as simple as forming a relationship, and the authors of this chapter clearly emphasize that. It takes interest, commitment, willingness to be available, an inclusive attitude, and the ability to be able to share rather than be possessive and protective of one's own domain. One of the most important mentor roles that I have had, that both students and other faculty appreciated, is including them on publications. This starts with providing an overview of the process, doing literature searches, reviewing the various publishing formats and online submissions, determining the different types of publications that one can submit, developing the content, and then managing the comments of the reviewers. Inexperienced faculty can be devastated by reviewer comments, especially when they feel they have "produced a masterpiece," whether in fact they have or have not. Through mentoring, students can have senior faculty input on their publications before they are ever submitted for review. This is turn will provide the student with an opportunity to learn how to mentor early in the process.

The American Association of Colleges of Nursing's (2006) *Essentials* document clearly differentiates between research-focused doctoral programs and DNP programs during which students engage in advanced practice nursing and gain the ability to provide leadership for evidence-based practice. This difference needs to be clearly known by DNP students before they enter the program. Some even decide to pursue both routes simultaneously or in sequence, understanding that both degrees can help to advance the creation and translation of knowledge into practice (Edwardson, 2010). Considering the newness of DNP programs, students may initially be uninformed on both the purpose and the process for acquiring the degree. Having a temporary mentor assigned prior to admission can facilitate this process and help to reduce stress once the student is enrolled—and we must recognize that any doctoral program is stressful!

REFERENCES

American Association of Colleges of Nursing (AACN). (2006). *The essentials of doctoral education for advanced nursing practice*. Retrieved from http://www.aacn.nche.edu/DNP/pdf/Essentials.pdf

Apold, S. (2008). The doctor of nursing practice: Looking back, moving forward. *Journal for Nurse Practitioners, 4*(2), 101–107.

Edwardson, S. (2010). Doctor of philosophy and doctor of nursing practice as complementary degrees. *Journal of Professional Nursing, 26*(3), 137–140.

Miller, J. (2008). The doctor of nursing practice: Recognizing a need or graying the line between doctor and nurse? *Medscape Journal of Medicine, 10*(11), 253. Retrieved from http://www.medscape.com/viewarticle/582269

Silva, M., & Ludwick, R. (2006). Ethics: Is the doctor of nursing practice ethical? *Online Journal of Issues in Nursing, 11*(2). Retrieved from www.nursingworld.org/MainMenuCategories/ANAMarketplace/ANAPeriodicals/OJIN/Columns/Ethics/DNPEthical.aspx

CRITICAL THINKING QUESTIONS

1. What are some strategies you can use to become an effective mentor?
2. Discuss the characteristics of an effective mentor for a DNP student or DNP graduate from an underrepresented group.
3. In what way would previous mentorship relationships need to be changed to meet the needs of more contemporary doctorally prepared advance practice nurses?
4. What are some specific issues about which the mentor must be aware and prepared to address?
5. Discuss relevant mentorship models that can be used for DNP students and DNP graduates.
6. How can mentorship style(s) be shaped or influenced by gender differences, cultural values or societal mores?
7. Apply a systems perspective to the need for mentorship in DNP students and DNPs: What is the state of practice now and what needs to happen to strengthen the practice of mentorship for the future?
8. Compare and contrast mentorship and collegial or peer support in doctorally prepared advanced nursing practice. Can one role and practice evolve into another, or are they mutually exclusive?
9. What are some outcomes you would expect to see from an effective mentoring relationship between colleagues?
10. To enhance equity for diverse cultural groups and increase their upward mobility in the profession of nursing, what responsibility does the profession have and what obligations do organizations have?

CHAPTER SEVENTEEN

Interdisciplinary and Interprofessional Collaboration

Essential for the Doctoral Advanced Practice Nurse

Julie Cowan Novak

INTRODUCTION

A series of Institute of Medicine (IOM) reports, *Crossing the Quality Chasm: A New Health System for the 21st century* (2001), *To Err is Human* (2000), and *Health Professions Education: A Bridge to Quality* (2003), were tipping points in the discourse related to patient safety and quality. The public reaction to these reports was significant. The reports catalyzed patient safety and quality research, improvement science, clinical translational science, and evidence-based practice. These IOM reports were foundational to the development of the Doctor of Nursing Practice degree. Health care summits across the United States resulted in common themes, including consumer-driven health care, basic universal health care for all, interoperability of electronic health records, new models of care for nurse-managed clinic systems, and interprofessional education, practice and research to promote collaboration (Rapala & Novak, 2007). In 2010, new health care reform legislation further supports this revolution.

SCOPE

This chapter will describe the development and sustainability of interprofessional partnerships for DNP program enrichment. Unique and traditional interprofessional education and interdisciplinary partners and effects on curricular redesign will be presented. Finally, interdisciplinary practice inquiry projects that build the evidence base and lead to documented outcomes, supporting the critical need for interprofessional and interdisciplinary collaboration will be discussed.

DEVELOPING INTERDISCIPLINARY PARTNERSHIPS FOR DNP PROGRAM ENRICHMENT

Academic

The academic patient safety call-to-arms occurred in 2003 when the IOM published *Health Professions Education: A Bridge to Quality.* Initially, the education report did not benefit from the media exposure of the earlier reports; education is not as sensational as lost lives. The root cause to any problem or issue is complex. The revolution in health care must not lose momentum in solving fundamental education-related patient safety, quality, and systems issues. Education as a root cause of these issues is losing lives once-removed (Rapala & Novak, 2007).

In addition to a common patient safety language, the IOM multidisciplinary group suggested a group of five core competencies that should be incorporated into the curriculum of all health care education programs. The five competencies are to: 1) provide patient-centered care; 2) to work in interdisciplinary teams; 3) to employ evidence-based practice; 4) to apply quality improvement; and 5) to utilize informatics (IOM, 2003).

Just as it is difficult for health care providers to respond to and balance a myriad of patient safety issues from medication reconciliation to information systems implementation, it is difficult for nursing academe to balance patient safety with operations, research, and teaching (Rapala & Novak, 2007). Stevens and Staley (2006), in their review of nursing response to IOM reports, state that these reports can serve as a blueprint for change.

Competencies related to the DNP *Essentials* (AACN, 2006), Quality, Safety, and Education of Nurses (QSEN), and Team Strategies and Tools to Enhance Performance and Patient Safety (TeamSTEPPS) (AHRQ, 2010) must be woven into the curriculum to address these core challenges. The TeamSTEPPS initiative is based on evidence derived from team performance, leveraging more than 25 years of research in military, aviation, nuclear power, business, and industry, to acquire team competencies. These team competencies affect knowledge (shared mental model), attitudes (mutual trust and team orientation), and performance (adaptability, accuracy, productivity, efficiency, and safety). Thus, a cadre of professionals who can participate in and lead team science (integrated multidisciplinary research teams), develop health homes, and integrate best current evidence with clinical expertise and patient/family references and values will be created for the effective delivery of health care (Stevens, 2009).

Health care providers of the 21st century must function effectively within nursing and interprofessional teams, fostering open communication, mutual respect, and shared decision making to achieve quality patient care. DNP programs must prepare the workforce for a complex health care environment, designing system-wide fixes. The siloed nature of professional schools and graduate programs with competing interests are barriers to collaboration. Joint curricular design replete with the opportunity for cross-walking core and cognate courses are essential. Interprofessional courses include genomics, systems, human factors influencing patient safety and quality, evidence-based practice, informatics, health economics, health policy, and public health principles. Coordination and collaboration are difficult to achieve due to physical location, competing priorities, and simple geography (IOM, 2003). Since the majority of educational and health care institutions were built prior to 1970, redesign of these facilities should promote opportunities for interdisciplinary collaboration and interprofessional education. Interprofessional simulation centers in universities and health care agencies provide an opportunity for DNP practice inquiry projects related to patient safety and quality, simulation and device design, competency development, outcomes management, and continuous learning.

Nurses must think more broadly about potential collaborators in solving the problems of the health care delivery system. Disciplines such as industrial engineering have much to offer as engineering principles are applied to information technology; system design; patient safety; medication administration and reconciliation; simulation; chronic disease management; and hospital and clinic development, design and renovation. The Doctor of Nursing Practice (DNP) was developed to reengineer health care (Novak, 2006) through designing accessible, effective, efficient, safe, high-quality health care delivery systems. The DNP addresses the complexity of the health care system head-on, including the information, knowledge and technology explosion; spiraling costs; and the need for a systems approach to create new models of care and solve existing health care dilemmas (Wall, Novak, & Wilkerson, 2005).

The DNP student brings core capabilities of health promotion, disease prevention, care management, patient safety, and care of the individual, family and community, as well as a biopsychosocial behavioral perspective, a population systems context, understanding of resource utilization, and a strong service orientation. Engineering students bring expertise in root cause analysis, systems design, device design, simulation, and human factors. Melding these entities yields a dynamic, synergistic, and innovative environment, where each partner brings affiliations and skills to improve care that is evidence based. This creates a horizontally and vertically integrated learning environment where not only the students benefit, but nursing and engineering faculty learn and create new educational and practice models (Rapala & Novak, 2007).

Governmental

Health policy didactic and residency courses are key elements of the DNP degree including, in-depth policy design, implementation, and evaluation. Interprofessional health policy courses for nursing, other health sciences, engineering, business, communications, and political science students provide an optimal setting for curricular enrichment, systems change, and effective advocacy and policy design. Residency experiences at the state and federal levels are invaluable. Enabling students to understand effective lobbying, cultivate relationships with key staff, work with professional organizations' legislative experts, share expertise through partnership development with legislators, gather data from constituents and stakeholders, provide testimony, assist in drafting legislation, and enact and evaluate policy are essential components of the program.

Promoting worldwide health is mankind's greatest challenge. The DNP and their interprofessional partners also have the potential to lead in the local-to-global health care policy arena. This requires an understanding of several global agencies, such as the World Health Organization, the Pan American Health Organization, the United Nations, the United Nations International Children's Emergency Fund (UNICEF), the World Bank, and the Centers for Disease Control (CDC) (Novak, in press).

All DNP practice inquiry projects should include health policy implications. For some projects, the relevant policy implications will integrate policy with ethics, research, and education. Exemplars include workforce and faculty shortages, funding for nursing education, care of the underserved, and barrier removal to increase access.

Nongovernmental Organizations for Global Service-Learning Projects

Nongovernmental organizations (NGOs) such as the Carter Center, the Bill and Melinda Gates Foundation, Christel House International, and the Johnson and Johnson Foundation, have supported global interprofessional service-learning projects for students in the health care disciplines. The Carter Center has three objectives: (1) to prevent and resolve conflicts, (2) to enhance freedom and democracy, and (3) to improve health (Carter Center, 2010). In the words of Carter Center cofounder and former U.S. President Jimmy Carter in his 1992 Nobel Peace Prize speech, "The bond of our common humanity is stronger than the devisiveness of our fears and prejudices. God gives us the capacity for choice. We can choose to alleviate suffering. We can choose to work together for peace. We can make these changes—we must" (Carter, 2002, para 39). The Bill and Melinda Gates Foundation has local, national, and global objectives. Globally, the Foundation focuses on reducing extreme poverty, improving health, and increasing public library access. Within Africa, the Foundation has had a profound effect on improving access to antiviral medications and the prevention and treatment for HIV/AIDS, TB, and malaria.

The author has partnered with Christel House International and the Johnson and Johnson Foundation to enact an ongoing interprofessional service-learning project in Cape Town, South Africa. Christel House International is a public charity that operates learning centers in impoverished neighborhoods with the goal of creating sustainable social and educational impact. Between 1999 and 2002, Christel House opened five learning centers in Mexico, India, South Africa, Venezuela, and the United States. Christel House K-12 Academy in Cape Town helps children break the cycle of poverty, realize their hopes and dreams and become self-sufficient, contributing members of society. Teams of nursing and medical students have partnered with local community leaders to provide school and family health promotion, HIV/AIDS, TB, and malaria prevention, intervention, and educational programs, and direct care in the Themba Care Orphanage and the Tafelsig Community Health Center. Service-learning research and community engagement projects are ongoing (Richards & Novak, 2010). DNP practice inquiry projects with interprofessional partners in the health sciences and engineering will take place in these sites in 2011 in phase four of this initiative. As nursing's status in second- and third-world countries varies widely, these initiatives and their interprofessional and interdisciplinary framework will provide a foundation for global DNP program development.

INTERPROFESSIONAL COLLABORATIVE RESEARCH

The focus of DNP Essential VII outcome is on the analysis of appropriate scientific data, the synthesis of concepts related to clinical prevention and population health to develop, implement, and evaluate interventions to address health promotion/disease prevention, and to evaluate care delivery models and/or strategies (AACN, 2006). The final practice inquiry project is a synthesis of theoretical concepts for program development combined with grounding in change theory, leadership theory, and concepts of program planning, implementation, and evaluation. Scholars at the Agency for Healthcare Research and Quality (2003) reported that it can take up to 20 years before scientific findings become part of practice at the bedside or community setting. The DNP program emphasis on interdisciplinary, evidence-based projects attempts to significantly decrease that lag time. DNP graduates have the ability to translate bench research and apply improvement science across health care settings.

This work is actualized in the DNP Scholarly Project. One exemplar would be community assessment, development, and sustainability factors for nurse-managed clinics as a system of care. These "Health Homes," led by Pediatric Nurse Practitioner/DNP students promote enhanced collaboration with academic partners including Community Pediatrics, Behavioral Health, and Dentistry and a new model of health care for 6,700 children enrolled in Head Start. The DNP plays an important role in the evaluation of new care delivery models, including identification of strategies that lead to positive outcomes. The DNP integrates principles of quality improvement, psychosocial, and cultural concepts and utilizes models and theoretical concepts to explain observed phenomena. Finally, the DNP utilizes principles of evidence-based practice and health care economics to evaluate care delivery models. An understanding of health economics and finance, including a cost analysis as a standard component of the final practice inquiry project, is essential. A practice inquiry exemplar might include an analysis of Medicare and Medicaid access and recommendations for system improvement or a gap analysis of county level health departments for national accreditation preparation that will be enacted by the Centers for Disease Control in 2011. These public health system improvements require effective interdisciplinary communication and collaboration.

The AACN (2006) criteria for the scholarly project describe a reflection of the breadth of education and synthesis of knowledge gained in the course of study. The projects demonstrate evidence of scholarship in other disciplines such as business, engineering, and pharmacology. The scholarly project is enriched through an interprofessional curriculum and interdisciplinary final project committees, ultimately resulting in collaborative peer-reviewed presentations, manuscript submissions, and other professional and lay publications.

SUMMARY

Doctor of Nursing Practice students and graduates face many exciting challenges in health care reform and in designing effective systems of health care delivery. These include being responsive to emerging needs and health issues in the local to global population and in developing interdisciplinary practice models that adhere to the principles of primary health care across settings in the context of a reengineered health care system. DNPs will mobilize research translation and dissemination, and practice implementation strategies to insure evidence-based practice as the norm rather than the exception (Novak, in press). They must use evidence-based models as a framework for local-to-global community public health partnerships and projects. These interdisciplinary and interprofessional initiatives can be tested and evaluated through DNP practice inquiry final projects, team science, and clinical translational research.

REFERENCES

Agency for Healthcare Research and Quality. (2003). *TeamSTEPPS*. Washington, DC. Retrieved from http://www.ahrq.gov/teamsteppstools/instructor/fundamentals/module3/igleadership.htm

American Association of Colleges of Nursing (AACN). (2006). *The essentials of doctoral education for advanced nursing practice*. Retrieved from http://www.aacn.nche.edu/DNP/pdf/Essentials.pdf

Carter Center. (2010). *About the center*. Retrieved from http://www.Cartercenter.org/about/index.html

Carter, J. (2002). *Nobel lecture.* Nobelprize.org. Retrieved from http://nobelprize.org/nobel_prizes/peace/laureates/2002/carter-lecture.html

Institute of Medicine (IOM). (2000). *To err is human: Building a safer health system.* Washington, DC: National Academy Press.

Institute of Medicine (IOM). (2001). *Crossing the quality chasm: A new health system for the 21st century.* Washington, DC: National Academy Press.

Institute of Medicine (IOM). (2003). *Health professions education: A bridge to quality.* Washington, DC: National Academy Press.

Novak, J. (2006). *The doctor of nursing practice: Reengineering healthcare.* New York, NY: The Helene Fuld Healthcare Trust.

Novak, J. (in press). Globalization and international health. In Nies, M. A., & McCwan, M. (Eds.), *Community health nursing: Promoting the health of populations.* St. Louis, MO: Elsevier.

Rapala, K., & Novak, J. (2007). Integrating patient safety into curriculum: The doctor of nursing practice. *Journal of Patient Safety and Quality Health Care,* March–April, 17–23.

Richards, E., & Novak, J. (2010). From Biloxi to Cape Town: Curricular integration of service learning. *Journal of Community Health Nursing, 27*(1), 46–50.

Stevens, K. R. (2009). *Essential competencies for evidence-cased practice in nursing* (2nd ed.). San Antonio, TX: Academic Center for Evidence-Based Practice, UTHSCSA.

Stevens, K., & Staley, J. (2006). The Quality Chasm reports, evidence-based practice and nursing's response to improve healthcare. *Nursing Outlook, 34*(2), 94–101.

Wall, B., Novak, J., & Wilkerson, S. (2005). The doctor of nursing practice: Reengineering health care. *Journal of Nursing Education, 44*(9), 393–403.

CHAPTER SEVENTEEN: Reflective Response

Grant Charles

There is an interesting underlying theme in Novak's chapter on interdisciplinary and interprofessional collaboration. Although not explicitly stated, by calling for increased collaboration amongst professions she challenges the way in which nursing (and by extension, other professions) has traditionally operated within the profession and with other disciplines. She raises some critical issues, which must be addressed if the health professions want to become more effective and efficient in their dealings with each other, with patients, and with communities. She rightfully identifies the price patients pay when members of the various health professions do not relate well to each other and when individual disciplines isolate and distance themselves from the people they serve. It has been well documented in a number of jurisdictions that when there is a lack of collaboration between the health professions, there is a corresponding increase in intervention errors and patient death (Kohn, Corrigan, & Donaldson, 2000; Romanow, 2002).

Novak correctly calls for increased attention to be paid to how relationships with other practitioners and with patients can be improved. However, she falls into the same trap that others do when writing in this area. She identifies where we should be going without really identifying why we struggle to get there. What is lacking from the chapter is a clear sense of how our professional training can hold us in place rather than helping us to develop new ways of being. Without a serious examination of our role in contributing to the current state of affairs, we risk changing only how we talk about collaboration and partnership rather than actually helping develop new ways of working with others. My response to Novak will focus on why we need to pay close attention to the points she raises regarding interprofessional practice and service learning, while at the same time calling for even further examination of not where we can go, but why we are not getting there.

Perhaps the best place to start in this response is to provide an overview of how we develop our identity as professionals. While a great deal has been written on the education of health care professionals, little attention has been paid to our individual identity development as professionals (Charles, Bainbridge, & Gilbert, 2010). It is our sense of who we are rather than just what we know that dictates how we interact with each other and with service users within the health care environment. Humans change over time. This change is dependent upon how we create meaning and form ideas about ourselves and our environment (Alexander, 2007; Valsiner, 2000). It is this process of determining meaning in interpersonal interactions that strongly influences who we become as individuals and professionals and in turn continues to influence how we relate to members of our own profession, other professionals, and the people for whom we provide services.

By adapting Valsiner's (2000) work on culture and human development, one can see that the development of our professional identity is dependent upon our interactions with the world around us. This occurs in three primary "locations" of development: intrapersonal, interpersonal, and community. These locations are, respectively, our own sense of self and personal history, our interpersonal interactions with others, and the social and cultural context within which we operate. There is an ongoing interplay occurring between these three locations. Interactions occur within each of these settings that provide opportunities for us to either maintain our current sense of self or to change (Valsiner). We become, in part, who we are in response to those with whom we interact either regularly or significantly. In terms of professional identity, the differences in the way various professions see the world develops through this ongoing interplay of varied experiences and worldviews of people working within each profession, the specific environments in which people operate, and the different historical and current contexts in which the various disciplines have developed.

This development of who we become as a member of a profession begins with our earliest entry-level training. While still under the influence of the broader context of society and personal relationships outside of their college or university, students are immersed in both academic and practice settings during the course of their professional training. Simply put, who we become in the course of our training is in part dictated by the environment in which we are trained and in part by the people with whom we interact. This is the foundation of most professional training. For example, if as nursing students we spend our time in our training primarily interacting with other nursing students, then as nurses we will likely assume the general values, attitudes, and knowledge modeled for us daily. In fact, if we do not incorporate these values, attitudes, and knowledge, then there is a good chance that we will not complete our training.

As we progress through our entry-level training, we increasingly see the world from the viewpoint of our profession. This may signal that we are becoming a member of our profession. It is easy to begin to think that the way our profession sees the world is the only "true" way to view it. This uniprofessional focus ensures the development of a worldview that has traditionally been seen as being appropriate to our profession. However, the lack of systematic exposure to other professions means that we do not have the opportunity to learn that there is more than one valid way of seeing the world. In fact, our training encourages loyalty to our own profession with the corresponding risk that we may reject, at least partially, the other ones.

It is this narrowing of perspectives that can create so many of the communication misunderstandings regularly seen between the various health professions (Charles, Bainbridge, & Gilbert, 2010). For example, how one interprets an interaction with a practitioner from another profession is dependent upon one's own profession's world view that is largely formed in each individual through professional training. If we have not had systematic exposure to other professions, then it is easy to assume that the way we see the world is "correct." Not only does one not automatically try to see the world from the other's perspective, but often we are not even aware that there is another perspective. It is easy to think that if a member of another profession does not agree with us, it is because they are wrong, misinformed, or maybe just not as well trained. When two people from different professions take this position when interacting with each other, it is quite understandable that there could be serious disagreement and conflict.

These clashes of world view can have serious negative outcomes for patients (Kohn et al., 2000; Romanow, 2002). These are, as mentioned, largely a consequence of how we train students in their entry-level programs. Unfortunately, we tend to take this early way we see the world into our practice. Unless successfully challenged, these ways of interacting with others continue and can easily be entrenched throughout our practice careers and through the acquisition of advanced-level degrees. Further education does not guarantee that we will become more open to the viewpoints of other professions. Indeed, there are powerful forces at play within the practice and academic communities that contribute to ongoing interprofessional difficulties.

There have been a number of barriers identified which inhibit the implementation of an interprofessional agenda within practice and academic sites (Charles, Bainbridge, Copeman-Stewart, Tiffin, & Kassam, 2006; Charles, Bainbridge, Copeman-Stewart, Kassam, & Tiffin, 2008; Paul & Peterson, 2001; Salhani & Charles, 2007). These include, as mentioned, different philosophies of working and values of the various professions (Loxley, 1997; Miller, Freeman, & Ross, 2001). Also, there can be a fear of deskilling or deprofessionalization (Loxley, 1997; Miller et al., 2001). The push for closed role boundaries and the protection of our own professional knowledge also contributes to the creation of barriers (Miller, et al., 2001). Other identified barriers include power differences between the professions, territoriality, and fear of domain infringement (Geva, Barsky, & Westernoff, 2000; Hornby & Atkins, 2000), role insecurity (Hornby & Atkins, 2000), and the perceived need for clinical freedom or autonomy (Loxley, 1997). The power of these barriers to hold us in our old ways of doing things should not be underestimated. Most of the health professions have struggled long and hard to find their place in the system and are loath to take any actions that would put them at risk, regardless of their stated commitment to collaborative practice. However, until we begin to address our part as individual practitioners and as members of a profession in contributing to the development and maintenance of these barriers, we cannot truly develop healthy interprofessional partnerships. Collaboration of this type means being willing to invite members of other professions into areas of our practice that we have traditionally claimed as our own. It also means being willing to accept that other ways of doing things can be as effective as the way we have traditionally done them.

Novak also mentions in her chapter how service-learning opportunities can contribute to the development of an improved health care delivery system. I strongly agree with her central message, although once again I would push the unspoken core concept of what she is saying to examine how these types of experience can help us find new ways of developing our sense of professional identity, thus changing how we interact with others. Service learning as a pedagogical approach has been developed as a way to respond to a perceived lack of reciprocal relationships between universities and communities (Checkoway, 1998; Kenny, Simon, Kiley-Brabeck, & Lerner, 2004; Lemieux & Allen, 2007; Ngai, 2006; Wilhite & Silver, 2005). There have been a number of benefits identified in service-learning projects for communities (see Gelmon, Holland, Seifer, Shinnamon, & Connnors, 1998) and universities (see Kenny et al., 2004) which I will not describe in this response. What I will focus on is how service learning can contribute to the development of professional identity for entry-level students and applies to new DNPs.

Service learning, similar to interprofessional collaboration, is an attempt to redefine how we interact with others. It is meant to break down the often rigid, one-way, top-down relationships that characterize traditional provider–patient interactions (Charles & Dharamsi, 2010). Community service learning has been developed in part as a response to a growing realization that while professional education produces good technical practitioners, it does not necessarily contribute to the development of socially responsible citizens. Student involvement in service-learning projects can help foster an applied, rather than an abstract sense of civic responsibility (Waterman, 1997). Benefits for students have been seen to include positive changes in moral development, civil responsibility, critical thinking, problem analysis, cultural awareness, and increased understanding of the connection between people and their social environments (Bordelon & Philips, 2007; Cone & Harris, 1996; Lemieux & Allen, 2007; Ngai, 2006; Roos et al., 2005). Perhaps most importantly, service-learning experiences teach students about the power of "patient voice." Community members are utilized as teachers and not solely recipients of services. This represents a significant shift in the relationship. The provider–patient partnership becomes reciprocal rather than unidirectional.

This shift in the relationship has tremendous potential for changing how we perceive ourselves as professionals and for how we interact with others. We now are beginning to understand the fact that we become who we are as professionals, in part, through our interactions with the people we serve (Alexander, 2008; Alexander & Charles, 2009; Garfat & Charles, 2007). Traditionally (and continuing till today), we have tended to see the provider–patient relationships as being one way. We give our skills and knowledge and they receive. Their role in this process is seen as being relatively passive. Our traditional way of interacting with patients has always ignored the true nature of relationships. Whether we want to acknowledge it or not, human relationships, even those of a professional nature, are bidirectional. There is always a two-way process in any human interaction (Valsiner, 2000). The motivation for trying to develop "professional" distance from those with whom we work is commendable. We have believed that this protects patients. However, what it can really do is dehumanize and invalidate them (and us) in the process. This is not healthy for anyone. Rather than denying the two-way nature of relationships, we need to challenge the underlying philosophy behind our interactions with patients and the reasons we provide service the way we do. The same holds true in our interactions with other professions.

There has to be room in our development of our professional identity to acknowledge the importance of mutuality in relationships. We need to begin to openly accept that if we want to work effectively with patients and other professions, then we need to develop a sense of shared relationship. This requires that we strive to ensure that there is room and opportunity for a joint investment in the relationship by each participant. This is not to say that we shift the focus from task to process, thus preventing a timely delivery of service. Rather, it is a call for an acceptance that a focus on reciprocity and mutuality can enrich the quality of the interaction and the outcome for both the patient and the provider.

All of this is to say that if we truly want to develop a healthier and more effective delivery system we need to challenge the way in which we interact with members of other professions and with the people we serve. We need to seriously examine how we develop our professional identities in order to identify those aspects of it that are holding back the development of reciprocal and respectful relationships with colleagues and patients. We need to seriously ask ourselves what it is in our profession's "worldview" and way of doing things that reinforces barriers and boundaries. We also need to appreciate that the other professions can help us achieve the goals of our profession rather than seeing them as a potential threat.

In order to do any of this, we have to reconceptualize how we train the entry level students, in this case, new BSN-to-DNPs (particularly), and post-master's DNPs too. It is not enough to change any single aspect of how we develop as professions. We must examine the interplay between professional identity development, the reciprocity of relationships with patients and other service providers, and the boundaries we create that, however well meaning, serve to distance ourselves from others. We cannot do this by simply calling for greater collaboration. We have to be willing to challenge our professional worldview. This is no easy task given the context within which we have developed and maintained our worldview. There can be no denying that many people will find this a risky proposition. However, if we do not do it, then the likelihood that we effect significant change in our delivery systems and patient outcomes is minimal.

I fully agree with Novak's call for increased interdisciplinary and interprofessional collaboration. As she has stated in her chapter "Doctor of Nursing Practice students and graduates face many exciting challenges in health care reform and in designing effective systems of health care delivery." (p. 351). However, I would take her comment one step further. As leaders in your profession, I would call upon you to become leaders in creating new ways of interacting with patients and other professionals. This involves challenging how advanced practice nurses or doctoral advanced practice nurses become who they become. This requires seriously questioning how nursing can not only contribute to an advancement of collaborative practice, but also how nursing also helps create the barriers that hinder or block these efforts. If change could be brought about simply by agreeing upon where we should be going, then we would all be already working in healthy and collaborative delivery and academic settings. Change is difficult and can only come about through the efforts of people willing not just to try to change the system, but also to try to change themselves. This is the essence of true leadership.

REFERENCES

Alexander, C. (2007). You are what you do. *Relational Child and Youth Care Practice*, 20(3), 17–21.

Alexander, C. (2008). Accepting gifts from youth: Reciprocity makes a difference. *Relational Child and Youth Care Practice*, 21(2), 27–35.

Alexander, C., & Charles, G. (2009). Caring, mutuality and reciprocity in social worker client relationships. *Journal of Social Work*, 9(1), 5–22.

Bordelon, T. D., & Phillips, I. (2007). Service learning: What students have to say. *Active Learning in Higher Education*, 7(2), 143–153.

Charles, G., Bainbridge, L., Copeman-Stewart, K., Tiffin, S., & Kassam, R. (2006). The Interprofessional Rural Program of British Columbia (IRPbc). *Journal of Interprofessional Care*, 20(1), 40–50.

Charles, G., Bainbridge, L., Copeman-Stewart, K., Kassam, R., & Tiffin, S. (2008). The impact of an interprofessional rural health care practice education experience on students and communities. *Journal of Allied Health*, 37, 127–131.

Charles, G., Bainbridge, L., & Gilbert, J. (2010). The UBC model of interprofessional education. *Journal of Interprofessional Care*, 24(1), 9–18.

Charles, G., & Dharamsi, S. (2010). Service learning, interprofessional education and the social work placement: Creating citizen practitioners. In E. Ralph (Ed.), *The practicum in professional education: Canadian perspectives* (pp. 69–87). Calgary, Canada: Detselig Enterprises, Ltd.

Checkoway, B. (1998). Reinventing the research university for public service. *Journal of Planning Literature*, 11, 307–319.

Cone, D., & Harris, S. (1996). Service-learning practice: Developing a theoretical framework. *Michigan Journal of Community Service Learning*, Fall, 31–43.

Garfat, T., & Charles, G. (2007). How am I who I am? Self in child and youth care. *Relational Child and Youth Care Practice*, 20(6), 6–16.

Gelmon, S., Holland, B., Seifer, S., Shinnamon, A., & Connnors, K. (1998). Community–university partnerships for mutual learning. *Michigan Journal of Community Service Learning*, 5, 97–107.

Geva, E., Barsky, A., & Westernoff, F. (2000). Developing a framework for interprofessional and diversity informed practice. In E. Geva, A. Barsky, & F. Westernoff (Eds.), *Interprofessional practice with diverse populations: Cases in point* (pp. 1–28). Westport, CT: Auburn House.

Hornby, S., & Atkins, J. (2000). *Collaborative care: Interprofessional, interagency and interpersonal* (2nd ed.). Malden, MA: Blackwell Science.

Kenny, M. E., Simon, L. A. K., Kiley-Brabeck, K., & Lerner, R. M. (2004). Introduction. In M. E. Kenny, L. A. K. Simon Kiley-Brabeck, & R. M. Lerner (Eds.), *Learning to serve: Promoting civil society through service learning*. Norwell, MA: Kluwer Academic Publishers.

Kohn, L. T., Corrigan, J. M., & Donaldson, M. S. (2000). *To err is human: Building a better health system*. Washington, DC: National Academy Press.

Lemieux, C. M., & Allen, P. D. (2007). Service learning in social work education: The state of knowledge, pedagogical practicalities, and practice conundrums. *Journal of Social Work Education*, 43(2), 309–325.

Loxley, A. (1997). *Collaboration in health and welfare: Working with difference*. London, UK: Jessica Kingsley Publications.

Miller, C., Freeman, M., & Ross, N. (2001). *Interprofessional practice in health and social care: Challenging the shared learning agenda.* London, UK: Arno.

Ngai, S. S. (2006). Service-learning, personal development, and social commitment: A case study of university students in Hong Kong. *Adolescence, 41*(161), 165–176.

Paul, S., & Peterson, C. Q. (2001). Interprofessional collaboration: Issues for practice and research. *Occupational Therapy, 15*(3/4), 1–12.

Romanow, R. J. (2002). *Building our values: The future of health care in Canada-final report.* Ottawa, ON: Commission on the Future of Health Care in Canada.

Roos, V., Temane, Q. M., Davis, L., Prinsloo, C. E., Kritzinger, A., Naude, E. et al. (2005). Service learning in a community context: Learners' perceptions of a challenging training paradigm. *South African Journal of Psychology, 35*(4), 703–716.

Salhani, D., & Charles, G. (2007). The dynamics of an interprofessional team: The interplay of child and youth care with other professions within a residential treatment milieu. *Relational Child and Youth Care Practice, 20*(4), 12–20.

Valsiner, J. (2000). *Culture and human development.* London, UK: Sage Publications.

Waterman, A. S. (1997). An overview of service-learning and the role of research and evaluation in service-learning programs. In A. S. Waterman (Ed.), *Service-learning: Applications from the research* (pp. 1–11). Mahwah, NJ: Lawrence Erlbaum Associates.

Wilhite, S. C., & Silver, P. T. (2005). A false dichotomy for higher education: Educating citizens vs. educating technicians. *National Civil Review*, Summer, 46–54.

CRITICAL THINKING QUESTIONS

1. Consider your own clinical practice experience. How much interprofessional communication do you employ?
2. Discuss whether you think nursing operates too much within its "nursing silo" or not?
3. Identify any way in which your DNP education curricula are structured for interdisciplinary experiences.
4. Who do you perceive will be your primary non-nursing doctorally prepared collaborators when you complete your degree and enter the workforce as a DNP graduate? Discuss how you might enhance this collaboration.
5. Give some thought to who you might select as possible preceptors in your DNP program and identify at least one non-nurse doctorally prepared mentor you might work with.
6. Discuss whether you believe BSN education does an adequate job teaching interprofessional and interdisciplinary collaboration.
7. Discuss whether you believe MSN education does an adequate job teaching interprofessional and interdisciplinary collaboration.
8. Identify one other health profession that you know the least about. Perform a Google search and discuss how you might collaborate with this health professional in a possible DNP-interprofessional role.
9. Go to the website of the *Journal of Interprofessional Care* (http://www.ingentaconnect.com/content/apl/cjic/2010/00000024/00000004;jsessionid=8phq1889mt5o8.alice). Retrieve an article from one of the current issues from your library and discuss the article's relevance to your future DNP role.
10. Devise a clinical research question that would involve the expertise of nursing and at least one other discipline.

CHAPTER EIGHTEEN

A New Level of Advocacy for Nurses in the Doctoral Advanced Nursing Practice Role

Louise S. Ward

INTRODUCTION

Doctorally prepared advanced practice nurses (DAPNs) must fully develop all the skills necessary to provide the best possible care within their roles. Research, leadership, teaching, and clinical practice are all areas for development as advanced practice nurses (APNs) achieve the doctorate. In this chapter, the term "doctorally prepared APN" will encompass all DNP or DrNP graduates, not only those practicing in traditional advanced clinical practice roles. Within each role of the doctorally prepared APN, these clinical experts must advance to a *new level of advocacy* in order to maximize their own role effectiveness.

Advocacy can be defined in several ways. Throughout their education and training, nurses are encouraged to be patient advocates. At the individual patient level, patient advocacy can be defined as "communicating with and informing patients, protecting patients, speaking out for patients, and building relationships with patients" (Hanks, 2010, p. 256). When studying policy, nurses learn to advocate for their profession and use the same skills employed on behalf of patients to promote professional practice or improve workplace environments (Green & Jordan, 2004). This chapter will present the case for DAPNs becoming advocates for socially responsible policies at the population level. For the purpose of this chapter, the definition of *advocacy* will be expanded to "strategies devised, actions taken, and solutions proposed to inform or influence local, state, or federal decision making" (Weiss, 2007, p. 1).

In their classic article on *Stages of Nursing's Political Development*, Cohen et al. (1996) outlined four stages through which the nursing profession is progressing. These stages also serve as a framework for individual nurses' development in the realm of political activism. APNs with doctoral degrees should be functioning at the highest stage to achieve the desired outcomes, not only for their careers, but also for their patients, staff, employers, and communities.

Doctorally prepared APNs must be ready to advocate for their patients at the most appropriate levels. In developing their doctoral role, APNs must learn to recognize political issues, frame problem statements, identify key stakeholders, and strategize to promote outcomes that best serve their patients, communities, and personal careers. They must understand not only policy development, but also the politics of changing policy at many levels.

BACKGROUND

Especially in its early history, professional nursing's past is one of political activism. Florence Nightingale, Lillian Wald, and others worked tirelessly against serious societal constraints to achieve their goals for nursing and for the populations they served (Conger & Johnson, 2000). As the field of medicine narrowed its focus to technological, individually oriented care, however, Conger and Johnson claim that nursing paralleled medicine's focus and withdrew politically. Although the profession, through the American Nurses Association (ANA), officially takes stands on societal issues, nursing education and practicing nurses have in recent years been relatively apolitical and noncontroversial. The current trend is to encourage renewed interest in policy for nurses, but research indicates that nursing students do not view political activism as related to their personal lives (Rains & Barton-Kriese, 2001). Once students graduate, they move forward with their careers within the constraints (as they see it) of existing policy. Perhaps one reason for the retreat of activism in nursing is that the field is so diverse that the only common feature that can be emphasized in nursing schools is nursing itself.

Traditional nursing education emphasizes *nursing*-focused policy and political action regarding nursing's scope of practice, funding for nursing education, and global support for general health-related policies initiated by others. This reflects the first two stages of nursing political development as described by Cohen et al. (1996), which are "buy in" and "self-interest." Of course, these two stages are necessary and important, and presumably the APN has already processed them through their exposure in undergraduate and master's education. Most APNs are also familiar with Stage 3, "Political Sophistication," in which coalitions are formed among nursing groups to be proactive on nursing issues (Cohen et al.). As leaders, however, it is essential that DAPNs become comfortable in Cohen and associates' fourth stage of political development.

Stage 4 involves actively taking the lead on a "broad range of health and social policy issues" (Cohen et al., 1996, p. 260). This stage looks beyond nursing to the world of social determinants of health and interdisciplinary strategizing to advance desired policy changes. Cohen et al. described the major step forward in Stage 4 as the fact that nurses are the instigators and leaders in proposing policy advances. Conger and Johnson (2000) further recommended that doctoral programs focus on policy analysis, research, and policy formulation, especially on behalf of those who have poor access to health care.

CALLS TO ACTION

The International Council of Nurses (ICN) has called on nurses to "play a strategic role in helping reduce environmental and lifestyle related health hazards" (ICN, 2007, p. 1) by working with governments and communities. Both the U.S. Centers for Disease Control (CDC, 2010) and the World Health Organization (WHO, 2010) are increasingly recognizing social determinants of health as important factors in health disparities. The ANA's 2005 *Code of Ethics with Interpretive Statements*, Section 9.4, specifically states:

> *9.4: Social reform*—Nurses can work individually as citizens or collectively through political action to bring about social change . . . . In these activities, health is understood as being broader than delivery and reimbursement systems, but extending to health-related sociocultural issues such as violation of human rights, homelessness, hunger, violence, and the stigma of illness.

In order to be current and relevant, DAPNs must look beyond the discipline of nursing and advanced practice issues, and beyond the health of their individual patients and practices, to address the larger social issues that affect them. The WHO's website on social determinants makes this very clear: *"Why treat people without changing what makes them sick?"* (WHO, 2010). This larger view of disease prevention makes it incumbent on APN leaders to be proactive in promoting equitable social policy (Rains & Barton-Kriese, 2001). Indeed, Browne and Tarlier (2008) called on nurse practitioners (NPs) to address the broader context of their patients' lives in order to fully realize the potential of the NP role.

THEORETICAL FRAMEWORK

Carnegie and Kiger (2009) proposed Critical Social Theory as a starting point for nursing in general and nurse leaders in particular. Critical Social Theory is implicitly political and emphasizes the political and ideological bases for social behavior. It focuses attention on the collective rather than the individual, and it seeks to identify oppression and misuse of power in order to facilitate the empowerment of disadvantaged populations.

Critical Social Theory integrates well with the ecological view of health determinants. In its 2003 report *Unequal Treatment*, the Institute of Medicine noted that the search for causes of health disparities must be expanded to include socioeconomic status, literacy, and health care access, in addition to biology (Smedley, Stith, & Nelson, 2003). This *ecological view* makes it clear that social disparities are associated with health disparities. Thus, inadequate housing, substandard education, and unemployment become legitimate concerns for the health professions. Rather than being a new paradigm for nursing, this view is really an affirmation of nursing's roots with Florence Nightingale and Lillian Wald, and an appropriate area of concern for APNs.

Advocacy at the level of ecological determinants is thus appropriate and expected for DAPNs, yet such advocacy raises ethical concerns about paternalism (Carnegie & Kiger, 2009). Policy and political action are always value laden and, indeed, it can be argued that this is especially true when based in Critical Social Theory. Just as the qualitative researcher must "bracket" preconceptions, so must DAPNs acknowledge and articulate their personal values before undertaking the task of advocating for social change. Articulating personal values assists participants to understand the potential to interpret events inaccurately due to those values, and thus guard against such inaccuracy (Carnegie & Kiger, 2009). Once personal values are articulated and bracketed, DAPNs can actively "hear" the concerns and priorities of their patients, giving legitimacy and direction to their activism.

Some authors posit that the withdrawal of nursing from social politics has contributed to health disparities in the United States (Browne, 2001; Carnegie & Kiger, 2009) and, if this premise is accepted, DAPNs can make substantial contributions to the health of the disadvantaged by reestablishing an activist stance. Political neutrality promotes social injustice by leaving unexamined the reasons for inequities and the role of the state in promoting disparities (Browne, 2001). At the doctoral level, APNs must articulate their political viewpoints and take the lead in promoting health care and social policies that are congruent with their views of the world.

To be effective change agents at this level, DAPNs in particular need to become more adept at working within the policy-making and political systems. A shift in approach from the static, politically neutral, traditional nursing stance to the dynamic, empowered, and impassioned activist approach requires developing new skills in policy and political analysis. Thus, doctorally prepared APNs should be prepared to become advocates for their patients at a new, more advanced level, and better position themselves to improve the health of aggregate populations with their clinical scholarship.

WHY DOCTORAL PREPARATION?

While any individual or group can become involved in advocacy for social change, it should be a *role expectation* of clinical nurses with DNP or DrNP degrees, and they should be specifically prepared for this role. DAPNs, because of their clinical practice, have an "insider's view" of patient concerns, barriers to care, and the larger social factors involved. Their doctoral education trains them to clearly articulate problems, speak, and write at an advanced level. In addition, DAPNs know how to analyze and interpret current research findings to support their cases and to conduct their own integrated clinical projects or research studies that can have policy relevance.

Doctor of Nursing Practice curricula, therefore, should include policy and political analysis skills, problem identification and articulation, and an introduction to the use of research and the media in policy advocacy. As with most education, these represent an incremental advance from the skills learned at the master's level, but the DAPN graduate will then have the confidence and background to make a difference at the policy level. This new level of advocacy should be threaded throughout the doctoral curriculum and into the final synthesis project or clinical/practice dissertation.

APPLICATION

What does this mean for the DAPN? Clinical practice will serve as a "trigger" for political action. When a patient who lives in public housing cannot keep medication cold because the refrigerator is broken, or the same patient cannot get rid of the household cat that aggravates her asthma because of a rat infestation, the DAPN is "triggered" to take political action with the housing authority. Doctoral preparation permits the APN to conduct scientifically strong, independent analysis of the prevalence of these problems and the relationships among the variables. Unavailability of nutritious snack options in schools will "trigger" the development of a parents' committee to demand change. Unavailability of nutritious food options in local stores can stimulate community action to request a farmers' market locally. The DANP is prepared to analyze current research on these issues and present them in understandable terms to the parties involved.

Work site injuries seen in the clinic can prompt the exploration with the employer into the need for safety training for workers or even the employment of an occupational health nurse. Unfair labor practices that jeopardize patients' health and safety will induce the DAPN to pursue policy change and OSHA inspections. A pattern of playground injuries seen in practice will activate a DAPN-led petition for safer equipment in the playground, and the lack of safe exercise options in a neighborhood will cause the DAPN to join with community groups for the development of after-school programs and options for adult exercise. Patients who are functionally illiterate will cause the DAPN to initiate not only appropriate instructional materials, but also adult literacy classes in the community. In all of these cases, the confidence that results from doctoral training enables the DAPN to analyze the situation, clearly state the problem, incorporate both independent analysis and existing research, and take a leadership role in the solution.

Within the activist approach, the focus expands from individual-level interventions (although these are certainly not abandoned!) to include aggregate and population-based interventions and advocacy. Not every injustice can be addressed by every doctorally prepared APN, but selective priorities can be set by each practitioner. Progress may start out slowly, but change will take place and health problems will be prevented through improved social conditions.

PROCESS

For years, nurses have made the assumption that policy will be directed at issues that are important (Catford, 2006). Unfortunately, we have failed to understand that policy makers are not experts in either health or health care and have many conflicting demands made on them. Policy makers can only make decisions based on the best information they have been given, and doctorally prepared APNs directly involved in practice are in a uniquely strong position to bridge that gap and help policy makers understand the issues. The first step in that process is to frame the issue under consideration as a problem (Catford, 2006).

The problem statement provides the rationale for policy change. A *problem* is not just an issue the profession would like to change; it is an issue that demands solution. Doctorally prepared APNs are in the ideal position to identify problems that affect their patients and their practices, and thus are "real"—grounded in experience, and accessible to policy makers. Using Critical Social Theory, this problem statement can be formulated to include overarching social determinants that must be improved in the long run. At the same time, the problem statement is ideally phrased to attract powerful coalition members.

Framing the problem statement to allow for a diversity of policy solutions can be challenging. Sometimes it seems clear to nurses that "repealing X law" (for example) is the issue to be argued. This approach is unappealing to policymakers because they are backed into a corner. When DAPNs can articulate the *problems resulting from X law* and why the resolution of those problems is advantageous, policy can be developed to solve the issue.

Excellent explanations of policy and political assessment, albeit often focused on the discipline of nursing rather than broader societal issues, are usually provided in nursing policy textbooks (e.g., Mason, Leavitt, & Chaffee, 2007), and the APN can perform these analyses for the identified problem. With a clear problem statement and policy analysis, DAPNs can then write a short (two-page) position statement on the issue. Ultimately this position statement can be used when meeting with staff members of legislators, but first, it is used to approach potential coalition members.

Coalitions, part of the political process of advocacy and stimulating change, are an important carry-over from Cohen et al.'s (1996) third stage of political development. The doctorally prepared APN now employs coalitions that encompass a much broader base to accomplish change in societal health determinants. In the examples given earlier, coalitions may be composed of parents, local storeowners, teachers, housing project residents, unions, and/or nonprofit organizations. Discussions and negotiations among such stakeholders may result in modifications in the original position statement.

Doctorally prepared APNs and their coalitions should also learn to be strategic in the use of the media to promote their cause. Sympathetic local media can be highly instrumental in influencing public opinion and setting the stage for change. Emphasizing the likely positive outcomes of the proposed change keeps the focus constructive and optimistic. While positioning the coalition for goal achievement, the DAPN should sim-ultaneously design and get ethics board approval for research to measure the outcomes of the successful advocacy. Both quantitative and qualitative designs may be appropriate for this purpose.

CONTRIBUTION

When doctorally prepared APNs take a stand to promote policies that respect and advocate for the most vulnerable populations, they will make contributions on many levels. To their practices and their patients, this advocacy will demonstrate true commit-ment to holism. Patients know that their employment status and housing conditions con-tribute to their health status; validation of this knowledge by their health care provider will be empowering and will open the door for true patient-centered care. Doctorally pre-pared APNs acknowledging the ecological view of health will begin to move the focus away from high-tech, pharmacologically oriented care toward primary prevention, which ultimately can reduce the burden of disease. Their advanced preparation will lay the foundation for the establishment of a *health system* that keeps people healthy, to augment the reforming the health *care* system that exists.

   National surveys have routinely demonstrated that nurses are widely respected and trusted by the U.S. public (Saad, 2009). By actively advocating on social issues, DAPNs will model social justice and a broad-based view of health that will enable not only the health care system, but also the public in general to see connections that will promote better health for all. Doctorally prepared APNs can renew the model originated by Florence Nightingale and lead the public in demanding needed reform.

SUMMARY

APNs with a terminal doctoral degree should achieve the highest level of political development in order to best serve their patients and communities. Doctorally prepared APNs owe it to their patients, profession, and selves to leave behind political neutrality and become activists in their approach to social policies that affect their patients' health. Advocacy and policy actions can be based on Critical Social Theory and aimed at changing social policy to support primary prevention and healthier populations. DAPNs will need to explore, articulate, and "bracket" their personal values to best serve their patients at this new level of advocacy. Clinical practice can serve as a "trigger" for identifying problems that need political attention. A clear problem state-ment will then facilitate both outreach to potential coalition members and political advocacy initiatives. APNs with the terminal degree should lead the way for nursing to reclaim its historical role of promoting social justice for the underserved and vulner-able populations in the United States.

REFERENCES

American Nurses' Association (ANA). (2005). *Code of ethics for nurses with interpretive statements.*
   [Online] Retrieved from http://nursingworld.org/ethics/code/protected_nwcoe813.htm#9.4
Browne, A. J. (2001). The influence of liberal political ideology on nursing science. *Nursing Inquiry,*
   8(2), 118–129.

Browne, A. J., & Tarlier, D. S. (2008). Examining the potential of nurse practitioners from a critical social justice perspective. *Nursing Inquiry, 15*(2), 83–93.

Carnegie, E., & Kiger, A. (2009). Being and doing politics: An outmoded model or 21st century reality? *Journal of Advanced Nursing, 65*(9), 1976–1984.

Catford, J. (2006). Creating political will: Moving from the science to the art of health promotion. *Health Promotion International, 21*(1), 1–4.

Centers for Disease Control (CDC). (2010). *Social determinants of health.* Retrieved from http://www.cdc.gov/socialdeterminants/

Cohen, S. S., Mason, D. J., Kovner, C., Leavitt, J. K., Pulcini, J., & Sochalski, J. (1996). Stages of nursing political development: Where we've been and where we ought to go. *Nursing Outlook, 44*(6), 259–266.

Conger, C., & Johnson, P. (2000). Integrating political involvement and nursing education. *Nurse Educator, 25*(2), 99–103.

Green, A., & Jordan, C. (2004). Common denominators: Shared governance and work place advocacy—Strategies for nurses to gain control over their practice. *Online Journal of Issues in Nursing, 9*(1), manuscript 6. Retrieved from www.nursingworld.org/MainMenuCategories/ANAMarketplace/ANAPeriodicals/OJIN/TableofContents/Volume92004/No1Jan04/SharedGovernanceandWorkPlaceAdvocacy.aspx

Hanks, R. G. (2010). Development and testing of an instrument to measure protective nursing advocacy. *Nursing Ethics, 17,* 255–267.

International Council of Nurses (ICN). (2007). *Position statement: Reducing environmental and lifestyle-related health hazards.* Retrieved from http://www.icn.ch/pshazards99.htm

Mason, D. J., Leavitt, J. K., & Chaffee, M. W. (2007). *Policy & politics in nursing and health care.* St. Louis, MO: Saunders.

Rains, J. W., & Barton-Kriese, P. (2001). Developing political competence: A comparative study across disciplines. *Public Health Nursing, 18*(4), 219–224.

Saad, L. (2009). *Honesty and ethics poll finds Congress' image tarnished.* Retrieved from http://www.gallup.com/poll/124625/Honesty-Ethics-Poll-Finds-Congress-Image-Tarnished.aspx

Smedley, B. D., Stith, A. Y., & Nelson, A. R. (2003). *Unequal treatment: Confronting racial and ethnic disparities in healthcare.* Washington, DC: The National Academies Press.

Weiss, H. B. (2007). From the director's desk: Advocacy and policy change. *The Evaluation Exchange,* 13, 1–2. Retrieved from http://www.hfrp.org/evaluation/the-evaluation-exchange/issue-archive/advocacy-and-policy-change/from-the-director-s-desk

World Health Organization (WHO). (2010). *Social determinants of health.* Retrieved from http://www.who.int/social_determinants/en/

CHAPTER EIGHTEEN: Reflective Response

Sheila M. Davis

INTRODUCTION: POLITICAL DEVELOPMENT

Ward challenges doctorally prepared advanced practice nurses (DAPNs) to move to a new level of advocacy to maximize their own role's effectiveness. In her review of Cohen's Stages of Nursing's Political Development (Cohen et al., 1996), Ward suggests that most advanced practice nurses are comfortable in the first two stages of political development—"buy in" and "self-interest"—and may have achieved the third stage of "political sophistication," but calls on advanced practice leaders to master the fourth stage of political development, "the instigators of policy change" (Cohen et al.). Looking beyond our discipline of nursing is critical. Unless pertaining to a particular issue that directly affects nurses (e.g., staffing or reimbursement), nurses and nursing professional organizations rarely are engaged on larger social issues that do adversely affect health, such as homelessness, poverty, and violence.

THEORETICAL FRAMEWORK

Ward's choice of Carnegie and Kiger's (2009) proposed Critical Social Theory as the framework for nursing and nursing leaders to engage in the political processes necessary for large-scale change is a sound one. One of the key elements of the theory is based on changing our focus from the patient to the collective, while identifying oppression and expanding our view of the causes of health disparities. Ward views this not as a paradigm shift for nursing, but as return to our roots in the views held by our nursing historical leaders, Florence Nightingale and Lillian Wald.

ROLE EXPECTATION

Ward views the incorporation of advocacy into practice as a role expectation for DAPNs. She argues that DAPNs are well positioned to become involved in advocacy for social change, and, therefore, the incorporation of policy and political analysis skills into a doctoral curriculum is critical to ensuring that nurses at the advanced practice doctoral level are able to fulfill this part of their role. The relative newness of the DNP and DrNP degrees, particularly in a time of health reform, provides a window for doctorally prepared advanced practice nurses to embrace advocacy as part of their expanding role.

APPLICATION AND PROCESS

Ward specifically discusses the application of advocacy to clinical practice by viewing clinical practice as a "trigger" for political action. The examples presented, lack of nutritious snack options in schools, work site and playground injuries, and lack of safe adult exercise programs—illustrate how a DAPN could utilize this "trigger" approach to identify a problem and take a leadership role in working toward a solution. Ward provides an overview of the process from the "trigger" identified in clinical practice to the development of a problem statement, the importance of the impact of policy and political analysis, and finally the culmination of the process in a position statement. These examples are important, because often, as we try and articulate how to move beyond our individual patient or community, there is no clear roadmap for how to actualize change. Using evidence-based practice as a backdrop through this process provides the DAPN with the critical evidence to support policy change.

CALL TO ACTION

Ward encourages the use of an existing nursing directive from our professional organization, the American Nurses Association's (ANA) *Code of Ethics with Interpretive Statement* (ANA, 2005). The broad view of social reform outlined in Section 9.4, as discussed by Ward, not only gives us license to broaden our view of political action to bring about social change, but extends our area of influence into areas of health-related, socio-cultural issues such as the violation of human rights, homelessness, hunger, violence, and the stigma of illness. By challenging nurses, specifically DAPNs, to action, Ward is calling for a higher level of accountability in a broader and more expansive view of health.

RECOMMENDATIONS FOR A STEP FURTHER

Utilizing Ward's call to action for DAPNs as a platform, I challenge us to go further by advocating for the adoption of health as a human right as a basis for nursing practice. Ward suggests that it is not a paradigm shift for nurses to utilize Critical Social Theory and puts an emphasis on the collective rather than the individual. I agree but suggest that it *is* the time to shift our paradigm in nursing, by incorporating a human rights approach to health.

Human rights is defined by Drevdahl and Dorcy (2007) as a subset of values within justice, a protection for both individuals and groups against actions that obstruct their freedoms or threaten human dignity. Human rights cover a broad range of issues including political, economic, and social rights. Gruskin, Mills, and Tarantola (2007) discuss the connection between health and human rights, "since the Nuremberg trials and the creation of the UN more than 50 years ago, interest in the association between health and human rights has grown" (p. 449).

There is a growing presence in the medical and public health literature, predominately pertaining to global health, of the link between health and human rights. Discussions of health as a human right are relatively limited in the nursing literature. It was briefly discussed by Kirkham and Browne (2006): "if health is a human right, the object of social justice becomes the health outcomes, not primarily equal access to health care services" (p. 328). Williams (2004) sees the value of health as a human right: "the human rights framework recognizes this dynamic relationship between fundamental human rights and health. It provides a language to describe the common experience of oppression among people in different parts of the world" (p. 76). We would benefit from a closer examination of the connections of health and human rights, and the broader implications of the many socio-cultural determinants of health.

The historical roots of social justice in nursing are rich and provide an important foundation from which to base a new paradigm, but a social justice approach to nursing has been limiting. Boutain (2005) provides a review of how social justice is described in the nursing literature in three predominant models: social, distributive, and market views of justice. Boutain (2005) acknowledges that "social justice definitions vary across disciplines and over time" and "social justice remains an elusive term that can be difficult to define and even more difficult to apply in practice" (p. 13).

A new level of advocacy for the doctoral advanced nursing practice role is critical, timely, and eloquently discussed by Ward. Doctorally prepared advanced practice nurses are embedded in all sectors of local, national, and global health systems and therefore, can have a far-reaching impact if mobilized. This is an opportunity to move beyond our historical roots of advocacy by simplifying our approach to health for all.

Viewing health as a human right provides a solid foundation from which to base nursing practice that is simple and does not become muddled in discussions of social, distributive, and market views of justice. The incorporation of advocacy into the DAPN role as an explicit role expectation, as Ward suggests, in my view lends itself to this timely paradigm shift. Doctorally prepared advanced practice nurses, well versed in complex health and delivery systems, are well positioned to take the lead on simplifying our approach to health as a basic human right.

REFERENCES

American Nurses Association (ANA). (2005). *Code of ethics for nurses with interpretive statements.* Retrieved from http://nursingworld.org/ethics/code/protected_nwcoe813.htm#9.4

Boutain, D. M. (2005). Social justice in nursing: A review of the literature. In M. de Chesnay (ed.), *Caring for the vulnerable: Perspectives in nursing theory, practice, and research* (p. 21–29). Sudbury, MA: Jones and Bartlett.

Carnegie, E., & Kiger, A. (2009). Being and doing politics: An outmoded model or 21st century reality? *Journal of Advanced Nursing, 65*(9), 1976–1984.

Cohen, S. S., Mason, D. J., Kovner, C., Leavitt, J. K., Pulcini, J., & Sochalski, J. (1996). Stages of nursing political development: Where we've been and where we ought to go. *Nursing Outlook, 44*(6), 259–266.

Drevdahl, D. J., & Dorcy, K. S. (2007). Exclusive inclusion: The violation of human rights and US immigration policy. *Advances in Nursing Science, 30*(4), 290–302.

Gruskin, S., Mills, E., & Tarantola, D. (2007). History, principles, and practice of health and human rights. *Lancet, 370*, 449–455.

Kirkham, S. R., & Browne, A. J. (2006). Toward a critical theoretical interpretation of social justice discourses in nursing. *Advances in Nursing Science, 29*(4), 324–339.

Williams, A. (2004) Nursing, health, and human rights: A framework for international collaboration. *Journal of the Association of Nurses in AIDS Care, 15*(3), 75–77.

CRITICAL THINKING QUESTIONS

1. Consider a problem that affects your patients' health that would benefit from policy change or advocacy. What individuals or groups would be natural allies in promoting that change?

2. What individuals or groups would be the strongest opponents?
3. What common ground can you find *or create* with the opponents stated from the above?
4. Which aspects are nonnegotiable and which are open to negotiation?
5. If the policy were changed in the desired manner, how would you measure success or failure of the change?
6. Can you project any unintended adverse sequelae of the policy change?
7. What personal values underpin your stance on the policy in question? How will you work with individuals who hold different values?
8. How does advanced research training enhance your ability to advocate for social policy change?
9. How does your advanced clinical expertise enable you to present more convincingly to policy makers?
10. What media approaches would be best suited for advancing the policy you advocate, and why?

CHAPTER NINETEEN

The Doctor of Nursing Practice Graduate and Use of the Title "Doctor"

Scott Oldfield

INTRODUCTION

Since the establishment of the first doctor of nursing practice program in 2001 at the University of Kentucky, there has been a steady increase in institutions offering and conferring the degree of Doctor of Nursing Practice (DNP/DrNP). According to the American Association of Colleges of Nursing (AACN) (2009), a total of 178 institutions offered doctoral nursing programs in the United States with 243 degree programs available in the fall of 2009. Of these, 120 were DNP programs (including one 1 DrNP program) established between 2001 and 2009. As the number of DNP programs has increased, so has the number of doctorally prepared nurses entering the work force equipped to function in leadership positions in a variety of settings. Recently, AACN (2010) released a report noting a total of 660 graduates from doctor of nursing programs in 2009 compared to 15 in 2002, a 44-fold increase.

The phenomenon of the professional doctorate in nursing has resulted in some uncertainty and confusion in both educational and clinical settings.[1] One of the more emotionally charged debates is the use of the title "doctor" by DNP graduates. *Doctor* is a title that is esteemed in both academia and health care. When a doctoral degree is conferred on an individual they are afforded the privilege of taking the title of doctor by his or her college or university. Despite this established tradition, the DNP graduate is faced with questions and sometimes skepticism regarding the academic rigor of the professional nursing doctorate compared to the traditional doctor of philosophy, placing into question the worthiness of the title doctor.

Another challenge for the doctorally prepared advanced practice nursing graduate adopting the title of doctor is the belief by many physicians that they have the sole proprietary rights to that title. Over the last decade, rhetoric from physicians has escalated with impassioned requests to protect and reserve the title of doctor for individuals practicing medicine. The American Medical Association (AMA) has led the charge, identifying patient confusion as impetus for promoting legislation for title protection:

> Whereas the growing trend of this title encroachment is of concern because patients will be confused when the titles of Doctor, Resident and Residency are applied to non-physicians who hold non-medical doctorates or to non-physicians in training.
>
> — *AMA, 2008b, para. 3*

These barriers to the utilization of the title doctor by doctorally prepared advanced practice nurses (DAPNs) are not insurmountable. First, a clear understanding of the term doctor and the development of doctoral education is necessary for an accurate historical viewpoint regarding the use of the title doctor. Second, tracing the trends in doctoral education within nursing will provide clarity regarding the place that the DNP degree holds within the nursing profession. Finally, a thorough review of the current environment in health care and society is necessary to formulate a successful response to detractors of the DNP graduate utilizing the title of doctor.

ETYMOLOGY AND DEFINITION OF "DOCTOR"

The term doctor originally derived from the Latin verb *docere*, which when translated means "to teach" (Skinner, 1970). According to the *Oxford Dictionary of Word Origins* (Cresswsell, 2010), until the end of the Middle Ages the term doctor primarily referred to individuals who authoritatively taught, such as early Christian theologians. Not until the 12th century and the formation of the European universities did the title take on formal academic significance. The University of Bologna, the oldest university in the western world, conferred the first doctorates in canon and civil law, and during the next century, additional doctorates were granted at other universities throughout Europe in medicine, grammar, logic, philosophy, and theology (Pace, 1909). It was not until the 15th century that individuals addressed as doctor referred specifically to a medical physician (Cresswsell, 2010).

At no point in modern history has the title doctor exclusively denoted a doctor of medicine. On the contrary, the term doctor has been inclusive of all individuals receiving a doctoral degree in any number of fields of study. According to *Stedman's Medical Dictionary* (Stedman, 2000) doctor is defined first as "a title conferred by a university on one who has followed a prescribed course of study, or given as a title of distinction; as doctor of medicine, laws, philosophy, etc.," and second, "a physician especially one upon whom has been conferred the degree of MD by a university or medical school" (p. 535). *Taber's Cyclopedic Medical Dictionary* (Venes, 2001) provides a similar definition with additional fields of study to include nursing: "the recipient of an advanced degree, such as doctor of medicine (MD), doctor of osteopathy (DO), doctor of philosophy (PhD), doctor of science (DSc), doctor of nursing science (DNS), doctor of dental medicine (DMD), doctor of education (Ed), or doctor of divinity (DD)" (Doctor, para. 1).

HISTORY OF DOCTORAL EDUCATION

The wide use of the doctor of philosophy (PhD) did not occur until the early 19th century; the predominant doctoral degrees prior to this point in history were nonresearch doctorates in the fields of law, medicine, and theology. The PhD originated in Germany and later spread to the United States with the first PhD awarded at Yale University in 1861 (Wellington, Bathmaker, Hunt, McCullough, & Sikes, 2005). By the 20th century, doctoral education evolved further with the emergence of the professional doctorate. According to the UK Council for Graduate Education (UKCGE) the professional doctorate is

> a programme of advanced study and research which, whilst satisfying the university criteria for the award of a doctorate, is designed to meet the specific needs of a professional group

external to the university, and which develops the capability of individuals within a professional context.

—UKCGE, 2002, p. 62

Taylor (2008) further defines the professional doctorate, when he states that the, "so-called 'professional' doctorates are doctorates that focus on embedding research in a reflective manner into a professional practice. They must meet the same core standards as 'traditional' doctorates in order to ensure the same high level of quality" (p. 80).

The origin of the modern professional doctorate can be found in the "ivy towers" of North America with the development of the EdD in the late 19th century at the University of Toronto. While the forerunners of the modern professional doctorate were primarily entry-level degrees into law, medicine, and theology, today's professional doctorate can be an entry-level or an advanced degree; the entry-level degree allowing entrance into a field of practice, while the advanced degree providing further professional education for individuals already practicing in their area of specialty. Institutions of higher education have been inundated with a myriad of health professional doctoral programs over the past 20 years. In addition to the DNP, several other fields within the health professions have developed doctoral programs. These doctorates include well established programs in dentistry (DDS/DMD), osteopathic medicine (DO), pharmacology (PharmD), and clinical psychology (PsyD), as well as fledgling allied health specialties in fields such as audiology (AuD), physical therapy (DPT), and occupational therapy (OTD) to name just a few (Snyder, 2006).

The professional doctorate has not remained isolated to the shores of North America; it has spread elsewhere throughout the Anglophone world (National Qualification Authority of Ireland [NQAI], 2006). The United Kingdom saw an increase in professional doctoral programs from 109 in 1998 to 192 in 2004 (UKCGE, 2005). The first professional doctorates in the United Kingdom were in the fields of engineering, education, and clinical psychology, followed by nursing and business administration. There are similarities and differences in the approach to the professional doctorate in the United Kingdom compared to the United States. One significant difference is the emphasis placed on knowledge development within the professional doctoral programs offered in the United Kingdom (Taylor, 2008). This is evidenced by the importance placed on research training for the professional doctoral student in the United Kingdom. According to the United Kingdom Economic & Social Research Council (2005):

> The ESRC considers that research training is important for all doctoral students (i.e., those studying for PhDs and for PDs) and that for students to be appropriately prepared to carry out research and produce a doctoral level dissertation, they require to be exposed to a range of research training similar to that set out in the Postgraduate Training Guidelines.
> *—United Kingdom Economic & Social Research Council,*
> *2005, Appendix 2, Research Training*
> *Requirements Section, para. 1*

A strong emphasis on empirical clinical research and the needed training is not fully supported in all of the professional doctoral programs in the United States, with nursing being no exception. This is demonstrated by that fact that only approximately 25% of the current DNP programs offers a course in nursing epistemology or philosophy of science (Dreher & Dahnke, 2010).

The development of professional doctoral programs can also be seen in other English-speaking countries including Australia, New Zealand, and Ireland, but this trend has not caught on in Continental Europe and has been met with skepticism. In

Sweden and Denmark, an industrial PhD similar in purpose and structure to a professional doctorate is offered, but ultimately it is just a variant of the PhD (NQAI, 2006). However, the University of Klagenfurt in Austria has developed a professional program at the doctoral level that may be a precursor to a professional doctorate (United Nations Educational, Scientific, and Cultural Organization—European Centre for Higher Education, 2004).

DOCTORAL EDUCATION IN NURSING: GRADUATES ACCUSTOMED TO THE TITLE 'Dr'

Doctoral education in nursing is a relatively new phenomenon. The origin of doctoral education in the United States has its origin at Columbia University's Teachers College with the creation of the Department of Nursing and Health in 1910. However, it was not until 1932 that the first doctoral nursing candidate, majoring in nursing education, received her degree of Doctor of Education (EdD). Two years later, in 1934, the first PhD in nursing was offered by New York University. In 1954, a third doctorate program in nursing was opened at the University of Pittsburgh with a PhD in clinical nursing and research. Not surprisingly, with the limited availability of doctoral nursing programs, the majority of nursing educators had doctoral degrees in other fields such as education or sociology. But in 1962, the federal government promoted the advancement of the nursing profession by initiating the indirect development of doctoral programs in nursing. The nurse scientist programs implemented by the government effectively increased doctoral nursing programs in the second half of the 20th century (Nichols & Chitty, 2005).

In 1979, a new doctorate of nursing was introduced by Case Western Reserve University. The Nursing Doctorate (ND) was intended for individuals who completed a bachelor's degree in something other than nursing, but later wanted to pursue a career as a nursing leader, whether in professional practice (later modified to include advanced practice too), research, or in an academic setting. The desire to develop a more clinically focused doctoral program in nursing led to the introduction of several additional degrees in the 1960s and 1970s, including the doctor of nursing (DNS), the doctor of nursing science (DNSc), and the doctor of science in nursing (DSN). As these programs matured, however, it became apparent that they were just variations of the research doctorate. By 2004, a total of 88 academic institutions were offering 96 doctoral programs in nursing, approximately 80% PhD programs and another 10% doctor of nursing science (DNS) programs. The remaining 10% of the programs in nursing included five ND, three DSN, one EdD, and one DNP (Pastor, Cimiotti, & Stone, 2004).

The end of the first decade of the 21st century has seen further change in doctoral nursing education. By the fall of 2009, the ND and DSN had been phased out altogether. The majority of DNS and DNSc programs had been converted to PhD programs with only one remaining DNSc offered at Yale University (it has since converted to a PhD) and three DSN programs in existence offered by Louisiana State University Health Science, CUNY-College of Staten Island, and The Sage Colleges. The majority of programs are either conferring PhD degrees or DNP degrees. From just 1 doctor of nursing practice program in 2004 to 120 in the fall of 2009, an explosion of the professional doctorate in nursing is changing the landscape of doctoral education in nursing (AACN, 2009).

In 2004, the AACN voted to require the DNP degree for entry level into advanced practice by 2015, touching off a lively debate among advanced practice nursing specialties with no true consensus reached. Several national nursing organizations have embraced the DNP degree, but are unwilling to designate the DNP as the sole educational option for the advanced practice nurse. The Nurse Practitioner Roundtable, comprised of several nurse practitioner organizations including American Academy of Nurse Practitioner (AANP), American College of Nurse Practitioners (ACNP), Association of Faculties of Pediatric Nurse Practitioners (AFPNP), National Association of Nurse Practitioners in Women's Health (NPWH), National Association of Pediatric Nurse Practitioners (NAPNAP), National Conference of Gerontological Nurse Practitioners (NCGNP), and National Organization of Nurse Practitioner Faculties (NONPF), offered a unified statement regarding nurse practitioner DNP education (2008). The DNP degree was endorsed, while at the same time the value of the current master's and higher degree nurse practitioner programs was acknowledged:

> Current master's and higher degree nurse practitioner programs prepare fully accountable clinicians to provide care to well individuals, patients with undifferentiated symptoms, and those with acute, complex chronic and/or critical illnesses. The DNP degree more accurately reflects current clinical competencies and includes preparation for the changing health care system. It is congruent with the intense rigorous education for nurse practitioners. This evolution is comparable to the clinical doctoral preparation for other health care professions.
> —*Nurse Practitioner Roundtable, 2008, Doctor of Nursing Practice section, para. 4*

The American Association of Nursing Anesthetists (AANA) also shares the belief that doctoral level education is in the best interest of the nursing profession, and in fact supports doctoral education for entry into the nurse anesthesia practice by 2025. However, the AANA is not acknowledging the DNP degree as the lone doctoral option, but are actually endorsing the awarding of *any doctoral degree*, creating more options for the nurse anesthetist. One such optional degree is the doctor of nursing anesthesia practice (DNAP), a non-nursing degree that has been approved by the Council of Accreditation of Nurse Anesthesia Educational Programs (COA) for nurse anesthesia programs that are not affiliated with a College of Nursing. The National Association of Clinical Nurse Specialists (NACNS) and the American College of Nurse Midwives (ACNM) have both taken a lukewarm stance on the DNP degree by neither endorsing nor opposing the DNP degree, but acknowledging it is one of the varieties of educational pathways for their members (ACNM, 2009; NACNS, 2009).

It has been theorized that the rapid proliferation of the DNP degree is a result of multiple factors within higher education and the health care industry. Rolfe and Davies (2009) suggest that the professional doctorate in nursing is a result of the dissatisfaction with the traditional PhD, which is perceived as producing individuals who are disconnected with nursing practice. Other factors that have been mentioned include a rapidly expanding knowledge base for practice, increasing complexity of patients, quality and safety of the care provided to patients, major shortages of doctorally prepared nursing faculty, and increasing educational expectations for the preparation of other health professionals (AACN, 2006a; Barry, 2009; Fulton, 2006). Irrespective of the catalysts driving the professional doctoral movement in nursing, the train has left the station at a blistering pace.

PROTECTION FOR THE TITLE "DOCTOR"

American Medical Association Resolutions

The professional doctorate in nursing has been met with skepticism and even fear among physicians who have voiced concern over the confusion that clients may experience when encountering a doctoral prepared nurse in the clinical setting, thus leading to a movement to protect the title of doctor and reserve this title to medical physicians, osteopathic physicians, and doctors of dental science.

The American Medical Association (AMA) responded to the rapid increase in the DNP programs with the submission of resolution 211 in May 2006 entitled "Need to Expose and Counter Nurse Doctoral Programs (NDP) Misrepresentation." The American Society of Anesthesiologists introduced this resolution making several unsubstantiated claims concerning the misrepresentation by nonmedical health care professionals and patient safety including:

- Whereas, confusion, injury and a breakdown of quality medical care would result from persons not trained as medical doctors and doctors of osteopathy misrepresenting themselves as "doctors" in clinical settings; and
- Whereas, at least one of the DNP programs is advertising its programs as "similar in concept to practice doctorates in other professions such as medicine (MD), law (JD), and dentistry (DDM)"; and
- Whereas, the quality of care rendered by individuals with a nurse doctoral degree is not equivalent to that of a physician (MD or DO); and
- Whereas, nurses and other nonphysician providers who hold doctoral degrees and identify themselves to patients as "doctors" will create confusion, jeopardize patient safety and erode the trust inherent in the true patient–physician relationship; and
- Whereas, patients led to believe that they are receiving care from a "doctor," who is not a physician (MD or DO), but the one who is a DNP may put their health at risk. (AMA, 2006, p. 1)

Based on the above concerns the resolution resolved:

- That it shall be the policy of our AMA that institutions offering advanced education in the healing arts and professions shall fully and accurately inform applicants and students of the educational programs and degrees offered by an institution and the limitations, if any, on the scope of practice under applicable state law for which the program prepares the student; and be it further
- That our AMA work jointly with state attorney generals to identify and prosecute those individuals who misrepresent themselves as physicians to their patients and mislead program applicants as to their future scope of practice (Directive to Take Action); and be it further
- That our AMA pursue all other appropriate legislative, regulatory and legal actions through the Scope of Practice Partnership, as well as actions within hospital staff organizations, to counter misrepresentation by nurse doctoral programs and their students and graduates, particularly in clinical settings (AMA, 2006a, p. 2).

The passing of resolution 211 on June 13, 2006 was countered quickly with the "AACN Talking Points in Response to the AMA's Resolution 211" (AACN, 2006b), released on June 22, 2006.

Several talking points were developed to counter the claims made by the AMA regarding misrepresentation by DNP graduates and programs. They include:

- Nursing and medicine are distinct health disciplines that prepare clinicians to assume different roles and meet different practice expectations. DNP programs prepare nurses for the highest level of nursing practice. They do not prepare nurses to be physicians. Transitioning to the DNP will not alter the current scope of practice for advanced practice nurses (APNs) as outlined in each state's Nurse Practice Act.

▪ No nursing schools offering the DNP are advertising these programs as a course of study to prepare physicians (AACN, 2006b, para. 2–3).

The argument for the use of the title "Doctor" by doctorally prepared nurses was concisely spelled out in the AACN's rebuttal to Resolution 211.

▪ The title of Doctor is common to many disciplines and is not the domain of any one group of health professionals. Many APNs currently hold doctoral degrees and are addressed as "Doctor," which is similar to how other expert practitioners in clinical areas are addressed, including clinical psychologists, dentists, and podiatrists. In all likelihood, APNs will retain their specialist titles after completing a doctoral program. For example, Nurse Practitioners will continue to be called Nurse Practitioners (AACN, 2006b, para. 4).

The AACN statement also stressed agreement with the AMA regarding the protection of the public by prosecuting individuals misrepresenting themselves as licensed health professionals and through the clear identification of credentials by actual health professionals providing direct patient care.

▪ Like the AMA, AACN recommends that action be taken against individuals who misrepresent themselves as physicians (or other health professionals) if they are not educated and licensed to assume that specific practice role. This concern extends to any unlicensed personnel who are referred to as "nurses" in physician's offices and other settings.
▪ AACN supports the AMA's recommendation to clearly identify a clinician's credentials both verbally and on name badges. This recommendation was included in the AACN's white paper on the *Hallmarks of the Professional Nursing Practice Environment* released in 2002. Consequently, DNP-prepared nurses would be expected to clearly display their credentials to insure that patients understand their preparation as a nursing provider, just as many APNs, physicians, and other clinicians currently do (AACN, 2002, p. 8; AACN, 2006b, para. 5–6).

In April 2008, the Illinois delegation of the AMA House of Delegates proposed a resolution entitled "Protection of the Titles 'Doctor,' 'Resident' and 'Residency,'" initially designated as resolution 303 but later renamed resolution 232. Issues of misrepresentation and patient safety were not addressed in this new resolution, but rather the potential confusion that could occur with nonphysician health care providers using the title doctor. The proposed resolution, therefore, resolved:

▪ That our AMA adopt that the title "Doctor," in a medical setting, apply only to physicians licensed to practice medicine in all its branches, dentists and podiatrists; and be it further
▪ That our AMA adopt policy that the title "Resident" apply only to individuals enrolled in physician, dentist or podiatrist training programs; and be it further

- That our AMA adopt policy that the title "Residency" apply only to physician, dentist or podiatrist training programs; and be it further
- That our AMA serves to protect, through legislation, the titles "Doctor," "Resident" and "Residency." (AMA, 2008b, p. 1)

Several organizations wrote letters of opposition to Resolution 303, including the American College of Clinical Pharmacy (ACCP), the American Chiropractic Association (ACA), the American Association of Naturopathic Physicians (AANP), and the American Nurses Association (ANA). Essentially, the predominant counterargument expressed by the opposing organizations was that the medical doctor has no proprietary right to the title doctor. The letter penned by the ANA stated, "the use of doctor is appropriate for these individuals who have earned the highest academic degrees conferred by a university and there is no legitimate reason to exclude nurses from this practice" (ANA, 2008, p. 2). The AMA approved amended Resolution 232 in June 2008 with the Texas delegation offering the introduction of felony language on the floor of the House of Delegates. The amended and adopted resolution 232 did not restrict the use of the title doctor by nonphysicians but it was resolved:

- That our AMA advocate that professionals in a clinical health care setting clearly and accurately identify to patients their qualifications and degree(s) attained, and develop model state legislation for implementation.
- That our AMA supports state legislation that would make it a felony to misrepresent oneself as a physician (MD/DO) (AMA, 2008a, p. 22).

Legislation Limiting the Use of "Doctor"

According to the most recent Pearson Report (2010), an annual state-by-state national overview of nurse practitioner legislation and health care issues, six states currently have legislated title protection for the title of doctor, and Arkansas and South Dakota have Medical Practice Acts placing limitations on the use of the title doctor. According to the Arkansas Medical Practice Act and Regulation established in 2001, unless licensed under the Medical Practice Act, the title doctor cannot be used in the provision of health care services. The legal use of the title doctor in South Dakota is a little more ambiguous. "Use of title and other acts constituting the practice of medicine may be cited to discourage use of Dr. title" (Pearson, 2010). Connecticut, Georgia, Maine, and Mississippi all have state statutory restrictions against a nurse practitioner with a doctorate being addressed as doctor. Although the Medical Practice Act in the state of Connecticut excludes nurse practitioners while rendering care under the collaboration of a licensed physician, the use of doctor is prohibited "with the intent to represent or in a manner that is likely to induce the belief that the person (1) practices medicine, (2) is licensed to practice medicine, or (3) may diagnose or treat any injury, deformity, ailment or disease for compensation, gain, or reward" (Pearson). In the state of Maine, the use of doctor is restricted to practitioners of allopathic and osteopathic medicine as well as chiropractors, naturopathic doctors, optometrists, and podiatrists. In the state of Mississippi, all health care providers are required by law to identify themselves to the public. Professional and academic credentials may be used after the name, but doctor may not be placed before the name. The remaining 42 states have no restrictions on the use of doctor by doctorally prepared nurse practitioners. However, 9 of the 42 states, Arizona, Illinois, New York, Ohio, Oklahoma, Oregon, Pennsylvania, Texas, and

Virginia, have no restrictions on the use of doctor as long as the nurse practitioner clearly is identified as an advanced practice nurse (Pearson).

International Perspectives

The attempt to limit the use of the title doctor is not exclusive to the United States. The 1991 Regulated Health Professionals Act, legislation enacted by the provincial government of Ontario, Canada, restricts the use of the title doctor in patient care settings. In an effort to avoid confusion among health care consumers, only members of the College of Chiropractors of Ontario, the Collage of Optometrists of Ontario, the College of Physicians and Surgeons of Ontario, the College of Psychologists of Ontario or the Royal College of Dental Surgeons of Ontario may be referred to as doctor in clinical settings (College of Audiologists and Speech–Language Pathologists of Ontario, 2003).

In the fall of 2009, John Mann, a member of the United Kingdom House of Commons, submitted a formal motion for debate in the House of Commons regarding title protection of the title doctor in the United Kingdom:

> That this House notes the title of doctor is not a protected title; further notes that practitioners of complementary medicine have an important role in health care, but believes that the title doctor implies a background in scientific orthodox medicine; further believes that the use of the term doctor by practitioners of complementary medicine is misleading and confusing; further believes that the array of other qualifications a trained orthodox doctor may hold can also be confusing; and calls on the Government either to protect the title of doctor for British Medical Association registered and suitably qualified practitioners, or to introduce a simple and popularly recognisable scheme that will distinguish between different traditions and levels of scientific evidence behind medicine.
> —*Mann, 2009, para. 1*

In Germany, known for its social formality, the law in place protecting the title of doctor is perhaps one of the most stringent. Stemming from a 1930s Nazi-era law, only people who earn PhDs or medical degrees *in Germany* are allowed to use the title of doctor. The law was modified in 2001 to extend the privilege to degree-holders from any country in the European Union. Any individual that identifies themselves as a doctor on German soil and has obtained his or her doctoral degree from a university outside the European Union can face up to a year in prison. Several Americans holding PhD's from universities in the United States have been under investigation for "title abuse." One of them was Ian Thomas Baldwin, a Cornell-educated researcher at the Max Planck Institute for Chemical, who elected to discontinue using the title "Prof. Dr. Baldwin" after being summoned by the local police. He now refers to himself as "Prof. Ian Thomas Baldwin, PhD, Cornell University" which is in compliance with German law (Whitlock & Smiley, 2008).

USE OF THE TITLE DOCTOR IN NURSING: THE DEBATE

The use of the title doctor by any individual receiving a doctoral degree, regardless of their area of study, is clearly established upon review of the etymology of the word doctor, the definition of the title doctor, and the history of the doctoral degree.

However, this centuries-old precedence has been placed into question by the medical establishment holding claims to what is essentially the slang use of the term 'doctor' to describe an individual holding a medical doctorate. Interestingly, in the AMA House of Delegates Preliminary Report of Reference Committee B (2008a), it was acknowledged "that any individual who has received a terminal degree in their area of study has the right to be called 'doctor.' However, the Reference Committee heard substantial and impassioned testimony in support of protecting the term 'doctor' in the medical setting to only refer to physicians" (p. 23).

The impassioned arguments offered in support of title protection have gone extensively unsubstantiated. Concerns for patient safety, one such argument initially offered, are simply not supported, and in fact the available data suggests that advance practice nurses provide quality care with equivalent outcomes as physicians in the primary care setting (Laurant et al., 2009). Another argument introduced by the AMA, the intentional misrepresentation of nonmedial health care providers as physicians, is also unfounded. According to a letter offered by the ACCP to the AMA in regards to resolution 232, "it is vital that patients fully understand the roles, responsibilities, scopes of practice, and credentials/qualifications of all health professionals involved in their care" (ACCP, 2008, p. 2). This belief is also embraced within nursing, and in fact the identification of a clinician's credentials was recommended in the AACN's white paper, *Hallmarks of the Professional Nursing Practice Environment* (ACCN, 2002).

More recently, proponents of limiting the title doctor in clinical settings have echoed concerns first arisen in academia stemming from concerns of degree creep (Siler & Randolph, 2006). With the rapid influx of professional doctoral programs and the variability among the programs offered, questions of academic rigor and standardization of the curriculum of clinical doctorate programs have been voiced (Miller, 2008). The profession of nursing has been proactive in addressing these concerns with the release of the AACN *Position Statement on the Practice Doctorate in Nursing* (AACN, 2004). In October 2004, this position statement attempted to clarify the purpose of the practice doctorate, including the identification of core content and core competencies, followed two years later by *The Essentials of Doctoral Education for Advanced Nursing Practice* (AACN, 2006a), clearly defining eight core competencies required for a DNP program. *The Essentials of Doctoral Education* was subsequently adopted by the Commission on Collegiate Nursing Education, the autonomous accrediting body of the AACN. Similarly, the National League for Nursing Accrediting Commission (NLNAC), the second accrediting agency for nursing education, also published standards and criteria of clinical doctorate programs in 2008, reflecting six standards complimenting the eight core competencies offered by AACN (NLNAC, 2008).

Issues of quality and standards are not exclusive to the United States, but are being debated in the United Kingdom as well, where there has been a rapid surge in professional doctorates. A variety of methods are being used in the United Kingdom to evaluate and assess the professional doctoral student. According to Taylor (2008), three primary approaches to assess the UK professional doctoral student include:

- *Coursework and dissertation*: normally by assignments (but also by short projects, group projects, presentations, and formal examinations) followed by a dissertation (showing an awareness of current research and, possibly, an addition to knowledge);
- *Portfolio assessment*: a range of assignments, often of varying length, which may or may not be based around a common theme (but without a formal dissertation or with a much reduced dissertation) and which show an awareness of research and, possibly, an addition to knowledge;

■ *Coursework and thesis*: relatively short assignments, followed by a major research project and thesis (normally requiring an addition to knowledge and the potential for publication) (p. 70).

Although Taylor attributes the diversity in the assessment process to the confusion experienced by many institutions of higher education, he also makes clear the positive contribution of the professional doctorate within doctoral studies. Upon conclusion of his paper, Taylor summarizes, "the importance of the professional doctorate in contributing to the extension of knowledge has been emphasised, based on rigorous research methods and with an expectation of dissemination through subsequent publications" (p. 85).

PRACTICAL RECOMMENDATIONS FOR THE DAPN

The final outcome of this transition in doctoral nursing education and the impact that this will have on nursing, the health care field, and society, the good and the bad, is being played out in real time with DNP graduates ultimately acting as change agents. DNP graduates are under a microscope as they take their newly acquired advanced nursing knowledge and develop roles in a variety of practice settings. If successful, a number of positive outcomes will transpire within institutions of higher learning and health care systems. Academically rigorous DNP programs are preparing nurses not only to function as doctoral advanced practice nurses in clinical and managerial settings, but as faculty in the colleges and departments of nursing addressing the nursing educator shortage (Dreher & Montgomery, 2009). Graduates of some professional doctoral nursing programs are also receiving the training necessary to conduct clinical research, adding to nursing knowledge. The DNP will also promote parity within multidisciplinary teams where nurses are working with colleagues in fields that require a doctorate as an entry-level degree.

According to Chism (2010), "First and foremost, DNP graduates, and others, need to educate themselves about their degree" (p. 222). The potential confusion created by the use of the title doctor by DNP graduates, whether it is in clinical settings or in academia, can either be viewed as a problem or an opportunity to educate others on the DNP degree and the value added by this advanced education. Every patient encounter affords the DAPN—*the opportunity to clearly link the title doctor with advanced practice nursing*. This can be accomplished by simply utilizing the title doctor prior to the name followed by the professional title, such as nurse practitioner or nurse anesthetist. An ongoing dialog with fellow nurses and other members of the multidisciplinary team regarding the education, title, and role of the DAPN will also help to garner support.

Familiarity of state law and regulations regarding the use of the title doctor is important for the DNP graduate to ensure compliance. In addition, keeping one's finger on the pulse of proposed federal and state legislation that could positively or negatively impact advanced nursing practice will allow for proactive steps to be taken. This is best accomplished when the nursing profession pools resources through state and national organizations. It is also suggested that one considers becoming a member of national and state advanced practice nursing organizations and coalitions which provide access to lobbyists working in the best interest of the profession of nursing, as well as provide real-time monitoring and updates on introduced bills that could impact practice, including the use of the title doctor. At the national level, the AANP is one such group that monitors federal bills and regulations that could influence nurse practitioner practice.

The AANP website has a legislation/practice section devoted to keeping their members updated on current legislation (http://www.aanp.org/AANPCMS2). The Pennsylvania Coalition of Nurse Practitioners is a state organization that also utilizes the Internet, using both a website and a listserve to provide members with legislative updates (http://www.pacnp.org/).

Finally, it is imperative for the DAPN to adopt Florence Nightingale's meticulous approach to data collection for the purpose of establishing empirical evidence substantiating the impact of the DNP degree on patient care and the profession of nursing. Just a few areas of potential interest and need for objective data include changes in autonomous practice, equitable third-party reimbursement, and improvement in patient access and care.

SUMMARY

The influx of professional doctoral programs being offered in nursing has resulted in uncertainty for individuals both in and out of the nursing profession. DAPNs are pioneers facing impediments to the acknowledgement of their academic accomplishments and their expert knowledge and skills. Nowhere is this more apparent than in the debate over the use of the title doctor.

The history of doctoral education is fluid and changing over time, with nursing education being no exception. From the first nursing doctorate conferred in the United States in 1932 to the various doctoral degree programs developed in the second half of the 20th century, including the ND, DNS, DNSc, and DSN (and a few others), there has been rapid growth in doctoral nursing education. The start of the 21st century has been marked by a new phenomenon in nursing education, the DNP. As of the fall of 2009, DNP program enrollments and graduations now exceed enrollments and graduations from traditional research-focused doctoral programs (Fang, Tracy, & Bednash, 2010). The growth of the professional doctorate in nursing is not exclusive to the United States, but has been observed in Australia, Canada, New Zealand, and the United Kingdom with similar growing pains observed.

The push for title protection of doctor has escalated with the increase in DAPNs over the first decade of the 21st century. The American Medical Association has taken its traditional paternalistic approach, adopting several resolutions to encourage the passing of legislation making it illegal for health care providers other than physicians, osteopaths, optometrists, and dentists to use the title of doctor. Ultimately, the AMA's characterization of the DAPN as an ill-educated individual loading up saddle bags full of roots, poisons, and a knife in order to head west and hang their shingle to practice medicine has gone unsubstantiated.[2] Any consumer confusion that may be created by the use of the title of doctor by advance practice nurses is an opportunity to educate the public of the role, responsibilities, scopes of practice, and professional credentials of the doctorally prepared advance practice nurse.

In an editorial written by Jean Barry (2009), confidence in the doctor of nursing practice degree is expressed. "The DNP is a terminal degree with a different focus than the PhD but very definitely equivalent in rigor and challenge. Graduates of DNP programs will have the highest level of nursing knowledge and expertise in the practice setting" (p. 100–101). With this view in mind, the doctor of nursing practice graduate needs to be proactive in securing and protecting a practice environment that allows for exceptional patient care, utilizing the full scope of the advanced practice nurse and the promotion of equality among health care providers. In addition, taking time to educate nursing colleagues and other health care providers will promote understanding and support within the health care industry, ensuring continued freedom to use the honorific title "doctor" and leading to change in the few states that currently restrict the use of the title by doctorally prepared nurses.

Although the title of doctor does not guarantee a level playing field, it is one less factor that can be raised in an attempt to maintain the stratification between various health care specialties. Finally, it is the responsibility and privilege of the doctor of nursing practice graduate to develop the role of the DAPN. In doing this, it is imperative that this new critical mass of DNP- (and some DrNP-) educated graduates help provide empirical evidence that will substantiate their importance to the nursing profession and society through the development of nursing science, education, and excellence in nursing care.

NOTES

1. Although the terms practice doctorate and clinical doctorate are used by various health care specialties to refer to nonresearch doctoral degrees, the author of this chapter will utilize the more general *professional doctorate* since it is inclusive of all nonresearch doctoral degrees regardless of the area of study.
2. In the late 1700s and early 1800s the United States experienced an expansion to the west. The westward settlers were often dependent upon traveling doctors that, more often than not, had never attended a medical school.

REFERENCES

American Association of Colleges of Nursing (AACN). (2002). *Hallmarks of the professional nursing practice environment*. Retrieved from http://www.aacn.nche.edu/publications/positions/hallmarkswp.pdf

American Association of Colleges of Nursing (AACN). (2004). *AACN position statement on the practice doctorate in nursing*. Retrieved from http://www.aacn.nche.edu/DNP/pdf/DNP.pdf

American Association of Colleges of Nursing (AACN). (2006a). *The essentials of doctoral education for advanced nursing practice*. Retrieved from http://www.aacn.nche.edu/DNP/pdf/Essentials.pdf

American Association of Colleges of Nursing (AACN). (2006b). *AACN talking points in response to the AMA's resolution 211*. Retrieved from http://www.aacn.nche.edu/dnp/pdf/amatalkingpoints.pdf

American Association of Colleges of Nursing (AACN). (2009). *Institutions offering doctoral programs in nursing and degrees conferred*. Retrieved from http://www.aacn.nche.edu/IDS/pdf/DOC.pdf

American Association of Colleges of Nursing (AACN). (2010). *The doctor of nursing practice: A report on progress*. Retrieved from http://www.aacn.nche.edu/DNP/pdf/DNPForum3-10.pdf

American College of Clinical Pharmacy (ACCP). (2008). *Communication to the American Medical Association regarding resolution 303*. Retrieved from http://www.psap.org/docs/positions/commentaries/ACCP_Response_to_AMA_Resolution_303-08.pdf

American College of Nurse Midwives (ACNM). (2009). *Position statement: Midwifery education and the doctor of nursing practice (DNP)*. Retrieved from http://www.midwife.org/documents/ACNMonDNP.pdf

American Medical Association (AMA). (2006). *Need to expose and counter nurse doctoral programs (DNP) misrepresentation*. Retrieved from http://www.pacnp.org/files/resolution__211_-_nursing_doctorate.pdf

American Medical Association (AMA). (2008a). *American Medical Association House of Delegates (A-08): Reports of Preference Committee B.* Retrieved from http://www.ama-assn.org/ama1/pub/upload/mm/471/annotatedb.doc

American Medical Association (AMA). (2008b). *Protection of the titles "doctor," "resident" and "residency."* Retrieved from http://www.ama-assn.org/ama1/pub/upload/mm/471/303.doc

American Nurses Association (ANA). (2008). *Communication to the American medical association regarding resolution 303.* Retrieved from http://www.nursingworld.org/FunctionalMenuCategories/MediaResources/PressReleases/2008PR/AMALetterTitles.aspx

Barry, J. (2009). To use or not to use: The clinical use of the title "doctor" by DNP graduates. *Journal of Nursing Administration, 39*(3), 99–102.

Chism, L. A. (2010). The Dr. Nurse: Overcoming title issues. In L. A. Chism (Ed.), *The doctor of nursing practice: A guidebook for role development and professional issues* (pp. 197–226). Sudbury, MA: Jones and Bartlett Publishers, LLC.

College of Audiologists and Speech–Language Pathologists of Ontario. (2003). *Use of the title "doctor."* Retrieved from http://deskref.caslpo.com/doctor_ps.doc

Cresswsell, J. (2010). Physician. *Oxford dictionary of word origins.* Retrieved from http://www.oxfordreference.com/views/ENRTY.html?subview=Main&entry=t292.e3720

Dreher, H. M., & Dahnke, M. D. (2010). Philosophy of science in a practice discipline. In M. Dahnke, & H. M. Dreher, *Philosophy of science for nursing practice: Concepts and application.* New York, NY: Springer.

Dreher, H. M., & Montgomery, K. E. (2009). Let's call it "doctoral" advanced practice nursing. *The Journal of Continuing Nursing Education, 40*(12), 530–531.

Fang, D., Tracy, C., & Bednash, G. (2010). *2009–2010 Enrollment and graduations in baccalaureate and graduate programs in nursing.* Washington, DC: American Association of Colleges of Nursing.

Fulton, J. S. (2006). Clinical doctorates: Meeting the public need? *Clinical Nurse Specialist, 20*(6), 266–267.

Laurant, M., Reeves, D., Hermens, R., Braspenning, J., Grol, R., & Sibbald, B. (2009). Substitution of doctors by nurses in primary care (review). In *The Cochrane Library 2009.* Retrieved from http://www.hss.state.ak.us/hspc/files/Primary_Care_Substitution.pdf

Mann, J. (2009). *Protection of the title of doctor.* Retrieved from http://edmi.parliament.uk/EDMi/EDMDetails.aspx?EDMID=38820

Miller, J. E. (2008). The doctor of nursing practice: Recognizing a need or praying the line between doctor and nurse? *Medscape Journal of Medicine, 10*(11), 253.

National Association of Clinical Nurse Specialists. (2009). *Position statement on nursing practice doctorate.* Retrieved from http://www.nacns.org/LinkClick.aspx?fileticket=TOZlongI258%3d&tabid=116

National League for Nursing Accrediting Commission (NLNAC). (2008). *NLNAC standards and criteria: Clinical doctorate.* Retrieved from http://www.nlnac.org/manuals/SC2008_DOCTORATE.pdf

National Qualifications Authority of Ireland (NQAI). (2006). *Review of professional doctorates.* Dublin: National Qualifications Authority of Ireland.

Nichols, E. F., & Chitty, K. K. (2005). Education patterns in nursing. In K. K. Chitty (Ed.), *Professional Nursing: Concepts & Challenges* (pp. 31–62). St. Louis, MO: Elsevier Saunders.

Nurse Practitioner Roundtable. (June, 2008). *Nurse practitioner DNP education, certification and titling: A unified statement.* Washington, DC: Author.

Pace, E. (1909). Doctor. In C. G. Herbermann, E. A. Pace, C. B. Pallen, T. J. Shahan, & J. J. Wynne (Eds) *The Catholic encyclopedia.* New York, NY: Robert Appleton Company. Retrieved from New Advent: http://www.newadvent.org/cathen/05072b.htm

Pastor, D. K., Cimiotti, J. P., & Stone, P. W. (2004). Doctoral preparation in nursing: What are the options? *Applied Nursing Research, 17*(2), 137–139.

Pearson, L. J. (2010). The Pearson Report. *American Journal for Nurse Practitioners, 14*(2), 49–53.

Rolfe, G., & Davies, R. (2009). Second generation professional doctorates in nursing. *International Journal of Nursing Studies, 46*, 1265–1273.

Siler, W. L., & Randolph, D. S. (2006). A clinical look at clinical doctorates. *Chronicle of Higher Education, 52*(46), 58.

Skinner, H. (1970). *Medical terms* (2nd ed.). New York, NY: Hafner.

Snyder, T. (2006). *Easy doctorates: Are all PhDs created equal?* Retrieved from http://www.doctorate-degree-phd-directory.com/Easy-Doctorates.htm

Stedman, T. L. (2000). *Stedman's medical dictionary* (26th ed.). Philadelphia, PA: Lippincott Williams & Wilkins.

Taylor, J. (2008). Quality and standards: The challenge of the professional doctorate. *Higher Education in Europe, 33*(1), 65–87.

UK Council for Graduate Education (UKCGE). (2002). *Professional doctorate.* Dudley, England: UKCBE. Retrieved from http://www.ukcge.ac.uk/OneStopCMS/Core/CrawlerResourceServer. aspx? resource=53BE34C8-EBDD-47E1-B1C7-F80B45D25E20&mode=link&guid=a57997aa5a9f4450b b141144a86634e6

UK Council for Graduate Education (UKCGE). (2005). *Professional doctorate awards in the UK.* Lichfield, UK: UKCBE. Retrieved from http://www.ukcge.ac.uk/Resources/UKCGE/Documents/PDF/ConfidentialityPhDTheses%202005.pdf

United Kingdom Economic & Social Research Council. (2005). *Postgraduate training guidelines: ESRC recognition of research training programmes: A guide to provision for postgraduate advanced course and research students in the social sciences* (4th ed.). Retrieved from http://www.esrcsocietyto-day.ac.uk/ESRCInfoCentre/Images/Postgraduate_Training_Guidelines_2005_tcm6-9062.pdf

United Nations Educational, Scientific, and Cultural Organization—European Centre for Higher Education. (2004). *Doctoral studies and qualifications in Europe and the United States: Status and prospects.* Bucharest: UNESCO. Retrieved from http://unesdoc.unesco.org/images/0013/001364/136456e.pdf

Venes, D. (2001). Doctor. *Taber's Online, Taber's cyclopedic medical dictionary* (21st ed.). Retrieved from http://www.tabers.com/tabersonline/ub/view/Tabers/143285/48/doctor?q=doctor.

Wellington, J., Bathmaker, A. M., Hunt, C., McCullough, G., & Sikes, P. (2005). *Succeeding with your doctorate.* London, UK: Sage.

Whitlock, C., & Smiley, S. (2008, March 14). Non-European PhDs in Germany find use of 'doktor' verboten. *The Washington Post.* Retrieved from http://www.washingtonpost.com/wp-dyn/content/article/2008/03/13/AR2008031304353.html

CHAPTER NINETEEN: Reflective Response 1

Owen C. Montgomery

I would like to congratulate (soon to be!) Dr. Scott Oldfield for his thorough, accurate, and historical review of the emotionally charged issue related to the use of the title "doctor" by advance practice nurses (APNs) who have completed a Doctor of Nursing Practice (DNP or DrNP) degree. His description of the evolution of the nursing profession's doctoral training leading up to the recent explosion of programs offering a DNP degree is critical to the understanding of a profession's "growing pains." In order for nursing as a profession to answer the challenge of the Institute of Medicine (IOM, 2003, 2005), the Joint Commission on the Accreditation of Healthcare Organizations (JCHO), and the National Research Council of the National Academies (2006) to reconceptualize health professions education to meet the needs of the health care delivery system, it is critical for nursing to continue to reevaluate and continue its evolution to meet the changing demands of the nation's complex health care system environment (AACN, 2006a; IOM, 2003, 2005)

Oldfield has given the reader a thousand-year lesson in the history of academic titles and in the emergence of multiple fields of education in the health professions. He does not give us the "thorough review" of the current environment of health care and society he says is required to respond to detractors of the use of the title doctor. However, his review of the etymology of the word "doctor," along with the history lesson, make a very convincing argument that "rigorously trained professionals" receiving their terminal degree, and "teaching" others using their now advanced knowledge in their field, deserve to be honored by being allowed to use the term "doctor."

Oldfield correctly identifies two very different challenges specific to the DNP graduate's use of the term "doctor." One challenge stems from the traditional doctorate graduates in nursing and other academic areas who have "earned" the right to be addressed as "doctor" based on the completion of their terminal degree, a major research project and the "addition to knowledge" (Taylor, 2008, p. 85). These faculty, mostly PhDs and EdDs, question the academic rigor of the new DNP degree. The second challenge is from the medical profession who are jealously protecting the tradition of reserving the title of "doctor" in clinical settings to graduates of allopathic, osteopathic, or dental schools.

With regard to the challenge from traditional graduates of doctoral programs, if the programs offering a DNP degree offer a terminal degree with a different focus than the PhD, but very definitely equivalent in rigor and challenge as suggested in the editorial by Barry (2009), then graduates will have attained the highest level of nursing knowledge and have a strong argument in using the academic title of "doctor" when given their terminal clinical degree. The core competencies of the AACN in the *Essentials of Doctoral Education for Advanced Nursing Practice* (2006a) must be diligently adhered to as well as the six standards of the clinical doctorate of the National League for Nursing Accrediting Commission (2008).

However, according to Oldfield, many DNP programs do not require a strong emphasis on empirical clinical research. Dreher and Dahnke (2010) document that only approximately 25% of DNP programs offer a course in nursing epistemology or philosophy of science, courses foundational to any kind of knowledge generation *or* evaluation of evidence. As the number of DNP programs and their graduates now outnumber the traditional nursing research doctoral programs and their graduates, academic nursing leaders must critically evaluate if DNP programs that do not require original research or a doctoral thesis are really demonstrating the rigor of their sister PhD or EdD programs? Is the DNP program expansion train "that has left the station at a blistering pace" on the right track? Are the conductors rigorous enough and the freight "weighty enough" for a terminal degree and to be called "doctor?" *In academia, the important word is "rigor" not "doctor."*

With regard to the challenge from the medical profession to graduates of DNP programs using the title "doctor" in their clinical activities, the title of "doctor" is a time honored one with, by Oldfield's account, over half a millennium of tradition suggesting that the well-trained and learned healers practicing their art in a clinical setting is a graduate of a rigorous professional training program in a allopathic or osteopathic medical or dental school. It is difficult, if not impossible, to write about this emotionally charged topic and not allow some of the emotion to seep into your writing. Oldfield is not immune and allowed himself to be drawn into the less than high-minded discussion with such phrases as "rhetoric from physicians," using "doctor" in reference to a medical degree graduate as "essentially the slang use of the term." The description of the American Medical's Association's (AMA) paternalistic characterization of the doctorally prepared APN as "an ill educated individual loading up saddle bags full of roots, poisons, and a knife in order to head west and hang their shingle to practice medicine" (p. 360) is the most colorful of these emotional phrases. This character is actually a description of *"Dr. Quinn: Medicine Woman,"* referring to an actual medical graduate of the first medical school in the world founded to educate women, the Female Medical College of Pennsylvania (founded 1850 in Philadelphia) I believe, despite the tradition, that the AMA and, especially, the Texas delegation should be embarrassed by both bringing this issue to the AMA house and even more by attaching the concept of a felony to the use of a title. *The 6 state house legislative efforts to protect the title of "doctor" are a waste of time and waste to tax payers' money.*

In contrast to Oldfield's defensiveness, the simple elegance of being correct is exemplified in the AACN's 2006 *Talking Points in Response to the AMA's Resolution 211.* The AACN document is thoughtful, professional, and high minded. The response states "Nursing and Medicine are distinct health disciplines that prepare clinicians to assume different roles" and "No Nursing School offering the DNP advertises their program as a course of study to become a physician" (AACN, 2006b, p. 1). This AACN document then simply states that the title of "doctor" is common to many disciplines and is not the domain of any one group of health professionals. A recent example of the real world confusion regarding the title "doctor" occurred following the untimely death of a beloved doctoral nursing faculty member, expert Nurse Practitioner, and friend Dr. Kathleen Falkenstein. Dr. Falkenstein dedicated her professional career to clinical practice, research, and education. In her obituary, the nationally recognized local newspaper chose initially to refer to Dr. Falkenstein as "Mrs." because they "usually reserve doctor for physicians unless they have been in academia for a long time." After several letters to the editor from medical and nursing colleagues alike, the paper *appropriately* corrected the obituary to 'Dr. Falkenstein.'

Nursing leadership should be asking if DNP graduates actually want to be called "doctor." Why would these 660 DNP graduates nationally in 2009 want to be misrepresented as "just a Doctor" when they are unique and pioneering nursing leaders. Why dilute their accomplishment by accepting the title used by over 1,000 times as many clinicians?

Dreher and Montgomery (2009) have concluded that we should refer to these doctor of nursing practice graduates as *Doctoral Advanced Practice Nurses.* Further, every patient encounter affords the doctorally prepared advanced practice nurse the opportunity to clearly link the title "doctor" with advance practice nursing (Chism, 2010). The pride of nursing is clearly apparent in the following quote:

> The caring tradition of nursing provides a superior foundation for the education of a woman's health care provider and differentiates our role from allopathic medical programs. The journey for such superiority commences with an empathic individual who seeks out a career in the healing arts through nursing school
>
> — *K. Montgomery, personal communication, July 1, 2010*

DNP graduates should embrace their nursing traditions. Oldfield correctly invoked Florence Nightingale's meticulous approach to data collection to substantiate the DNP's impact on nursing. According to the AACN (2006a), DNPs should use their doctoral status to represent nursing in multidisciplinary teams on equal footing with other academic doctoral graduates. One clear example of such type of collaboration is the transdisciplinary model of Women's Health Education at Drexel University:

> At Drexel University, the College of Medicine and the College of Nursing and Health Professions have designed and developed an education curriculum and multidisciplinary forum to support a transdisciplinary model of women's health care. This innovative primary care model has obstetrics and gynecology medical students, women's health nurse practitioner students, physician assistant students, and nurse-midwifery students together in a collaborative setting. The program fosters development of team-building skills across disciplines to improve communication, reduce medical errors, and improve the quality of patient care
>
> — *Unpublished material, Owen C. Montgomery, PI*

To completely answer the IOM (2003) challenge, DNPs must help teach the next generation of health practitioners, medical and nursing alike. *In summary, the most important title for the DNP graduate should not be the title of "Doctor" but the title of "Nurse"!*

REFERENCES

American Association of Colleges of Nursing (AACN). (2006a). *The essentials of doctoral education for advanced nursing practice.* Retrieved from http://www.aacn.nche.edu/DNP/pdf/Essentials.pdf

American Association of Colleges of Nursing (AACN). (2006b). *AACN talking points in response to the AMA's resolution 211.* Retrieved from http://www.aacn.nche.edu/dnp/pdf/amatalking-points.pdf

American Medical Association (AMA). (2006). *Need to expose and counter nurse doctoral programs (NDP) misrepresentation.* Retrieved from http://www.pacnp.org/files/resolution__211_-_nursing_doctorate.pdf

Barry, J. (2009). To use or not to use: The clinical use of the title "doctor" by DNP graduates. *Journal of Nursing Administration, 39*(3), 99–102.

Chism, L. A. (2010). The Dr. Nurse: Overcoming title issues. In L. A. Chism (Ed.), *The doctor of nursing practice: A guidebook for role development and professional issues* (pp. 197–226). Sudbury, MA: Jones and Bartlett.

Dreher, H. M., & Dahnke, M. D. (2010). Philosophy of science in a practice discipline. In M. D. Dahnke & H. M. Dreher, *Philosophy of science for nursing practice: Concepts and application.* New York, NY: Springer.

Dreher, H. M., & Montgomery, K. (2009). Let's call it "doctoral" advanced practice nursing. *Journal of Continuing Education in Nursing, 40*(12), 530–531.

Institute of Medicine of the Natural Academies. (2003). *Health professions education: A bridge to quality.* Washington, DC: National Academies Press.

Institute of Medicine of the Natural Academies. (2005). *Advancing the nation's health needs: NIH research training programs.* Washington, DC: National Academies Press.

National Research Council of the National Academies. (2006). *Advancing the nation's health needs: NIH research training programs.* Washington, DC: National Academies Press.

National League for Nursing Accrediting Commission. (2008). *NLNAC standards and criteria: Clinical doctorate.* Retrieved from http://www.nlnac.org/manuals/SC2008DOCTORATE.pdf

Taylor, J. (2008). Quality and standards: The challenge of the professional doctorate. *Higher Education in Europe, 33*(1), 65–87.

Jason E. Miller

The use of the title "doctor," as the author has duly explained, by doctoral advanced practice nurses (APNs) in a clinical setting is a very hot topic at present. Physicians and APNs have expressed antithetical viewpoints concerning APNs using the title "doctor" in a health care setting. These two professions, that would do best to complement and enhance each other in the name of patient care, are engaged in a battle that some would argue is merely one of semantics while others would argue puts patient safety at stake. The concern, however, is not without merit and is an important and valid one in need of resolve.

The author has delivered an informative analysis on the origins and history of the term "doctor," beginning with its Latin precursor, *docere*. The author correctly states that the physician community does not have a meritorious argument for the exclusive use of the generalized term "doctor;" however, as I will demonstrate in this response, the author has not presented a compelling argument for the use of the title "doctor" by APNs while engaged in patient care. The real argument here does not concern the general term but rather the specific use of the title in a specific setting.

The patient confusion argument forms the crux of the American Medical Association's (AMAs) opposition to the usage of the title "doctor" by APNs in practice, and its resultant call for title protection (AMA, 2008). Moreover, with popular media printing, direct quotes such as "'We're constantly having to prove ourselves,' said Chicago nurse practitioner Amanda Cockrell, 32, who tells patients she's just like a doctor 'except for the pay'" (Johnson, 2010, para. 7), the likelihood of patient confusion, sans title protection, is significant. In fact, the author even seems to acknowledge "[t]he potential confusion created by the use of the title 'doctor' by DNP graduates..." (p. 359). The author welcomes this challenge as an opportunity to link the title "doctor" with advanced practice nursing. I agree that the opportunity is ripe for introducing patients to this growing practitioner type, but respectfully disagree with the author's proposed method.

The author proposes use of the title "doctor," then the practitioner's name, and finally the applicable professional title, such as nurse practitioner, as sort of a tagline at the end. This method would result as follows: Dr. Susan Jones, CRNA. Unfortunately, I do not believe that this solution clears the hurdle of patient confusion. Rather, I feel an approach that places the emphasis on the actual degree conveyed, including the level, would far better ameliorate patient confusion and work to convey to the general public the growing number of doctoral-trained APNs. I therefore propose a variant of the method set forth by Maj. Leonard Gruppo in his editorial arguing for doctoral level training for physician assistants (Gruppo, 2005). Gruppo (2005) addressed the issue of patient confusion not by arguing for the use of the title "doctor," but rather against it, advising instead that "[w]e must teach doctoral PAs not to introduce themselves as 'doctor' and not to wear name tags that say, 'Doctor Jones'" (p. 6).

Following Gruppo's proposal removes the term "doctor" in its entirety and would simply list the degree as follows: Susan Jones, DNP, CRNA. I propose a variant on Gruppo's approach with respect to doctoral-trained APNs that would appear as follows: Susan Jones, doctoral CRNA. This modified approach retains the use of the term "doctor" by modifying the professional title, in the present example, CRNA, with the adjective "doctoral." I believe that this is the best approach to further the interests of doctoral APNs without creating unnecessary patient confusion.

As expressed by organizations such as the AMA (2006), and as acknowledged by the author, patient confusion is a very real concern. While the author delivers a very detailed analysis of the etymology and definition of the term "doctor," the author has attempted to downplay the significance of patient perception by noting the nonmedical origins of the general term "doctor," further emphasizing that "[i]t was not until the 15th century that individuals addressed as 'doctor' referred specifically to a medical physician" (p. 350). The scope of the author's argument extends broadly to use of the general term and spans back to the Middle Ages. The author does not, however, adequately counter the 600 years of relatively exclusive attribution of the title "doctor" to physicians, specifically in the health care setting, and the resultant patient expectations attached to such specific usage.

Expectations of a term's usage and meaning have not, historically, been left without consideration. For purposes of analogy, a reverse parallel can be found in the legal concept of trademark genericity. Trademark genericity occurs when common usage causes a distinctive trademark to become generic over time (Harvard, n.d.). Courts have thrust thermos, cellophane, and aspirin into the public domain as a result of the generalized use of those once-specific terms (Harvard, n.d.). As demonstrated in the realm of trademark law, historically, the courts have placed such a high level of regard on public perception as to essentially permit a trademark to become a common noun.

Trademark genericity demonstrates how a very specific term can gain common meaning through general usage, based upon public perception of the term. Why, then, could the opposite not hold true whereby a common term can, through extensive and exclusive usage in a specific setting, garner a specific public perception with respect to that specific setting? The present question involves not a trademark but a title. The extensive and nearly exclusive usage of that title in that specific setting results not in genericity but rather specificity. Public perception of the use of the title "doctor" in a health care setting has, therefore, culminated in "title specificity" of the term in that specific setting. Where a trademark can lose its uniqueness through general use, the specific use of the title doctor in a clinical setting has resulted in a public expectation and thus "title specificity" has occurred. The common element to these two reverse parallels is public perception and expectation. Where is public perception and expectation more relevant, more pertinent, than in health care?

This "title specificity" begs for protection of the title, at least until such time that public knowledge of doctoral APNs has reached the point where the use of the title doctor by doctoral APNs in a clinical setting will not assail patient expectations and lead to unnecessary confusion and all of its ill consequences.

Figure 19.1 summarizes this concept of "title specificity," starting with use of the "generic term." This point in the cycle relates to the early stages of the etymology and definition of the term "doctor," described by the author, up through sometime during the 15th century, just prior to when the term first saw usage to refer to physicians. The second point in the cycle then represents this initial point of specific usage during the 15th century. The third point is representative of the period from the 15th century moving forward until the use of the term "doctor" in a patient care setting became synonymous

FIGURE 19.1
The cycle of title specificity toward the use of "Doctor"

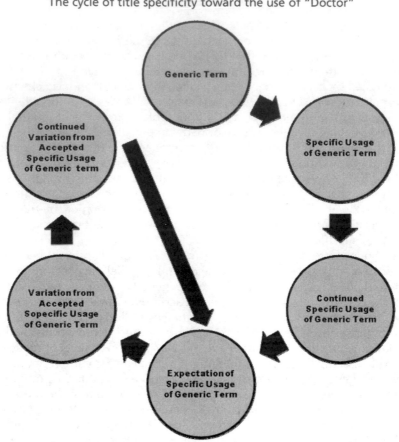

with physicians, which is illustrated by the fourth point. The fourth point, for physicians in a clinical setting, results in "title specificity." The fifth point is where we are today with the proliferation of doctoral-trained APNs, while the sixth point represents some unknown time in the future. It is through points five and six of the cycle where the risk for patient confusion is high. The goal of the doctoral APN community should be to go from the sixth point to the fourth point by educating patients of this growing practitioner type. The overriding concern through this transition must be the interest of the patients. The best way to achieve this goal, for the time being, is, in my opinion, by denoting the degree level only and not through direct use of the title "doctor" in a clinical setting. Through time, without appropriate title protection, as additional doctoral practitioners transition into and through the cycle, this "title specificity" will erode until such a point that the title "doctor" will no longer elicit a specific patient perception and expectation, with patient confusion being the unfortunate by-product. Physicians want to avoid this erosion altogether while doctoral APNs seemingly want to join in under this "title specificity." Only a cautious transition through points five and six, anchored by appropriate title protection, can ultimately lead to the acceptance of doctoral APNs as "doctors" without causing undue patient confusion and without potentially opening the door to virtually any health care professional using the title "doctor" in a clinical setting without restriction via erosion of established "title specificity(ies)."

Considering the brevity of existence of the DNP, as compared to 600 years of use of the title "doctor" by physicians in a health care setting, what solution minimizes patient confusion yet affords doctoral-trained APNs the opportunity to educate patients of the growing number of doctoral APNs? My take on Gruppo's method permits doctoral APNs to convey the level of degree without creating unnecessary patient confusion. States that have not already done so should enact title protection statutes to ensure against patient confusion during this transition phase. A model act that the individual states could adopt would be a great solution to ensure uniformity across state lines. Such legislation and model act could be written to sunset unless re-codified at some point in the future so that the topic can be revisited after doctoral APNs have become more thoroughly established. This approach would also work to sooth the concerns of the physician community and build an amiable connection between physicians and doctoral APNs.

REFERENCES

American Medical Association (AMA). (2006). *American Medical Association. Resolution 211 (A-06).* Retrieved from http://www.pacnp.org/files/resolution__211_-_nursing_doctorate.pdf

American Medical Association (AMA). (2008). *American Medical Association House of Delegates (A-08): Reports of reference committee B.* Retrieved from http://www.ama-assn.org/ama1/pub/upload/mm/471/annotatedb.doc

Harvard Cyber Law. (n. d.). *Overview of trademark law.* Retrieved from http://cyber.law.harvard.edu/metaschool/fisher/domain/tm.htm

Gruppo, Jr., & Maj, L. Q. (2005), Clinical doctorate degrees—Are we ready? [editorial]. *Perspective on Physician Assistant Education, 16*(1), 5–7.

Johnson, C. K. (2010). *Doc deficit? Nurses' role may grow in 28 states.* Retrieved from http://www.msnbc.msn.com/id/36472308/

CRITICAL THINKING QUESTIONS

1. What conclusions can be ascertained regarding the use of the title "doctor" by DAPNs based on the etymology and definition of the title "doctor?"
2. With the relatively short history of doctoral nursing education, what significance does the doctor of nursing practice degree have on the present and future profession of nursing?
3. Should the doctor of nursing practice degree be an entry-level degree or an advanced degree? Explain.
4. What role should the DAPN have in both practice and academia?
5. With the shortage of nursing educators, what role does the doctorally prepared advance practice nurse play in filling the gap in the education of future nurses?
6. In what capacity does a nurse with a doctor of nursing practice degree participate in the furthering of nursing science?
7. How does a doctor of nursing practice degree provide parity in a multidisciplinary practice setting?

8. What are some proactive steps that can be taken by a DAPN to ensure the use of the title of "doctor" is available to them?
9. How can physicians and other health care professionals be engaged in a productive dialog regarding the roles, responsibilities, and scope of practice of the DAPN?
10. What empirical measurements can be tracked by the DAPN to validate their value to nursing, health care, and society?

CHAPTER TWENTY

Enhancing the Doctoral Advanced Practice Role With Reflective Practice

Graham Stew

> *By three methods we may learn wisdom: first, by reflection, which is the noblest;*
> *second by imitation, which is the easiest; and third by experience,*
> *which is the bitterest.*
> —*Confucius*

INTRODUCTION

This chapter is addressed to you, the advanced practice nurse (APN) studying at a doctoral level, and will explore the concept of reflective practice and its relevance for you and your work. It will examine definitions of reflective practice and how the art and science of nursing can be combined with reflection to produce praxis—advanced nursing practice based upon scholarship, expertise, and critical thinking. The teaching of reflective practice appears to be more predominant in nursing curricula outside of the United States, and so some of these concepts may be new to you. However, this chapter will hopefully remind you that there is no end point to learning, and that reflection can support further exploration of your practice.

WHAT IS REFLECTION AND REFLECTIVE PRACTICE?

The challenge for most writers in this field is to agree on a satisfactory definition of reflection, and the literature is full of worthy attempts. Despite differences in these texts and the plethora of definitions, one dominant assumption among these writers is that reflection is worthwhile and can enhance practice. In the context of learning, reflection is a generic term for intellectual and affective activities in which individuals engage their experience to create and clarify meaning in terms of self, which results in a changed conceptual perspective (Boud, Keogh, & Walker, 1985). John Dewey (1938) summarized the process: "... we learn by doing and realizing what came of what we did" (p. 12). Is it simply learning from experience?

Over the years, experienced nursing professionals like yourselves have developed practical knowledge and working intelligence as you made sense of your work in theoretical ways (Schön, 1983). Much of this learning has been subconscious, meaning that you may know more than you consciously realize. Through reflection, this tacit knowledge (or knowing-in-action) can be made conscious and explicit (Argyris & Schön, 1974). Taylor (2000) defined reflection as "the throwing back of thoughts and memories, in cognitive acts such as thinking, contemplation, meditation and any other form of attentive consideration, in order to make sense of them, and to make contextually appropriate changes if they are required" (p. 3). This definition allows for a wide variety of thinking as the basis for reflection, and it is similar to many other explanations by suggesting that reflective thinking is a rational process that produces positive change (Boud et al., 1985; Boyd & Fales, 1983; Mezirow, 1981).

In simple terms, reflection enables you to learn from experience through a systematic process of thinking. You are probably already familiar with Kolb's (1984) well-known learning cycle, which is helpful here (Figure 20.1).

Unless the individual moves through all four stages of this cycle:

1. The actual experience
2. Reflecting upon it
3. Relating these reflections to existing knowledge and creating a new perspective on the experience
4. Returning to the practice setting ready to test new understandings

then conscious learning in its fullest sense has not occurred.

Kuiper and Pesut (2004) defined reflection as a metacognitive process that supports thinking about one's own thinking related to an experience and within a conceptual framework. Jarvis (1992) distinguishes reflective practice from thoughtful practice and suggests a reflective practitioner is one who is able to "problematise many situations of professional performance so they can become potential learning" (p. 180). How to *problematize* practice? The challenge for experienced practitioners like yourselves is to

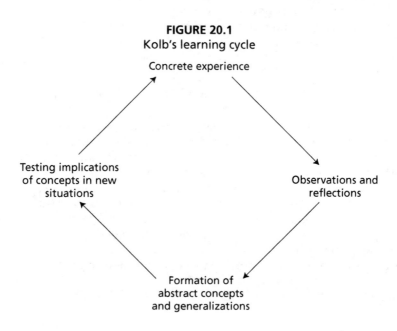

FIGURE 20.1
Kolb's learning cycle

Concrete experience

Testing implications
of concepts in new
situations

Observations and
reflections

Formation of
abstract concepts
and generalizations

somehow make the familiar strange, and to become aware of (and question) many of your assumptions about practice. This process of unpacking existing knowledge can facilitate *unlearning* many aspects of previous practice, which then opens up possibilities for fresh learning. Unlearning can require a significant break with previous modes of understanding, doing, and being (Rushmer & Davies, 2004). This intellectual work of change can naturally create tensions between *outside-in* or research knowledge, and *inside-out* or practice knowledge (Hargreaves, Earl, Moore, & Manning, 2001). Nevertheless, changes in understanding that do not lead to changes in practice are meaningless, while changes in practice that are not associated with changes in understanding will not lead to meaningful or lasting improvement (MacDonald, 2002). As advanced practitioners, aspects of your practice can be so familiar that you may spend a good deal of time on *automatic pilot*, hardly aware of your responses to routine situations. Is this intuitive expertise at work, or is it simply unthinking ritual?

WHY BOTHER TO REFLECT?

So why, you may be asking, should you bother to reflect? After all, your skills and knowledge have been developed over many years, and your clinical practice has probably achieved a high standard. In my experience, ANPs who undertake doctoral study face the unsettling tasks of examining their practice and of challenging many things they once took for granted. This unpacking of assumptions and questioning of the evidence base for your practice can be acutely uncomfortable, as customary ways of working over the years are exposed as perhaps having little justification or theoretical foundation. It is here that reflection can come to the rescue. Some comments from my United Kingdom students on the professional doctorate in nursing program may give you a sense of their experience of reflection:

> I question why we do things more in practice, and reflection has opened up a totally new concept of what nursing means to me
>
> I cannot believe how many assumptions I held about my practice ... stripping these away has been scary but enlightening and empowering!
>
> I ponder and question everything now; nothing is taken for granted, unless I can give myself a sound rationale for doing that. It's not comfortable, but I now see how necessary it is

I suggest that as a doctor of nursing practice graduate you will be expected to extend the boundaries of professional knowledge and practice, and that this contrasts with the role of the MSN graduate, whose role is to demonstrate mastery of the discipline. Because of this increased expectation of the *doctoral advanced practice nurse*, the skills of reflective practice become even more essential (Dreher & Montgomery, 2009; Teekman, 2000).

In striving to develop and enhance your nursing practice, the function of critical reflective inquiry is to "... correct and improve the practice through self-reflection and criticism and ... [to] generate models of 'good practice'" (Kim, 1999, p. 1206). By bringing together head, hands, and heart (understanding, application, and emotion), you can develop practical wisdom, or *phronesis. Phronesis* is the ability to consider one's actions in order to deliver change, especially to enhance the quality of one's practice, and the key to unlocking this practitioner wisdom is reflection, and the key to reflection is self-awareness.

WHAT IS SELF-AWARENESS?

Reflection involves sensitive introspection, and thus, a vital aspect of reflective practice is self-awareness. Self-awareness is central to the process of reflection and can be defined as the:

> ... process [over time] of noticing and exploring aspects of the self, whether behavioural, psychological or physical with the intention of developing personal and interpersonal understanding . . . . To become more aware of and to have a deeper understanding of ourselves is to have a sharper and clearer picture of what is happening to others.
>
> —*Burnard, 2002, pp. 30–1*

Thus, self-awareness is the foundation for reflective practice as the outcomes from being self-aware underpin the whole process. When self-aware, you become conscious of your beliefs, values, qualities, strengths, and limitations. In other words, self-awareness involves an honest examination of who you think you are. It allows you to see yourself in a particular context and identify how your presence and actions affect a situation. Through self-awareness, we are able to learn how to consciously use ourselves in interactions with others (Forbes, 2008). Burnard (2002) states that being self-aware enables us to "... select therapeutic interventions from a range of options so that the patient or client benefits more completely. If we are blind to ourselves we are also blind to our choices. We are blind, then, to caring and therapeutic choices that we could make on behalf of our patients" (p. 36). Associated with self-awareness is mindfulness, which can be deceptively simple. It is moment to moment awareness, being totally in the present. Experiences and sensations are observed as they are experienced, without being caught up in the mental events that usually follow sensations. Thoughts and feelings are noted and acknowledged as they arise, but judgment and analysis is avoided (Kabat-Zinn, 2005). If reflection is a necessary prerequisite for learning, then mindfulness is a prerequisite for experience. It represents a simple awareness of what is present from one moment to the next. By being totally present to whatever arises in your practice, you can respond appropriately and authentically to the needs of your patients and the situation. As a doctor of nursing practice student, mindful self-awareness also assists you with identifying your own learning needs and the ways in which your learning needs can be met. It is then involved in your evaluation of whether those needs have been met.

HOW DO YOU REFLECT ON PRACTICE?

Donald Schön (1987) noted differences between *reflection-on-action* happening after practice, and *reflection-in-action* happening in the moment of practice. For example, as a clinical situation unfolds around you, you may be thinking on your feet and making apparently instant decisions (reflection-in-action), and then later, thinking over what happened in order to make sense of it (reflection-on-action). In this way, Schön (1983) argued that each practitioner builds a situational repertoire that is forever being expanded and modified to meet new situations. Often, the alternations from practice to theory and back to practice, and so on are so fast that it seems like one integrated process, and

> ... it is this entire process of reflection-in-action which is central to the 'art' by which practitioners sometimes deal well with situations of uncertainty, instability, uniqueness, and value conflict.
>
> —*Schön, 1983, p. 50*

As a doctoral advanced nurse practitioner/clinician, you have accumulated a huge practice repertoire of knowledge, skills, and actions, most of which you may be largely unaware. In short, as an expert, you possess "... a deep background understanding of clinical situations based upon many past paradigm cases" (Benner, 1984, p. 294). In your clinical setting, you may practice *intuitively*, which probably involves a complex recognition of patterns within the situation, to which you can respond without conscious deliberation. You *just know* what needs to be done, and when called upon to explain your actions, you can be at a loss to provide a rational justification.

This is where structured reflection can help to *unpack* your tacit knowledge, bring it into awareness, and explicate it for others. There are many published models of reflection to use (e.g., Atkins & Murphy, 1993; Johns, 2004, 2007; Taylor, 2000), but three simple questions can be used to explore any event or experience: *What?, So What? and Now what?* This sequence of questioning moves us through the processes of description, analysis, and synthesis. If you wish, please work through the critical questions at the end of this chapter, which will guide you through this process and which are relevant for all levels of reflection. These simple questions are based upon Johns' (2007) model of structured reflection shown in Exhibit 20.1.

Christopher Johns (Johns & Freshwater, 2005) recognizes the differences between traditional models of *reflection-on-experience*, and his own approach to *mindful practice* or reflection as a way of being, noting that:

> Reflection-on-experience is typified as a cognitive approach to reflection, that is, as something someone does. In contrast, mindful practice most typifies reflection as a way of being: a way that honours the intuitive and holistic nature of experience.
> —*Johns & Freshwater, 2005, p. 7*

Thus, Johns and Freshwater's definition of reflection is focused not so much on our personal cognitive knowledge about our own practice, as on knowledge of the *self* itself.

> Reflection is being mindful of self, either within or after experience, as if a window through which the practitioner can view and focus self within the context of a particular experience, in

EXHIBIT 20.1 Johns' Model of Structured Reflection, 15th Edition

- Bring the mind home.
- Focus on a description that seems significant in some way.
- What particular issues seem significant to pay attention to?
- How were others feeling and what made them feel that way?
- How was I feeling and what made me feel that way?
- What was I trying to achieve and did I respond effectively?
- What were the consequences of my actions on the patient, others, myself?
- What factors influenced the way I was feeling, thinking, and responding?
- What knowledge did or might have informed me?
- To what extent did I act for the best and in tune with my values?
- How does this situation connect with previous experience?
- How might I respond more effectively given this situation again?
- What would be the consequences of alternative actions for the patient, others, myself?
- What factors might constrain me acting in new ways?
- How do I *NOW* feel about this experience?
- Am I more able to support myself and others better as a consequence?
- Am I more able to realize desirable practice?

Reprinted with permission from Sage Publications, Johns, C. (2007). Toward easing suffering through reflection. *Journal of Holistic Nursing*, 25(3), 204–210.

order to confront, understand and move toward resolving contradiction between one's vision and actual practice.

—*Johns, 2004, p. 3*

It can be seen then, that earlier models of structured reflection focused on cognitive *learning from experience*, whereas more recently, writers have depicted reflection as a *way of being* in practice that is a shift from epistemology to ontology (Johns & Freshwater, 2005).

Many nurses (in my experience) complain that their work situation allows very little space and time for reflection: "we're just too busy ... patients can't wait for us to reflect!" My response would be that reflective practice does not demand extra time or energy, but an altered relationship to one's work. Although in many settings, groups of nurses reflect together on specific clinical incidents and may keep reflective journals to assist in making sense of their experience; however, these structured methods are not always necessary. I encourage all my doctoral nursing students in the United Kingdom to maintain a reflective research journal that helps to capture their changing thoughts and feelings as they progress through their program. The journal entries act as an excellent resource for student/supervisor meetings, a guide for the reflective elements of their final thesis, and also a way to reinforce the students' reflexivity throughout the research process. If you (as a doctoral APRN) can make sense of your practice as you go about your daily work using systematic and thoughtful reflection, not only will this reflection increase your personal understanding, it will also likely result in your continued professional growth and self-empowerment.

WHAT ABOUT NURSING KNOWLEDGE?

You may be asking yourself—"It's all very nice being reflective, but what about the development of nursing knowledge?" The dominant paradigm for nursing knowledge over the last few decades has been one of *technical rationality*, supported by the rise in research-based practice. The term *technical rationality* originated with Habermas (1970) and was employed by Schön (1983) to refer to the dominance of theory over practice (and hence of theorists over practitioners).

The development of nursing science has been the result of a one-way flow of information from researchers through academic journals and textbooks, to nursing practitioners. Grounded in *technical rationality*, new developments in nursing practice have been driven by the findings of scientific (usually quantitative) research studies and the writing of theorists (Rolfe, 2006). Hypothetico-deductive positivist models of research, working from the general to the specific, generate *middle-range* or *grand* theories to be translated into everyday practice. In actual fact, they produce evidence *of* or *from* phenomena, and not evidence *for* practice, as is usually assumed. Such assumptions are an act of belief, and give *evidence-based practice* a spurious respectability. Nursing theory created by academics away from the clinical setting (on the *high, hard ground* of technical rationality) cannot be easily incorporated into practice (in the *swampy lowlands*), in the same way that oil and water cannot mix. The incommensurability between these two discourses or worldviews has led to the *theory–practice gap*, much discussed and lamented by educationalists and practitioners alike. Although some nursing theories are developed retroductively from practice, the gap still exists because they are not returned for testing or implementation in their own original setting (the *practice–theory–practice gap*).

This problem, however, can be addressed through reflective inquiry, which turns technical rationality on its head by starting with the individual nurse's experience, and then *unpacking* it to discover what can be learned and applied in future situations. Reflection, therefore, offers an alternative, inductive approach to learning and knowledge generation. It challenges the usual hierarchy of evidence by shifting the emphasis from the findings of large-scale research studies to the knowledge generated by individual practitioners from their own practice, thereby promoting practitioners to the status of researchers and theorists in their own right (Rolfe, Freshwater, & Jasper, 2001).

Central to this process is a specific practice event experienced uniquely by individuals, from which a number of more abstract generalizations may be derived. It is consistent with the essence of nursing, where no two clinical situations are ever the same. Through exploring specific incidents in practice and generating new theoretical perspectives, other types of knowledge that are essential to you as a doctoral advanced nurse practitioner can be utilized and valued. In addition to *propositional* knowledge (from published research and textbooks), you use *personal* knowledge (self-awareness and ethical values), and *practice* knowledge (the cumulative wealth of experience from previous clinical situations). All three types of knowing are embedded in the expert nurse's everyday practice in order to provide high-quality and holistic patient/client care, and this combination of different ways of knowing and their application to practice can be termed *praxis*.

Praxis or *doing action* effectively dissolves the traditional theory–practice gap by making theory and practice mutually dependent upon one another. Nursing praxis is a bringing together of theory and practice that involves a continual process of hypothesizing and testing out new ideas and of modifying practice according to the results. Therefore, I would argue that all practitioners are not only *theorists*, but also *researchers*, engaged in numerous pieces of *action research* and the generation of informal theory. In its everyday use, the phrase "research-based practice" limits the knowledge deemed acceptable for practice. However, reflective nurse practitioners can access other types of knowledge through the kind of critical inquiry that takes place within nursing praxis. Practice knowledge created through reflection can be judged by its own criteria—its relevance and value to care—rather than any external criteria normally reserved for positivist research. Such research may have a sample of 1, and might not be generalizable beyond that single person. Nevertheless, it is still valid research and represents what Rolfe and Gardner (2005) called a nursing science of the unique, concerned with *persons* rather than *people*.

As a consequence, distinctions between research and practice and between the generation and application of knowledge merge into one. Theory does not determine practice, but is generated from practice. In fact, the process is circular with practice generating theory and theory modifying practice, which generates new theory and so on. Nursing praxis is a fusion of knowing and doing, in which research is incorporated into everyday practice, and in which theory and practice become two sides of the same coin. The doctoral APN is thus not *just a nurse with a lot of experience*, but instead a practitioner who can freely move between different ways of knowing and who is able to select and transform knowledge appropriate to the situation. Trusting your intuitive personal and practice knowledge requires courage and conviction, because it requires a shift from reliance on abstract, propositional thinking to thinking based on clinical reasoning related to concrete experiences. Do you have the ability to pay attention to and learn from everyday practice with the aim of realizing the optimal standard of care for your patients? This artistry, in my opinion, is the hallmark of an advanced and expert practitioner, and also denotes doctoral level practice. The resulting science and art of nursing are then woven into a rich tapestry of practice, which honors the intuitive and holistic nature of experience.

PARADIGM WARS?

The dominant discourse or paradigm in nursing has been, and remains, the *natural science* approach of evidence-based practice and the randomized controlled trial. So long as this positivist worldview dominates contemporary science, it will probably continue to hold sway in nursing. And yet, the profession would be enriched if it could also accommodate the *human science* tradition. Mitchell and Cody (1992) summarized their overview of human science with the assertion that the

> ... lived experience, the world as experience, meaning, and understanding are all aspects of a unitary process of human life and cannot be adequately described, explained, or analyzed through objectification, measurement, or reduction
>
> —*Mitchell and Cody, 1992, p. 55*

Watson (1999a) has identified similar philosophical and conceptual foundations for human science, adding that human science epistemology "... allows not only for empirics, but for advancement of esthetics, ethical values, intuition, and process of discovery" (p. 16). Essentially, human science aims at knowledge development that enhances understanding of the multidimensional meanings inherent in human existence, rather than that which seeks to explain, predict, and control human phenomena, as in the natural science tradition.

Nurse scholars such as Newman (1986), Paterson and Zderad (1988), Parse (1981, 1998), and others have promoted human science perspectives in the interests of humanistic nursing. Can we combine nursing science with the artistry of nursing? Self-awareness and mindful reflection can be the way forward to producing thoughtful, innovative, and critical practice. It is when the nurse is in this place of personal wisdom, gaining new and deeper insights, that a caring moment becomes more possible (Watson, 1979, 1999b).

SUMMARY

Reflective practice is something more than thoughtful practice. It is that form of practice which seeks to problematize many situations of professional performance, so that they can become potential learning situations and you, as a doctoral advanced nurse practitioner, can continue to learn, grow, and develop in and through your practice. As you journey through your doctoral program, you will be developing the qualities related to this level of study—critical thinking and reflexive self-awareness—in addition to extensive specialist knowledge, practical research skills, and scholarship. Doctoral study involves mastering procedures not only for generating knowledge, but also for becoming aware of different ways of knowing and of the limits of knowledge. It means tolerating uncertainty and realizing that all knowledge is provisional, and that we can be certain of nothing in science (Popper, 1969). It is this shift in the breadth and depth of intellectual perspective that distinguishes master's from doctoral level study, from MSN-prepared APRN to the doctoral DNP or DrNP graduate.

The reflective *skill set* of the doctorally prepared APN includes challenging assumptions about evidence, learning to think and write reflexively, developing your own characteristic voice, and producing practice-based knowledge. Your professional identity and self-awareness will be transformed through your doctoral journey, and both your practice and your research will be underpinned by sensitive and insightful reflection. By developing both *praxis* (mindful action) and *phronesis* (practical wisdom), you can expand your concepts of what constitutes knowledge and reality. As doctorally prepared nurse scholars (whether in direct practice roles or not) you will have the skills of generating nursing knowledge from practice, and mindful, reflective awareness will enable you to achieve excellence in your own professional nursing performance. This approach honors your patients, yourself and your profession. Do you not owe it to your patients, yourselves, and your profession?!

REFERENCES

Argyris, M., & Schön, D. (1974). *Theory in practice: Increasing professional effectiveness.* San Francisco, CA: Jossey-Bass.

Atkins, S., & Murphy, K. (1993). Reflection: A review of the literature. *Journal of Advanced Nursing, 18*(8), 1188–1192.

Benner, P. (1984). *From novice to expert: Excellence and power in clinical nursing practice.* Menlo Park, CA: Addison-Wesley.

Boud, D., Keogh, R., & Walker, D. (1985). *Reflection: Turning experience into learning.* London, UK: Kogan Page.

Boyd, E. M., & Fales, A. W. (1983). Reflective learning: Key to learning from experience. *Journal of Humanistic Psychology, 23*(2), 99–117.

Burnard, P. (2002). *Learning human skills: An experiential and reflective guide for nurses and health care professionals* (4th ed.) Oxford, UK: Butterworth Heinemann.

Dewey, J. (1938). *Experience and education.* New York, NY: Macmillan.

Dreher, H. M., & Montgomery, K. E. (2009). Let's call it "doctoral" advanced practice nursing. *The Journal of Continuing Nursing Education, 40*(12), 530–531.

Forbes, J. (2008). Reflexivity in professional doctoral research. *Reflective Practice, 9*(4), 449–460.

Habermas, J. (1970). Technology and science as 'ideology', in *Toward a Rational Society* (Shapiro, J. Trans.) Boston, MA: Beacon Press.

Hargreaves, A., Earl, L., Moore, S., & Manning, S. (2001). *Learning to change: Teaching beyond subjects and standards.* San Francisco, CA: Jossey-Bass.

Jarvis, P. (1992). Reflective practice and nursing. *Nurse Education Today, 12,* 174–181.

Johns, C. (2004). *Becoming a reflective practitioner* (2nd ed.), Oxford, UK: Blackwell Publishing.

Johns, C. (2007). Toward easing suffering through reflection. *Journal of Holistic Nursing, 25*(3), 204–210.

Johns, C., & Freshwater, D. (2005). *Transforming nursing through reflective practice* (2nd ed.). Oxford, UK: Blackwell Publishing.

Kabat-Zinn, J. (2005). *Coming to our senses: Healing ourselves and the world through mindfulness.* London, UK: Piatkus Books.

Kim, H. S. (1999). Critical reflective inquiry for knowledge development in nursing practice. *Journal of Advanced Nursing, 29*(5), 1205–1212.

Kolb, D. A. (1984). *Experiential learning—Experience as the source of learning and development.* New Jersey, NJ: Prentice-Hall.

Kuiper, R. A., & Pesut, D. J. (2004). Promoting cognitive and metacognitive reflective clinical reasoning skills in nursing practice: Self-regulated learning theory. *Journal of Advanced Nursing, 45*(4), 381–391.

MacDonald, G. (2002). Transformative unlearning: Safety, discernment and communities of learning. *Nursing Inquiry, 9*(3), 170–178.

Mezirow, J. (1981). A critical theory of adult learning and education. *Adult Education, 32*(1), 3–24.

Mitchell, G. J., & Cody, W. K. (1992). Nursing knowledge and human science: Ontological and epistemological considerations. *Nursing Science Quarterly, 5,* 54–61.

Newman, M. (1986). *Health as expanding consciousness.* St. Louis, MO: Mosby.

Parse, R. R. (1981). *Man-living-health: A theory of nursing.* New York, NY: Wiley.

Parse, R. R. (1998). *The human becoming school of thought: A perspective for nurses and other health professionals.* Thousand Oaks, CA: Sage.

Paterson, J. G., & Zderad, L. T. (1988). *Humanistic nursing.* New York, NY: National League for Nursing Press.

Popper, K. (1969). *Conjectures and refutations.* London, UK: Routledge & Kegan Paul.

Rolfe, G. (2006). Nursing praxis and the science of the unique. *Nursing Science Quarterly, 19*(1), 39–43.

Rolfe, G., & Gardner, L. (2005). 'Do not ask who I am…': Confession, emancipation and (self)-management through reflection. *Journal of Nursing Management, 14,* 593–600.

Rolfe, G., Freshwater, D., & Jasper, M. (2001). *Critical reflection for nursing and the helping professions: A user's guide.* New York, NY: Palgrave.

Rushmer, R., & Davies, H. T. O. (2004). Unlearning in health care. *Quality and Safety in Health Care, 13*(Suppl II), ii10–ii15.

Schön, D. A. (1983). *The reflective practitioner.* London, UK: Temple Smith.

Schön, D. (1987). *Educating the reflective practitioner.* London, UK: Jossey-Bass.

Taylor, B. (2000). *Reflective practice: A guide for nurses and midwives.* Buckingham, UK: Open University Press.

Teekman, B. (2000). Exploring reflective thinking in nursing practice. *Journal of Advanced Nursing, 31*(5), 1125–1135.

Watson, J. (1979). *Nursing: The philosophy and science of caring.* Boston, MA: Little & Brown.

Watson, J. (1999a). *Nursing: Human science and human care.* Sudbury, MA: Jones & Bartlett.

Watson, J. (1999b). *Postmodern nursing and beyond.* New York, NY: Churchill Livingstone.

CHAPTER TWENTY: Reflective Response

Rosalie O. Mainous

Reflection should be a component of all nursing practice, but it is essential for doctoral prepared advanced practice nurses. As expert clinicians, consumers of research, and skilled in evidence-based practice, those with the professional doctorate must utilize reflection to bring together what is known, what is clinically relevant, and what can be improved upon.

This author identifies several key components of reflective practice. Self-awareness is essential, as is the unlearning of old ways of doing to allow for a new paradigm to emerge. It is purposeful, rational and leads to positive change. Those who are pursuing a doctorate in nursing practice must examine the "old" practice and apply a new skill set, while reflecting upon progress in improved patient outcomes. Mindfulness is also a component, that is, being in the moment and totally present to the clinical scenario faced. The conceptualization of mindfulness becomes murky later in the chapter while citing Johns and Freshwater (2005), when the author distinguishes between reflection and mindful practice. I would agree with the author's earlier proposition.

The author describes the way most new knowledge reaches the bedside. It has been driven by the work of theorists and researchers, working from the general to the specific with the generation of middle range theories. These theories are then tested clinically, and may be altered or give rise to new theoretical constructs. However, while some theories are developed in a practice vacuum, many are now developed by interprofessional teams that include clinical researchers, practicing clinicians, and a cadre of scientists from a variety of disciplines. The theory–practice gap, which does exist, is due in part to the underuse of new knowledge and of translation of science to the bedside, now a national priority. This process becomes circular. Researchers (PhDs) trained in specific research methodologies together with expert practitioners (DNPs) pose a clinical question for testing; practitioners test the theory in the clinical setting and then reflect on the findings; the findings are evaluated through the lens of an experienced clinician at which point the team makes sense of the findings and determines what can be translated back to the bedside as evidence for practice. This is somewhat different from what the author proposes; that is, that all practitioners are theorists and researchers.

The author points out the importance of clinician knowledge and expertise which should be recognized by the theorists and researchers as valuable and a unique contribution to science. I agree. Some clinical knowledge is created through reflective practice. This author points out the inevitable merging of traditional research as the generation of new knowledge with reflective practice and its contribution to the body of evolving science for the discipline. This movement has been fully conceptualized in the newly emerging field of Synthesis Science, that of the language and methodology of evidence-based practice. In evidence-based practice models, while randomized controlled trials are seen as the gold standard, many other forms of knowledge are accepted including clinician expertise (which in best practice should derive in part from reflection) to qualitative findings. Schön (1987), the father of reflective practice, suggests that an epistemology of practice that traditionally has had a positivist slant, termed *technical rationality,* now incorporate the experience of the practitioner, which is evident in many different models of evidence-based practice. According to Kinsella (2007), Schön's position of adding reflective practice to the understanding of a clinical scenario does not denigrate traditional research knowledge, but instead is additive and has important ramifications for those applying it to practice. Reflective practice together with evidence-based practice has been suggested to be the two skills necessary to form a model of professional thinking (Bannigan & Moores, 2009).

As with any pedagogical strategy, it must be leveled appropriate to the student population. Just as pharmacology is taught one way and with a specific set of outcomes to be achieved at the baccalaureate level, it becomes more complex with different outcomes and different teaching strategies at the master's level. Reflection as a strategy for mastery differs for every level of nursing practice. Reflection for the doctoral advanced practice nurse will be at a high level and incorporate several ways of knowing.

REFERENCES

Bannigan, K., & Moores, A. (2009). A model of professional thinking: Integrating reflective practice and evidence based practice. *Canadian Journal of Occupational Therapy, 76*(5), 342–350.

Johns, C., & Freshwater, D. (2005). *Transforming nursing through reflective practice* (2nd ed.). Oxford, UK: Blackwell.

Kinsella, E. A. (2007). Technical rationality in Schön's reflective practice: Dichotomous of non-dualistic epistemological position. *Nursing Philosophy, 8,* 102–113.

Schön, D. (1987). *Educating the reflective practitioner.* London, UK: Jossey-Bass.

CRITICAL THINKING QUESTIONS

1. Identify a situation or incident in your recent clinical experience that was significant, powerful, or memorable in some way *(either positively or negatively).* Tell the story briefly, either in writing or verbally within your group. What happened? *(What?)*
2. What were you thinking and feeling? Why did you act or not act as you did?
3. What was good and bad about the experience?
4. What factors influenced your decisions and actions?
5. What sense can you make of the situation? *(So what?)*
6. What else could you have done, and what would have been the result?
7. How has your practice changed as a result of this experience?
8. If a similar situation arises again, what will you do? *(Now what?)*
9. What have you learned from this experience?
10. How can you share this learning with others? Is it nursing knowledge?

CHAPTER TWENTY-ONE

Enhancing a Doctor of Nursing Practice Degree with a Mandatory Study-Abroad Program

H. Michael Dreher, Mary Ellen Smith Glasgow, Vicki D. Lachman,
Scott Oldfield, and Cynthia Gifford-Hollingsworth

INTRODUCTION

While study-abroad attendance at the undergraduate level is increasing in the United States (after decreasing post 9/11), still only an extremely small number of students ultimately study abroad, and there is no real data on the number of undergraduate nursing students who participate (Conant, 2010). At the graduate level, there is an absence in the literature of study-abroad programs that focus exclusively on graduate nursing students. In 2006, Drexel University started what is perhaps the very first mandatory study-abroad program for any nursing program in the United States which focuses its two-week study-abroad program on its doctor of nursing practice program. This chapter describes the program and describes the experience of both faculty and students who have participated in the program in London and Dublin.

WHY STUDY ABROAD FOR DOCTORAL NURSING STUDENTS?

In an increasingly geopolitical, global-oriented world, it is incumbent that that the most educated health professionals, including doctoral-prepared clinicians, scientists, and scholars, have the kinds of real-world experiences that will give them the best context for discussing the international implications of health issues and in making informed decisions about health policy and practice. Indeed, the rise of the SARS virus (Dreher et al., 2004) and the emergence of the H1N1 flu virus (Gardner, 2009) are vivid recent examples of why nurses, now more than ever, know that the health of someone on one continent may have a direct impact on the health of citizens on another.

Increasingly, international higher education is big business. Foreign students contribute more than $12 billion to the U.S. economy each year, with the United States currently by far the largest host country, with more than a quarter of the world's foreign students (Altbach, 2004). Even with the global recession, global education is still growing (Redden, 2009a). However, while the Institute of International Education in 2008 reported an 8% increase in American students studying abroad (2006/2007 data), the overall proportion of American undergraduates in 4-year institutions studying abroad has been reported as very low, 0.2% (Altbach) to 3% (Cushner & Karim, 2004).

Furthermore, in this 2006–2007 report, only 5.1% of all study abroad was among students in health profession majors. For over a decade, there have been suggestions that internationalizing the nursing curriculum is essential to prepare nurses for the challenges of the 21st century (Zorn, 1996). One critique is that current nursing curricula fail to properly acknowledge the global environment (Duffy, 2001), and that any significant movement to more formally globalize nursing curricula in the United States has been largely absent. A review of the literature identified several recent peer-reviewed articles describing U.S.-based study-abroad programs (Christoffersen, 2008; Fennell, 2009; Johanson, 2006; Levine, 2009; Parker, Locsin, & Longo, 2006; Saenz & Holcomb, 2009), but there were no study-abroad programs that focused on graduate nursing students exclusively, much less doctoral students. Nevertheless, in 2006, our forward thinking doctoral nursing faculty were convinced that a short-term formal study-abroad experience would be an innovative enhancement to our doctor of nursing practice program. It would prepare our students to better face the contemporary global problems that highly educated nursing and other health professionals will increasingly be challenged to solve. This chapter will provide practical information related to the approval and funding process necessary to implement these types of programs and, given the lack of graduate (or doctoral) nursing study-abroad programs described in the literature, highlight the perspectives of both faculty and students who participated in the program.

THE DREXEL DOCTOR OF NURSING PRACTICE PROGRAM'S INTERNATIONAL STUDY-ABROAD PROGRAM

Why Was it Created?

The initial idea for the program began with the Doctoral Nursing Department Chair who became aware our LeBow College of Business sent their MBA students abroad for one week as part of the standard curriculum. With a new Provost on campus seriously interested in promoting the Drexel brand more internationally, and with a renewed focus on encouraging international programs for both undergraduate and graduate students, it seemed plausible that our new doctoral program could also embed a study-abroad program in the curriculum. Further, if master's students were spending one week abroad, it seemed logical that doctoral students should stay longer.

The Drexel DrNP[1] program's international study-abroad program was thus first conceived in early 2006, and the first doctoral nursing students and faculty participated in the inaugural program in London in April 2007. The DrNP International Study Abroad Program is a two-week intensive program that is offered in the second year of study. It takes place during the student's last quarter of study (spring quarter) prior to completing all formal doctoral coursework and beginning dissertation seminar in the subsequent summer quarter. Because our DrNP program was designed for the working adult, with classes one day a week, a two-week program was deemed the most feasible. While a two-week study-abroad program may not seem like a long time, indeed short-term study-abroad programs (from 2 to 8 weeks in duration) now predominate, attracting 55% of all study-abroad students (Institute of International Education, 2008), and standards for short-term study-abroad programs are now being published in the literature (Redden, 2009b). In retrospect, our new doctor of nursing practice curriculum was well positioned to both integrate and accommodate a short-term study-abroad program. The first course in the 3-year part-time doctoral program was *The Politics of Health: Implications for Nursing*

Practice, and there was a desire by the course chair and the doctoral faculty to include content on how doctoral-prepared nurses should and could participate more fully in dialogue and activism regarding international health issues (Dreher, Lachman, Smith Glasgow, & Ward, 2008). This idea of a two-week program seemed ideal and indeed feasible, and in consultation with the MBA program, we immediately found a campus-based graduate program model that provided design guidance.

Why is the Program "Mandatory"?

One of the very first decisions we made was, that *if* we decided to truly implement the program, it would be mandatory, not optional. Our view was rooted in fairly egalitarian ideals. At the undergraduate level, too often study abroad becomes an "elite" activity for privileged students. This is widely recognized and has been perpetuated by international standards for study abroad, which carry high social prestige (Fry, 1984). While our first 11 doctoral students all worked full time; they certainly had financial obligations beyond the typical undergraduate, and some even had children in college (the mean age of the first class was 43). Still we calculated that an affordable program could be created; however, we felt that if the activity were optional, we likely would not have full participation. Thus, the goals of making our doctor of nursing practice program even more innovative with an emphasis on global learning would not be complete. Further, the department chair did not see administratively how we could operate our DrNP program cost effectively or coherently with some students going abroad and others not. Because this program was conceived after our first class matriculated in September 2005, we approached students in January 2006 and chose to move forward with the proposal only if all 11 students agreed to participate. Initially, only 10 of 11 students wanted to participate. But with some coaxing the one recalcitrant student agreed, and thus we began what turned into a full year of planning in order to get the graduate study-abroad program designed, approved, funded, and then scheduled.

How is the Program Funded?

The germination of this idea came at an opportune time for the DrNP program. The Drexel annual budget planning process for the following academic year usually begins each February and this allowed strategic time to create and submit a proposal to the Associate Dean for Doctoral Education and Research, to the College Dean, and to the university Provost using the standard budget procedures. There were two strategies taken that were critical to rapid and ultimate approval in our first cycle submission. *First* this new graduate study-abroad program really matched the new evolving mission of the university to enhance its international image and reputation; one way was by increasing study-abroad offerings to students. Our particular emphasis on graduate students, specifically doctoral students, was deemed highly innovative in the approval process. *Second,* the department chair proposed using a creative financing procedure which would make the offering more palatable to prospective students, who might at first glance think they could never afford to both attend a three-year doctoral nursing program (with all the normal costs typical students are likely to incur) *and* participate in a 14-day study-abroad program which would certainly require them to take time off from work. We knew *the idea* of a mandatory study program would be attractive to students who were looking for a distinctive doctor of nursing practice doctoral program, but in the end the idea has to become "real" to the prospective student. Since funding our doctoral study-abroad program involved funding both student and faculty travel, each will be discussed separately.

FUNDING DOCTORAL STUDENTS STUDYING ABROAD

To make the program both attractive and "doable" for prospective students, the decision was made to take the full cost of the program (airfare, housing, events, health insurance, and administrative costs) and to divide the total cost of the program to each individual student into a DrNP International Study Fee paid in eight separate quarterly payments. Because Drexel is on quarters, this allowed the first-year students to make a payment of some $450 over 4 quarters in year one and two, and thus attend the study-abroad program in their 7th quarter (spring quarter) in year two. Upon their return, they do make one final payment in the summer quarter.[2] If the students are on financial aid (and many of them are), their International Study Fee is considered part of their financial aid package *since the program is mandatory*. This is a very critical point. If it were optional, financial aid would not cover it. We have now followed this procedure for four years, and it has been very effective. Even students who are not on financial aid do not view the quarterly charge as excessive. With a new Provost and new billing procedures, the program is now starting to bill over 12 quarters (the full three year program of study) and this new procedure to bill over three years, rather than two, will need to be evaluated. It will reduce the quarterly payment, but it does have intra-College budgetary implications that will need to be tracked.

Certainly the International Study Fee is a creative way to provide for the financing of doctoral students to attend the program. Their 8-quarter (or 12) fee goes into a designated college account whereby the Department Chair can then fund group airfares annually, shared apartment accommodations abroad (two students share one apartment and single upgrades at the individual student's expense are usually available), costs for all tours, events, additional local guest scholars for the two courses that are offered abroad each year, and the administrative fee charges by our partner, the London-based Foundation for International Education (FIE). Because Drexel University was one of the founding schools to participate in FIE's London program, they had experience with Drexel University and our quarter system. However, the Drexel DrNP program was not just FIE's first short-term study-abroad program they sponsored, but also the first graduate *and* first doctoral program they hosted.

FUNDING ACCOMPANYING DOCTORAL FACULTY ABROAD

While the quarterly international study fee indeed covers the expenses for the participating doctoral students, it does not cover the expenses of the participating faculty. Doctoral study-abroad programs are inherently different from undergraduate study program programs, and may even be different from most master's study-abroad programs. It would be inconceivable to simply place a full cohort of doctoral students in another institution abroad and have them taught completely by external faculty. While this is the model for most undergraduate study-abroad programs (especially language study-abroad programs) (Institute of International Education, 2007), our doctoral students follow a certain prescribed curriculum; and our own faculty (by rotating which courses are scheduled to be taught abroad) rotate going abroad. Indeed, our study-abroad program was not exclusively designed for our students, *but its mission was also designed to benefit our doctoral nursing faculty scholars as well.* By also including a faculty objective for our program, traveling teaching faculty are then able to make international contacts that could lead to global collaborations that, in turn, could further enhance Drexel's international image and reputation. In preparation for each year's program, selected teaching faculty secure local scholars to come into the classroom as guest speakers to enhance each course's content.

Our emphasis on the international benefits to our teaching faculty is one real difference in undergraduate versus graduate study abroad. Second, securing guest scholars for rotating different doctoral level courses is an activity that cannot easily be outsourced to another host school or institution. Recruiting scholars with a very specific type of expertise or area of scholarship requires that our own traveling faculty (they know a year in advance what courses are going to be offered abroad and who will be teaching them) make international connections and, through their network of referrals, approach the best local or regional university scholars and invite them to speak. Because we have a two-week program with one course offered usually 9–12 Monday through Thursday, and the second class 1:30–4:30 pm[3] (Fridays are reserved for class field trips and the weekends are free for students and faculty), typically there generally are two guest speakers per class per week. Additionally, we have been successful at arranging a full day off campus at another host institution (Dublin Trinity College, Kingston University/ St. George's of London, and the University of Brighton). As mentioned previously, since Drexel operates on a 10-week quarter system, students attend class on campus in week 1 and 10 only, and weeks 3 and 4 are typically entirely abroad. Thus, the students are not on campus in Philadelphia for the other 6 weeks and all 30 quarter class hours are met using this model.

Because Drexel's DrNP program relies on its own doctoral faculty traveling abroad to both teach, network, and act as semiformal guides for student activities (undergraduate students must be chaperoned and supervised to a larger degree than graduate students to avoid risks to the university), there must be a separate budget for faculty expenses (housing, food, and travel). The Drexel DrNP program typically sends two or three faculty abroad each year with each class of students. For our fourth program in London in 2010, there was a new day program at the University of Brighton with their professional doctoral students and faculty, and this was our first experience with our DrNP students networking with other international students in professional nursing and other health related doctoral programs.[4]

Courses taught abroad are selected by the Department Chair as part of the annual nursing teaching schedule procedures. Doctoral nursing courses are purposefully rotated so a diverse set of faculty can take part in the experience. While there is no standard procedure for faculty selection (for example by seniority), the philosophy of the department chair has been mostly to use the experience to reward highly productive faculty who have been awarded tenure, received a major grant, or had exceptionally high teaching evaluations in the doctoral program. If the international mission of a university is important to its respective Department Chair and College Dean, then annual requests to fund this particular faculty activity (airfare, accomodations, and food) will become part of the normal budget process.

THE DrNP-IN-LONDON PROGRAM: A FACULTY PERSPECTIVE

London is a cosmopolitan historical city rich in health care and public health history. Therefore, setting up meaningful extracurricular adventures with opportunities for learning with FIE was easy. The study-abroad experience in London began the first weekend upon arrival. Since this is a doctoral study-abroad program, a decision to eschew the typical dorm experience used for undergraduates was made, and the doctoral students were housed instead in an affordable hotel/apartment in Kensington within easy walking distance to all FIE facilities. After an overnight Friday transcontinental flight, a very light day-one schedule was recommended. Students were given a brief late afternoon orientation to the FIE facilities and a quick overview of the neighborhood. On day two, both students and faculty attended a guided walking tour of the Kensington neighborhood, including an intriguing view of the homes of John Stuart Mill and Robert Browning, as well as Kensington Palace and Hyde Park. A Sunday afternoon guided coach tour of London gave us an overview of greater London, including some of the beautiful historical sites such as Westminster Abby, Tower of London, and House of Parliament. London is the home of the Florence Nightingale Museum which holds a unique collection of artifacts clearly depicting the life of this notable woman, and students were provided tickets to attend this museum on their own. During a Medical Walking Tour (especially designed for us by a historian at FIE) later in the program, students and faculty covered the streets of London's medical quarter and beyond, giving us views of the old hospitals for sick children and poor immigrants. A day trip to Cambridge granted a view of an ancient university city with college buildings of all architectural styles and meadows leading down to the river Cam. Their King's College Chapel has some of the finest Gothic fan vaulting in England. The theater opportunities on London's West End rival New York City, and the students and faculty attended dramatic performances of *Blood Brothers* at the Phoenix Theatre and *Billy Elliot* at Victoria Palace Theatre. In year two, students and faculty were also given a tour of the Royal College of Surgeons, which included a view of the Hunterian Collection, an outstanding collection of over 3,500 natural history specimens assembled by the surgeon and anatomist John Hunter. One benefit of working with FIE is that they have traditionally provided complimentary admission to teaching faculty to all scheduled events and provided a private office, computer support, and cell phones to the faculty as well.

Coursework formally began on the first Monday after arrival. The speakers who visited our classrooms were selected to bring to students the "England view" on a variety of topics, just as the sites provided them with a flavor of England's architecture, arts, and history. The following was a sample year-one itinerary and roster of speakers in our all day visit to Kingston University and St. George's University of London:

- *Dignity in everyday nursing practice*—Dr. Ann Gallagher, Senior Research Fellow
- *Nursing leadership in the modern NHS*—Ms. Jayne Quigley, Head of Nursing, Leadership Development, St. George's Healthcare NHS Trust
- *Leading nursing in a London Hospital*—Dr. Geraldine Walters, Director of Nursing, St. George's Healthcare NHS Trust and Visiting Professor, Buckinghamshire Chilterns University College
- *Leading and researching nursing in a multiprofessional faculty*—Ms. Kath Start, Deputy Dean and Head of School of Nursing, Faculty of Health and Social Care Sciences
- *The nurse consultant role in critical care*—Ms. Deborah Dawson, Nurse Consultant in Critical Care, St. George's Healthcare NHS Trust

The students and faculty were also privileged to have a lively discussion of educational differences in doctoral education with Professor Fiona Ross, Dean of the Faculty of Health and Social Care Sciences.

Over two years, speakers in one of the two courses taught abroad, Clinical and Applied Ethics in Nursing Practice (which has been taught twice), have included Dr. Verena Tschudin, then a Reader and Director of the International Centre for

Nursing Ethics (ICNE), who spoke on "International dimensions of nursing ethics," as well as "Human rights issues: Women and nurses," and Dr. Paul Wainwright, Professor, Kingston University and St. George's University of London on "Research ethics in the UK." In addition, there was the eminent international biomedical ethics scholar Professor Donna Dickenson, who won the Fourth International Spinoza Lens Award 2006 for Ethics (the first woman to win this award). She used a very dynamic reflective questioning style with the doctoral students. In the 2007 session, she selected assigned readings from her new book, *Property in the Body: Feminist Perspectives* (Dickenson, 2007), and in 2008 the program focused on her most recent book *Body Shopping: The Economy Fueled by Flesh & Blood* (Dickenson, 2008). In 2008, the doctoral students also had the opportunity to take part in an interactive presentation with Dr. Christopher Johns. Dr. Johns (2006) is recognized internationally as a pioneer of reflective practice within nursing and health care. During this half-day session, students gained a thorough understanding of the true meaning of reflection, its application in health care practice settings, and how to incorporate reflective practice into their future roles as doctoral-prepared nurses and clinical scholars.

All of the educational sessions and extracurricular activities were designed to give students a deeper understanding of a different perspective on nursing and health related ethical, legal, and educational issues the UK faces. Students typically get the course syllabi a couple of weeks before the quarter begins, so they might complete most of their readings prior to traveling abroad. What we have clearly gleaned is that *reading* about socialized medicine, nursing education, or reflective practice is not the same as hearing and experiencing the strengths and problems with these very different systems. The evaluations repeatedly have supported our decision to immerse our doctoral students, including some who have never been abroad, in this different world.

The DrNP-in-London Program: A Doctoral Student's Perspective

"As I boarded the Virgin Atlantic Boeing 747 in the spring of 2008, I was filled with anticipation. Weeks leading up to our departure, I poured over the itinerary and gathered as much travel information as I could about London and the surrounding countryside. Despite my best intentions to sleep during the flight, I diligently read the course material while we flew over the Atlantic. But my eyes periodically drifted from my articles on ethics and pedagogy sitting on my tray table to the clouds out my window as I daydreamed about the time yet to be spent 5,700 kilometers across the ocean. With an hour remaining in the flight some skeptical thoughts also interrupted my pleasant escape. Although the required experience abroad was one of the intriguing elements of the Drexel University DrNP degree, I harbored a small amount of doubt regarding the impact this experience was going to have in changing how I viewed the world around me. Our itinerary allowed for two full days of acclimation prior to the start of class. I spent my first day familiarizing myself with the local surroundings. Nestled in west London, our accommodations off Gloucester Road in the Borough of Kensington were equal distance between Hyde Park and Kensington Palace and the nearest tube stop and the building housing the classrooms. The neighborhood streets were lined with several foreign embassies and a variety of eclectic restaurants, including several "Gastro Pubs" which I frequented often during my two-week stay. The next day we took a walking tour of Kensington in the morning and a bus tour of London in the afternoon, which truly gave me the lay of the land. That evening, as I sat preparing for the following day's classes, I stared out my hotel window at the street lights below, once again daydreaming about the experiences yet to be had. I awoke the following morning to the start of a two week journey filled with discovery in and out of the classroom. In addition to the intellectual rigor fostered by the Drexel faculty and readily embraced by my peers, something I had grown to expect over the last year in the DrNP program, I was challenged by several guest lecturers specializing in the field of nursing ethics. Dr. Wainwright provided a perspective on research ethics, not entirely unfamiliar, but still unique to the United Kingdom. Dr. Gallagher lectured on virtue ethics, inviting a dialogue impossible not to join. We also had the honor of having Dr. Dickenson, who spoke on reproductive ethics, and much of the concepts she presented that morning in late April were ideas shared from her soon-to-be-published book. Particularly memorable was a pleasant train ride to the University of Bedfordshire, north of London, to hear Professor Christopher Johns, author of several books including *Engaging Reflection in Practice: A Narrative Approach* (2006), used the previous semester prior to our London experience. Dr. Johns lectured as if he was telling a story, a format many of the British lecturers seemed to follow. We were encouraged to discuss our own personal experiences, and by the end of our time together, a tapestry of our reflections had been woven together as a testament to the power of reflective practice. Hearing from, interacting with, and then being escorted through the reflective process was far more enriching than my previous attempt at reading his book and then attempting to synthesize reflective practice into my everyday life. A visit to the St. George's Healthcare National Health Service Trust main campus in Tooting, southwest London, one of the United Kingdom's largest teaching hospitals and associated with the renowned St. George's University of London, provided an opportunity to observe and compare a socialized health care system to our own capitalistic health care system in the States. Perhaps the highlight of the visit for me was speaking with the nursing staff on their vascular unit. I was encouraged to find far more similarities than differences in the management of clients with vascular disease. It was also refreshing to see the importance placed on the nursing contribution to the care of the patient. By the completion of the visit I had a true appreciation for the National Health Services and the attempt to provide every citizen with availability and access to primary health care. The remainder of the time not taken up with academic and professional pursuits was spent with my classmates touring Cambridge, exploring the culture, people, and historical sites of London, including a fascinating medical walking tour and a visit to the Florence Nightingale Museum. On the last day of my London adventure I took a walk into Hyde Park, a stroll I became quite fond of over the previous two weeks. As I slowly walked along the edge of Round Pond, my mind was no longer consumed with daydreams of anticipated future experiences or skepticism. Instead, it was filled with the knowledge, experiences and memories obtained from the past two weeks. Knowledge gleaned from the exceptional guest lecturers who so willingly shared their expertise. Experiences fostering an international perspective of nursing, and a realization of the responsibility I bear to my profession that goes beyond the door of my institution and is not limited by borders. And memories of people and places that I will carry with me for the rest of my life."

Scott Oldfield, DrNP (c), CRNP, Vascular Surgery Clinic, Geisinger Medical Center, Danville, Pennsylvania. Drexel University, class of 2006.

THE DrNP-IN-DUBLIN PROGRAM: A FACULTY PERSPECTIVE

In London, students learned to love the city. In Dublin, students learned to love and appreciate the people of Ireland. Initially, many of the students were less than enthusiastic about having their study-abroad experience in Ireland. They wanted to go to a country that they perceived as culturally sophisticated and known for its theatre and museums. Instead, they were introduced to a country that had its own charm, unique culture, and rich history. Our study tour guide in 2009, Colin Hogan, was an American graduate student from Chicago studying at the Dublin School of Business. Colin helped students and faculty navigate the city as well as shared his experiences as an international student.

Again after a short Saturday orientation, the second day in Ireland began with a medical walking tour conducted by Pat Liddy, a well-known Dublin historian, author, and artist who has developed a unique walking tour service for Dublin. Indeed, we were the first medical walking tour that Mr. Liddy ever conducted. On this tour alone students learned about the Irish Healthcare System, the potato famine, religious oppression, women's health care, and the political and religious landscape's affect on childbearing rights, as well as had a visit to the Rotunda Hospital which specializes in women's health and midwifery services. The hospital, founded in 1745, was the original Dublin Lying-In Hospital and maternity training hospital, the first of its kind in Europe. There the students had an opportunity to have a question and answer session with the nursing administrator on call, and began to get a glimpse of nursing education and nursing practice in Ireland.

Two doctoral courses were offered during the Dublin study-abroad experience: "Legal Issues Confronting Nursing Faculty and Administrators" and "Qualitative Methods for Clinical Nursing Inquiry." Irish guest lecturers were invited to classes to present the "Irish Perspective" on assigned topics and readings. The legal issues course used a case-based approach to examine the multitude of legal and ethical issues that confront the contemporary nursing faculty member in the classroom, in clinical settings, or in situations in their professional role as a faculty member. A lecturer from the University of Limerick discussed basic Irish nursing education from both a historical and current perspective. Students and faculty learned that Ireland moved swiftly to the BSN entry only in the 1990s, and unlike the United States, undergraduate nursing students specialize early on in their education in one of five specialties: general population, intellectual disabilities, psychiatric mental health, midwifery, and child nursing.

The program also consisted of a day at Trinity College School of Nursing and Midwifery, which provided an opportunity to interact with their doctoral students and faculty and also to hear a lecture on our host country's health system, always an integral part of our program. Drexel students attended a presentation on the PhD Program in nursing and midwifery outlining the school's research resources, and they attended a PhD proposal defense. Trinity students heard a similar Drexel DrNP Program presentation. All students were then able to compare and contrast institutional research infrastructure, including release time, research support, and incentives, as well as the differences related to research start-up packages and salary incentives, which were greater for Drexel. While doctoral nursing education was relatively new to Trinity College, the institution had a wide and historic international legacy, educating both Oscar Wilde and James Joyce, among others.

Trinity College provided a wealth of guest scholars for our qualitative methods course and a wider discussion of graduate nursing education in Ireland. Guest lecture topics included:

- *Ethical considerations in qualitative research*—using a study on women's experiences of carrying a fetus with an abnormality as an exemplar;
- *Qualitative research data collection strategies*—using a study on women's experiences of myocardial infarction as an exemplar;
- *Mixing data, design and analysis: Triangulation as a qualitative research strategy*—using examples from studies on student midwives' views of their education and quality of life at end of life care; and
- *Qualitative sampling issues: Field notes, memoing, and interviewing*, focusing on a grounded theory approach and using a study on sexuality in mental health nursing as an exemplar.

Unlike the prevailing paradigm in the United States, Trinity College of Nursing and Midwifery faculty are trying to hone their quantitative research program, while American nursing faculty are still grappling with balancing qualitative and quantitative research as equal partners. These presentations provided valuable opportunities for discussion, as the Drexel DrNP program is a hybrid nursing doctorate, and all doctoral candidates complete a clinical dissertation. Thus, the PhD students at Trinity and the DrNP students from Drexel appreciated and benefited from exploration of each other's research projects during our day visit.

In the context of their multicultural study-abroad education, students and faculty experienced such activities as the "Unmanageable Revolutionaries: Women in Irish History Walking Tour," a Dublin Literary Pub Crawl, and an incredible night of tragic drama attending Arthur Miller's "All My Sons" at the famed Gate Theater in Dublin. During the Irish women's history tour, it was startlingly apparent to us that the accomplishments of Irish women were sadly missing as a major aspect of Irish history. Foreign domination, a historically patriarchal society, religious oppression, and lack of childbearing rights appear to have largely contributed to Irish women's invisibility in Irish history. This walking tour alone led to great discussion about the Irish role of women and of women's right globally that permeated the classroom. Having attended the London program once and now the Dublin program, each was uniquely different, while both were incredibly rewarding for students and faculty.

The DrNP-in-Dublin Program: A Doctoral Student's Perspective

"As an adult doctoral student with multiple responsibilities, including a full time career and family, the thought of adding an international study abroad program seemed daunting. As the time neared, however, with all the planning and packing upon us, the excitement grew. Spending two weeks in Ireland with my 11 other peers, learning about health care and health care education, as well as taking two courses would soon be a reality, and not just a paragraph on paper, as a small blurb describing the DrNP program. The courses selected to be taken in Ireland were oriented to qualitative research methods and legal issues in nursing academia, both very appropriate for courses for study abroad. I do not think we could have experienced and learned more about qualitative research in any better way than with the opportunities we were given in Ireland. We had multiple qualitative research-ers, all well established in their fields, come to the Dublin School of Business and give us lectures about their own research, as well as various methods utilized in their research. Each lecturer was well prepared and willing to entertain questions from each of us. Also, after the lectures, our professor from Drexel would summarize and clarify any questions raised during the morning's session and prepare us for the next day. I think we were each impressed how each lecturer brought to us a living classroom from which we were able to absorb much more than if we had just read their articles and discussed them in class in Philadelphia. We also spent a day at Trinity College with the Doctoral Nursing students in the morning and in the after-noon learned about their educational system, types of research being pursued by the students, and strengths of their program. During lunch, there were informal opportu-nities to share personal experiences with doctoral education and our own research interests with the Trinity students and faculty. We discussed the differences between the US and Ireland, as well as the differences between Drexel University and Trinity College. Many of us also visited the *Book of Kells* and Trinity Library that same day. In our time off, we enjoyed taking in the sights and tastes of Ireland. Each of us wandered in our own directions, some of us taking in Howth, Belfast, Galway, the Cliffs of Moher, and Cork, to name a few. We enjoyed watching football and rugby from the local taverns, and of course had to spend some time in the Temple Bar Area listening to Irish music and enjoying the Guinness (we were doctoral students!). As a group, we visited Glendalough and the Wicklow mountains on our last day in Ireland. We even got used to the rainy damp weather and appreciated the beautiful days we had, as well. The country of Ireland is beautiful, and the people could not have been more welcoming. The camaraderie among many of us was enhanced significantly, and was a bonus to everything else we experienced and learned on this short, but expansive learning experience. Many other programs *encou-rage* their students to study abroad, but we were privileged that this was a mandatory part of our curriculum. I know some of my classmates clearly underestimated the impact this trip would have on our lives. I am sure if it were only optional, our chief nursing officer colleague, for example, would have said she could not afford to leave her high-powered position for two weeks. Instead she had to go and, indeed, had a ball. For any doctoral students studying abroad, it will most likely be an unforgettable, life altering experience, well worth the inconveniences it may cause in the life of a doctoral student."

Cynthia Gifford Hollingsworth, DrNP (c), MSN, CRNP, CPNP, Surgical Research Nurse Supervisor, Department of Surgery, College of Medicine, Drexel University, class of 2007.

WHAT WE LEARNED FROM BOTH EXPERIENCES

When Drexel planned and implemented the mandatory two-week study-abroad experi-ence, the faculty was not clear on the direct impact that such an experience would have on the overall student's global and doctoral educational experience. In year one, faculty were immediately and pleasantly surprised how deep an impression the study-abroad experience had on the students, both personally and professionally. Simply based on assessments from our first-year faculty, students, and FIE partners in London, the study program became a standard part of our DrNP curriculum, and we advertised it as "mandatory" for our second class of 2006.

During the first 4 years of this program, we know that many of our students had never even been abroad, and others who had traveled abroad had not visited London or Dublin. This is actually not surprising when one recognizes that our most typical doctoral nursing student is a woman in her forties often managing families, education, and a full-time career. Although some students were reticent about going abroad due to family responsibilities, most adapted quite well and enjoyed the experience immensely. Students not only learned course content, but were able to experience a different culture for a two-week period and be exposed to a different health care system, educational system, research viewpoint, and perspective. In Ireland, students were quite interested to learn about the religious oppression of the Irish people and its effects even today. Many modern Irish who themselves had not experienced oppression still spoke about the psychological pain of oppression in their normal dialogue with the students. Many of the students identified with these feelings and their pain resonated with them. In London, students were able to experience an incredibly massive, cosmopolitan city that probably provided a more diverse cultural experience, but certainly less intimate and personal, than Dublin. The faculty were particularly observant of the impact Ireland had on many of our students who were of Irish descent and in the country for the first time.

Overall, the DrNP study-abroad experience provides students with an opportunity to experience another country studying abroad, and learning another culture while maintaining a full-time or part-time employment in the states. Our doctoral students, who are generally studying part-time, had an opportunity to immerse themselves in their studies for a two-week period and also bond as a group, becoming familiar with each other as individuals, students, and professionals. Students also learned about London or Dublin in the classroom and out in the field without the immediate pressures of family and work. They learned that largely Anglophilic London and Dublin are indeed very different from their own American culture, and that despite having an accent, or having a different educational system or health care system, we are still at the core more alike than different.

SUMMARY

After 4 years and now planning our fifth study-abroad program (which will add a 4-day experience in Edinburgh, Scotland when our students attend the *2nd International Conference on the Professional Doctorate* in 2011 as part of their London program), it is clear that this innovation has become an integral part of our curriculum. Even with the downturn in the economy, we have been able to modestly increase the quarterly fee each year (e.g., one year due to increased fuel charges and another due to fluctuating currency exchange rates). Our intention was never to be based solely in London, although partnering with the London-based FIE has made the job of planning such a short-term study-abroad program much easier. It takes an incredible amount of planning to put a high-level, scholarly program together. We have been adamant that this is not a "vacation" but truly a study-abroad experience. Therefore, the meticulous planning of scholars to come to our foreign-based classrooms takes enormous networking and, indeed, we compensate our visiting classroom scholars with modest honoraria. We still debate to what extent this is a "cultural immersion" experience. We tried to take our program to Madrid one year, but unfortunately there was a scarcity of scholars fluent in English who could guest lecture for us on much focused topics. We also found the accommodations and suburban location of the host school unacceptable. Indeed, graduate students, and particularly doctoral students, will not want to be treated as undergraduates or thrown in with them in the same type of accommodations. The majority of our students work full-time, so they do typically have discretionary income that will allow them to pay a little more for more upscale accommodations and amenities. The department chair actually flew to Dublin to inspect the facilities, and we likewise had a faculty member spend a day in Madrid to assure us our experiences would have a high likelihood of succeeding. This was critically important to us, especially when considering new, unproven venues.

Finally, we have learned that the amount of time necessary to plan such a program requires *more time* for graduate students than undergraduates. Our MBA colleagues have confirmed this with us. Therefore, one of our doctoral nursing faculty serves as a DrNP Study Abroad Facilitator and works in concert with the Chair each year to plan the micro-details of the program. The department chair has typically gone in the first year of a new venue so the second-year experience can be highly fine tuned, but this is not necessarily permanent practice. But when a department chair is walking in Dublin with a fellow faculty member who says, "Wow, I am so privileged to be here," then the expectations that these faculty will indeed use their new international experiences to network, collaborate, and ultimately increase their global scholarly reputations (and hence to our College and University) is alive (and well worth the investment).

After 4 years, our overall evaluation has been that this mandatory international experience is an important and distinctive part of our doctor of nursing practice program. Further, our faculty has just approved a similar two-week format for our forthcoming PhD program which will be tailored for the PhD student. We hope to match our PhD students with an international faculty mentor in our host city and have the DrNP and PhD students share one course and take another separately. This will likely necessitate sending an additional faculty member annually and adjusting our budget accordingly. London and Dublin now seem very solid alternating sites for us, but we are anxious to experiment and have our students and faculty explore the globe more. One of our host institutions is now considering developing a reciprocal experience for their doctoral nursing students with Drexel. We suggest this short-term model could be easily replicated by international doctoral nursing students coming to the United States and certainly for other U.S.-based doctoral nursing programs. With the rise of globalization, it is critical that nursing students, particularly doctoral-educated clinical nursing scholars, have an enhanced understanding of international health issues. Participation in a mandatory study-abroad program for doctoral nursing students is one way to accomplish this. So when the article *"So What Did You Learn in London"* was republished on the internet recently (Redden, 2007), it caught both our students' and faculty's eyes, and we think the answer is, "a lot."

Postscript: This chapter is dedicated to the memory of Dr. Kathy P. Falkenstein (December 7, 1952 to June 4, 2010), who accompanied traveling students and faculty to London in 2007 and Dublin in 2009.

NOTES

1. The Drexel DrNP is a hybrid professional doctorate combining advanced nursing practice with the conduct of clinical research, and all students complete a clinical dissertation (Dreher, Donnelly, & Naremore, 2005).
2. For the first class, the students were simply required to make 8 quarterly payments which began the subsequent quarter after the program was approved. Starting with the second class (2006), students began making quarterly payments immediately upon matriculation.

3. We specifically give students a lunch break of 1.5 hours between classes to better reflect the UK/European culture which takes a more leisurely attitude toward gastronomy. Predictably, the first class asked to decrease the mealtime to get out of class early and the faculty refused. Our longer lunch meal times in the end are usually evaluated favorably.
4. Much to our dismay, the active volcanoes in Iceland in April 2010 delayed our students study abroad program by a week, and so we skyped in most all of our planned speakers as students completed week one (much to their dismay) on campus. Students did attend week two in London and many stayed abroad longer after the formal program ended.

REFERENCES

Altbach, P. (2004). Higher education crosses borders. *Change, 36,* 18–25.

Christoffersen, J. E. (2008). Leading a study-abroad group of nursing students in Nicaragua: A first-timer's account. *Nursing Forum, 43,* 238–246.

Conant, E. (2010, September 12). Students without borders: Why more college kids are choosing to travel—alone—to far flung locales. *Newsweek.com.* Retrieved from http://education.newsweek.com/2010/09/12/students-find-study-abroad-adventure.html

Cushner, K., & Karim, A. (2004). Study abroad at the university level. In D. Landis, J. M. Bennett, & M. J. Bennett (Eds.), *Handbook of intercultural training* (3rd ed., pp. 289–308). Los Angeles, CA: Sage.

Dickenson, D. (2007). *Property in the body: Feminist perspectives.* Cambridge, UK: Cambridge University Press.

Dickenson, D. (2008). *Body shopping: The economy fuelled by flesh & blood.* Oxford, UK: Oneworld.

Dreher, H. M., Dean, J. L., Moriarty, D., Kaiser, R., Willard, R., O'Donnell, S. et al., (2004). What you need to know about SARS now. *Nursing 2004: The Journal of Clinical Excellence, 34,* 58–63.

Dreher, H. M., Donnelly, G., & Naremore, R. (2005). Reflections on the DNP and an alternate practice doctorate model: The Drexel DrNP. *Online Journal of Issues in Nursing, 11,* 1. Retrieved from http://www.nursingworld.org/MainMenuCategories/ANAMarketplace/ANAPeriodicals/OJIN/TableofContents/Volume112006/No1Jan06/ArticlePreviousTopic/tpc28_716031.aspx

Dreher, H. M., Lachman, V. D., Smith Glasgow, M. E., & Ward, L. S. (2008). *Educating the global clinical scholar: The first doctoral nursing program to institute a mandatory study abroad program.* AACN Doctoral Education Conference, Captiva Island, FL, January 2008.

Duffy, M. E. (2001). A critique of cultural education in nursing. *Journal of Advanced Nursing, 36,* 487–495.

Fennell, R. (2009). The impact of an international health study abroad program on university students from the United States. *Global Health Promotion, 16,* 17–23.

Fry, G. (1984). The economic and political impact of study abroad. *Comparative Education Review, 28,* 203–220.

Gardner, A. (2009). Pandemic (H1N1) update—The role of nurses. *Australian Nursing Journal, 17,* 5, 7.

Institute of International Education. (2007). Current trends in U.S. study abroad and the impact of strategic diversity initiatives. *IIE Study Abroad White Paper, Meeting America's Global Education Challenge.* Retrieved from http://www.iienetwork.org/file_depot/0-10000000/0-10000/1710/folder/62450/IIE+Study+Abroad+White+Paper+I.pdf

Institute of International Education. (2008). *Open door 2008 data tables.* Retrieved from http://opendoors.iienetwork.org/page/131530/

Johanson, L. (2006). The implementation of a study abroad course for nursing. *Nurse Educator, 31,* 129–131.

Johns, C. (2006). *Engaging reflection in practice: A narrative approach.* Hoboken, NJ: Wiley-Blackwell.

Levine, M. (2009). Transforming experiences: Nursing education and international immersion programs. *Journal of Professional Nursing, 25,* 156–169.

Parker, M., Locsin, R., & Longo, J. (2006). Global communities and healthcare transition: Analysis of a study-abroad course to Thailand. *International Journal for Human Caring, 10,* 86–87.

Redden, E. (2007). So what did you learn in London? *insidehighered.com*. Retrieved from http://insidehighered.com/news/2007/06/01/research

Redden, E. (2009a). In global recession, global ed still growing. *insidehighered.com*. Retrieved from http://insidehighered.com/layout/set/print/news/2009/29/international

Redden, E. (2009b). Standards for short-term study abroad. *insidehighered.com*. Retrieved from http://www.insidehighered.com/news/2009/01/30/standards

Saenz, K., & Holcomb, L. (2009). Essential tools for a study abroad nursing course. *Educator, 34*, 172–175.

Zorn, C. (1996). The long-term impact on nursing students participating in international education. *Journal of Professional Nursing, 12*, 106–110.

CHAPTER TWENTY-ONE: Reflective Response

Ann Bartley Williams

Study abroad programs have become *de rigueur* in recent years, with many American universities and colleges declaring that every student should have an international educational experience before graduation. Given that U.S. institutions host multitudes of foreign students, the growing interest in providing our own young scholars with a broader worldview is welcome.

As noted by Dr. Dreher and colleagues, most of these new programs serve undergraduates and there are no data describing the extent to which undergraduate nursing students participate. Given the demanding and relatively inflexible demands of a preservice nursing curriculum, it is likely that few nursing students are able to take advantage of the new international opportunities. There is a similar lack of information about graduate nursing programs abroad; to the best of my knowledge, the Drexel group is the sole nursing doctoral program with a mandatory study abroad component.

Competence in a foreign language has long been mandatory for doctoral programs in the humanities and social sciences. Further, it is not uncommon for humanities and social science doctoral students to spend a significant part of their training conducting research outside of the United States. In contrast, foreign language study is not required for advanced nursing degrees, and most master's- and doctoral-level scholarship concerns domestic, U.S. health issues. By instituting a mandatory study abroad experience for DrNP students, the Drexel faculty is breaking new ground in higher nursing education.

The Drexel group's rationale for *offering* short-term formal study abroad was that the experience would prepare their DrNP graduates to better face contemporary global problems. The rationale for *mandating* the experience was that if the program were optional, the full cohort of DrNP candidates would not participate, and the program would be elitist to the extent that students with greater work, family, and financial responsibilities would opt out. Requiring participation was an unusual and bold move, but the requirement seems to have been well-accepted. In this report, the authors do not discuss what, if any, arrangements are possible, should the time abroad truly represent a hardship under special circumstances for individual students.

Exposure to a wide range of cultures and societies is commonly regarded as admirable, but more targeted and specific goals are needed to drive course development, implementation, and evaluation. Students in the health professions usually focus early in their careers on mastering clinical skills and are eager to have clinical experiences abroad. Often, they seek opportunities to be of service and to work in resource-limited settings. The challenge in creating programs to answer these needs include the relatively limited skills of beginning practitioners, the limited amount of time available to spend out of the United States, the material and physical demands on faculty, host country practice standards and regulations, and requirements of U.S. accrediting bodies for structured clinical education.

Graduate nursing students with mature clinical careers, such as DrNP candidates, may be less interested in hands-on clinical education abroad than in the opportunity to learn first hand about nursing issues, policies, and the context of care in other countries. The program designed by the Drexel faculty brings courses from the Drexel curriculum, along with the faculty responsible for those courses, to sites abroad where the usual course experience is enriched by lectures from local scholars and field trips. Research methods, policy, ethics, and health systems courses lend themselves well to transplantation.

Student course requirements are not discussed in this chapter, but are the key to ensuring a substantive educational experience. Reflective journals and diaries can suggest a structure for student observations during the time abroad and support thoughtful review and summation upon return. Coursework such as case studies and papers should link the core theoretical content, which would be the same wherever the course were offered, with the contextual content presented by the international site.

Among developed and wealthy countries, the United States is perhaps unique in the parochialism of its educational system. The lack of foreign language competence among American students unfortunately limits the range and depth of experiences available to them outside of our borders. The Drexel program takes advantage of the Anglophone world, sending students and faculty to English speaking countries. However, given the fact that the vast majority of educated people in other countries speak English as a second language, and usually quite well, programs such as this need not be geographically limited.

The Drexel program views the opportunity to teach at their international sites as a positive benefit for faculty, which is almost certainly true. Teaching abroad offers faculty an opportunity to enhance their own scholarship and to build their network of international collaborators. On the other hand, spending two weeks with a small group of student travelers, many of whom are out of the country for the first time, is a significant responsibility. The most mature and sophisticated individuals may become quite disoriented and dependent in a completely unfamiliar setting. Interpersonal tensions within the group can escalate and require skilled attention. And, of course, emergencies, large and small, occur. The opportunity to teach abroad is a wonderful opportunity, but it is also a great deal of work.

Designing a day-to-day class schedule that remains true to the course goals, while taking full advantage of the foreign resources, is a pedagogical challenge. The better integrated the theory and context, the richer the learning experience. To do this, the faculty must become experts in the application and relevance of their course material to the host country. That expertise will grow as individual faculty members repeat the course, developing their network of local experts and collaborators. Drexel's policy of rotating the opportunity to teach abroad, motivated by a desire to share the opportunity with as many members of the faculty as possible, could limit the long-term development of deeper understanding and collaboration.

Evaluation of educational programs is a challenge, especially given the long-term and sometimes generic goals. When time and money are short, sustaining a mandatory study abroad program for DrNP students is going to require evidence of effectiveness. Narrative feedback from student and faculty participants tells us that individuals found the experience rewarding, perhaps even life changing. But, how does one demonstrate that the students who participate in a study abroad program are "better prepared to face global health problems?" A prospective evaluation of the subsequent career decisions and accomplishments of this cohort would be a significant contribution to the discipline of nursing education.

CRITICAL THINKING QUESTIONS

1. How important is it to you to be educated with a "global nursing scholar framework?"
2. Describe a couple of international nursing/health-related issues of which you believe you would have better comprehension of if only you had more life-experience/experiential exposure to them.
3. How has international travel helped your global IQ, or have you had limited or no international travel experiences?
4. Undergraduate study-abroad models have proliferated. Should graduate study abroad be as prevalent? Why or why not?
5. Our research indicates there is a shortage of nursing study-abroad opportunities. Why is this so and what could be done about it?
6. If you had to design an international clinical practicum in your DNP degree, what would it entail?
7. Americans, even educated ones, are notoriously monolingual. Do you speak a second language, and what value to international health in the context of your career trajectory would being proficient in a second language be?
8. Describe how a lack of study-abroad opportunities for nurses, particularly doctoral graduate nursing students, impacts the health of the average global citizen. Or does it?
9. What did you learn from the narrative experiences of the two Drexel DrNP students who described their study-abroad program in London and Dublin?
10. How might you go about helping implement a similar study-abroad program in your own doctor of nursing practice program?

CHAPTER TWENTY-TWO

The New DNP Certification Exam

Yes? No? You Decide

Bobbie Posmontier

INTRODUCTION

In August of 2000, Mary Mundinger, who was both President of the Council for the Advancement of Comprehensive Care (CACC) and Dean of Columbia University School of Nursing invited educational leaders in Nursing and Medicine to discuss the future role and preparation of advanced practice registered nurses (APRNs) (National Board of Medical Examiners [NBNE], 2009). The work of this first conference resulted in suggesting the Doctor of Nursing Practice degree as the entry-level degree for the APRN of and set the stage for the eventual development of a DNP certification exam by the joint efforts of the NBNE and the CACC (Mundinger, 2008a). Since the administration of the first DNP certification examination in 2008, however, a storm of controversy has ensued regarding its value (Mundinger, 2008b). In order to understand the controversy, this chapter will review its major components and explore the arguments for and against the DNP certification examination.

WHAT IS THE DNP EXAMINATION?

The NBME and CACC proposed a voluntary two-tiered examination to assess clinical knowledge, diagnostic skills, and independent clinical management of patients across the lifespan in a variety of health care settings in order to validate advanced DNP clinical competencies (American Board of Comprehensive Care [ABCC], 2009). The purpose of this voluntary examination was to provide an extra level of standardized assurance of safety and competency to the public and other medical professions (NBME, 2009). Once the examination was passed, the ABCC would then designate the DNP as a diplomate in Comprehensive Care (DCC) by the American Board of Comprehensive Care and permit use of the title "doctor" in clinical practice (Landro, 2008; Mundinger, 2009).

The examination consists of questions that evaluate the diplomate candidate's ability to assess the severity of disease, make clinical judgments, and manage patient-centered mainstream high-impact diseases (ABCC, 2009). Although the examination was mainly designed to test the advanced clinical skills of adult and family nurse practitioners with a DNP, other APRNs with a DNP degree were also invited to sit for the examination if they believed they have mastered the examination's content.

The actual 2-day examination is based in part on Step 3 of the United States Medical Licensing Examination (USMLE). It consists of two 5-hour tests administered in 60-minute blocks allowing 90 seconds per question (ABCC, 2009). The examination is comprised of two dimensions including: (1) 336 multiple-choice questions that require action-oriented clinical decisions and judgment for normal development and disease, and (2) a series of dynamic interactive patient vignettes that evaluate the diplomate candidate's ability to apply knowledge and to manage a variety of patient problems across various health care settings along a simulated-time format. Acting as primary health care providers, diplomate candidates manipulate simulated time in a variety of acute or chronic patient cases by advancing the computer clock to find out results of diagnostic tests, procedures, and patient conditions so that additional assessments, treatment orders, consultations, and interventions can be formulated. Diplomate candidates are allotted 25 minutes to complete each patient vignette, and scoring is based on algorithms derived from codified policies of experienced health care providers.

Diplomate candidates are expected to possess advanced-level knowledge in normal development, mechanisms of disease, and general principles of patient-care management (ABCC, 2009). In addition, they are expected to provide evidence of an in-depth understanding of disorders of the blood and of the central nervous, mental, skin, musculoskeletal, respiratory, cardiovascular, gastrointestinal, renal and urinary, male and female reproductive, endocrine, and immunologic systems. The diplomate candidate is also expected to demonstrate expertise across a variety of clinical tasks including the ability to perform history and physical assessments, order appropriate diagnostic tests, formulate diagnoses and prognoses, order appropriate medications, perform health maintenance, understand disease prevention, provide clinical interventions, communicate with multidisciplinary health care team members, demonstrate an understanding of legal and ethical issues, and demonstrate an understanding of patient-care management across a variety of health care settings.

Three eligibility criteria are required to sit for the examination: national certification as an APRN, graduation from an accredited DNP program, and recognition or licensure by a state board of nursing as an APRN (ABCC, 2010b). Although the DNP examination was not designed to replace national certification or guide curriculum development, the NBME and CACC consider it an additional assurance to the public of a high level of clinical competency and safety of the DNP graduate. A controversial issue that has not been fully addressed is whether future non-DNP-educated doctoral APRNs with a different doctorate degree (e.g., PhD) may be eligible to sit for the examination, because at present they are not eligible.

ARGUMENTS FOR THE DNP EXAMINATION

Proponents of the DNP certification examination argue that it was never designed to evaluate clinical expertise among nonclinical DNP graduates (administrative and education tracks) (NBME, 2009). According to the NBME and CACC, the DNP examination was designed to assure the public that clinical DNP graduates function within the boundaries of their practice as well as meet the standards of their profession. They further assert that evaluation reflecting national standards of practice is the only mechanism that can ensure safe and high-quality patient care.

According to proponents of the DNP examination, the line between physician and DNP practice is very clear, because the context and scope of the examination is different than the three-step USMLE examination for physician certification (NBME, 2009). Unlike the physician USMLE examination, the DNP certification examination is a shorter examination, does not require prior formal clinical skills assessment, and does not require prior fundamental scientific knowledge as required by physician certification candidates. Because the DNP certification examination should reflect the same level of clinical acumen as primary care physicians, proponents also defend the choice of the NBME as the developer of the examination (Kane, 2009; Mundinger, 2007).

In contrast to physician certification, proponents also argue that the DNP examination more comprehensively evaluates the training of DNPs in patient care coordination to facilitate access to care and meet health care disparities (NBME, 2009). Unlike physicians, DNPs represent a new generation of primary care providers who not only manage complex illnesses in hospitals, emergency departments, and outpatient offices, but also coordinate care among various health care providers and health care settings, and provide preventive services that encompass contextual components such as social and family support and cost-effective health care (Kane, 2009; Landro, 2008). Rather than replicating the physician USMLE examination, the DNP examination contains different dimensions of the USMLE Step 3 that reflect advanced nursing practice. Mundinger (2009) argues that opposition to the examination may be fueled in part from physicians who worry that competition from DNP diplomates may lower their income and prestige.

Proponents of the DNP examination assert that concerns about physician regulation of APRN practice are unfounded (Mundinger, 2008a or 2008b; NBME, 2009). Justification for this position is based on the fact that the DNP examination is only one component of the certification process. In order to receive a diplomate status, DNPs must also possess national certification as an APRN, graduate from an accredited DNP program, and be recognized or licensed by a state board of nursing as an APRN, all of which are governed almost exclusively by nursing associations (with the exception of the Certified Nurse Midwife which is governed by the American College of Nurse Midwives). In addition, the DNP examination may actually assist in better defining the boundaries between doctoral advanced practice nursing and medicine.

The DNP examination represents expert input from both nursing and medicine professionals; these both support a multidisciplinary health care team approach that better serves the needs of primary care patients. According to the NBME and the CACC, future health care will require the collaboration of multidisciplinary health care teams whose individual members possess a variety of educational backgrounds and clinical expertise to meet the health care gaps created by an increasing shortage of primary care providers (Mundinger, Starck, Hathaway, Shaver, & Woods, 2009). Nonphysician primary care providers such as DNP's are vital to reduce the fragmentation and inefficiency of patient care, especially among the medically underserved. Without a sufficient pool of primary care providers, proponents of the DNP examination assert that there will be increased cost, decreased quality of care, and decreased patient satisfaction. They further argue that the increased use of DNPs will require additional assurance that DNPs have met national standards of care expected of all primary care disciplines. Each primary care discipline, however, will need to define its boundaries and standards in patient-care management. With the ultimate goals of patient safety and excellent health care, the NBME and CACC promoted the development of the DNP examination to provide evidence of high-quality standardized assessment of DNPs who practice within the boundaries of their profession and provide care that is complementary to other primary health care professions. The NBME and CACC also view the DNP examination as complementary to the goals of uniform regulation of APRN practice via LACE (licensing, accreditation, certification, education), which emphasizes the achievement of competency-based standards of practice (American Psychiatric Nurses Association, 2010).

Proponents of the DNP examination also assert that the DNP examination reflects more in-depth knowledge, training, and skills than master's-prepared APRNs, and that this distinction is necessary to assure the public of safe and high-quality care (Landro, 2008). In contrast to opponents' negative views regarding the broadness of the examination, the ABCC asserts that the DNP certification examination was designed to be broad in scope to reflect the DNP diplomates' complex advanced practice knowledge, skills, and decision making (ABCC, 2009). Finally, according to proponents, the DNP examination, which is based on standards endorsed by medicine, assures the public that the DNP diplomate is not a second-tier professional (Landro, 2008).

Although some opponents argue that there is no distinct difference between master's-prepared and doctorally prepared APRNs, proponents argue that DNPs invest more time in education beyond the master's level to prepare them to act as leaders in translating research into practice and to address the faculty shortage (McGrath & Piques, 2009). According to proponents, each represents a distinct level of practice reflected in their essential components (see Table 22.1). While master's-prepared APRNs are more focused on a specific populations such as pediatric or women's health care in limited health care settings, the DNP is more focused on complex diagnosis, coordination of care, and management of individuals across a variety of health care settings (Landro, 2008). In addition, their extended training in medical practice and management is more similar to primary-care physicians than to master's-prepared APRNs (Mundinger, 2009).

Compared to master's-prepared APRNs, who focus mainly on *understanding* theories of practice and health care policies, DNPs are expected to take *leadership* in translating theoretical knowledge into clinical practice, changing health care policy, organizing and facilitating financing of health care to eliminate health care disparities, and improving the overall quality of care to benefit patients (AACN, 1996, 2006). In contrast to master's-prepared APRNs who are expected to *utilize* evidence-based nursing in practice, DNPs are expected to *synthesize, translate, disseminate,* and *integrate* new evidence-based knowledge into practice. Although master's-prepared APRNs are educated to *deliver culturally sensitive care, promote health,* and *prevent disease* for specific patient populations, DNPs focus on improving the nation's health by *integrating* and *institutionalizing evidence-based nursing knowledge* for disease prevention and health promotion for individuals and populations. The DNP also takes health care management one step further by not only managing complex illnesses and conducting individual and systemic assessments, but by evaluating links between individuals, populations, and health care financing and policy.

According to the American Nurses Credentialing Center (ANCC), a majority of nurses are in favor of the DNP certification exam (ANCC, 2010). In an ANCC survey of 4,284 nurses, where 71% were currently practicing as an APRN, respondents were asked, "What do you envision as the desired future for certification of nurses holding the DNP degree in the year 2015?" While 60% expressed the desire for a single endpoint examination, 40% expressed the desire for staged examinations where testing would occur at one or more midpoints during master's preparation with a final endpoint DNP examination.

H. Michael Dreher, Chair of the Doctoral Nursing Department at Drexel University, which has had a DrNP program since 2005, stated support for the exam, reporting "While there is a great deal of opposition to this DNP exam, I am for it. I do not think it was prudent for the AACN to include the executive role in the DNP degree construction and exclude the educator role. Therefore, the DNP exam emphasizes the clinical practitioner role and any credible credential that Doctor of Nursing Practice graduates can

TABLE 22.1
***Essentials* of DNP versus MSN Preparation for APRNs**

DNP Preparation (Adapted from *The Essentials of Doctoral Education for Advanced Nursing Practice*, AACN, 2006)	MSN Preparation (Adapted from *The Essentials of Master's Education for Advanced Practice Nursing*, AACN, 1996)
I. Theoretical Foundations for Practice—act as leaders to use the conceptual scientific foundation of nursing to translate knowledge into clinical practice to benefit patients in all practice environments.	I. Theoretical Foundations of Nursing Practice—critiques, utilizes and evaluates theory within practice
II. Organizational and Systems Leadership for Quality Improvement and Systems Thinking—taking the lead in changing policy, organization and financing of health care to eliminate health disparities, improve quality and safety, and evaluate cost effectiveness of care.	II. Understanding policy, organization, and financing of health care
III. Clinical Scholarship and Analytical Methods for Evidence-Based Practice—synthesizes knowledge, translates research into practice, disseminates knowledge, and integrates new knowledge into practice.	III. Research-utilization of evidence-based nursing.
IV. Information Systems/Technology and Patient Care Technology for the Improvement and Transformation of Health Care.	IV. Ethics—understand principles, personal values, beliefs to frame nursing practice
V. Health Care Policy for Advocacy in Health Care—involves influencing policy design and development, analysis of policy, and political activism to decrease health care disparities, improve quality of care, and influence health care financing in all levels of government.	V. Understanding how health care policy is organized and delivered
VI. Inter-professional Collaboration for Improving Patient and Population Health Outcomes—facilitates interdisciplinary collaboration.	VI. Professional role development to operationalize theoretical principles and norms of specialty
VII. Clinical Prevention and Population Health for Improving the Nation's Health—leaders in integrating and institutionalizing evidence- based prevention for individuals and populations.	VII. Human diversity and social issues to deliver culturally sensitive care to patients. Health promotion and disease prevention for specific patient population
VIII. Advanced Nursing Practice—address complex medical management across a variety of health care settings; able to manage more complex illness, conducts individual and systemic assessments, evaluates links between individual, population, health care financing and policy.	VIII. Advanced health/physical assessment, physiology and pathophysiology, pharmacology

obtain that can differentiate their practice beyond the MSN is worthy of at least further trial and study" (Dr. H. Michael Dreher personal communication, May 10, 2010). Dreher and Montgomery (2009) also suggest that the new term "doctoral advanced practice nursing" be used to differentiate "master's-level advanced practice nursing," and one could infer that this DNP exam may perhaps validate clinical practice beyond current masters APRN competencies.

In summary, proponents refute the criticisms of the DNP examination by asserting:

- It was never designed for nonclinical DNPs;
- The boundaries between physician practice and even doctoral advanced practice nursing are quite clear;
- Concerns of physician regulation of NP practice are unfounded;
- Multidisciplinary health care teams with clear professional boundaries represent the future of primary care to meet the needs of the underserved;
- The DNP certification is necessary to assure the public of high standards of care; and
- The DNP examination is worthy of further trial and study.

In addition, proponents assert that the DNP certification examination supports the uniform regulation of APRN practice via licensing, accreditation, certification, and education. Finally, proponents assert there is a distinct difference between the practice of master's- and DNP-prepared APRNs.

ARGUMENTS AGAINST THE DNP EXAMINATION

The most salient arguments against the DNP certification examination question the validity of the examination for nonclinically based DNPs such as administrators and educators. In addition, nonclinically based APRN administrators and educators earning a DNP are only required to be actively certified by the ANCC in their respective roles. Those who oppose the examination cite the 50% pass rate achieved by 45 examinees in 2008 and the 57% pass rate among 19 examinees in 2009 to bolster the argument against its validity (ABCC, 2010c). The American Association of Nurse Practitioners (AANP), American College of Nurse Practitioners (ACNP), and some specialty groups of the American Medical Association have publicly expressed their opposition to the DNP examination (Guadagnino & Mundinger, 2008; Hoyt & Proehl, 2009). Because those DNPs who pass the examination will use the title "doctor," some argue that the boundaries between medicine and nursing have been blurred to an extent that will cause public confusion. In addition, the use of the USMLE as the template for the DNP exam has raised some concerns that the public will be misled to think that DNP certification is equivalent to physician certification. Some opponents also express concern that NBME credentialing will ultimately result in physician regulation of APRN practice, because the NBME is viewed as a medical credentialing agency (NONPF, 2008).

Opponents also argue that there are already psychometrically sound national certifying exams for APRNs and question the utility of an additional certification examination (Counts & Dempster, 2008; Stanik-Hutt, 2008). They further argue that the DNP certification examination is based on the practice of medicine and does not measure APRN expertise. Unlike current national certifying examinations for APRNs, opponents believe that the DNP examination is extraneous and unrelated to advanced practice nursing. NONPF (2008), which designed a population-based academic curriculum for the DNP, issued a statement that the individual-based DNP certification examination from the NBME is too broad to assess competency among DNP graduates with differing roles and specialties. This statement was also endorsed by six other organizations representing nurse practitioners including the American Academy of Nurse Practitioners, American College of Nurse Practitioners, Association of Faculties of Pediatric Nurse Practitioners, National Association of Nurse Practitioners in Women's Health, National

Association of Pediatric Nurse Practitioners, and National Conference of Gerontological Nurse Practitioners (Johnson, 2008).

Several physicians have expressed concern regarding the ability of the DNP to practice independently (Guadagnino & Mundinger, 2008). In addition, some physicians have raised concerns that unsupervised DNP diplomates will ultimately decrease patient safety and quality of care. Some opponents also argue that there is no research to substantiate that DNP certification improves patient care (Michalski, Sagan, Moore, Bednash, & Rosseter, 2006). Finally, opponents argue that adding another layer of certification will dissuade nurses from becoming APRNs and further decrease the pool of available primary-care providers (NONPF, 2008).

In summary, opponents argue that the DNP certification examination is irrelevant to nonclinical DNP graduates and DNP graduates who do not have expertise in family and adult advanced nursing practice. Further, opponents believe it:

- Blurs the lines between physician and doctoral advanced nursing practice (Guadagnino & Mundinger, 2008; Hoyt & Proehl, 2009);
- May result in physician regulation of advanced nursing practice (NONPF, 2008);
- Is unnecessary as a plethora of psychometrically sound national certifying examinations already exist (Counts & Dempster, 2008; NONPF, 2008);
- Is too broad to assess competency among DNP graduates with differing roles and specialties (NONPF, 2008);
- Could result in decreased safety and quality of care (Guadagnino & Mundinger, 2008);
- May dissuade nurses from becoming APRNs (NONPF, 2008); and
- May add an extraneous certification examination that may increase barriers to practice (NONPF, 2008).

WHERE DO WE GO FROM HERE?

We are currently sitting at another crossroads in nursing history where proponents and opponents of the DNP competency examination are currently unable to find a middle ground between their two divergent positions. The nursing profession has continually experienced "growing pains" since the days of Florence Nightingale. While some innovations have flourished, others have failed, and yet others have undergone metamorphosis through lively dialogue. For example, when the National League for Nursing refused to give nurse midwives a special niche during their 1954 convention, a group of 20 nurse midwives formed the American College of Nurse Midwifery (ACNM) (Rooks, 1997). Despite the alienation that nurse midwives felt from the nursing profession in the 1950s, today State Boards of Nursing, the Advanced Practice Registered Nurse Consensus Group, and the ACNM are working side-by-side with other professional nursing organizations on *The Consensus Model for Advanced Practice Registered Nurses* (APRN Consensus Work Group & the National Council of State Boards of Nursing APRN Advisory Committee, 2008).

Representatives from both groups will need to come to the negotiating table to decide on the values they hold in common and work to achieve high standards of quality and safety from a common vision. Do they both agree that they need to meet the growing needs for primary care, remove barriers to practice, and better define practice as separate yet complementary to medicine? Do they agree with the majority of nurses in the ANCC survey who support a DNP certification examination? Both groups will need to discuss their differences and find a path that meets their diverse needs. Representatives from both groups will need to better define and determine the difference in competencies between the DNP and the master's-prepared APRN so that the purpose of a national DNP certification examination is clearer. They will need to address whether a competency examination endorsed by medicine is necessary for public confidence in DNP practice.

If both groups can agree on the value of the DNP certification exam, they will need to address the reasons for its low pass rate. Because the DNP certification examination is currently designed to evaluate the competence of DNPs from adult and family practice, representatives from both groups may need to discuss the possibility of revising or developing other specialty versions of examination so that it is a more valid measure of other clinical APRN specialties. In addition, both groups will also need to discuss the possibility of revising the DNP competency examination to better reflect the population-based focus of the DNP curriculum.

SUMMARY

As the doctoral APRN moves into the future, the nursing profession and individual APRN specialties will need to define the competencies that result in the highest-quality care for patients and their families, as well as set them apart from the practice of medicine. Both opponents and proponents of the DNP competency examination are needed at the negotiating table to explore what is ultimately best for patient care. Because properly managed interpersonal conflict can result in opportunities for new learning and growth, the opinions of both sides may be needed to drive the growth of doctoral APRN practice to its fullest potential. So now, after having read this chapter, are you for the new DNP certification exam? Yes? No? Perhaps you want to think it about it more . . . and then decide.

REFERENCES

American Association of Colleges of Nursing (AACN). (1996). *The essentials of masters education for advanced practice nursing.* Retrieved from http://www.aacn.nche.edu/Education/pdf/MasEssentials96.pdf

American Association of Colleges of Nursing (AACN). (2006). *The essentials of doctoral education for advanced nursing practice.* Retrieved from http://www.aacn.nche.edu/DNP/pdf/Essentials.pdf

American Board of Comprehensive Care. (2009). *Examination content for DNP certification examination.* Retrieved from http://www.abcc.dnpcert.org/09DNPpractice.pdf

American Board of Comprehensive Care. (2010a). *About the ABCC and the CACC.* Retrieved from http://www.abcc.dnpcert.org/about.shtml

American Board of Comprehensive Care. (2010b). *Eligibility requirements.* Retrieved from http://www.abcc.dnpcert.org/overview.shtml

American Board of Comprehensive Care. (2010c). *2009 Certification examination performance data.* Retrieved from http://www.abcc.dnpcert.org/exam_performance.shtml

American Nurses Credentialing Center. (2010). *ANCC DNP survey results released.* Retrieved from http://198.65.134.123/Headlines/DNPSurveyResults.aspx

American Psychiatric Nurses Association. (2010). *An introduction to LACE.* Retrieved from http://www.apna.org/i4a/pages/index.cfm?pageid=3498

APRN Consensus Work Group & the National Council of State Boards of Nursing APRN Advisory Committee. (2008). *Consensus model for APRN regulation: licensure, accreditation, certification & education.* Retrieved from http://www.aacn.nche.edu/Education/pdf/APRNReport.pdf

Counts, M., & Dempster, J. (2008, April 4). Letter to the Editor sent to the *Wall Street Journal*. *American Academy of Nurse Practitioners.* Retrieved from http://www.aanp.org/NR/rdonlyres/9A676C85-022C-460B-9FCD-63361829DF8A/0/wsjletter0408.pdf

Dreher, H. M., & Montgomery, K. E. (2009). Let's call it "doctoral" advanced practice nursing. *The Journal of Continuing Nursing Education, 40*(12), 530–531.

Guadagnino, C., & Mundinger, M. (2008). Growing role of nurse practitioners. *Physician News Digest.* Retrieved from http://www.lifeupenn.org/Growing%20role%20of%20nurse%20practitioners.pdf

Hoyt, S., & Proehl, J. (2009). Weighing in on the DNP examination. *Advanced Emergency Nursing Journal, 31*(4), 261–263.

Johnson, P. J. (2008). The DNP* storm. *Neonatal Network, 27*(5), 297–298.

Kane, R. (2009). The advanced practice nurse: An answer to the primary care challenge. *Clinical Scholars Review, 1*(1), 37–28.

Landro, L. (2008, April 2). Making room for Dr. nurse. *Wall Street Journal.* Retrieved from http://online.wsj.com/public/article_print/SB120710036831882059.html

McGrath, J. M., & Piques, A. (2009). The past, the present, and the prospective student: Is there a recipe for the DNP? *Journal of Perinatal and Neonatal Nursing, 23*(3), 207–212.

Michalski, K., Sagan, C., Moore, K., Bednash, G., & Rosseter, R. (2006). Readers and authors respond to "Introducing the Doctor of Nursing Practice." Retrieved from http://www.medscape.com/viewarticle/543596

Mundinger, M. (2007, November 28). Who will be your doctor? *Forbes.com.* Retrieved from http://www.forbes.com/2007/11/27/nurses-doctors-practice-oped-cx_mom_1128nurses.html?partner=alerts

Mundinger, M. (2008a). Certification is the answer: What is the question? *Clinical Scholars Review, 1*(1), 3–4.

Mundinger, M. (2008b). American Board of Comprehensive Care Certification (ABCC): Too close to medicine? *Clinical Scholars Review, 1*(2), 67.

Mundinger, M. (2009). The clinical doctorate 15 years hence. *Clinical Scholars Review, 2*(2), 35–36.

Mundinger, M. O., Starck, P., Hathaway, D., Shaver, J., & Woods, N. F. (2009). The ABCs of the doctor of nursing practice: Assessing resources, building a culture of clinical scholarship, curricular models. *Journal of Professional Nursing, 25*(2), 69–74.

National Board of Medical Examiners. (2009). *Development of a certifying examination for doctors of nursing practice.* Retrieved from http://www.nbme.org/PDF/NBME-Development-of-DNP-Cert-Exam.PDF

National Organization of Nurse Practitioner Faculties. (2008). *Nurse practitioner DNP education, certification and titling: A unified statement.* Retrieved from http://www.nonpf.com/associations/10789/files/DNPUnifiedStatement0608.pdf

Rooks, J. (1997). *Midwifery and childbirth in America.* Philadelphia, PA: Temple University Press.

Stanik-Hutt, J. (2008). Debunking the need to certify the DNP degree. *The Journal for Nurse Practitioners, 4*(10), 739.

CHAPTER TWENTY-TWO: Reflective Response 1

Janice Smolowitz

In this chapter, Dr. Posmontier reviews the history, context, and commentary about the American Board of Comprehensive Care (ABCC) examination as a basis for understanding and exploring the current controversy that surrounds this examination. As an advanced practice registered nurse (APRN), educator, and Diplomate of Comprehensive Care (DCC), I was struck by the author's consistent reference to this voluntary certification as the "DNP examination." I believe that using the term "DNP Examination" contributes to the controversy and obscures the purpose of the examination. Although only graduates of DNP degree programs may qualify to take the ABCC examination, it is not the "DNP examination." The ABCC examination is designed to test the knowledge of doctorally prepared APRNs who specialize in the provision of comprehensive care (Starck, 2010).

Over the past few years, there has been a rapid proliferation of DNP degree programs. These programs focus on direct and indirect care. The majority of programs do not prepare students to take the ABCC examination, which tests knowledge of the provision of comprehensive care. DNP APRNs who focus on the provision of comprehensive care have educational preparation beyond that of a master's-prepared adult or family nurse practitioner. They are expert clinicians who are knowledgeable about individuals' health care needs across the lifespan, practice in all clinical settings, analyze and interpret evidence as the basis for health care choices, and engage patients in collaborative relationships in the provision of continuous, coordinated services that include health promotion, disease prevention, and definitive disease management (Smolowitz, Honig, & Reinisch, 2010). DNP APRNs who successfully complete the certification examination are designated as DCCs to identify the area of specialization (ABCC, n.d.; Council for the Advancement of Comprehensive Care, n.d.).

When discussing the examination, Dr. Posmontier addresses differences between master's- and doctorally prepared APRNs utilizing the American Association of Colleges of Nursing's (AACN) *Essentials* (2006). She notes that proponents of the examination argue that DNPs invest more time in education to prepare themselves as leaders in translating research into practice and to address the faculty shortage. When considering the AACN *Essentials* (2006) and the ABCC examination, discussion should solely focus on *Essential VIII: Advanced Nursing Practice* (AACN, 2006). According to Essential VIII, increased health care sophistication has resulted in nursing specialization to ensure competence in complex practice areas. DNP programs provide specialty preparation in one area of nursing practice and integrate additional practice experiences throughout the program to provide learning experiences in a variety of patient care settings. The ABCC examination specifically tests knowledge of health and illness *across the lifespan and clinical settings*, providing mechanisms by which DNP graduates of programs that focus on comprehensive care can validate their additional clinical expertise.

Dr. Posmontier describes some of the debate surrounding who is qualified to take the ABCC examination using current APRN titles. Discussion should instead focus on shaping the future of DNP education to prepare graduates to meet society's needs. Looking to the future, the ABCC examination should be utilized as a mechanism for testing knowledge of comprehensive care for APRNs as explicated in the *Consensus Model for APRN Regulation: Licensure, Accreditation, Certification and Education* (LACE) (APRN Consensus Work Group & the National Council of State Boards of Nursing APRN Advisory Committee, 2008). According to LACE criteria, individuals will be licensed as independent practitioners in one of the four APRN roles within at least one of the identified population foci. Practice specialization will occur within the established population. According to this model, a DNP APRN in the role of a certified nurse practitioner, who specializes in cross-site health care, and is educated to provide care for individuals across the lifespan, could choose to sit for the ABCC examination to demonstrate competency.

While I appreciate the varying viewpoints presented by Dr. Posmontier, I was deeply distressed by the number of opinions offered by members of the medical and nursing community, which were presented as fact. Statements have been made about the development of the examination and its implications for the nursing profession. This examination is built on the principle that health care professionals who deliver similar clinical services should be held to the same standards. At the present time, it is not possible to conduct a practice analysis of comprehensive care, as too few APRNs are formally educated or clearly identified to perform this. Although the ABCC examination blueprint is not based on an APRN practice analysis, the items in the test pool have been validated using a standardized process by National Board of Medical Examiner (NBME) psychometricians and APRNs appointed by Council for the Advancement of Comprehensive Care (Starck, 2010).

Dr. Posmontier discusses the 50% pass rate achieved by 45 examinees in 2008 and the 57% pass rate among 19 examinees in 2009. These facts have been used to support the argument that this is not a valid examination. There is another interpretation of these data. The first two examinations are considered beta tests. Very few DNP programs focused on comprehensive care have been developed, and the curriculum is not standardized. Moreover, this interpretation is not without precedent. According to Donald Melnick, MD, President, NBME, only 8 of 15 physicians who took the first NBME examination in 1916 passed. Dr. Melnick has also stated that over the years this exam has been a driver for better medical education (Starck, 2010).

In summary, the ABCC examination (not the DNP examination) is not controlled by physicians. It does, however, reflect DNP APRN competency in a clinical specialty. The ABCC examination measures the common clinical knowledge of comprehensive care providers developed for DNP-prepared clinicians by similarly DNP-prepared clinicians.

REFERENCES

American Association of Colleges of Nursing (AACN). (2006). *The essentials of doctoral education for advanced nursing practice.* Retrieved from http://www.aacn.nche.edu/dnp/pdf/Essentials.pdf
American Board of Comprehensive Care (ABCC). (n.d.). *About the ABCC and the CACC.* Retrieved from http://www.abcc.dnpcert.org/about.shtml

APRN Consensus Work Group & the National Council of State Boards of Nursing APRN Advisory Committee. (2008). *Consensus model for APRN regulation: Licensure, accreditation, certification & education.* Retrieved from http://www.aacn.nche.edu/Education/pdf/APRNReport.pdf

Council for the Advancement of Comprehensive Care. (n.d.). Home page. Retrieved from http://caccnet.org/

Smolowitz, J., Honig, J., & Reinisch, C. (2010). *Writing DNP clinical case Narratives: Demonstrating and evaluating competency in comprehensive care.* New York, NY: Springer.

Starck, P. (2010). DNP comprehensive care certification: What are the issues? *Clinical Scholars Review, 3*(2), 59–63.

CHAPTER TWENTY-TWO: Reflective Response 2

Geraldine M. Budd

Nurse practitioners (NPs) and other advanced practice nurses (APRNs) are committed to providing safe, independent, and high-quality patient care. This is why the American Association of Colleges of Nursing (AACN) voted in 2004 to endorse the Doctor of Nursing Practice (DNP) degree. This is also why the DNP exam was developed for APRNs. While the DNP degree is a positive move for the nursing profession, the DNP exam is not. Below, I outline the reasons why I believe this is so.

Currently, only 23 states allow for completely independent NP practice (Pearson, 2010); all other states require some type of physician supervision of NPs. Most nursing authorities recognize that physician supervision limits the scope of NPs to provide care to patients in a high-quality and cost-efficient manner. In contrast, some physicians and policy makers believe that NP supervision or collaboration with physicians is needed because NPs have less education and, therefore, a high potential to deliver unsafe or inferior care when compared to physicians (Flanagan, 1998; Freudenheim, 1997; Winslow, 1997).

Twenty years of data have demonstrated that NP care is superior or similar to that of physician care (American Academy of Nurse Practitioners, 2007/2010). The most notable study was led by Dr. Mary Mundinger, Dean of the Columbia University School of Nursing (Mundinger et al., 2000) and a strong advocate of independent NP practice. This nursing leader has led a multifaceted quest to ensure that NPs obtain the right to practice independently. Her accomplishments include beginning an independent NP practice at Columbia University and spearheading a major media campaign to promote it (Flanagan, 1998). Dr. Mundinger was also an early supporter of the DNP as the standard degree for NP practice and she opened one of the first DNP programs (first a DrNP) in the country at Columbia University. Then, in 2008, she joined forces with established medicine to bring forth the DNP exam. This final step sets Dr. Mundinger apart from other nursing leaders advocating for independent NP practice. It represents a backward- rather than a forward-thinking move for nursing. Patterning an exam for NPs after a medical exam and having the National Board of Medical Examiners (NBME) involved in the administration of this exam brings nursing full circle back to being subservient and controlled by medicine. Most nursing experts and national organizations (National Organization for Nurse Practitioner Faculties, American Academy of Nurse Practitioners, National Conference of Gerontological Nurse Practitioners, and American College of Nurse Practitioners among others) strive to consistently paint a "separate but equal to physicians" view of NPs and APRNs. All members of the health care team work together to do what is best for the patient. Their roles and objectives may differ, however. For NPs and APRNs the major emphasis is on safe and effective care that stresses patient–provider communication and health promotion education, while physicians generally adhere to more of a disease cure model. That said, NPs—as APRNs in some states—diagnose

435

and treat medical problems. Barbara Safriet (1994) of the Yale law faculty has written extensively about physicians limiting APRN practice and points out that physicians have tried to establish themselves as the sole overseers of the treatment of all human illness and suffering. Providing limits to what other providers can do with patients is generally seen by those in the legal world as *restraint of trade*. That physicians, desire to restrain the trade of other providers, in this case NPs and APRNs, must serve as a reminder that physicians often have a lack of interdisciplinary perspective on training and practice, and instead focus on protecting their "turf" (Safriet).

Certification is now required for NP licensure in 46 states. To be eligible for advanced practice certification, a registered nurse must hold a master's or higher degree in nursing and must have been prepared to provide care to a specified population (e.g., adults, families, children, acute-care patients). These criteria are outlined in an important document, the *Consensus Model for APRN Regulation: Licensure, Accreditation, Certification & Education* (APRN Consensus Work Group & the National Council of State Boards of Nursing APRN Advisory Committee, 2008). Over 50 nursing organizations collaborated to develop this landmark work, outlining the essential components of certification and education, and clearly describing a process of ensuring APRN competency that is controlled by the nursing profession. In addition to the *Consensus Model for APRN Regulation* (2008), the AACN is closely monitoring the issues related to movement to the DNP for APRNs. This group is providing frequent updates to the nursing community and has begun the process of accrediting DNP programs. It is clear that as education for NPs and APRNs moves to a DNP-only model, certifying bodies will respond and adapt to their requirements for sitting for exams.

In 2008, seven NP organizations, representing education and practice, developed an *NP DNP Education, Certification and Titling: A Unified Statement* (Nurse Practitioner Roundtable, June 2008). The consensus of that group best represents what nursing has previously—and should currently and in the future—stood firm on:

> Certification examinations for nurse practitioners are based upon sound scientific principles of advanced nursing practice and knowledge. These examinations are developed from the discipline of nursing and do not draw from another discipline's examination or examination mechanism.
>
> —*Nurse Practitioner Roundtable, 2008, p. 2*

It will be interesting to follow this issue as it continues to percolate in the profession.

REFERENCES

American Academy of Nurse Practitioners. (2007/2010). Quality of nurse practitioner practice. Retrieved from http://www.aanp.org/NR/rdonlyres/34E7FF57-E071-4014-B554-FF02B82FF2F2/0/QualityofNPPractice4pages.pdf

APRN Consensus Work Group & the National Council of State Boards of Nursing APRN Advisory Committee. (2008). *Consensus model for APRN regulation: Licensure, accreditation, certification, and education*. Retrieved from http://www.aacn.nche.edu/Education/pdf/APRNReport.pdf

Flanagan, L. (1998). Nursing practitioners: Growing competition for family physicians? *Family Practice Management, 5*(9), 34–36, 41–43.

Freudenheim, M. (1997, September 30). Nurses increasingly becoming primary-care physicians/Health-care industry sees innovation as another way to cut costs. *New York Times.com*. Retrieved from http://www.nytimes.com/1997/09/30/business/as-nurses-take-on-primary-care-physicians-are-sounding-alarms.html?ref=nursing_and_nurses

Mundinger, M. O., Kane, R. L., Lenz, E. R., Totten, A. M., Cleary, P. D., Friedewald, W. T. et al. (2000). Primary care outcomes in patients treated by nurse practitioners or physicians. *Journal of the American Medical Association, 283,* 59–68.

Nurse Practitioner Roundtable. (2008). *Nurse practitioner DNP education, certification and titling: A unified statement.* Washington, DC: Author.

Pearson, L. (2010). *The Pearson Report 2010: The annual state-by-state national overview of nurse practitioner legislation and healthcare issues* [online by subscription only at http://www.pearsonreport.com/]. Summary retrieved from http://www.pearsonreport.com/overview

Safriet, B. J. (1994). Impediments to progress in health care workforce policy: License and practice laws. *Inquiry, 31,* 310–317.

Winslow, R. (1997, February 7). Nurses to take doctor duties, Oxford says. *The Wall Street Journal,* p. A3.

CRITICAL THINKING QUESTIONS

1. What are the major differences between master's and doctoral-level certifications?
2. What do you think are pros and cons of the NBME's designing the DNP certification examination? Would another certifying body be more appropriate and why?
3. What are the major factors that differentiate the DNP practice from physician-based primary care practice?
4. Does the DNP certification examination promote or obstruct multidisciplinary collaboration? Why?
5. Does the DNP certification examination enhance public confidence? Why or why not? What is your rationale?
6. How can the current 50% pass rate support the arguments of both opponents and proponents of the DNP certification examination?
7. Would another layer of certification dissuade or encourage nurses from becoming APRNs? What is your rationale?
8. How could you argue that DNP certification improves patient care?
9. How would you answer the criticism that there are already enough psychometrically sound APRN certification examinations?
10. What are your thoughts about the appropriateness of the DNP certification examination for APRN specialties other than family and adult advanced nursing practice? How would you answer the criticism that the examination is not appropriate for specialty APRNs such as pediatric and women's health care APRNs?

CHAPTER TWENTY-THREE

Advising Doctor of Nursing Practice "Clinicians" How Their Role Will Evolve with a Practice Doctorate

Perspectives from a 30-Year Nurse Practitioner

Joan Rosen Bloch

INTRODUCTION

How similar or different will advanced practice nurses who are DNP/DrNP[1] graduates be compared to Master of Science in Nursing (MSN) graduates? Will roles be different for advanced practice nurses who formally had MSNs and build upon that with their doctorate in nursing practice? How will they differ? Will the roles evolve by inductive or deductive development—or perhaps a combination of both? What determining factors will shape the roles of advanced practice-registered nurses (APRNs) with different "levels" of education preparation? Must we be prescriptive and restrictive, at this point jeopardizing the flexibility and creativity of professional roles that may evolve? Perhaps, with requisite skills and knowledge offered at the doctoral level, empowered nurses can build upon their prior education and practice experiences, and let their professional journey grow in a flexible way that best serves three main stakeholders: the profession of nursing, health care systems, and, of course, the people served by both the profession of nursing and systems of health care.

MUST THE ROLE BE DEFINED AT THIS TIME? WHAT IS THE VISION?

If you are reading this chapter and seeking direction of how either your role will be shaped differently, or how, as an educator, you can facilitate shaping the role of your doctor of nursing practice (DNP) students in ways that are different from the MSN student, you probably are reading this introduction and wondering if the above paragraph has created "double talk" with no clear vision. You are probably right. If you think you will find a clear role description that separately delineates APRN roles based on the MSN and DNP degrees, pause right now ... because ... the vision is being shaped *now* by all of us. We (you and us) are the next generation of what Dunphy, Youngkin, and Smith (2004) coined as the "rebels, renegades, and trailblazers" (p. 25) of nursing's future. The rebels, renegades, and trailblazers of yesteryear shaped the current myriad of APRN roles as we know them today. Yet, as you read in previous chapters of this book, formalization of the APRN role into the construct as we now know it took multiple decades. Remember, Loretta Ford, EdD, RN, PNP, FAAN, the pioneer of the nurse practitioner movement, met tremendous resistance from the discipline of nursing as she forged forward with her visionary model of nursing practice with the nurse practitioner role (Ford, 1997). (See earlier chapters to learn more about the history of the APRN role as we know it today. Carefully consider the barriers that those bold and brave nurses confronted. Are there parallels today?)

Shaping the future role possibilities of a nursing workforce with practice doctorates occurring in the years to come rests with all of us. Not only is this a time of creativity, but a time for critical evaluation of why one is considering the DNP degree and not the traditional PhD. Deep, honest reflection of this basic question should yield great insights to guide a myriad of possibilities that should enhance the nursing profession's tripartite contributions (practice, research, and education) for the greater good of society. History has shown us that the boundaries of practice are pliable and flexible enough to change with time and context to meet the needs of all stakeholders (Aiken & Fagin, 1992; Joel, 2004; Stanley, 2005). Passage to this new millennium with the nursing practice doctorate presents new opportunities for the profession of nursing to empower those most passionate about nursing, who have the perseverance to pursue and accomplish a terminal degree marked in their disciplinary home in nursing. The practice doctorate *must* differ from the traditional PhD to take the nurse on a trajectory beyond the "research walls" of academia in which the PhD is expected to advance nursing science as a full-time research scholar (Bloch, 2005; McGrath & Piques, 2009). Yet, while the degree is separate, but equal, nursing doctorate graduates *must* work together for the greater good of nursing and health care. With health care reform under the Barack Obama presidency, this is an opportune time for nursing. Nursing is central to the key policy issues and has the ability to shape health care reform (Fairman, 2010). Nursing made great strides in the last half of the 20th century, with profound role successes in practice as APRNs and in academia as PhD scholars. The fight for the development and acceptance of nursing PhD programs and the APRN role did not happen overnight, but took more than a quarter century (McGrath & Piques). While the work of the last century emphasized getting our foothold into academia and into independent practice arenas where we are now more visible to other "players" (i.e., beyond those of our patients who were cared for by nurses), the profession is now well positioned to participate in shaping and improving the health and health care system of our nation.

Unity and coalitions between all those in nursing, regardless of all degrees and the "alphabet soup of credentials" within the nursing profession are necessary. As we forge ahead into this millennium and allow our insights from our disciplinary lens to be shared and heard at interdisciplinary forums, we must take this opportunity to work together to try to repair our health care system which is in a dire state of crisis. While the infant mortality rate in the United States ranks 30th compared to all other nations (MacDorman & Mathews, 2009), and while we are about the wealthiest country in the world, it is quite apparent that our health care system is broken and desperately needs help. With the success of nursing roles (the independent role of APRNs in practice and PhD scholars in academia), it is exciting that the evolving practice doctorate has been embraced nationally, and in record speed. This is evidenced by the results of the American Association of Colleges in Nursing (AACN) 2009 survey, revealing that there were already 120 DNP/DrNP programs with another 161 planned (AACN, 2010). Clearly, there is a need for another level of expertise that builds upon MSN education in practice, despite a clear prescription for the role in the marketplace for the DNP graduate. As McGrath and Piques (2009) explain, nursing's commitment to this practice doctorate reveals our commitment to advancing health care by educating a generation of very motivated nurses to create unprecedented opportunities within a multilayered, complex health care environment. Thus, the future roles will be shaped by the expertise the DNP brings to health care practice and policy.

MSN VERSUS DNP: WHICH IS BETTER ENTRY INTO APRN CLINICAL PRACTICE?

Should the DNP be required for entry into APRN practice by 2015 as the AACN has proclaimed (AACN, 2004)? With the formation of this new academic doctorate degree, there has been ferocious debate among nursing leadership about restructuring APRN educational curriculum, certification, and licensure related to APRN practice. With much confusion mounted by uncertainty leading to rumors, concerns, and dissension, the leaders of key nursing organizations that were stakeholders in current and future roles for APRNs formed a group to work hard to reach consensus. This group works to bring unity so that nursing as a whole can move forward together as a united entity, to work with the larger community and improve the health of this nation (APRN Consensus Work Group, 2008). While during the mid-1990s to 2003 organizations made individual and collaborative efforts to address the myriad of regulatory APRN issues, it was not until 2003 when they all came together. After a six-year period, they reached an agreement on a consensus model for APRN regulation. The model established guidelines for titling, education, certification, accreditation, and licensing for the four clinical APRN roles—certified registered nurse anesthetists (CRNAs), certified nurse midwives (CNMs), clinical nurse specialists (CNSs), and certified nurse practitioners (CNPs).This model, endorsed by 44 national nursing organizations, is a great feat for nursing; for in addition to developing nationally recognized standards for APRN regulation, the consensus model clarified the role and scope of APRNs, which assists policy makers and the lay public with understanding the key roles of APRNs (Stanley, Werner, & Apple, 2009).

For details about the consensus model, referred to by the acronym LACE (Licensure, Accreditation, Certification, and Education), the reader is directed to the cited article by Stanley et al. (2009). However, it is imperative to understand that the LACE model *does not repute the value of MSN as entry into APRN clinical practice*. While AACN and other organizations recommend the practice doctorate for clinical APRN roles, there is currently no movement to actually restrict APRN licensure and certification only to DNP graduates. Dr. Anne O'Sullivan, a member of the consensus group and former president of the National Organization of Nurse Practitioner Faculties (NONPF), in her report on April 18, 2010 at NONPF's annual conference held in Washington, DC, clarified, on behalf of the consensus group, that there is no current plan to dissolve the MSN degree requirement as the entry degree for APRN practice. She emphasized that there is absolutely no evidence that the public would be better served by changing the MSN-required degree to a DNP degree as entry into clinical APRN practice. On the contrary, it was emphasized that there is a plethora of evidence documenting the positive impact that master's prepared APRNs have had on improving health outcomes among diverse populations with various health conditions throughout the United States (Joel, 2004; Stanley, 2005). So, why should entry into APRN practice be changed from requiring an MSN degree to a DNP degree?

The two officially recognized accreditation agencies for nursing by the U.S. Secretary of Education, The National League for Nursing Accrediting Commission

(NLNAC) and Commission on Collegiate Nursing Education (CCNE), have clarified that they will continue to accredit master's-level educational programs, and their standards have not changed to require doctoral preparation for nurse practitioner programs. Although the AACN's (2006) document, *The Essentials of Doctoral Education for Advanced Nursing Practice*, recommends 2015 as a date for transition from master's to DNP degree programs for APRN education, they have clarified that this date was only a recommendation (NONPF, 2010).

WILL THE PRACTICE DOCTORATE EDUCATIONAL JOURNEY PROVIDE ADDITIONAL KNOWLEDGE AND SKILLS TO CHANGE THE CLINICIAN ROLE?

The DNP is an academic degree, not a specific prescribed clinical role. At the current time, it is designed to build upon former academic nursing degrees to enhance and provide knowledge above and beyond that provided at the MSN and Bachelor of Science in Nursing (BSN) levels. With a practice doctorate, however, it is anticipated that current advanced practice clinical nursing roles will be enhanced so that doctoral advanced practice nurses can apply new knowledge and skills to improve health and health care systems. The AACN's (2006) aforementioned key document, *The Essentials of Doctoral Education for Advanced Nursing Practice*, outlines and defines eight foundational outcome competencies for graduates of practice doctorate programs. These eight foundational competencies were previously cited in Chapter 4 and throughout this text. Educators use these competencies as the key roadmap to create innovative and integrated curricula to meet these competencies.

With critical evaluation of these competencies, one should be able to identify that there are developmental components of these competencies that are woven throughout nursing curricula from undergraduate to doctoral levels. For example, at the undergraduate level, required basic science courses introduce BSN students to scientific underpinnings of practice, and clinical rotations based in hospitals introduce BSN students to complex systems. Yet, professional roles differ developmentally. At the baccalaureate level, professional role development requires understanding the role of the nurse. Upon graduating with a MSN degree, the professional role is developmentally focused on their "new" advanced nursing practice role, a role different from their BSN nursing role.[2]

Problematic for issues of nursing leadership and advancement in today's complex health care systems is that the current curricula for master's educational programs are filled to capacity with little room for additional courses with additional content (Newland, 2010). Therefore, the practice doctorate is a natural next step for clinicians who want more from their professional role. Thus, DNP curricula, by design, include higher-level and expanded content. At the current time, most practice doctorate students enter DNP programs with a master's degree built upon AACN's (1996) *The Essentials of Master's Education for Advanced Practice Nursing*. Dr. Jamesetta Newland, the editor-in-chief of *The Nurse Practitioner: The American Journal of Primary Healthcare* and a Fellow of the American Academy of Nurse Practitioners (FAANP), articulates and justifies the need for additional education with the formation of a practice doctorate. She argues that leadership skills must be part of the curriculum, and not dependent on acquisition of these skills as "on the job training" often "under fire." To meet the extensive learning objectives for today's practice as an APRN, the typical length of an MSN nursing program is insufficient and argues for more education for ANPs and for recognition of the additional education as a practice doctorate. She states:

> Why should nursing not have a practice doctorate as do other major health care professions? ... The DNP is a practice doctorate conceived to prepare advanced clinical leaders in developing the skills necessary to bring about change within the health care organization to improve quality of care and health outcomes.
>
> —*Newland, 2010, p. 5*

AN ECOLOGIC EDUCATIONAL FRAMEWORK APPROACH TO THE PRACTICE DOCTORATE

The goal held by many educators is that future roles for DNP graduates will be based in practice (Bloch, 2005; Boland, Treston, & O'Sullivan, 2010; Newland, 2010). Curricula are designed to allow the doctoral educational journey to be one of professional growth and empowerment that builds upon clinical experience and expertise shaped prior to MSN preparation. It can be viewed as an advanced version of the "novice to expert" APRN role for which one finds oneself upon completion of one's MSN degree. With this novice to expert construct applied in advanced nursing practice, the goal for the DNP role is that DNP graduates are positioned (with their new doctoral level knowledge) to seize opportunities as they come by using this academic credential (DNP) to open doors, to be creative, and help transform their workplace or the health care system in which they seek employment. This theme was confirmed in a descriptive longitudinal study of 22 DNP graduates from the University of Washington. The graduates emphasized that their doctoral work enhanced their practice roles in multiple ways, increasing parity with physician colleagues with better skills and opportunities to translate research to practice and policy (Brown & Kaplan, 2010). Students who are deciding between a practice doctorate (DNP) or a research doctorate (PhD) should decipher where they really see their role: (1) entrenched in the real world of health care practice, or (2) behind the "ivy towers" entrenched in curriculum development and the conduct of research in the pursuit of advancing nursing knowledge requiring competition for research grants. Yet, these two worlds must intersect, for those with DNPs have an important academic role educating future APRNs. Therefore, such a dichotomy is not so neats and the nursing discipline should look at other disciplines (e.g., medicine, dentistry, law) where the practitioners and researchers often move between both worlds. Merged communities of researchers and practitioners are essential for effective feedback loops of knowledge dissemination and translation necessary for evidence-based practice and practice-based evidence (Lyons, 2009).

Conceptualizing the possibilities of DNP roles and their subsequent impact on health and health care can be understood by an ecological education framework emphasizing how the DNP academic degree is built upon the BSN and MSN academic degrees. Within an ecologic framework, a systems perspective is viewed, consisting of the health care system and various but distinct nursing systems, integrating within this larger system with complex microlevels and macrolevels. This synergy of systems demands multidisciplinary participants having educational competencies that allow progression from entry to expert levels, preparing the practitioner with developmental knowledge and skill sets transferable to practicing within complex health care systems.

The BSN degree provides core competencies for entry into practice. The MSN degree builds upon this and allows the professional nurse to focus in a particular specialty area of nursing. In general terms, the specialization can be within the systems of nursing education, administration, or clinical practice. For APRN clinical specialties, there are regulatory licensures and professional certifications required for specific APRN clinical practice (see Chapter 3). While the historical evolution of APRN roles and resulting regulatory requirements dependent on first obtaining professional certification occurred over several decades, MSN education today is more prescriptive and shorter than those in the 1970s that produced the "rebels, renegades, and trailblazers" of yesteryear. Specific MSN programs differ dependent on the knowledge and skills acquisition for the specific specialty APRN practice. For example, MSN nurse-anesthetist programs are quite different from the pediatric nurse practitioner and nurse midwifery programs. At the completion of a master's degree, advanced practice nurses have a concrete idea of what their clinical role will be as an MSN-prepared APRN; they chose their specialty area. Their studies were focused on their specific specialty role and socialization to that specialty APRN role. Their classroom and clinical practicum experiences were therefore tailored to meet learning goals for their clinical specialty APRN role.

PATHWAYS TO POTENTIAL DNP ROLES

With a leap of faith, a love of clinical nursing, and a passion for learning, practice doctorate students are ripe for an empowering journey in academia. Acquiring a terminal degree provides opportunities for individualized tailored learning experiences that build upon their particular clinical specialty interest within the greater context of their doctoral courses. Intensive advisement from doctoral faculty facilitates this process and simultaneously creates a synergistic relationship between doctoral faculty and doctoral students. Thus, doctoral education differs dramatically from master's APRN-prescribed education.

Glowing as it sounds, what about the practicalities? What exactly will the graduate do? Will employers want to hire, and even pay more for a practice doctorates? Well, this line of reasoning has never interfered with the attainment of higher academic degrees. Do students pursue PhDs in the humanities because of potential salaries? A PhD in early American Victorian romance literature surely was not a ticket to becoming a millionaire; however, it may have provided the particular individual with an irreplaceable intellectual satisfaction above and beyond any other. Should clinical nurses not have advanced educational opportunities that permit them to build upon what they already know, and occupy professional roles that can advance practice, perhaps in ways in which the PhD graduate cannot? The evidence is solid that nurses, staff nurses, *and* APNs often take a salary reduction after obtaining a PhD and transitioning to faculty positions (Yucca & Witt, 2009). Imagine, clinical nurses can advance their academic degree and remain in practice. Perhaps their income will change — maybe for a higher rate, but not necessarily; however, their opportunities will expand. If a position requires independent thinking, creativity, innovation, and leadership, it is only the nature of the applicant with the best credentials who is most likely to get it. It may be the academic degree that differentiates the applicants. Thus, having a DNP degree should trump an MSN degree if all other qualifications are equal.

TABLE 23.1
Student Tips for Success for Creating Your New and Expanded Doctor of Nursing Practice Role

Tips	Examples
1. Use your educational journey to build upon your prior professional experiences. Critically evaluate your knowledge deficits and how your prior professional settings may have limited your exposures and experiences.	▓ Knowledge is power. Empower your future opportunities by gaining more knowledge. Put yourself in settings that you may not have had access to before.
	▓ Go to community policy meetings or shadow top "administrators or policy makers" to broaden your perspectives of the micro- and macroenvironments.
	▓ Take courses not exposed to before (e.g., finances, basic science, advanced informatics); something that will give you an advantage in the area in which you seek your role development.
2. Take this educational journey as an opportunity to expand your horizons. Explore different role options and use the opportunity of your "student" status to shadow experts in those roles.	▓ Reach out to a Centers for Disease Control and Prevention (CDC) official working in your area of interest. Perhaps you can visit the CDC and schedule a focused visit that meets your individually created objectives. You can "test out" such a position to see if that is what you may want to work towards.
3. Peer-mentor your classmates and let yourself be peer-mentored by your classmates.	▓ Strong bonds are created during doctoral studies, especially when you are the ones shaping the future roles of nurses with practice doctorates. Learn the strengths that each of you has and how you may collaborate in a way that builds on what each of you can "bring to the table."
4. Intra-disciplinary and inter-disciplinary collaboration will be essential for the success of your new role. Remember: professional relationships are built on trust, honest communication, and integrity. Professional behaviors built on these qualities will enhance your ability to serve as a positive role model of the practice doctorate (Chism, 2009). This may be your best asset after your title of *Doctor* opens new doors.	▓ As the first generation with practice doctorates, you serve as a role model. Your professionalism and ethical nursing practice must prevail at the highest standards. Others will be testing you; if you pass, opportunities will be presented. If you use your doctoral degree unwisely to wield power and control, you will meet much resistance. (Houdin, Naylor, & Haller, 2004; McGrath & Piques, 2009).
5. Lastly, never complain about the costs of your doctoral degree. When you negotiate your role and compensation, do your homework. Know your market worth and do not expect your future employer to pay more just for the *doctor* title unless you can *articulate* the returns on their investment will be above and beyond what is being offered. Seeking a practice doctorate was your choice!	▓ "Attitude, attitude, attitude" is critical in the workplace environment. Attitudes reflecting gratitude for the opportunities your employer has provided will win support when you propose your award winning ideas. Attitudes of resentment that you are undervalued and underpaid contaminate workplace morale. If you truly believe that is your situation, it is time to "move on" and, equipped with your practice doctorate, find a different role for you.

Graduates of practice doctorate programs have already entered the marketplace across the nation. NONPF has embraced the DNP degree as a key role for clinical educators. As senior nurse practitioner faculty have begun to retire, new faculty prepared with DNPs are now actively involved in preparing the next generation of nurse practitioners, and their involvement in NONPF is apparent. NONPF's white paper titled *Criteria for NP Scholarly Projects in the Practice Doctorate Program* (2007) identifies the pedagogy that supports these projects, and the list in this white paper illustrates how some clinicians developed additional knowledge and skills beyond their MSN to complete such projects. A sample of scholarly project examples from NONPF's white paper can be found at the following website: http://www.nonpf.com/associations/10789/files/ScholarlyProject Criteria.pdf

SUMMARY: EMBARKING ON PRACTICE DOCTORAL STUDIES—ADVICE FOR YOUR FUTURE ROLES

As a 30-year veteran nurse practitioner who embarked on returning to academia for advanced nursing degrees in 1981 (MSN) and 1997 (PhD), I offer some advice. Keep an open mind and take the educational opportunity to learn about ways in which your contribution to the greater good of society can grow through your potential roles as a nurse. The beauty of returning to an academic center is that you are exposed not only to new knowledge from the courses you are enrolled in, but you are also exposed to others within nursing and outside of nursing who will expand your network for future opportunities directly and indirectly; perhaps directly by being offered an employment opportunity by someone you have met along this journey, or indirectly by exposing you to new types of employment opportunities you would have never considered before. As shown in Table 23.1, I have created "tips for success" that are developed from my 30 years of integrated experiences as a practicing nurse practitioner and educator.

Embarking on journeys for new academic degrees that resulted in new roles has always further strengthened my love and devotion to the discipline of nursing. Little did I know about the actual roles I would eventually assume at the completion of my first academic degree; however, I successfully found roles I did not imagine before. These new roles, enabled by my newly acquired academic degrees, provided me with immensely satisfying professional opportunities and growth. Thus, my advice to those considering embarking on a journey for a practice doctorate is to take a leap of faith with an open mind and enjoy the doctoral journey.

NOTES

1. The use of DNP is inclusive of the DrNP and any other letters that signify the nursing practice doctorate.
2. Advanced nursing practice (ANP) is used for all MSN roles and includes specific clinical APRN roles. There are excellent resources that address the specific roles for APRNs, two of which are referenced in this chapter, Stanley (2009) and Joel (2008). These books discuss very specific issues which are important as the APRN begins their journey in a new advanced role. The assumption of this chapter is that the DNP role is built from the entry educational level into APRN practice, and so these specifics are not addressed here.

REFERENCES

American Association of Colleges of Nursing (AACN). (1996). *The essentials of master's education for advanced practice nursing.* Washington, DC: Author.

American Association of Colleges of Nursing (AACN). (2004). *AACN position statement on the practice doctorate in nursing October 2004.* Retrieved from http://www.aacn.nche.edu/DNP/pdf/DNP.pdf

American Association of Colleges of Nursing (AACN). (2006). *The essentials of doctoral education for advanced nursing practice.* Retrieved from http://www.aacn.nche.edu/DNP/pdf/Essentials.pdf

American Association of Colleges of Nursing (AACN). (2010). *The doctor of nursing practice: A report on progress.* Power point slides from the 2010 annual conference. Retrieved from http://www.aacn.nche.edu/DNP/pdf/DNPForum3-10.pdf

Aiken, L., & Fagin, C. (1992). *Charting nursing's future: Agenda for the 1990s.* Philadelphia, PA: J.B. Lippincott Company.

APRN Consensus Work Group & National Council of State Boards of Nursing APRN Advisory Committee. (2008). *Consensus model for APRN regulation: Licensure, accreditation, certification & education.* Retrieved from http://aacn.nche.edu/education/pdf/APRNReport.pdf

Bloch, J. (2005). The doctor of nursing practice (DNP): Need for more dialogue. [Letter to the Editor]. *Online Journal of Nursing Issues, 10*(3). Retrieved from http://www.nursingworld.org/ojin/admin/toc.htm

Boland, B. A., Treston, J., & O'Sullivan, A. L. (2010). Whether you seek a DNP program that offers online, full-time, or part-time options, prospective students should know what to look for when pursuing this esteemed degree. *The Nurse Practitioner, 35*(4), 37–41.

Brown, M. A., & Kaplan, L. (2010). *Opening doors: The practice degree that changes practice.* Poster session presented at the 36th Annual Meeting of the National Organization of Nurse Practitioner Faculties, Washington, DC.

Chism, L. A. (2009). *The doctor of nursing practice: A guidebook for role development and professional issues.* Sudbury, MA: Jones and Bartlett.

Dunphy, L. M., Youngkin, E. Q., & Smith, N. K. (2004). Advanced practice nursing: Doing what had to be done—radicals, renegades, and rebels. In L. A. Joel, *Advanced practice nursing: Essentials for role development* (pp. 3–30). Philadelphia, PA: F. A. Davis.

Fairman, J. A. (2010) Historic and historical opportunities: Nurse practitioners and the opportunities of health reform. In E. M. Sullivan-Marx, D. O. McGivern, J. A. Fairman, & S. A. Greenberg (Eds.), *Nurse practitioners: The evolution and future of advanced practice* (pp. 3–14). New York, NY: Springer.

Ford, L. (1997). A voice from the past: 30 fascinating years as a nurse practitioner. *Clinical Excellence for Nurse Practitioners, 1*(1), 3–6.

Houdin, A. D., Naylor, M. D., & Haller, D. G. (2004). Physician–nurse collaboration in research in the 21st century. *Journal of Clinical Oncology, 22*(5), 774–776.

Joel, L. A. (2004). *Advanced practice nursing: Essentials for role development.* Philadelphia, PA: F. A. Davis Company.

Lyons, J. S. (2009). Knowledge creation through total clinical outcomes management: A practice-based evidence solution to address some of the challenges of knowledge translation. *Journal of Canadian Child and Adolescent Psychiatry, 18*(1), 38–45.

MacDorman, M. F., & Mathews, T. J. (2009). Behind international rankings of infant mortality: How the United States compares with Europe. *NCHS Data Brief, 28*, 1–8.

McGrath, J. M., & Piques, A. (2009). The past, the present, and the prospective student. *Journal of Perinatal and Neonatal Nursing, 23*(3), 207–212.

Newland, J. A. (2010). In defense of the DNP. *The Nurse Practitioner: The American Journal of Primary Healthcare, 35*(4), 5.

National Organization of Nurse Practitioner Faculties. (2007). *Criteria for NP scholarly projects in the practice doctorate program.* Retrieved from http://www.nonpf.com/associations/10789/files/ScholarlyProjectCriteria.pdf

National Organization of Nurse Practitioner Faculties. (2010). *APRN consensus model frequently asked questions*. Retrieved from http://www.nonpf.com/associations/10789/files/FAQsfinal2010.pdf

Stanley, J. M. (2005). *Advanced practice nursing* (2nd ed.). Philadelphia, PA: F. A. Davis.

Stanley, J. M., Werner, K. E., & Apple, K. (2009). Positioning advanced practice registered nurses for health care reform: Consensus on APRN regulation. *Journal of Professional Nursing, 25*(6), 340–348.

Yucca, C. B., & Witt, R. (2009). Leveraging higher salaries for nursing faculty. *Journal of Professional Nursing, 25*(3), 151–155.

CHAPTER TWENTY-THREE: Reflective Response

Carol Savrin

Dr. Bloch begins her chapter by asking if the advanced practice nurse (APN) role will be different as we begin to educate APNs at the DNP level. She then indicates that "We" are the change and that "We" are the people who are going to shape the role of the future. I most heartily agree with her assessment. If one looks at the history of the nurse practitioner role, one will see that the role has been evolving and changing ever since it was envisioned by Loretta Ford in the 1960s. The advanced practice roles developed out of a need that was identified and nurses were the ones who stepped in to fill the need. In the case of the nurse anesthetist, the job was being done by the surgeons, but since they had a greater interest in the surgery than in the anesthesia, the job was not being done well (Diers, 1991). The midwife role was initially brought here from England and filled a need in rural and underserved areas where people could not afford a doctor to assist with delivery. With the advent of the World War I, there were not enough English midwives who either came to or stayed in the United States, and so the Frontier Nursing Service under Mary Breckenridge began to train nurse midwives to fill the need (FNS, 2000). In the second reflective response in Chapter 3, Dr. Zuzelo writes that Dr. Hildegard Peplau is credited with first coining the term 'Clinical Nurse Specialist' in 1938 to describe "an advanced practice nurse with expertise in nursing practice in the care of complex patients" (p. 96). The final advanced practice role to develop was the nurse practitioner role, which began in the 1960s and 1970s in direct response to a shortage of primary care physicians in the underserved areas, especially the rural areas of the country. Traditionally, the role is agreed to have begun with the continuing education program developed by Loretta Ford and Henry Silver in Colorado in 1965–1966 (Ford, 1967).

All of the advanced practice roles have been fluid. They have changed over the years, and have evolved as society changed and as the need changed. The latest development in the APN role is that it is evolving globally. The individual culture of the local entity clearly shapes the role, so that the APN role in Botswana is different from the APN role in Singapore, which is different from the APN role in South Korea. While students might find it comforting to be told by current educators exactly what the role will be in the future, that is not how nursing has evolved, nor is it how the APN role has evolved. There was a point in time when nurses were not allowed to take blood pressures, and clearly that has changed over time. To paraphrase the overly quoted Gandhi (b. 1869, d. 1948), we have to "be the change that you want to see in the world,"[1] or in our case, the change we want to see in the NP world.

Interestingly, to some extent, the DNP or practice doctorate role has to wait for society to catch up with the responsibilities and embrace the role. When Rozella Schlotfeldt first envisioned the practice doctorate in the 1970s (Schlotfeldt, 1973), society was not ready for nurses to be educated at a doctoral level and people did not understand the role. It took many years for people to understand and embrace the role and the concept of a practice doctorate. Dr. Schlotfeldt envisioned that the ND (nursing doctorate) would affirm nursing's place as a profession and with recognition within the health care profession and as an important discipline. She envisioned the practice doctorate as very different from the PhD or research doctorate. The ND has evolved into the current DNP and all the schools that once had ND programs have revised them to DNP programs; however, the initial concept has not varied greatly. Nurses with a DNP put research into practice rather than practice a program of research. Translational research is the hallmark of the DNP.

Whether APNs are educated at the MSN or DNP level is currently highly controversial, with cost being a major issue in the discussion. However, whether they are educated at the MSN or DNP level, they will continue to evolve and will continue to meet a need within society. Dr. Bloch indicates that the current DNP is "designed to build upon former academic nursing degrees to enhance and provide knowledge beyond that provided at the BSN and MSN level" (p. 410). In fact, currently, that is true of most programs. That is partially because we have thousands of APNs who are desirous of further education and have embraced the DNP with enthusiasm. Additionally, many schools have found it easier to establish a post-master's DNP prior to the establishment of a post-baccalaureate DNP. It remains to be seen if in the future the DNP becomes a post-baccalaureate program only, as the AACN has suggested, or if the MSN will continue to be offered for the basic APN education and the DNP offered for a more extensive advanced education.

I have postulated that internationally the role of the APN developmentally can be described as paralleling the stages that are described in Erikson's stages of growth and development (Savrin, 2009). It is interesting to theorize that a similar Eriksonian pattern can be ascribed to the development of the APN role in the United States related to the educational level. It is possible that students must progress from the stage of:

1. Trust (perhaps, in their educators); to
2. Autonomy (for themselves); to
3. Initiative (making changes in their own environment); to
4. Industry (making changes in the health care environment); to
5. Intimacy (with the rest of the providers in the health care environment); and to
6. Identity (formation of a new identity of the APN role).

If one looks at the APN role and education in this manner, it may be surmised that the MSN education encompasses the first three stages and the DNP encompasses the final three stages for this development.

To argue for education at the DNP level, all APNs should learn about culture and behavior of organizations, the role of policy in the provision of health care, and the business of health care. It is possible that the APN in the initial stages must spend so much time learning about the pathophysiology, diagnosis and treatment of diseases, and the pharmacological and nonpharmacological treatment of diseases, that they are not ready to incorporate the organizational systems, the policy issues, and the business aspects into their practice settings. At this time, the post-MSN DNP is therefore transformational in changing the thinking patterns and enhancing the approach to APN practice for those folks who choose to pursue it. The post-MSN DNP students have: (1) mastered the diagnosis and treatment of the patients they see; (2) are ready to incorporate research into practice as a way of thinking; (3) to enhance practice through creating coalitions with other health care providers; and (4) working together to change the policies that govern the health care environment. I agree with Dr. Bloch that we are embarking on a journey with the practice doctorate, and that we all need to embrace the journey and see where it takes us.

NOTE

1. Quote widely cited.

REFERENCES

Diers, D. (1991). Nurse midwives and nurse anesthetists: The cutting edge in specialist practice. In L. H. Aiken, & C. M. Fagan (Eds.), *Charting nursing's future: Agenda for the 1990's* (pp. 159–180). New York, NY: Lippincott.

Ford, L., & Silver, H. (1967). The expanded role of the nurse in child care. *Nursing Outlook, 15,* 43–45. *Care, 19,* 38A–39A.

Frontier Nursing Service. (2000). *The frontier nursing service: A history.* Wendover, KY: Frontier Nursing Service Inc.

Savrin, C. (2009). Growth and development of the nurse practitioner role around the globe. *Journal of Pediatric Health Care, 23*(5), 310–314.

Schlotfeldt, R. (1973). Planning for progress. *Nursing Outlook, 21,* 766–769.

CRITICAL THINKING QUESTIONS

1. Reflect deeply within yourself and identify at least three reasons you are considering a doctoral degree in nursing.
2. Identify how you hope your professional role would change as a DNP graduate.
3. Consider the barriers that those bold and brave nurse practitioners of yesteryear confronted as the role evolved. Discuss the parallels today with the new DNP academic degree.
4. Discuss the leadership knowledge and skills you feel you need as you translate your insights from practice during this time of national health reform.
5. Explain the roles and responsibilities of DNP graduate APRNs in evidence-based practice and practice-based evidence.
6. In what ways would your skills need to be enhanced to meet the AACN's essential outcome competency "Information Systems/Technology and Patient Care Technology for the Improvement and Transformation of Health Care?"
7. Describe your position, with its rationale, in the debate of which academic degree should be entry into APRN practice: the MSN versus the DNP.
8. Identify strategies (at least two) to ensure the development of another academic degree in nursing, the DNP, helps to unify and strengthen the worlds of nursing research and practice.
9. Develop a sample of a formal memorandum of understanding between you, in your role as a DNP with a colleague, a research nurse with a PhD, for knowledge dissemination, translation, and implementation collaboration.
10. Using the AACN's eight outcome competences for DNP education, write a new job description in your clinical setting for yourself with the enhanced knowledge and skills you will gain with a DNP.

CHAPTER TWENTY-FOUR

Today, Tomorrow, and in the Future

What Roles Are Next for Nurses Engaged in Doctoral Advanced Nursing Practice?

H. Michael Dreher and Mary Ellen Smith Glasgow

INTRODUCTION

Despite the plethora of still surging numbers of the new doctor of nursing practice (DNP) programs, the impact these graduates will ultimately have on the U.S. health care system remains largely unknown. This is perhaps both disconcerting and opportunistic. There is need for data that support the improved health outcomes of aggregate populations if the role of the DNP graduate is to be supported by the free market and by consumers. Beyond the work of Mundinger and coleagues (2000) that supports this new degree's likelihood of having a positive impact on health outcomes, not initially having substantive pilot data for the DNP degree presents a challenge to the profession. It is now up to the new cadre of DNP graduates and educators to indeed prove the worth of this new degree. We are optimistic that in time work on proving the degree's worth will be done, and the innovation of the DNP degree will be affirmed. This concluding chapter takes a summary view of the four primary doctoral advanced practice roles we have delineated in this text—Practitioner, Clinical Executive, Educator, and Clinical Scientist. We will reflect on what the DNP degree is today and what it will likely look tomorrow, as programs already in existence are beginning to tweak their curricula after having conducted their first round of program evaluations with their first batch of graduates now entering the workforce. Finally, we will look at the future. We will make some creative projections about where this degree might lead the new graduate. As we move further into the 21st century and the unfolding decade of health reform ahead of us, our projections evolve out of Toffler's (1971) groundbreaking 1970s work *Future Shock*, Naisbitt's (1982) *Megatrends* from the 1980s, and from the 1990s to today, with the contemporary work of Harvard Business School professor and innovation guru Clayton Christensen, who first coined the term *disruptive innovation* (Christensen, 1997; Christensen, Grossman, & Hwang, 2008). These futuristic works from over several decades form the footprints for this degree's ultimate future. These luminaries and social critics of society, and our progress and future, serve as models for our own predictions about the roles *that are next*, perhaps, for the DNP graduate. It should be an exciting journey!

THE DOCTORAL ADVANCED NURSING PRACTICE-EDUCATED "PRACTITIONER"

When *U.S. News and World Report* featured a doctorally prepared RN on the cover of its January 2005 issue with the title "Who needs doctors: Your future physician might not be an MD—and you may be better off!"—indeed a Pandora's box was opened, and the rush to anoint an alternate supply of primary care providers in the United States was ushered in, but retrospectively in a most controversial way (Fischman, 2005). That was in 2005, and now 5 years later, we have grown from less than 10 DNP programs to some 200-plus programs either in operation in 2010 or in the planning stages (American Association of Colleges of Nursing [AACN], 2010)! We are certain that the designers of this degree (a Dean's Task Force at the American Association of Colleges of Nursing) had no idea this would be the projected growth of this new degree. Indeed, in 2010, the number of DNP programs is predicted to surpass the number of PhD programs in nursing that degree has been around since 1934 (Dreher, 2009a). With this truly large number of DNP programs now producing new doctorally prepared *practitioners* (referring broadly to nurse practitioners, nurse midwives, nurse anesthetists, and clinical nurse specialists) for the health care market, the real questions are who is going to employ them and *will they perform differently* than if they were instead master's-prepared advanced practice nurses?

Recently, the term *doctoral advanced practice nursing* (Dreher & Montgomery, 2009) (the acronym 'DAPRN' is used in this text) has been proposed to better differentiate the practice of a DNP/DrNP graduate from the practice of a traditional master's-prepared clinician or practitioner. We think this is critical, because if there are no new, real, identifiable skills that a new doctorally prepared practitioner possesses, then why should advanced practice registered nurses (APRNs) have pursued the doctorate, and why should the market place pay these health care professionals any more money? So our first challenge to the profession and in particular to the DNP educator and graduate, is to be very clear about what additional skills *beyond the MSN* the DNP graduate is going to acquire. It is our view that the emergence of new roles for the DNP-prepared practitioner will be dependent on a critical mass of graduates presenting new prospective employers with measurable claims of what they have acquired during their doctoral education. For this reason, we do believe there will be both: (a) programs that will quickly produce quality graduates (the programs that are very adept at producing clinicians ready to practice at the doctorally advanced practice level); and, unfortunately, also (b) programs that will do a very poor job of this. We are particularly concerned about the impact of programs that poorly differentiate graduates with the master's versus the doctoral degree, and whether graduates hired from weak programs will leave their new employers skeptical of graduates with this new degree. Indeed, in a recent issue of *The Academic Nurse* (the journal of Columbia University's School of Nursing and its Alumni), the proliferation of DNP degrees that are easy to obtain "without studying clinical care or research" was identified as a cause of concern (Ten Years of Progress, 2010, p. 24).

To combat this, we encourage DNP students, especially new DNP students reading this text early in their curriculum, to challenge the faculty to make sure you are getting more of what the *Essentials of Doctoral Education for Advanced Nursing Practice* (AACN, 2006) refers to in Essential VIII as *Advanced Nursing Practice* (p. 16). In other words, for the post-master's DNP student—you already are an *advanced practice nurse* and now matriculating to become a *doctoral advanced practice nurse*—what in your respective curriculum fits specifically into this box? Are you getting additional content in practice? Are you building on what you already know? Is your program leveraging technology to give you additional experience with standardized patients or informatics skills to track and document patient assessments and outcomes in near real time? We hear that family nurse practitioner graduates from master's programs indicate they wish they had more advanced skills at differential diagnosis and more in-depth, cadaver-based anatomy in which to better support their case presentations during grand rounds with other interdisciplinary colleagues (often interns, residents, and other medical professionals). Perhaps most importantly, we firmly believe that DAPRNs ought to be the most skilled at implementing social/behavioral interventions for their primary care patients. Do you have a course that focuses on or includes this content? We challenge you *to challenge your faculty* to be clear about what additional skill sets your DNP program is going to need to help you achieve. For BSN-to-DNP program students the challenge is similar, but different. Here the question is what didactic curriculum can be clearly differentiated as truly doctoral advanced nursing practice content and what would typically belong to a traditional MSN practitioner's program? Whether you are a post-master's (entering with an earned master's degree) or an entry-level DNP student (entering with a BSN), we know these may be difficult questions for new programs to answer. However, only by creating a different kind of graduate will the degree and the permanence of the DNP graduate in the market place take hold and graduates likely be compensated additionally and equitably for the higher education they possess.

In his book *Future Shock*, Toffler coined the term *information overload*. Certainly, this was one of the many reasons given for the formation of the DNP degree. With technological advances in society increasing exponentially, it was often assumed that in order to master more information, the APRN in a typical master's program needed more courses and more credit hours to maintain competency. Even though many master's programs in many disciplines typically are completed in 30 semester credits, many MSN programs, especially those preparing advanced practitioners, vastly exceeded 30 credits. Thus, one rationale for creating the DNP degree was to avoid any further master's "credit creep" and to recognize that the current length of the MSN degrees was already heading toward typical credits awarded for a doctorate (AACN, 2006). Therefore, a powerful argument for degree credit parity was made for the creation of this doctoral degree instead of again just adding more additional master's credits and courses (Dracup & Bryan-Brown, 2005). We agree that information overload, possibly a problem for society even pre-Toffler, remains a contemporary issue for the DNP student and gradu-ate. Upon reflection, in some ways the pace of new knowledge has probably not changed since 1970. However, today's DNP student and graduate increasingly faces, perhaps more than ever, the legal burden (not to mention the ethical obligation) to "keep up-to-date" to maintain expected practice competencies. We would even go as far as to surmise that the DNP graduate, especially the practitioner who may often be working side-by-side in clinic environments with other doctorally prepared clinicians, may have an additional burden to project and demonstrate that their practice skill set is superior to APRN colleagues who only have a master's degree.

One of the precepts of *Megatrends* from the 1980s was that "We are moving in the dual direction of high tech/high touch, matching each new technology with a compensa-tory human response" (Naisbitt, 1982, p. 1). We think the future DNP practitioner is going to be more technology oriented than even today. Indeed, it is the doctorally prepared clin-ician who is the most adept at knowledge management and who will likely become the most expert clinician (Dreher, 2009b). The question for today's DNP student is what kind of focus on technology does your curriculum include? Are you learning how to manage the massive amount of information input you need to evaluate and discriminate among in order to stay abreast of your particular field? This means going much further than subscribing to and reading the right journals in your discipline. It is about using technology devices that can comb new articles and findings in one's field electronically, and having them sent directly to one's iPhone, Blackberry, PDA, or perhaps to the next generation device that has not even been identified yet. Indeed, one such program (PubMed) already does this and was described by Cornelius, Childs, and Wilson in chapter 14. We do not know today what kind of technology competencies will be required for doctoral advanced practice nurses to maintain the kind of expert practice required of them in the future. But today we already see clinicians in progressive practices walking out of patient rooms with Dictaphones in hand, dictating their notes in real time using DragonFly, probably the leading voice recognition software on the market today in health care practices. What about you? What is your technology quotient? Are you a "techie"? If not, are you at least competent with the latest health care support technology? More importantly, how do you envision your future practice, and how do you plan to "keep up" and be competitive with your other health care professional colleagues? Already it is increasingly recognized that baccalaureate and master's nursing education has become adept in their emphasis on technology in health care. Similarly, at the doctoral level, we believe this is a prime area where DNP graduates can show a level of technology mastery above and beyond what the other health care practitioners from other disciplines commonly use. Again, look at your own DNP curriculum. Is the technology support you will need for doctoral advanced nursing practice there?

H. M. Dreher, the first author of this chapter, was privileged to attend the Harvard Macy Institute's Program for Leading Innovations in Healthcare and Education at the Harvard Business School and Harvard Medical School in 2007. The week-long program was led by the guru of innovation, Clayton Christensen, DBA (Doctor of Business Administration, Harvard). With an audience largely comprised of physician educators from medical schools from around the world (but with some nursing faculty and other related disciplines also in attendance), Dr. Christensen startled the attendees one morning by announcing that physicians should stop their turf battles over who should provide primary care. Of course my ears pricked up with this discussion (as I am sure did the ears of the several other nurses in attendance), and he went on to say that there were already nonphysician primary care providers such as nurse practitioners and physician assistants who have already demonstrated they can provide a high level of primary care effectively. Moreover, he thought many physicians were simply underused for the vast education and expertise they possess. He encouraged physicians to focus less on simple diagnosis and treatment of common disorders, which other disciplines could manage more cost effectively, and instead focus on the next horizons of medical specialty practice and science. Dr. Christensen's 2009 book (with Grossman & Hwang), *The Innovator's Prescription: A Disruptive Solution for Health Care*, even states "...nurse practitioners (and other physician extenders) practicing in retail clinics, should disrupt the precision medicine portion of the physician's practice" (p. 112). I found the discussion absolutely exhilarating, and as a department chair of a DrNP program, I was convinced that my own graduates were absolutely positioning themselves to be this new kind of expert, nonphysician, primary care provider he was applauding. So at least the Harvard Business School is sympathetic to the work product of nurse practitioners and other advanced practice clinicians (we however dislike the term *physician extender*), even if the American Medical Association (AMA) is not. Indeed, they continue to oppose, in particular, the new practice of the DNP graduate and their use of *Doctor* (described by Oldfield in chapter 19). Further, there is even a new

AMA (2009) policy paper warning about the spread and encroachment of nonphysician primary care providers. However, one must not assume all physicians are against doctorally prepared advanced practice nurses. From our view, the AMA perceives the DNP graduate and practitioner who will call themselves doctor to be a real threat to their sphere of influence and their power and authority as experts on health care, and also, most certainly, as a financial threat.

We continue to be uncertain of the future of the Diplomat in Comprehensive Care exam (the DNP exam or the 'ABCC exam' as Dr. Smolowitz in the chapter 23 response prefers). While we believe it will help better differentiate the DNP graduate from the master's-prepared APRN, the numbers of individuals who have passed this exam in its first 2 years is incredibly small. Moreover, the broad opposition to it within the profession is substantial, including the then-President of the American College of Nurse Practitioners, Dr. Julie Stanik-Hutt (2008). We actually see most of the opposition coming from PhD-prepared nurse practitioners who probably feel left out because, without a DNP degree, they cannot take the exam. This is a fair argument, but in the end, a PhD is a research-intensive degree, and its aim has never been to improve the clinical skills of master's-prepared advanced practice nurses. It remains to be seen whether "patients and payers will recognize this subset of DNP graduates (Diplomates of Comprehensive Care) are the clinical experts of choice" as Dean Mary Mundinger and the Columbia University School of Nursing faculty suggests (Ten Years of Progress, 2010, p. 25).

Nevertheless, we think it is more prudent for doctoral advanced practice practitioners to work from a positive frame of reference and to find ways to explore collaboration with physicians, particularly with those who do respect the practice of highly educated advanced practice nurses. We encourage you to seek out these sympathetic physician partners and to work with them and to establish successful partnerships. One of our first DrNP graduates indeed runs a primary care practice with an MD colleague, and she is a full partner in the joint practice. She did not have that kind of practice arrangement *prior* to having her DrNP degree. So this is clear indication of the kind of leverage the new doctoral advanced practice nurse may exert today and perhaps more commonly in the future. Indeed, it is the expert role modeling of today's practice DNP graduates and their demonstration of advanced knowledge, skill, expertise, and ability that will go a long way toward paving the way for future graduates who may themselves secure full partnership primary practice positions with physicians and other health care providers.

Finally, we envision primary care primary practices comprised completely of DNP prepared practitioners. It is not hard to imagine a practice being set up with full partners (founders and highly experienced doctoral advanced practice nurses) and employing new associate partners as new graduates are hired with an expanding practice. We envision new associate partners working their way up the ladder to full partner and then enjoying the benefits of a jointly managed nursing primary care practice, much like what happens in the legal field. We especially predict that these types of doctoral nursing primary care practices could be competitive for contracts to provide health services, especially to vulnerable populations where physicians just do not want to practice. These environments might include prisons, nurse-managed primary community health care centers, inner city and rural health care clinics, and other areas. Banded together, we predict that a practice of DNP graduates (how about a cadre of transdisciplinary nurse practitioners, nurse midwives, and clinical nurse specialists?) could negotiate real autonomy and provide expert primary health care in a diversity of health care agencies and venues. And with certified nurse midwives finally winning 100%

reimbursement under Medicare (since 1988 they have only been reimbursed at 65% of the rate paid to a physician for the same services) for disabled and senior women needing reproductive health services and maternity care, maybe even the payment models for advanced practice nursing care are moving in the right direction (Summers, 2010). However, a quirk in the Medicare law still prevents APRNs from "signing home health plans of care and from certifying Medicare patients for the home health benefit" (Conant, 2010, p. 18). Nevertheless, with the new 2010 Patient Protection and Affordable Care Act, and real health care reform now scheduled to roll out over the next decade or so, the future is bright for doctoral advanced practice nurses, especially if they creatively and innovatively design efficient models of health care delivery. We are really optimistic about what the DNP practitioner/clinician graduate can contribute. Are you?

THE DOCTORAL ADVANCED NURSING PRACTICE-EDUCATED "CLINICAL EXECUTIVE"

Given that fundamental change is needed in the U.S. health care delivery system to improve quality care (Institute of Medicine, 2001), the doctoral advanced nursing practice educated *clinical executive* (Chief Nursing Officers, Vice Presidents, and other executive-level nurse leaders) will be called upon to address emergent and challenging issues for nursing practice, as well as to create opportunities that will shape and implement innovative changes in the health care system. Today, the doctoral level clinical executive is in short supply. Future doctoral-level nurse administrators and executive leaders will also be charged to improve health and health care outcomes through evidence-based practice in diverse clinical and health care settings. The clinical executive with doctoral advanced nursing practice education emphasizes evidence-based approaches for quality and safety improvement in practice settings, applies research methods to decision making, and translates credible research findings to increase the effectiveness of both direct and indirect nursing practice. Some of the specific competencies outlined in the *Essentials* documents for the DNP clinical executive include: using sophisticated, conceptual, and analytical skills in evaluating the links between clinical, organizational, fiscal, and policy issues; establishing processes for interorganizational collaboration for the achievement of organizational goals; designing patient-centered care delivery systems or policy-level delivery models; collaborating effectively with legal counsel and financial officers around issues related to legal and regulatory guidelines; and demonstrating advanced levels of clinical judgment, cultural sensitivity, and systems thinking (AACN, 2006). The clinical executive track of the DNP degree offers numerous courses on leadership theories, the process of leadership, and leadership as it pertains to a health care setting. The practicum experiences for the clinical executive student provide an opportunity for the student to apply leadership theories in health care settings. More importantly, the program of study allows students to further develop their own leadership through introspection, coursework, clinical work, and mentorship. These types of educational experiences can be elemental, as the clinical executive tries to execute and provide for more quality health care.

Furthermore, it will be critical for the DNP curriculum to have a heavy emphasis on business ethics as well as clinical ethics. The clinical executive may be one of a few individuals in senior leadership with a true understanding of the complexity of patient care, nurses' roles/responsibilities, and the requisite human and fiscal resources required for positive clinical outcomes. As the voice of nurses in the organization, the clinical executive needs to have political capital—a good reputation and irreproachable ethics. In order to fulfill one's fiduciary responsibilities, the clinical executive must also be knowledgeable and vigilant with regard to fiscal accountability.

Doctoral level nurse executives will be called upon to bring their respective organizations to a better position than where they found it. Ideally, the doctoral advanced nursing practice-educated clinical executive will: (1) earn the trust of one's organization; (2) be deeply engaged with nursing staff and/or employees; (3) earn legitimacy and mobilize one's own people around a focused agenda; (4) devote considerable efforts to developing one's employees and building the organization's collective leadership capabilities; and (5) strive for high performance in the organization while delicately balancing a high commitment to the institution (Eisenstat, Beer, Foote, Fredberg, & Norrgren, 2008). These requisite leadership skills, coupled with the knowledge to influence health care outcomes, afford doctoral-level clinical executives an opportunity to effect change like no other time in nursing's history.

At the end of the day, it is all about leadership. The clinical executive of tomorrow, with a doctoral advanced nursing practice education, plays a pivotal role in supporting an autonomous and professional nursing practice culture. Successful implementation of an empowered environment rests with the nurse leader's ability to create a constructive atmosphere, which involves the implementation of supportive infrastructures that encompass accountability, pursuit of excellence, and open communication. In this way, clinical nurses are allowed the autonomy to make decisions and foster practices in accordance with professional nursing standards. Thus, a progressive nurse leader can shape an institution through one's value system and passion for nursing. With this model, innovative care models will develop and flourish (Upenieks, 2003).

High-performing organizations and/or those organizations that aspire to become high-performing organizations will closely scrutinize leadership capacity (Wells & Hejna, 2009). Hospitals and health care institutions will be among them. Magnet hospitals, designated facilities that have been certified by the American Nurses Credentialing Center for their excellence in nursing practice, will continue to be recognized as institutions with superior measures of nursing job satisfaction and patient outcomes because of their distinguished organizational characteristics. These institutions will maintain well-qualified nurse executives in an organizational structure that emphasizes open participatory management and will use professional practice models for the delivery of nursing care. Strong leadership and advocacy for nursing offers an autonomous, self-managed, self-governed climate that allows nurses to fully practice their clinical expertise. In addition, there is a framework for professional career development and education opportunities for nurses to increase their level of clinical expertise or restructure their nursing career focus (Upenieks, 2003).

As clinical executives acquire doctoral-level knowledge and competencies in greater numbers and with health care reform now rolling out, nurse leaders will be asked to participate on hospital boards, lead organizations, and provide consultation on various practice models and initiatives. The doctoral-level nurse executive will have the requisite knowledge, experience, and competencies to skillfully manage an array of complex organizational issues. In the future, we will see clinical executives with doctoral advanced nursing practice education in greater numbers as senior health care executives such as Chief Executive Officer, Chief Operating Officer, or Chair of the Board of Trustees, as organizations begin to realize their value. As DNP-educated nurse executives improve health and health care outcomes through evidence-based practice, utilize knowledge related to evidence-based approaches for quality and safety improvement, and apply research processes to decision making, we will see innovation like never before.

THE DOCTORAL ADVANCED NURSING PRACTICE-EDUCATED "EDUCATOR"

To meet current and projected nursing shortages, nursing education programs need to increase their capacity by approximately 90%. However, these programs are faced with a *severe shortage of faculty*, making it difficult to expand. Furthermore, the already small pool of qualified faculty is rapidly shrinking—almost one-third are over the age of 55 (Benner, Sutphen, Leonard, & Day, 2009). The current system of doctoral education in nursing does not have the capacity to prepare the number of graduates necessary to replace retiring faculty and does not have a sufficient number of nurse researchers to generate knowledge for the discipline (Potempa, Redman, & Anderson, 2008). According to the Robert Wood Johnson Foundation (2007), a large percentage of senior nursing faculty members will retire over the next 5 years, and half the current nursing faculty are likely to retire by 2016. Therefore, in the United States, the nursing profession is at important crossroads that could determine the direction of nursing education and knowledge development. Recent reports of the AACN indicate that there has been a 176% ($N = 3,291$) increase in student enrollment in DNP programs, from 1,874 students in 2007 to 5,165 students in 2009 (Fang, Tracy, & Bednash, 2010; Raines, 2010). The PhD programs have remained stagnant with an increase in student enrollment of only 0.10% ($N = 3$) from 3,973 students in 2007 to 3,976 students in 2008, but it has increased 5.1% from 2008 to 2009 (Fang et al., 2010; Raines, 2010). These data indicate the trend for PhD enrollment is unknown. Further, when one pauses and reflects on the fact that the profession is poised to lose half of its faculty by 2016, many of whom are PhD prepared, the question remains whether there will be sufficient doctoral-level nursing faculty? Equally important, will DNP graduates really be prepared to assume competent nurse educator roles? Who will generate the knowledge of the discipline? Furthermore, the current system does not encourage young men and women to embrace the faculty role or the conduct of research.

Today, many nursing faculty are divorced from clinical practice. Current expectations of the tripartite nursing faculty role in relation to teaching, scholarship, and service are not realistic in advancing nursing science, clinical practice, or education. Nursing faculty juggle large teaching and service loads while attempting to engage in scholarship. For those nursing faculty who are actively involved in research, the juggling act is even more pronounced. In addition, few nursing faculty have formal practice appointments as part of their faculty role that allows them to stay clinically updated to perform their teaching. For example, many nurse practitioner, nurse midwifery, and nurse anesthesia faculty have outside practice obligations to maintain their clinical hours/expertise for specialty certification in addition to their full-time faculty appointments. Many advanced practice nurse faculty opt for this financial arrangement in order to gain additional compensation given the low salaries of nursing faculty. Efforts to recruit future faculty will continue to be futile unless faculty salaries are increased and brought in line with clinical salaries and teaching positions in other disciplines (Benner et al., 2009). Going forward, nursing faculty salaries must be reevaluated in order to compete with nonacademic positions available to doctoral-level nursing professionals. Nursing leaders need to look to their academic colleagues in male-dominated professions, such as business, engineering, and law, to seek solutions related to faculty compensation. Another recommendation is to tie market salaries to accreditation and create formal academic clinical partnerships and practice arrangements in an effort to increase salaries and inform clinical teaching.

We are also concerned about whether doctoral advanced practice nurses with DNPs who have academic appointments will ever be tenured? If the faculty nurse practitioner, for instance, needs to practice to maintain certification as well as conduct research in order to get tenure, how will this happen? We see two unfortunate scenarios. In scenario A, the faculty nurse practitioner is not allowed on the tenure track at research-intensive or research-extensive universities, because she did not complete a clinical dissertation or DNP thesis or was not allowed to conduct empirical research. In this case, vast numbers of faculty nurse practitioners will be excluded from full membership in the academy or the professoriate. In scenario B, the DNP graduate *is* allowed on the tenure track at the above universities, but because this faculty nurse practitioner now has to produce the level of scholarship necessary for tenure *and* practice—not just for recertification, but to be competent and current in the graduate classroom—this faculty member is set up for failure. There are unfortunately no easy answers for this dilemma, but it is a serious one and it needs to be addressed.

With the introduction of a new critical mass of nursing educators with the DNP degree, the profession has an opportunity to reexamine the various roles of nurse faculty and create a model that encourages faculty to master one or two areas rather than the current "jack all trades" approach. The authors suggest three professorial roles: Nurse Scientist, Educator Clinician, and Clinician Educator. Nursing education must redefine the expectations of the nursing faculty with a primary focus on research, teaching, or clinical. *The Doctoral Advanced Nursing Practice-educated Educator is in a unique position to serve in the Educator Clinician role or Clinician Educator role, as they are able to integrate the knowledge they present in the classroom with a clinical practice context.* The question remains, however: Will they get the educational theory and didactic content needed in order to be successful in the classroom? With over 30% of DNP graduates now going into academia, will DNP programs create options that do not entail extra courses or more tuition for doctoral advanced practice nurses who want to teach other advanced practice students (Zungolo, 2009)?

As Potempa and Tilden (2004) have identified, the role of the "nurse scientist" is critical to generating knowledge in our discipline. Nursing deans need to find ways to better support research-intensive nursing faculty, perhaps with more realistic teaching loads and service obligations in return for high scholarly productivity. Rather than have research-active faculty engaged in clinical teaching, for example, research-active faculty would be better served to spend their time teaching nursing research at all levels (undergraduate, master's, and doctoral) and mentoring students in the conduct of research. In doing so, we create an environment that fosters the mission of scholarly productivity and knowledge development for nursing faculty. Having research-focused faculty teach both undergraduate and graduate students fosters the desire of young students to obtain a research doctorate and conduct nursing research. The role of the nurse scientist requires a change in expectations related to workload, faculty investment, research start-up funds, and a requisite reward system for scholarly productivity. It is our assumption that the nursing faculty members who are focused on research will be much more productive than faculty members required to participate in traditional tripartite (teaching, service, and scholarship) roles. With the appropriate education and training on the conduct of research, both DNP and PhD nursing graduates have the potential to contribute to the empirical evidence base of nursing. Furthermore, with the NIH in 2009 opening up some grant mechanisms to DNP graduates, it is very likely that some practice doctorate graduates (likely a small minority) might even become nurse scientists, too. Again, physicians, largely with no training in research methods during medical school, routinely submit research grants to the National Institutes of Health. It is welcoming to see that the NIH is recognizing and welcoming research proposals from a wider audience.

The Carnegie Foundation for the Advancement of Teaching recently released the results of the first national nursing education study in 30 years (Benner et al., 2009). The study *Educating Nurses: A Call for Radical Transformation* explores the strengths and weaknesses in nursing education and identifies the most effective practices for teaching nursing and argues convincingly that nursing education must be reconstructed. Based on this study, there is a need to address the specific educational demands of teaching the complex practice of nursing and reconnect with the practice context of the nursing discipline. The DNP-prepared educator has the clinical knowledge and educational foundation to address these critical issues noted in The Carnegie Study. Further, the study recommended that nursing educators make four shifts in their thinking about teaching and in their approaches to fostering student learning for the future:

1. *From a focus on covering decontextualized knowledge to an emphasis on teaching for a sense of salience, situated cognition, and action in particular situations.*
   Many faculty organize their classes around lists of abstract theory, giving their students little or no indication about how to integrate the knowledge they present into practice. Nursing faculty should help students learn to apply nursing knowledge and science.
2. *From a sharp separation of clinical and classroom teaching to an integration of the two.*
   Traditionally, there has been a sharp divide between classroom and clinical teaching. When faculty provide only simple, rudimentary examples or test students on elemental competencies, they may not be helping students to prepare for diverse, complex, real-life, stressful clinical situations.
3. *From an emphasis on critical thinking to an emphasis on clinical reasoning and multiple ways of thinking.*
   Critical thinking alone cannot develop students' perceptual acuity or clinical imagination. Clinical imagination, which requires students to grasp the nature of patients' needs as they change over time, is needed, as well as critical, creative, and scientific reasoning.
4. *From an emphasis on professional socialization to an emphasis on formation.*
   Experiential learning environments across the nursing curriculum are needed to support formation. Nursing education must focus on the formation of professional identity rather than on socialization (Benner et al.).

When one ponders the radical transformation that will be required for nursing education in the 21st century, the authors assert that the reconstruction of nursing education and a reconnection to practice will only be achieved by a diverse group of doctorally prepared faculty, namely the Nurse Scientist, Educator Clinician, and Clinician Educator. The doctoral advanced nursing practice trained educator is well suited to integrate the classroom content and the practice context. An innovative DNP program curriculum is needed that truly combines the practice emphasis with education-related content and their practical integration. To our knowledge, only Case Western Reserve University (Educational Leadership) and Drexel University (Educator Track) provide this combined approach. The AACN has not endorsed the practice of the educator in the same way they embraced the practice of the clinical executive within the design of the DNP degree. We cannot mandate doctoral advanced practice nurses who are interested in faculty roles to take additional electives or a minor, with focus on the education-related content, *in addition* to the DNP practice content for individuals interested in the faculty role. We are facing a critical nursing faculty shortage that will impact the entire profession and we need to let go of time-honored traditions, such as the current nursing education model that separates theory from practice, the need for extensive clinical practice before matriculating in doctoral programs, and the heavy teaching and service requirements of research-intensive doctoral-prepared faculty in order to move the discipline forward (Tilden & Potempa, 2003). Lastly, the nurse educator role needs to be included in all doctoral programs in order for the nursing profession to meet current and projected nursing shortages.

THE DOCTORAL ADVANCED NURSING PRACTICE-EDUCATED "CLINICAL SCIENTIST"

As was described in chapter 8, the advanced practice role of the clinical scientist is unique to Drexel University, although we know there are many master's-prepared nurses across the country currently working in the clinical trials field who are matriculating in various DNP programs. We are also aware of DNP graduates that are running clinical trials and submitting research proposals as primary investigators. Chiefly, this new role is a DNP degree innovation designed to support both: (1) the clinical nurse scientist in the largely clinical trials/pharmaceutical research industry; and (2) as a more intensive clinical research track option for DNP/DrNP students who want an even more enhanced focus on research than what is typical in a DNP curriculum. With health care remaining a growing field, even during this economic recession, there is no reason to believe that an aging baby boomer population will not demand even higher quality health care services. That means the drive for more research, more funding for new drugs and devices, and more innovation will continue. The implementation of contemporary health care legislation now being implemented in the Obama Administration is about to excelerate, but it is clear that the climate for even more cost-effective health care innovation is here. *Innovation* is indeed a timely concept nursing needs to embrace more fully. In November of 2009, President Obama announced his new "Educate to Innovate" campaign, and in his remarks he said,

> The key to meeting these challenges—improving our health and well being, harnessing clean energy, protecting our security, and succeeding in the global economy—will be reaffirming and strengthening America's role as the world's engine of scientific discovery and technological innovation. And that leadership tomorrow depends on how we educate our students today, especially in those fields that hold the promise of producing future innovations and innovators.
>
> —*Obama, 2009, p. 1, para 8*

A doctorally educated clinical nursing scientist in the clinical trials industry should be a force for new innovation, specifically for nursing sensitive health care outcomes. Indeed a 2005 editorial in the journal *Expert Review of Medical Devices* titled "Nursing and Biomedical Engineering Transdisciplinary Clinical Trials Collaboration" states,

> Given the research training in design, methods and statistical analyses that nurses gain during doctoral study, there is no plausible reason why doctorally-prepared nurses should be excluded from the role of PIs in the testing of noninvasive devices commonly used in nursing practice, such as gastric and postpyloric feeding tubes, pulse oximeters, capnography and tonometry instruments, bedside monitors, wound management systems, kinetic beds, thermometers, endotracheal tubes, suctioning devices, nutritional support therapies and medication delivery systems
>
> —*Mick and Ackerman, 2005, p. 131*[1]

This is actually a very powerful argument for the doctorally educated expert nurse clinician to be trained in the methods of conducting clinical research and not just the evaluation, translation, and dissemination of clinical research that has for some reason become the restricted domain of the DNP prepared nurse in most DNP programs. Building on the strong clinical background of experienced APRNs who are now entering post-master's DNP/DrNP programs, Mick and Ackerman further state:

> Even more compelling is the argument that doctorally-prepared nurse practitioners in the USA, who possess physician-equivalent diagnostic, interventional and prescriptive authority, are better qualified, in some instances, to carry out clinical research than physician colleagues who may not have engaged in any discrete research training during medical school or residency. Development of role autonomy in medical diagnosis and decision making is a hallmark of the nurse practitioner curricula.
>
> —*Mick and Ackerman, 2005, p. 131*[1]

We fully agree and think this last statement really embraces what ideally the DNP, doctorally educated APRN (and seasoned clinician) should be able to do.

In the Drexel University DrNP curriculum, Clinical Scientist Track students have several curricular options. First, all students complete a doctoral clinical practicum that pertains to the students' approved clinical research question. In Chapter 8 one of the clinical research questions that a Drexel University Clinical Scientist Track student is using as a basis for her clinical dissertation was described. Second, Clinical Scientist Track students also complete a doctoral role practicum where each student in this track is matched with a funded nursing scientist in the department. A faculty/student learning contract is completed that outlines the kind of clinical research goals the student wants to achieve. Almost always, one of the doctoral role practicum outcomes is a publishable joint manuscript with the student as first author and faculty as second author. If the faculty member has an ongoing clinical research study, the doctoral student is mentored in some aspect of the conduct of the study. In addition, each DrNP student completes two cognates in their track. Cognates are more than just electives. They must directly support the doctoral student's course of study and align with career goals. Several Clinical Scientist Track students have completed a three-course sequence, post-master's certificate in Epidemiology and Biostatistics offered by our School of Public Health. We highly encourage all students in this track to complete this certificate program. Others have taken statistical electives offered by our Department of Physical Therapy. Some have completed independent study courses with professors in their clinical research area. The overall goal for students in this track is to obtain the highest proficiency in clinical research methods as is possible in a doctor of nursing practice curriculum that simultaneously has an equal emphasis on *practice.*

So where do we see DNP students with sound clinical research skills flourishing in the clinical trials/pharmaceutical research industry? To best answer this question, we asked Dr. Diane Mick, the coauthor cited in the 2005 article who encouraged more doctorally prepared APRNs for the clinical trials/medical device industry. In an interview she stated,

> Now in the second decade of the 21st century, the clinical trials industry continues to grow and become more complex. Due to increased research and development opportunities, there is an ongoing need for doctorally-prepared nurse scientists who can serve as principal investigators for clinical trials. By virtue of educational preparation as advanced practice nurses, nurse scientists have the same diagnostic, therapeutic, and prescriptive privileges as many physicians. Nurses have the additional advantage of possessing strong experiential

backgrounds with insight into clinical problems in need of solutions at the bedside. Clinician end-users, such as nurses, can provide recommendations for improvements to industry-sponsored devices, and may have a degree of influence on whether a clinical service or an institution ultimately will adopt the device or pharmaceutical agent for use in practice. From this perspective, nursing involvement in clinical trials research can be characterized as a win-win-win situation. Nurses at both the staff and advanced practice level help to improve health care by moving medical devices and pharmaceuticals from the laboratory to patients who need them. Industry benefits by having their products evaluated in real-time in real patient care situations. Patients benefit from the use of innovative devices and medications to improve and sustain their health.

—*Dr. Diane Mick, personal communication June 28, 2010*

Finally, what about the DNP student, whether in a Clinical Scientist Track or not, who wants to pursue a post-doctoral research fellowship? Is this possible? This question is already very controversial. We have heard doctoral educators at the annual AACN Doctoral Nursing Education Conference stand and offer the following arguments: "Certainly, if DNP grads want retraining and more education in the conduct of research, then they should be eligible to apply and complete a post-doctoral research fellowship. That's precisely what physicians do, since their degree does not formally include research" or "No way! The DNP is not a research degree, and post-doctoral students must come with a PhD in hand." We actually do not like such black and white arguments, and think the solution is more in the middle. In other words, if the DNP or DrNP graduate has completed a strong clinical research project (whether a clinical dissertation, practice dissertation, or other type of research project), we strongly endorse the idea that each student applicant be evaluated individually. While DNP graduates seeking to pursue a post-doctoral research fellowship will not likely become the norm, why close the door? While we dislike the overused phrase "think out of the box," it does apply here. True, physicians do not normally complete a research project during their MD degree (in the United Kingdom some actually do), but if they get the "research bug" as medical students, they generally take an elective in clinical research during their medical training or spend an extra year in a clinical research fellowship in their field of interest. The Howard Hughes Medical Institute (2010), for example, sponsors a Medical Fellows Program, and they advertise the program as a year of full-time biomedical research for medical, dental, and veterinary students. Because the DNP is a professional doctorate like the MD (Doctor of Medicine), DDS (Doctor of Dental Science), and DVM (Doctor of Veterinary Medicine), why not create such options for DNP students or integrate them into clinical research fellows programs traditionally open to physicians and other professional doctorate programs? With the NIH now allowing doctor of nursing practice graduates to compete for Mentored Patient-Oriented Research Career Development Awards (Parent K-23) as of December 2009, perhaps institutional post-doctoral fellowships will follow and at least evaluate individual DNP/DrNP applicants. We suggest this be examined seriously, especially because full-time post-doctoral research fellowship enrollment (part-time study is not the norm) dropped 6.1% from 2008 to 2009 (Fang et al., 2010). This drop in post-doctoral enrollment seems to confirm Potempa, Redman, and Anderson's (2008) concerns about our capacity to replace our retiring nurse scientists.

Yes, this *is* very different from what nursing has done in the past. But with stagnant enrollments and graduations from nursing PhD programs (2008–2009 PhD graduations increased by only 2.2% or 12 more graduates nationally!), there must be more than one pipeline to the production of nursing knowledge for the discipline (AACN, 2009; Dreher, 2009c; Fang et al., 2010; Smith Glasgow & Dreher, 2010). There ought to be new options for DNP students and graduates who get the "research bug," too, and we are very forthright that the option for these types of graduates *ought not* to be to "go back and get a PhD." Further, with there being such an enormous shortage of nursing faculty with even one doctorate, we are very skeptical of suggesting dual DNP/PhD programs due to their increased length, time commitment, and cost. Is the MD/PhD model something nursing really wants to embrace? We surmise only time will tell. The Clinical Scientist Track is an alternate preparation for such graduates seeking more refined research skills and experiences. We encourage DNP programs, especially those that formally permit an empirical clinical research project, to create more Clinical Scientist Track options, both for students interested in the clinical trial industry and for those who for whatever reason just cannot complete a PhD, but who still seek to acquire real, practical clinical research skills.

SUMMARY

Clayton Christensen, heralded as the guru of innovation, describes disruptive innovation as a "process by which a product or service takes root initially in simple applications at the bottom of a market and then relentlessly moves 'up market,' eventually displacing established competitors" (2009, p. 1). Indeed, in 2006, some nursing scholars, using this term first coined for the business world, described the new DNP degree as a disruptive innovation (Hathaway, Jacob, Stegbauer, Thompson, & Graff, 2006). We largely concur, although we are among a cadre of doctoral nursing educators who would like to see the DNP degree shaped for the future more by: a broader representation of nursing faculty in the academy; by the outcome data that will emerge as scholars study these graduates and their impact on the health care system; and by the rapidly changing health care consumer marketplace, rather than by various nursing accreditors. There is already evidence widespread in the literature that accrediting agencies in the health professions are actually stifling degree innovation with their desire for conformity and regulation (Dreher, 2008; Melnyk & Davidson, 2009; Neal, 2008; Stewart, 2009). With some 30 million or more individuals coming into the U.S. health care system in the next 5 years, we think DNP graduates are particularly positioned to capitalize on this opportunity to provide more high-quality, effective primary care.

We do express concern that with the transition to the entry-level doctorate for advanced practice and possible dissolution of the master's degree over time, there may be a decline in overall numbers of new nurse practitioners entering practice. There are others expressing this concern (Bloch, 2007; Dreher & Gardner, 2009; Ford, 2008). The good news is that the Obama Administration in June 2010 announced: (1) $30 million dollars in 2010 to begin training an additional 600 nurse practitioners, including providing incentives for part-time students to become full time and complete their education sooner; and (2) $15 million dollars to establish 10 new nurse practitioner-led clinics, which assist in the training of nurse practitioners, are staffed by nurse practitioners, and provide comprehensive primary health care services to populations living in medically underserved communities (HealthReform.Gov, 2010). As our medical and health system starts to shift more visibly to a preventive care model, we think highly educated nurses, particularly doctoral advanced practice nurses, have an opportunity to seize the day. We wholeheartedly believe that the doctoral advanced practice nurse of today, tomorrow, and the future will be the primary generator of "practice knowledge" and "practice-based evidence nursing knowledge" that focuses on finding solutions to real clinical, educational, or organizational problems in the field (clinic, classroom, or executive suite) (Dreher, 2010). Yes, we foresee doctoral advanced practice nurses creating new practice knowledge and practice evidence for our discipline, and then efficiently translating and disseminating it to practice. All nurses engaged in any type of doctoral advanced nursing practice, however, will need to be more visible, daring, innovative, data driven, and outcome oriented. The proof of the ultimate merit of this degree will be proven by what these new graduates accomplish. The distinctive role of the DAPRN or DAPN, no matter the setting or job description, will likely challenge a lot of assumptions. Do not let conventional thinking or history or glass ceilings get in your way.

THE FUTURE OF NURSING: LEADING CHANGE, ADVANCING HEALTH

Committee on the Robert Wood Johnson Foundation Initiative on the Future of Nursing at the Institute of Medicine chaired by Donna E. Shalala, President of the University of Miami, was released. Highlights of this report with relevance for this text include:

1. Include a nurse educator role in all master's and doctoral programs;
2. Increase emphasis on global health and knowledge development at all educational levels;
3. Cultivate disciplinary knowledge across all levels of curricula based on an understanding of the science of the discipline and the scientific process;
4. Develop "scientifically aware" nurse clinicians who will collaborate with nurse scientists to move research to the bedside. Focus on "Evidence-Creating Nursing," the direct collaboration between nurse clinicians and nurse scientists.
5. Re-engineer the Doctor of Nursing Practice (DNP) to include the conduct of research in the form of a practice dissertation (Smith Glasgow, Dunphy, & Mainous, 2010, G8-G9).

NOTE

1. Quote reproduced from *Expert Rev. Medical Devices*, 2(1), 131–133 with permission of Expert Reviews LTD.

REFERENCES

American Association of Colleges of Nursing (AACN). (2006). *Essentials of doctoral education for advanced nursing practice*. Retrieved from http://www.aacn.nche.edu/DNP/pdf/Essentials.pdf

American Association of Colleges of Nursing (AACN). (2008). *Enrollment growth in U.S. nursing colleges and universities hits an 8-year low according to new data released by AACN*. Retrieved from http://www.aacn.nche.edu/Media/NewsReleases/2008/EnrlGrowth.html

American Association of Colleges of Nursing (AACN). (2009). *2009 Annual report advancing higher education in nursing*. Retrieved from http://www.aacn.nche.edu/DNP/DNPProgramList.htm

American Association of Colleges of Nursing (AACN). (2010). *Doctor of nursing practice (DNP) programs*, September 2010. Retrieved from http://www.aacn.nche.edu/DNP/DNPProgramList.htm

American Medical Association. (2009). *AMA Scope of Practice Data Sets: Nurse practitioners*. Chicago, IL: Author.

Benner, P., Sutphen, M., Leonard, V., & Day, L. (2009). *Educating nurses: A call for radical transformation*. Stanford, CA: The Carnegie Foundation for the Advancement of Teaching.

Bloch, J. (2007). *The DNP/DrNP degree as entry into NP practice: Is this nursing's answer to eliminate disparities in health care access for vulnerable populations?* Paper presented at The Practice Doctorate: Where is it Headed? The First National Conference on The Doctor of Nursing Practice: Meanings and Models, Annapolis, Maryland, March 28–30, 2007.

Christensen, C. (1997). *The innovator's dilemma: When new technologies cause great firms to fail.* Cambridge, MA: Harvard Business Press.

Christensen, C. (2009). *Clayton Christensen, Key concepts—Disruptive innovation.* Retrieved from http://www.claytonchristensen.com/disruptive_innovation.html

Christensen, C., Grossman, J., & Hwang, J. (2008). *The innovator's prescription: A disruptive solution for health care.* New York, NY: McGraw-Hill Professional.

Conant, R. (2010). Headlines from the hill: Lawmakers need to hear from nurses on home health care. *American Nurse Today, 5*(7), 18.

Dracup, K., & Bryan-Brown, C. (2005). Doctor of nursing practice: MRI or total body scan. *American Journal of Critical Care, 14*(4), 278–281.

Dreher, H. M. (2008). Innovation in nursing education: Preparing for the future of nursing practice. *Holistic Nursing Practice, 22*(2), 77–80.

Dreher, H. M. (2009a). *The doctor of nursing practice degree in the U.S.: History & politics, problems & progress.* Paper presented at the International Conference on Professional Doctorates, London, England, November 9–10, 2009.

Dreher, H. M. (2009b). How do RNs today best stay informed? Do we need knowledge management? *Holistic Nursing Practice, 23*(5), 263–266.

Dreher, H. M. (2009c). Education for advanced practice: The question: Is the PhD or DNP the right degree model for future advanced practice nurses? L. Joel, *Advanced practice nursing: Essentials for role development* (2nd ed.), (pp. 58–71). Philadelphia, PA: FA Davis.

Dreher, H. M. (2010). Next steps toward practice knowledge development: An emerging epistemology in nursing. In M. D. Dahnke, & H. M. Dreher, *Philosophy of science for nursing practice: Concepts and application.* New York, NY: Springer.

Dreher, H. M., & Gardner, M. (2009). *With the rise of the DNP, who will conduct primary care research?* Paper presented at the Second National Conference on the Doctor of Nursing Practice: The Dialogue Continues..., Hilton Head Island, South Carolina, March 24–27, 2010.

Dreher, H. M., & Montgomery, K. (2009). Let's call it "doctoral" advanced practice nursing. *The Journal of Continuing Education in Nursing, 40*(12), 1–2.

Eisenstat, R., Beer, M., Foote, N., Fredberg, T., & Norrgren, F. (2008). The uncompromising leader. *Harvard Business Review, 86*(7–8), 50–57.

Fang, D., Tracy, C., & Bednash, G. D. (2010). *2009–2010 Enrollment and graduations in baccalaureate and graduate programs in nursing.* Washington, DC: American Association of Colleges of Nursing.

Fischman, J. (2005). Who will take care of you? *U.S. World News & Report,* January, 25, 2005.

Ford, J. (2008). Editorial: DNP a bad idea. *Advanceweb.com.* Retrieved from http://community.advanceweb.com/blogs/np_1/archive/2008/07/23/editorial-on-dnp.aspx

Hathaway, D., Jacob, S., Stegbauer, C., Thompson, C., & Graff, C. (2006). The practice doctorate: Perspectives of early adopters. *Journal of Nursing Education, 45*(12), 487–496.

HealthReform.Gov. (2010). *Fact sheet: Creating jobs and increasing the number of primary care providers.* U.S. Department of Health & Human Services. Retrieved from http://www.healthreform.gov/newsroom/primarycareworkforce.html

Howard Hughes Medical Institute. (2010). *Research training fellowships for medical students.* Retrieved from http://www.nap.edu/catalog/12956.html

Institute of Medicine. (2001). *Crossing the quality chasm: A new health system for the 21st century.* Washington, DC: National Academies Press.

Institute of Medicine. (2010). *The Future of Nursing: Leading Change, Advancing Health.* Committee on the Robert Wood Johnson Foundation Initiative on the Future of Nursing at the Institute of Medicine. Washington, DC: National Academy of Sciences. Retrieved from http://www.nap.edu/catalog/12956.html

Melnyk, B., & Davidson, S. (2009). Creating a culture of innovation in nursing education through shared vision, leadership, interdisciplinary partnerships, and positive deviance. *Nursing Administration Quarterly, 33*(4), 288–295.

Mick, D., & Ackerman, M. (2005). Nursing and biomedical engineering transdisciplinary clinical trials collaboration. *Expert Review of Medical Devices, 2*(1), 131–133.

Mundinger, M., Kane, R., Lenz, E., Totten, A., Tsai, W., Cleary, P. et al. (2000). Primary care outcomes in patients treated by nurse practitioners or physicians: A randomized trial. *Journal of the American Medical Association, 283,* 59–68.

Neal, A. (2008). Seeking higher-ed accountability: Ending federal accreditation. *Change: The Magazine of Higher Education Regulation,* Sept–Oct, 25–29.

Naisbitt, J. (1982). *Megatrends.* New York, NY: Warner Books.

Obama, B. (2009). Remarks by the President on the "Education To Innovate" Campaign. Retrieved from http://www.whitehouse.gov/the-press-office/remarks-president-education-innovate-campaign

Potempa, K. M., & Tilden, V. (2004). Building high impact science: The dean as innovator. *Journal of Nursing Education, 43*(11), 502–505.

Potempa, K. M., Redman, R. W., & Anderson, C. A. (2008). Capacity for the advancement of nursing science: Issues and challenges. *Journal of Professional Nursing, 24*(6), 329–336.

Raines, C. F. (2010). *The doctor of nursing practice: A report on progress.* American Association of Colleges of Nursing. Retrieved from http://www.aacn.nche.edu/dnp/pdf/DNPForum3-10.pdf

Robert Wood Johnson Foundation. (2007). *Charting nursing's future.* Retrieved from http://www.rwjf.org/files/publications/other/nursingfuture4.pdf

Smith Glasgow, M. E., & Dreher, H. M. (2010). The future of oncology nursing science: Who will generate the knowledge? *Oncology Nursing Forum, 37*(4), 393–396.

Smith Glasgow, M. E., Dunphy, L. M., & Mainous, R. O. (2010). *Innovative nursing educational curriculum for the 21st century. In The Future of Nursing: Leading Change, Advancing Health.* Committee on the Robert Wood Johnson Foundation Initiative on the Future of Nursing at the Institute of Medicine. Washington, DC: National Academy of Sciences, (pp. G8–G12). Retrieved from http://www.nap.edu/catalog/12956.html

Stanik-Hutt, J. (2008). Debunking the need to certify the DNP degree. *The Journal for Nurse Practitioners, 4*(10), 739.

Stewart, D. (2009). *Challenges and opportunities for the professional doctorate: A North American perspective.* Paper presented at the European Conference on the Professional Doctorate, London, England, November 5–6, 2009.

Summers, L. (2010). How the health care reform law affects APRNs. *The American Nurse, 42*(3), 16.

Ten years of progress: The council for the advancement of comprehensive care. (2010, Spring). *The Academic Nurse: The Journal of Columbia University School of Nursing and its Alumni,* 20–27.

Tilden, V., & Potempa, K. (2003). The impact of nursing science: A litmus test. *Nursing Research, 52*(5), 275.

Toffler, A. (1971). *Future shock.* New York, NY: Bantam Books.

Upenieks, V. V. (2003). What constitutes effective leadership? Perceptions of magnet and non-magnet nurse leaders. *JONA: The Journal of Nursing Administration, 33*(9), 456–467.

Wells, W., & Hejna, W. (2009). Developing leadership talent in healthcare organizations. *Healthcare Financial Management, 63*(1), 66–69.

Zungolo, E. (2009). *The DNP and the faculty role: Issues and challenges.* Paper presented at the Second National Conference on the Doctor of Nursing Practice: The Dialogue Continues..., Hilton Head Island, South Carolina, March 24–27, 2009.

CHAPTER TWENTY-FOUR: Reflective Response

Suzanne S. Prevost

This final chapter by Dreher and Smith Glasgow raises several important questions and challenges for faculty, graduates, and employers of doctorally prepared advanced practice nurses. The rapid expansion of Doctor of Nursing Practice (DNP) programs, from less than 10 in 2005 to greater than 120 in 2010 (AACN, 2009), demonstrates the broad acceptance of this phenomenon by nursing faculty and administrators across the United States. Likewise, the exploding volume of DNP student applications and enrollment provides evidence that this movement is enthusiastically embraced by students and practicing nurses, as well as those in academe. It is both intriguing and challenging to observe such a positive response to a nursing innovation with minimal evidence to support its effectiveness.

Why are we moving forward with such blind faith? Perhaps this reaction is based on the widespread acceptance of the inadequacies of our existing health care delivery systems and the consensus that we need new models of health care delivery and better-prepared knowledge workers on the front lines. We must, however, instill a sense of urgency among DNP faculty and students to work cohesively and intentionally to build this body of evidence. The authors suggest that the emergence of new DNP roles will depend upon graduates presenting employers with measurable claims of what they have acquired in their education. I would challenge these graduates to go beyond measurable claims to the presentation of significant results. In this case, significance is not limited to statistical significance but might be equally compelling in the form of clinical or economic significance.

I applaud Drs. Dreher and Smith Glasgow for their clear delineation of the four doctoral advanced practice roles of practitioner, clinical executive, educator, and clinical scientist in this text, as well as their expression of these roles in the curricula at Drexel University. While the practitioner and clinical executive roles are widely accepted, considerable controversy remains regarding whether clinical doctoral programs can provide sufficient preparation for nurse educators and clinical scientists (AACN, 2006; Clinton & Sperhac, 2009; Florczak, 2010).

The rapid development of doctoral level advanced practitioner programs across the United States demonstrates the growing national sentiment favoring this level of preparation for advanced practitioners. Yet, a few nurse leaders still contend that master's-level preparation is sufficient for advanced practice registered nurses (APRNs) (IOM, 2010). The variability in DNP program quality, specifically in relation to the level and intensity of advanced clinical practice experiences, is indeed a valid concern and probably contributes to this debate. Most faculty and administrators of DNP programs are planning for and documenting adherence to the minimum clinical hour requirements set forth in the 2006 AACN *Essentials* document as they prepare their graduates for certification exams and prepare their programs for accreditation visits. However, the specific nature of those clinical experiences, the content within them, and the levels of supervision are widely divergent. More specific delineation of what constitutes minimal clinical experiences for master's level advanced practice nurses versus the evolving expectations for doctoral level advanced practice nurses would certainly be beneficial.

The value of doctoral preparation for clinical executives seems to be less controversial. A totally new skill set is required to succeed in current and future executive level leadership positions. Our history of promoting the most beloved nurse clinicians into such leadership positions will not serve the profession well in environments of increasing competition to produce clinical and financial outcomes consistent with constantly rising benchmark targets. Dreher and Smith Glasgow advocate for a combined high-tech/high-touch approach in the preparation of practitioners. This combination is equally important for clinical executives. Advanced competencies in emotional intelligence, appreciative inquiry, and motivation must be combined with a high degree of technologic proficiency, financial acumen, and political savvy. Awareness and understanding of, and adaptability to new technologies will be essential because these decisions and applications increasingly influence system efficiencies and the financial bottom line. I agree with the authors that these leaders will not be limited to traditional positions in nursing administration but will also be well suited for a variety of chief executive and interdisciplinary leadership positions, as well as offices and board positions in professional organizations and community service agencies. DNP faculty should challenge these students to dream big and invest at least a portion of their clinical practicum hours in mentored leadership experiences beyond nursing administration.

Expectations regarding the role of DNP graduates as educators have evolved over the past decade. Early in the development of DNP programs, many opponents expressed the concern that DNP programs would divert potential PhD candidates and therefore contribute to the growing shortage of nursing faculty (Meleis & Dracup, 2005). Of course, this concern was predicated on the assumption that DNP graduates could not or should not be considered for nursing faculty positions. It is important to note that the AACN *Essentials* document states, "... the basic DNP curriculum does not prepare the graduate for a faculty teaching role any more than the PhD curriculum does. Graduates of either program planning a faculty career will need (additional) preparation ..." (AACN, 2006, p. 7).

As DNP programs proliferate, the DNP-prepared advanced nursing practice educator who is actively engaged in practice will clearly be the candidate of choice to fill these DNP faculty positions. Likewise, these practitioners will be better prepared to teach undergraduate nursing students, especially in clinical settings, than many PhD-prepared researchers. In more recent publications, including the just released 2010 report from the Institute of Medicine titled *A Summary of the February 2010 Forum on the Future of Nursing*, some nurse leaders advocate for the recognition of nursing education as a specialized area within advanced nursing practice which could be taught in DNP tracks specifically designed for educators. The authors of this chapter are leading this charge by offering such a program.

Dreher and Smith Glasgow raise important questions regarding workload expectations and compensation for these advanced practitioner educators. At the University of Kentucky, we value such individuals as essential leaders in both our teaching and practice initiatives. We are currently refining our model of compensation for these faculty members. In addition to incorporating practice hours into the faculty workload, we are planning to provide higher rates of compensation for practice activities consistent with the market salaries for other practitioners in our region.

The role of clinical scientists is probably the most controversial option for doctoral advanced practice nurses. For decades, many nurses have been instrumental members of clinical research teams, especially in teams conducting pharmaceutical and medical device trials. Unfortunately, these study coordinators are rarely given high-level decision-making authority, nor are they usually given substantive credit or compensation in the dissemination of patents or other products of those studies. Formal and specific doctoral preparation will help to legitimize this important nursing role. The Clinical Scientist Track described in this chapter is innovative and fills an important niche in health-oriented research and development.

Dreher and Smith Glasgow raise two additional questions that merit discussion. Should DNP graduates be considered for postdoctoral research fellowships? And, will they achieve tenure in the academy? The answers to these questions may also be embedded in Christensen's notion of "disruptive innovation." Early in the DNP movement, the most common response to both questions was "No." Similarly, 10 years ago, most nursing faculty responded "No," when asked whether nursing courses could be taught effectively online. Time changes things. As Christensen would say, when the disruptive DNP innovation moves up market it will displace the established competitors. Or in this case, it will gain the respect of the new majority rather than be inhibited by those who cling to traditional models of nursing practice, education, and research.

Health care and education are changing rapidly. Nursing educators and practitioners must keep an open mind and search for new solutions to keep pace and succeed in such dynamic environments. The potential for success in postdoctoral fellowships and the tenure process may be influenced more by individual intellect, talent, and persistence than the type of doctoral program if all candidates are given equal consideration and opportunities. I encourage DNP students and graduates to go forth, lead clinical innovations, and document the evidence to show the world their important contributions. I also challenge established nursing leaders to reframe our traditional definitions of significance, productivity, and effectiveness to embrace and support these "disruptive" yet progressive practitioners, clinical executives, educators, and clinical scientists.

REFERENCES

American Association of Colleges of Nursing (AACN). (2006). *Essentials of doctoral education for advanced nursing practice.* Retrieved from http://www.aacn.nche.edu/DNP/pdf/Essentials.pdf

American Association of Colleges of Nursing (AACN). (2009). *Doctor of nursing practice (DNP) programs.* Retrieved from http://www.aacn.nche.edu/DNP/DNPProgramList.htm

Clinton, P., & Sperhac, A. M. (2009). The DNP and unintended consequences: An opportunity for dialogue. *Journal of Pediatric Health Care, 23*(5), 348–351.

Florczak, K. L. (2010). Research and the doctor of nursing practice: A cause for consternation. *Nursing Science Quarterly, 23*(1), 13–17.

Institute of Medicine (IOM). (2010). *A summary of the February 2010 forum on the future of nursing education.* Washington, DC: The National Academies Press.

Meleis, A., & Dracup, K. (2005). The case against the DNP: History, timing, substance, and marginalization. *The Online Journal of Issues in Nursing, 10*(3). Retrieved from http://www.nursingworld.org/MainMenuCategories/ANAMarketplace/ANAPeriodicals/OJIN/TableofContents/Volume102005/No3Sept05/tpc28_216026.aspx

CRITICAL THINKING QUESTIONS

1. What core competencies differentiate the master's-prepared advanced practice nurse from the doctoral advanced practice nurse?
2. How should DNP programs incorporate technology and knowledge management in their respective curricula?
3. Christensen, Grossman, and Hwang in *The Innovator's Prescription: A Disruptive Solution for Health Care* (2009) state "... nurse practitioners practicing in retail clinics, should disrupt the precision medicine portion of the physician's practice." Discuss the role of a nurse practitioner in retail clinics and other forms of disruptive innovation.
4. Describe the role of the doctoral advanced nursing practice *"Clinical Executive"* of the future. What specific competencies does the doctoral advanced nursing practice *"Clinical Executive"* require?
5. How can a progressive doctoral-level nurse leader shape an institution through one's value system and passion for nursing?
6. Today, many nursing faculty are divorced from clinical practice. How can the doctoral advanced nursing practice "Educator" change the current system and reconnect with the practice context of the nursing discipline?
7. What are the benefits and risks of the doctoral advanced nursing practice "Educator" in academia? Please cite benefits and risks to the individual DNP educator and to the nursing profession as a whole.
8. Describe how the academy can develop the productive nurse scientist of the future.
9. What are the possibilities for the doctoral advanced nursing practice "Clinical Scientist in the clinical trials/pharmaceutical research industry?
10. What effect will the transition to the entry-level doctorate for advanced practice and the dissolution of the master's degree over time have on the nursing profession?

Index